AF520495

ANIMAL NUTRITION

ANIMAL NUTRITION

Advances & Developments

Chief Editor
DR. (Mrs.) USHA R. MEHRA
Editors
DR. PUTAN SINGH
DR. A.K. VERMA

2012

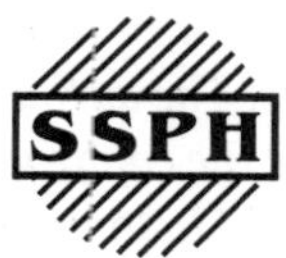

SATISH SERIAL PUBLISHING HOUSE
403, Express Tower, Commercial Complex, Azadpur, Delhi-110033 (INDIA)
Phone : 011-27672852, Fax : 91-11-27672046
E-mail : info@satishserial.com, hkjain1975@yahoo.com
Website : www.satishserial.com

Published by :

SATISH SERIAL PUBLISHING HOUSE
403, Express Tower, Commercial Complex, Azadpur, Delhi-110033 (INDIA)
Phone : 011-27672852 Fax : 91-11-27672046
E-mail : info@satishserial.com, hkjain1975@yahoo.com

ISBN 81-89304-89-5

Typeset at: Harminder *for* Laxmi Art Creation
Printed at: Salasar Imaging Systems, Delhi-110035

Preface

The feeding practices in developing countries including most of the South-East-Asian region are different, where the animals are fed, largely on crop residues and other agro-industrial by-products. Most of the books on animal nutrition describe feeding practices prevalent in agriculturally advanced western countries implying the use of good quality fodders and cereals. The livestock production systems as adopted in western countries are not appropriate for main of the developing countries. Therefore, there is a much felt need for a text book of advanced animal nutrition, for students from Asian and other developing countries.

This book is the result of multiauthor efforts. The contributors were invited for their expertise on the topics and professional involvement. Since the various chapters have been contributed by several authors, some repetition or overlapping of information was inevitable.

This book attempts at providing a clear thorough and up-dated information fundamental to animal nutrition as well as its application in developing countries in an easily accessible manner. This volume is intended to serve as a text-book for reference for the more advanced workers of animal science. Some topics of peripheral interest only which are usually included in animal nutrition texts have been omitted. Each topic is discussed from a multidisciplinary angle to aid and assist understanding and not merely as a routine to fulfill the requirement of syllabi.

The chapters in this book are arranged in a logical progression each of which is a manageable "package" for discernible readers. In any event, with a book of this type there is always a question of how much and what type of detail to present to the readers. The author's preconception of the audience for the book may or may not be correct. Consequently, it is a matter of picking and choosing what to include or exclude.

The first chapter is devoted to acquaint the reader, with the livestock farming practices in developing countries of the world. Emerging areas such as application of biotechnology to improve the nutritive value of low grade roughages is discussed at full length. Two chapters deal with the energy metabolism of ruminants and describe in detail the calorimetric techniques including respiration calorimetry. Recent trends in protein nutrition are given a wide coverage. Matters of practical interest for example the utilization of agro-industrial by-products as feed resources is discussed in detail.

Many chapters are devoted to special topics to provide full and comprehensive information such as immunological aspects in animal nutrition, and feeding behaviour of farm animal, which are not usually covered in some books and lectures. The nutrition and feeding in tropics of various species of domestic animals such as cattle, buffalo, goat and pig are described in detail. Special mention has been made of the feeding of equines and livestock in the hills. Yak and Mithun are the little known Asian animals though both have an economic future and are becoming familiar in the international sphere of animal science. These animals have potential to be developed and utilized for human benefit.

As the demand of dog as companion animal is increasing in human life a chapter on nutrition and feeding of pet animals has been introduced. Special mention has been made on the topic of advanced poultry nutrition.

In changing scenario of animal nutrition some recent topics like purine derivatives to determine microbial protein supply in ruminants, role of herbal feed additives in animal nutrition, role of protected fat in the diet of high yielding dairy animals, assessing quality and safety of animal feeds as well as quality assurance for livestock production are also included.

I am grateful to all my friends, colleagues and the contributors for making this book a success. I am thankful for their ungrudging help in this publication. I would like to specially thank Dr. D.V. Reddy, Prof, and Head, Department of Animal Nutrition, Rajiv Gandhi College of Veterinary and Animal Sciences, Pondicherry for his suggestions and comments on many chapters.

All Constructive suggestion and comments are invited form the readers so as to make the book more useful in future.

Usha R. Mehra

List of Contributors

1. **A.K. Verma,** Principal Scientist & In-charge, Swine Production Farm, Indian Veterinary Research Institute, Izatnagar-243 122 (U.P.), India.
2. **A. Sahoo,** Principal Scientist and Head, Animal Nutrition Central Sheep wool Research Institute Avikanagar, India.
3. **A. Thulasi,** Senior Scientist Animal Nutrition division, National Institute of Animal Nutrition and Physiology Adugodi, Bangalore-560030, India.
4. **A.B. Mandal,** Principal Scientist, Animal Nutrition, Central Avian Research Institute, Izatnagar-243 122 (U.P.), India.
5. **A.K. Patra,** Department of Animal Nutrition, West Bengal University of Animal and Fishery Sciences, 37, K.B. Sarani, Belgachia, Kolkata-700 037 (W.B.), India.
6. **A.K. Pattanaik,** Senior Scientist, Division of Animal Nutrition, Indian Veterinary Research Institute, Izatnagar-243 122, (U.P.), India
7. **A.K. Srivastava,** Director, National Dairy Research Institute, Karnal - 132 001, Haryana, India.
8. **Anamika Mishra,** Scientist, Animal Genetics and Breeding, High Security Animal Disease Laboratory, Indian Veterinary Research Institute, Anand Nagar, Bhopal-462 021 (M.P.), India.
9. **Ani Bency Jacob,** Veterinary Surgeon, Department of Animal Husbandry, Government of Kerala, Kerala, India.
10. **Ashwin A. Raut,** Senior Scientist, Animal Biotechnology, High Security Animal Disease Laboratory, Indian Veterinary Research Institute, Anand Nagar, Bhopal-462 021 (M.P.), India.
11. **Asit Das,** Senior Scientist, Wildlife Section, Indian Veterinary Research Institute, Izatnagar-243 122 (U.P.), India.

12. **B.C. Das,** Senior Scientist, Division of Physiology and Climatology, Indian Veterinary Research Institute, Izatnagar-243 122 (U.P.), India.
13. **C.S. Prasad,** Vice-Chancellor, Dr. Punjabrao Deshmukh Agriculture University, Akola, Maharashtra, India.
14. **D. Nagalakshmi,** Associate Professor, Department of Animal Nutrition, College of Veterinary Science, Sri Venkateswara Veterinary University, Rajendranagar, Hyderabad-500 030 (A.P.), India.
15. **D. Swarup,** Director, Central Institute for Research on Goats, Makhdoom, Farah-281 122, (U.P.), India.
16. **D.N. Kamra,** Director, Centre of Advanced Faculty Training in Animal Nutrition and Head, Division of Animal Nutrition, Indian Veterinary Research Institute, Izatnagar-243 122 (U.P.), India.
17. **D.T. Pal,** Senior Scientist, National Institute of Animal Nutrition and Physiology, Adugodi, Bangalore-560 030, India.
18. **D.V. Reddy,** Professor & Head, Department of Animal Nutrition, Rajiv Gandhi College of Veterinary and Animal Sciences (Pondicherry University), Puducherry-605 014, India.
19. **E.R. Ørskov,** Director, International Feed Resources Unit, The Macaulay Institute, Craigiebuckler, Aberdeen, U.K.
20. **Gerhard Flachowsky,** Institute of Animal Nutrition, Friedrich-Loeffler-Institute (FLI), Federal Research Institute for Animal Health, Bundesallee 50, D-38116, Braunschweig.
21. **Gyanendra Singh,** Senior Scientist, Division of Physiology and Climatology, Indian Veterinary Research Institute, Izatnagar-243 122 (U.P.), India.
22. **H. Rahman,** Joint Director, ICAR Research Complex for NEH Region Sikkim Centre, Tadong, Gangtok-737 102, Sikkim, India.
23. **I.A. Wright,** ILRI Regional Representative Asia, Regional Office for South Asia, CG Block, NASC Complex, New Delhi-110 012, India.
24. **J.C. Macrae,** J.C., Former Head, Physiology Division. The Rowett Research Institute, Aberdeen, U.K.
25. **J.M. Brockway,** J.M., Former Principal Scientific officer. The Rowett Research Insititute, Aberdeen, U.K.
26. **J.P. Sehgal,** Principal Scientist, National Dairy Research Insitute, Karnal-132 001, Haryana, India.
27. **Jayant Lohakare,** Full Time Faculty, College of Animal Life Sciences Kangwon National University KNU Ave 1, Chunchon-200 701, South Korea.
28. **K.K. Baruah,** Director, National Research Centre on Yak, Dirang, West Kameng Dist.-790 101, Arunachal Pradesh, India.

29. **K.K. Mishra,** Veterinary Officer, Agricultural Technology Information Centre (ATIC), Indian Veterinary Research Institute, Izatnagar-243 122, (U.P.), India.
30. **K.K. Singhal,** Principal Scientist, Dairy Cattle Nutrition Division, National Dairy Research Institute, Karnal-132 001, Haryana, India.
31. **K.T. Sampath,** Director, National Institute of Animal Nutrition and Physiology, Adugodi, Bangalore-560 030.
32. **K.Y. Deshpande,** SMS (Animal Science), KVK, SKUAST-J, Rajouri-185 131 (J&K), India.
33. **Kiran Kumari,** Research Scholar, College of Veterinary Science and Animal Husbandry Anjora, Durg-491 001
34. **M. Chandrasekharaiah,** Senior Scientist, National Institute of Animal Nutrition and Physiology, Adugodi, Bangalore-560 030.
35. **M. Wadhwa,** Senior Biochemist Department of Animal Nutrition, Guru Angad Dev Veterinary and Animal Science University, Ludhiana.
36. **M.K. Tripathi,** Senior Scientist, Central Institute for Research on Goats, Makhdoom, Farah-281 122 (U.P.), India.
37. **M.P.S. Bakshi,** Former Head, Department of Animal Nutrition, Guru Angad Dev Veterinary and Animal Science University, Ludhiana.
38. **Michael Blummel,** Animal Nutritionist c/o ICRISAT, Patancheru, Hyderabad, India.
39. **Mohini Saini,** Senior Scientist, Wildlife Section, Indian Veterinary Research Institute, Izatnagar-243 122 (U.P.), India.
40. **N. Haque,** Principal Scientist (Animal Nutrition), National Research Centre on Mithun, Jharnapani, Medziphema, P.O. Medziphema, Dist. Dimapur-797106, Nagaland, India.
41. **N.K.S. Gowda,** Senior Scientist, National Institute of Animal Nutrition and Physiology, Adugodi, Bangalore-560 030.
42. **N.N. Pathak** (Former Director, Central Institute for Research on Buffaloes, Hisar), 113 B, Vatika, Sun City Vistar, Bareilly-243 122 (U.P.), India.
43. **Narayan Dutta,** Senior Scientist, Division of Animal Nutrition, Indian Veterinary Research Institute, Izatnagar-243 122 (U.P.), India.
44. **Neeta Agarwal,** Tech. Officer (T-9), Animal Nutrition Division, Indian Veterinary Research Institute, Izatnagar-243 122 (U.P.), India.
45. **O.K. Raina,** Senior Scientist, Veterinary Parasitology, Indian Veterinary Research Institute, Izatnagar-243 122 (U.P.), India.
46. **P.K. Naik,** Senior Scientist, (Animal Nutrition) ICAR Research Complex for Goa, Ela, Old Goa-403 402, Goa, India.

47. **P.S. Banerjee,** Senior Scientist, Veterinary Parasitology, Indian Veterinary Research Institute, Izatnagar-243 122 (U.P.), India.
48. **Putan Singh,** Principal Scientist, Division of Animal Nutrition, Indian Veterinary Research Institute, Izatnagar-243 122 (U.P.), India.
49. **R.R. Shukla,** Former Prof., Vallabhbhai Patel Chest Institute, University of Delhi, Delhi, India.
50. **R.S. Dass,** Principal Scientist, Division of Animal Nutrition, Indian Veterinary Research Institute, Izatnagar-243 122 (U.P.), India.
51. **Raina Pathak,** College of Veterinary Science and Animal Husbandry, Anjora, Durg-491 001, India.
52. **S. Anandan,** Senior Scientist, Animal Nutrition, National Institute of Animal Nutrition and Physiology Adugodi, Bangalore-560 030, India.
53. **S. Nanda,** P.G. Scholar, College of Veterinary Science and Animal Husbandry Anjora, Durg-491 001.
54. **S. Swarnkar,** P.G. Scholar, College of Veterinary Science and Animal Husbandry Anjora, Durg-491 001.
55. **(Mrs.) Saroj Toppo,** Senior Scientist, ICAR Research Complex for NEH Region Sikkim Centre, Tadong, Gangtok-737 102, Sikkim, India.
56. **S.C. Gupta,** Principal Scientist, Veterinary Parasitology, Indian Veterinary Research Institute, Izatnagar-243 122 (U.P.), India.
57. **S.K. Mishra,** Ph.D, Scholar, Division of Dairy Microbiology, National Diary Research Insitute, Karnal, Haryana-132 001.
58. **S.K. Ranjhan,** Director, Hind Agro Industries Limited, Aligarh-202 122, India.
59. **S.K. Sirohi,** Senior Scientist, National Dairy Research Institute, Karnal-132 001, Haryana, India.
60. **S.P. Tiwari,** Professor and Head, Animal Nutrition, College of Veterinary Science and Animal Husbandry, Anjora, Durg-491 001, India
61. **S.V. Rama Rao,** Principal Scientist, Project Directorate on Poultry, Rajendranagar, Hyderabad-500 030 (A.P.), India.
62. **Tribhuwan Sharma,** Professor and Head Department of Animal Nutrition, Rajasthan Agriculture University Beechwal, Bikaner-334 402.
63. **U.K. Mishra,** Director of Instructions, IGKV, Raipur (C.G.).
64. **(Mrs.) Usha R. Mehra,** Scientist Emeritus, Division of Animal Nutrition, Indian Veterinary Research Institute, Izatnagar-243 122 (U.P.), India.

Contents

Animal Nutrition, 2012
eds. Dr. (Mrs.) Usha R. Mehra et al., pp. 1-28
Satish Serial Publishing House e-mail : info@satishserial.com; website : www.satishserial.com

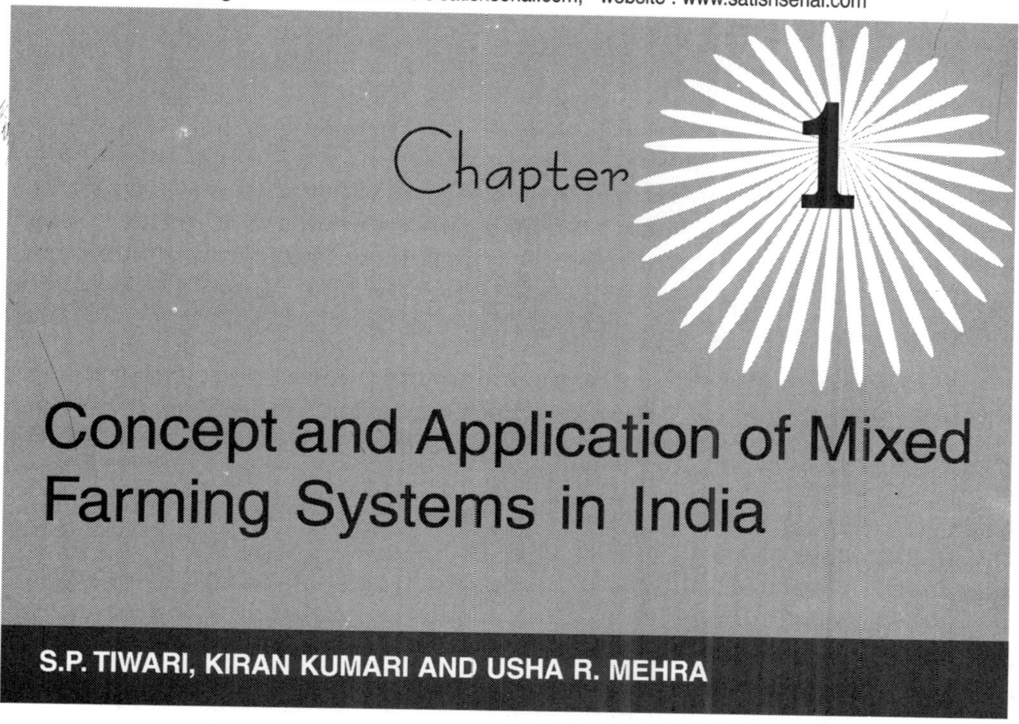

Chapter 1

Concept and Application of Mixed Farming Systems in India

S.P. TIWARI, KIRAN KUMARI AND USHA R. MEHRA

The concepts associated with integrated farming systems (IFS) are practiced by numerous farmers throughout the globe. A common characteristic of these systems is that they invariably have a combination of crop and livestock enterprises and in some cases may include combinations of aquaculture and trees. The definition of IFS is varied and dependent on the context. Agbonlabor *et al.* (2003) defined the concept as a type of mixed farming system that combines crop and livestock enterprises in a supplementary and/ or complementary manner. Okigbo (1995) defines these systems as a mixed farming system that consists of at least two separate but logically interdependent parts of a crop and livestock enterprises. Contrasting these definitions Radhammani *et al.* (2003) describes IFS's as a component of farming systems which takes into account the concepts of minimizing risk, increasing production and profits whilst improving the utilization of organic wastes and crop residues. Jayanthi *et al.* (2000) based on experiences from Tamil Nadu, India, described these systems as a mixed animal crop system where the animal component is often raised on agricultural waste products while the animal is used to cultivate the soil and provide manure to be used as fertilizer and fuel. Edwards (1997) narrowly defined the system as an aquaculture system that is integrated with livestock and in which fresh animal waste is used to feed fish. It is clear from the above that there are synergies and complementarily between enterprise that comprise a crop and animal component that form the basis of the concept of IFS (Radhammani *et al.*, 2003). In this respect integration usually occurs when outputs (usually by-products) of one enterprise are used as inputs by another within the context of the farming system. The difference between mixed farming and integrated farming is that enterprises in the integrated farming system are mutually supportive and depend on each other (Csavas, 1992).

It is clear from the above discussion that the primary objective of the IFS is to maintain production of food and other goods and services that contribute to food security and income generation. Other functions that are just as important are achieving environmental sustainability and contributing to ecosystem services. This would imply that these systems have components that incorporate the concepts of multifunctionality. Multifunctionality is interpreted in terms of multiple roles assigned to agriculture. In the framework of multifunctionality agriculture as an activity is entrusted with performing four main functions in society, namely, food security and environmental, economic and social functions. In general, increasing the number of functions tends to increase the stability of agriculture and land use (Price 2000).

Integrated Farming Systems

Integrated farming systems are effectively systems that have traditionally been undertaken by farmers in countries that include Indonesia, China, Malaysia, Vietnam, Rwanda and Thailand. However, in many countries these traditional systems have been replaced by the establishment of commercial cash and staple crop production systems that have been promoted by governments.

Continuous production of crops without external inputs reduce the ability of the soil resource base to both provide and retain nutrients which often results in a decline in productivity (Noble and Ruaysoongnern 2002). In addition, the reliance upon a few crops in combination with a high risk of crop failure due to a range of factors (i.e. disease, drought) exposes farmers to a high degree of variability with respect to yields and income and therefore risk (Ashby 2001). Further, some authors indicate that commercial farming systems are a threat to the environment through a loss of genetic diversity and the possible negative impacts of these systems and their associated inputs (Ashby 2001).

Integrated farming systems are often viewed as a sustainable alternative to commercial farming systems particularly on marginal lands with the objective of reversing resource degradation and stabilizing farm incomes. Lightfoot and Minnick (1991) reported that the integration of trees into these systems offers income security and ecological protection. Added to this, the use of diverse plants and animals broadens possible sources of income generation. The generation of wastes and by-products from these entities are transferred between enterprises, thereby reducing the need for external inputs such as feeds and crop nutrients (Little and Edwards, 2003). Animals on a farm provide inputs to other enterprises and constitute a source of meat and milk, a means of savings, and a source of social status (Schierre et al, 2002; Little and Edwards 2003).

Diversification of farming activities should invariably improve the utilization of labor, reduce unemployment in areas where there is a surplus of underutilized labour and provide a source of living for those households that operate their farm as a full time occupation (van Brakel et al. 2003). Based on evidence and synthesis of published literature, the important characteristics of the integrated farming system that differentiated if from commercial farming systems are presented in Table 1. The table presents differences that exist between farming systems that include the high degree of diversity of genetic species in the integrated farming systems and enterprises and practices, which are employed to attain the household objectives. The synergy between enterprises increases with on-farm diversity and is fundamental to the integrated farming system concept. The commercial system cannot be moved to the direction of the integrated system if there are no synergies between enterprises through the integration of activities. Therefore, the distinction between the integrated farming system and the commercial farming system is not absolute, but is rather a matter of degree of integration of resources in the farm system (Tipraqsa, 2006).

The Role of Integrated Farming Systems in Agriculture

Within the published literature there are two main areas that have been intensively studied, namely 1. studies that assess the financial viability of IFS through the analysis of farm budgets; and 2. studies that optimize resource allocation.

Financial viability: On farm trials in which farmers incomes form the basis of research have found that the incorporation of trees and vegetables crops are highly lucrative (Ashby 2001). The study in Tamil Nadu was designed to assess the financial viability of a poultry and fish culture system. The study concluded that under the prevailing conditions, higher incomes and on farm labor use can be achieved by integrating different enterprises on the farm. Similarly, the integration of poultry, fish and mushroom with rice cultivation over a five-year period. The study concluded that the integrated system that included the aforementioned three components increased net farm incomes and on-farm labor when compared with the conventional rice cropping system. Radhamani et al. (2003) also reviewed several studies on the financial viability of integrated farming system and concluded that they positively influenced the economic viability of these systems. The results from these structured studies that received regular inputs such as genetic resources, labor, irrigation and information are somewhat removed from reality. In most cases the availability of and access to these inputs is variable and is often contingent on factors that are beyond the control of the farmer.

Table 1 : Relative characteristics comparison of the integrated farming system with the commercial farming system (Tipraqsa, 2006)

Aspects and properties of systems	Farm type	
	Integrated	Commercial
Biophysical characteristics		
1. Farm age	Young	Old
2. Irrigation infrastructures	Many	Few
3. Diversity (of crops, animals & enterprises)	High	Low
Socio-economic characteristics		
4. Farming area owned by the household	Large	Small
5. Family labour	Much	Little
6. Labour saving technologies (tractors, water pumps)	Few	Many
7. Hired labour	Much	Little
8. Off-farm income	Much	Little
Outputs		
9. Productivity	High	Low
10. Soil fertility	High	Low
11. Financial profitability (gross farm income)	High	Low
12. Flexibility of product use[a]	Much	Little
13. Diversity (of activities, products & income sources)	High	Low
14. Stability[b]	High	Low

[a]The flexibility of product use refers to the availability of alternative ways of product disposal such as home consumption instead of sales (Dillon and McConnell 1997). [b]System stability refers to the absence or minimization of year-to-year fluctuations in either production or value of output. It also implies either stability in input costs, yields and prices or counterbalancing movements in these influences on values of output (Dillon and McConnell 1997).

Dalsgaard and Oficial (1997) outlined an approach to model, describe, analyze and quantify the productive and ecological characteristics of the agro ecosystem at the level of the farm. The study employed a range of techniques (bio resource flow diagrams, farm transects, direct observation, field measurements, farm records and informal discussion) to develop a model and compare it with the commercial farming system. The comparative analysis suggested that diversification and integration of resource management can be productive, profitable and manageable, given access to labor and secure tenure. Similarly in the Cameroon, Ngambeki et al. (1992) demonstrated the profitability of the system by integrating livestock into a crop based farming through increased financial benefits and a better use of intermediate farm resources such as manure, draft power, and crop residues.

A significant number of studies have been undertaken into the financial viability of IFS. Pant (2002) assessed the potential and economic viability of integrated agriculture-aquaculture (IAA) systems under three different agro-ecological zones namely: drought prone, rain-fed lowland, and rolling land. An assessment of 234 farm households practicing IAA revealed that enterprise compositions within the IAA system varied between the three agro-ecological setting, yet rice paddy, fruit, vegetables, chicken, ducks, and aquaculture enterprises were common on all farms. In all agro ecologies, livestock production was extensive due to limited use of supplementary feed. In the drought-prone agro-ecology, rice yields were 2.5 t ha^{-1}, approximately double that of rain-fed lowlands. The study also reported that farm households in the lowlands responded to demands in nearby market by producing significantly higher amounts of fruit and vegetables than the other two agro-ecologies. Among the different agro-ecologies, the rain-fed lowland had the lowest gross farm income.

Allocation of resources: A further aspect that has been comprehensively studied is the aspect of resource allocation within the context of IFS. Schiere *et al.* (2002) studied the role of livestock and provided criteria for the sustainability of integrating livestock into a crop production system, which was then used for scenario analyses. The study used linear programming (LP) to optimally allocate resources over time and space. The results of the scenario studies illustrated options and trade-offs between different crop and livestock combinations in terms of their sustainability criteria. The study concluded that livestock are essential for the sustainability of the system. In southern Nigeria, Agbonlahor *et al.* (2003) determined the optimal resource allocation for farm planning that both satisfy productivity requirements to meet economic profitability and continued soil fertility to achieve sustainability. The study employed a LP approach to determine the optimal resource use. The study concluded that a sustainable system is possible in this area through the integration of poultry and crop enterprises.

In the lowland areas of Tamil Nadu, India, Jayanthi *et al.* (2000) estimated the water use efficiency of systems by integrating crops, poultry, pigeon, fish, and mushroom cultivation. The results indicated that integrated farming requires less water per unit of production than mono cropping systems. In Malaysia, the contribution of aquaculture has the potential to increase present farm income 3.3 times if resources are allocated optimally to fish culture and broiler meat enterprises. In Thailand, an appropriate technology was developed to reduce water loss from farm ponds in IFS floating materials (foam, bamboo, and dry coconut) in the farm ponds. The studies suggested that the foam and bamboo are suitable for this purpose, whereas dry coconut husks were not.

Resource degradation in rice farming systems in Thailand endangers food security, but the systems may become more sustainable by combining them with aquaculture and livestock farm enterprises by capitalization of their synergies in resource use and re-use, i.e. by adopting integrated farming systems. Most empirical studies that assess this potential have focused on a few specific aspects, but not on the multiple social, economic, and ecological functions of resource integration. In Northeast Thailand integrated farming systems were found to outperform the normal or commercial farming systems in all four dimensions of a multifunctional agriculture: food security, environmental functions, economic functions, and social functions. The findings support the notion that diversification and integration of resources on farms is feasible in both economic and ecological terms. The analyses indicated that integrated farming does not, however, diminish the need for external inputs. High start-up cost might constrain farmers from switching to integrated farming and from exploiting the benefits of resource integration.

Different Types of Mixed Farming Systems

Crop-Livestock farming system

In the conventional system, the crop residues are fed to the cattle and the cattle dung (FYM) are put back to the field as manure or used as fuel. With increasing demand of fuel in rural areas, most of the available bulky organic manure is being consumed as fuel even though it is very good source of many of the plant nutrient (Table 2 & 3).

Table 2 : Contents of major nutrients in some manures (expressed as % on DM basis)

Bulky organic manures	N	P_2O_5	K_2O
Farmyard	0.5	0.3	0.5
Compost (rural)	0.5	0.5	1.0
Cow dung	1.5	0.5	0.5
Cow dung slurry from biogas plant	1.8	1.0	1.0
Sheep and Goat dung	3.0	1.0	2.1
Buffalo dung	1.5	1.0	1.0
Pig dung	3.0	2.5	2.0
Poultry litter	3.0	2.5	1.5

(Biswas and Mukherjee, 1989)

Table 3 : Contents of secondary and micro – nutrient elements in animal excreta and sludge (on oven-dry basis)

Material	CaO (%)	MgO (%)	Cu (ppm)	Zn (ppm)	Mn (ppm)	Fe (ppm)
Cow dung	0.37	0.33	16	177	155	3000
Pig dung	0.21	0.54	73	202	189	5000
Horse dung	0.26	0.49	14	35	139	2770
Camel dung	0.70	0.46	13	20	71	1620
Poultry dung	2.28	1.38	25	158	277	2780
Sludge (activated)	5.00	20.10	02	305	115	2490

(Biswas and Mukherjee, 1989)

Tiwari (1993) reported that these organic sources could be utilized both as fuel and manure by incorporating the biogas technology in the system. In doing so, the dung as well as the farm wastes could be used to produce biogas and resulting slurry becomes enriched manure containing 1.8 per cent N and 1 per cent each of P_2O_5 and K_2O (Table 2). The slurry could also be used as fish feed. Better benefit would accrue if the slurry could be incorporated in the soil, immediately after application, since the loss of nitrogen was very much reduced (Table 4) as compared to leaving the slurry on the surface.

Table 4 : Nitrogen losses in manure affected by application method.

Method of application	Type of manure	Nitrogen loss* (%)
Broadcast without incorporation	Solid	15-30
	Liquid	10-25
Broadcast with incorporation	Solid	1-5
	Liquid	1-5
Injection (Knifing)	Liquid	0-2

* Numbers do not include losses from storage. (Sutton, 1985).

The human excreta were considered to be a very good source of biogas (Tiwari, 1993). Though, the benefit of biogas technology is well known, it is not being widely used because of location specific technological and adoption problems.

Crop- Livestock- Forestry farming system

The farming system involved crop, livestock and forestry as depicted in Fig 1. Inclusion of the forestry in the crop-livestock farming system was considered to provide feed and the grazing ground for the livestock and in return the forest could get back the livestock droppings as manure. However, grazing must not exceed the optimum level for increasing the productivity of the forest. The role of forest cover in the integration was to reduce runoff and soil erosion, increase ground water recharge, function as CO_2 sink and to preserve the environment.

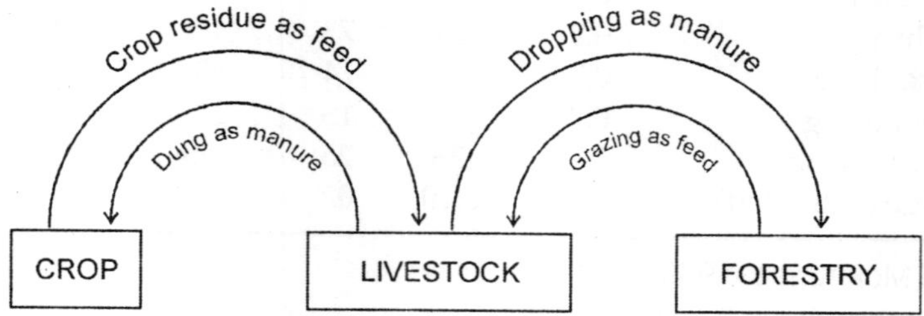

Fig. 1 : Crop – Livestock - Forestry system

Flooded Rice - Poultry - Fishery farming system

In integrated farming system, involving flooded rice, poultry and fisheries, a high degree of complementarities was achieved as shown in Fig 2. The potential area in India under rice-fish system was found to be 4.5 mha. Fishes grown in ponded rice field provide utilizable source of N to the crop by excreting amino-N as NH_3. It has been observed that yield of rice increased when fish was cultured along with rice (Table 5).

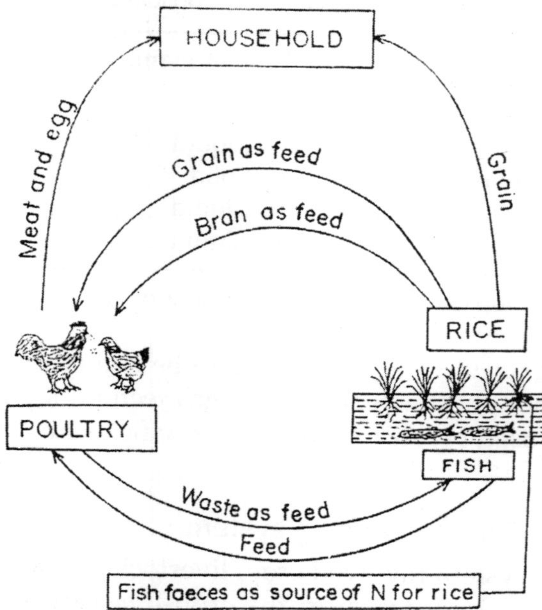

Fig. 2 : Crop – Poultry – Fishery farming system

Table 5 : Paddy yield with and without fish in Girdih (Bihar)

Treatment	Block	Paddy (Dry wt.) (Maunds/Acre)	Straw (Dry wt.) (Maunds/Acre)
Paddy alone	I	24.95	25.16
	II	14.93	20.34
Paddy + fish	I	26.57	28.00
	II	21.41	29.60

To increase the productivity of the system, it is necessary to select rice and fish genotypes which are compatible and fit in the system (Tiwari, 1993). There are many advantages of such system. It has been reported that rice-fish agro ecosystem increased nitrogen uptake by rice while increasing the organic carbon content of soil. The fish prevents and controls certain plant diseases and reduces the incidence of pests and weeds.

There has been rapid increase in poultry farming in India. The poultry could be effectively integrated in the rice-fish farming system. The compositions of poultry wastes (Table 6) indicate that it is a very good source of fish feed.

Table 6 : Constituents of Poultry waste.

Constituents	DM (% range)
Crude protein	18-40
Lignin	07-16
Urea, creatine and other nitrogenous compounds	03-10
Uric acid	28-55
Ammonia	08-15
Calcium	1.5-08
Phosphorus	1.2-2.6
Potassium	02-03

(Muller, 1980).

The small fish grown in rice field was very good poultry feed. The rice bran and grain and grain could also be used as poultry feed. Beside this, poultry also acted as insect suppressant. Movement of poultry and fish in ponded rice made the soil softer and increased dissolved oxygen in water.

Rice - Poultry – Fishery - Livestock system

Suitable enterprises from the systems already described were combined together to form another integrated farming system (Fig. 3), which was more labour intensive, economically sound and environmentally safe. In such an integrated system, dependence on inorganic fertilizer was greatly reduced by utilizing different organic sources available in the system. This, however, required the development of suitable methods of management of organic manures to increase the efficiency of various nutrient elements present in them.

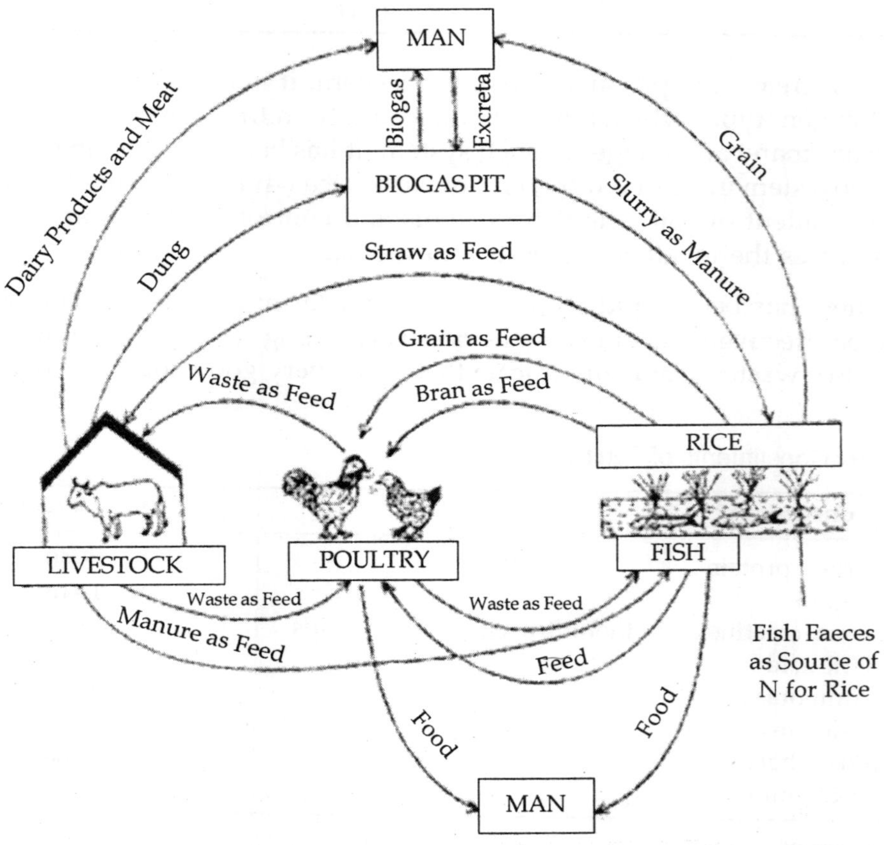

Labour Intensive Integrated Farming Economically Sound and Environmentally Safe

Fig. 3 : Crop - Livestock - Poultry - Fishery farming system

Dependence on inorganic manure was further reduced when manuring is practiced by introducing a suitable short duration crop for the purpose. Experiments had shown that almost same yield of rice was obtained by supplying nitrogen through green manure as in organic and organic sources. In this integrated system, fish production depends primarily on the livestock waste of the farm. Fish fed directly from manure as through formation of protein rich zooplankton, phytoplankton and macrophytes. For increasing productivity of the ponded ecosystem based on livestock manure, it was desirable to have an estimate of nitrogen to phosphorus ratio of livestock manure, because nitrogen was more likely to be limited than phosphorus for bacterial growth and phytoplankton formation. It was so since nitrogen is more volatile than phosphorus and thus more rapidly lost from the ponds. Since the amount and composition of livestock feaces and urine varied widely with total live weight, age and feed characteristics, climate and management.

Manures, added to fishpond, varied in their efficiency to produce fish biomass. It was observed that the manure obtained from one dairy cow produced 100-200 kg/year of fish biomass where as manure from the broiler produced 3-4 kg/year of fish biomass (Table 7).

Table 7 : Fish biomass production from manure

Source of manure	Biomass production (kg/ year)
One dairy cow	100-220
One beef cattle	90-160
One sheep	10-17
One pig	15-40
One laying hen	6-8
One turkey	7-8
One replacement bird	4-5
One broiler	3-4

(Muller, 1980).

Other farming systems

Farming which combines crop production with livestock raising is called Mixed Farming. In each area farming system changes according to the climate, economical status of the farmer and the resources available with the farmers. Singh (1961) described mixed farming as a combination of livestock enterprises (milch cattle, sheep, goats and pigs), bee-keeping, fish rearing *etc.*, with arable farming to secure optimum resource use and yield maximum income to farmers.

Talib and Singh (1961) highlighted the regional variations in the pattern of mixed farming based on the type and quality of livestock in Aulant, Mirka and Lodhi Nangal villages in Punjab. The results showed that the buffaloes were proportionately more in number in Mirka and Lodhi Nangal, while cows were more numerous in Aulant. The number of goats and sheep were insignificant in all the three villages but a cross-section of farmers in one or two villages; undergo poultry farming on a limited scale. Madhava Swamy (1985) studied the impact on additional income and employment potential due to inclusion of subsidiary occupations such as dairying, poultry and sheep rearing to the crop farming. He suggested that the optimum size of a diversified farming unit should be up to 4-5 milch cattle or 30 sheep or 500 poultry birds to lead a moderate standard of living and also to cross the poverty line. Singh and Sharma (1988) identified five different farming systems for the small farmers in Mid-Western region of Uttar Pradesh, *viz.*, (i) crop farming, (ii) crop + dairy farming, (iii) crop + goat farming, (iv) crop + dairy + goat farming and (v) crop + dairy + poultry farming system. Singh *et al.* (1990) evaluated the economics of buffaloes and crossbred cows under mixed farming systems in the semi-arid tract of Haryana and revealed that mixed farming with three cross bred cows was more profitable as compared to mixed farming with three buffaloes. In another report (Deoghare *et al.*, 1991) described four different farming systems were identified in Karnal district (Haryana) that includes (i) crop farming (ii) crop + poultry farming (iii) crop + dairy farming (iv) crop + dairy + poultry farming systems, of which crop + dairy + poultry farming system was found to be superior in income generation. Chaudhry and Chaudhry (1992) evaluated the possibilities of increasing net farm income by including labour intensive dairy enterprises and vegetables along with crops under existing levels of technology in Pakistan. The results suggested that the dairy animals (buffaloes) were found to be an essential part of farm plans for securing increased net cash returns, providing employment for family's excess labour and served as excess labour and served as useful outlet for crop byproducts, which would otherwise go waste.

Integration of arable farming with any combination of dairying, sheep, goat, poultry, piggery, bee-keeping, fish culture, vegetables cultivation, horticulture and mushroom cultivation for yielding additional income, besides providing additional employment opportunities to the surplus family labour especially in the case of small and marginal farmers have been advocated by Khatkar *et al.* (1991). In Mid-Western Uttar Pradesh, Singh *et al.* (1991a) identified six farming systems *viz,* i) crop farming, ii) crop + dairy farming, iii) crop + goat farming, iv) crop + dairy + goat farming, v) crop + goat + poultry farming and vi) crop + piggery farming and concluded that wherever dairy constituted a component of farming system; it has appeared as a major source of income. Sastry *et al.* (1992) identified various livestock keeping systems of landless and land owning households in a Southern Indian province with cows and followers; buffaloes and followers; bullocks; goats; sheep; mixed herd of large ruminants; mixed flock of small ruminants; mixed herd/flock of large and small ruminants and with no livestock.

Income and Employment Generation

Majority of the studies conducted to assess income and employment generation through livestock activities in the country were confined only to milch animals and diversification of farming systems with milch animals. Less attention had been paid to study the influence of other livestock enterprises *viz.* goat, bullock, poultry *etc.* in different farming systems on rural income and employment generation. This underlined the need for a detailed examination to assess the income and employment generated by the livestock under different farming systems.

Income

Panneerselvam (1974) described the gross income, as the total value of products received from crop enterprises, livestock enterprises, hiring out of animals, sale of animals, income from sale of products of perennial crops, off farm-income and income from non-farm sources. Mishra *et al.* (1978) studied the production economics of milch goats (12 Beetle and 12 Alpine X Beetel does and 1 Saanen buck) in the village Dwellings on 1.5 acres of land under stall-feeding and intensive management system for a year at the NDRI, Karnal. A resident labour input was provided to the unit. Green fodder grown at the farm (1.5 acres) was supplied to the goats mixed with wheat *bhusa*. The monthly income and expenditure statement revealed a net income of Rs 81 per month.

Sardana and Panghal (1984) estimated the net return at the existing level of technology and resource use, without buffalo as Rs 3133 and Rs 6804 on introducing one buffalo in the production plan with an increase of 117.18 per cent at Bhiwani district in Haryana. Saini and Singh (1985) calculated that the diversification of arable farming with livestock activities resulted in an increase in income ranging from 12.21 per cent to 54.15 per cent. Singh *et al.* (1985) found that the dairy farming on per unit area basis was more profitable than crop farming. It promised an average return of Rs 4792 and Rs 4638 per acre in group I (land holding above 5 acres) and group II (land holdings of 5 acres and below) households in the sub-urban and Rs 2305 and Rs 2290 in the rural villages of Punjab, respectively. Madhava Swamy (1985) observed that the net returns were higher by Rs 620, Rs 5198 and Rs 1598 in diversified farms of dairying, poultry and sheep rearing, respectively over the crop enterprise farm in Karnool district of Andhra Pradesh. Kumar *et al.* (1985) calculated the average gross annual income from goat rearing on the small (Rs 4242), medium (Rs 4965) and large (Rs. 5824) flocks from 120 goat-rearing households. The study involved 12 villages in Mahendragarh and Bhiwani districts of Haryana. A study on farming pattern of sheep breeders was conducted in 8 villages of ORP of the Central Sheep and Wool Research Institute, Avikanager in Rajasthan to work out the economics of crop and livestock farming adopted by the farmers in the area (Singh, 1987). Livestock contributed 47% and agriculture 43% to the total income of these breeders.

Sheep, goats and bovines contributed 11.9, 22.3 and 23.2 %, respectively to the total income (Table 8).

Table 8 : Comparative gross income from livestock and agriculture

Farming	Sources of income	Gross income (%)	Income (Rs)
Sheep	Wool	3.10	
	Milk	0.55	11.9
	Lamb sale	7.14	
	Manure	1.06	
Goat	Milk	11.70	
	Kids sale	8.24	22.3
	Manure	2.32	
Bovines	Milk	19.12	
	Animal sale	1.15	23.2
	manure	2.97	
Agriculture			42.6

(Singh, 1987)

Bhogal *et al.* (1988) concluded that dairying contributes significantly to the total family income and employment of small and marginal farmers and agricultural labours of Western Uttar Pradesh but the contribution was more substantial in the later cases. Singh *et al.* (1990) studied the levels of income on small and marginal farms (Table 9) under various farming systems in mid-western region of Uttar Pradesh. Using the linear programming technique they observed crop activities as the most dominant and their contribution to existing income as 62% followed by off- farm activities (25%) and goat enterprise (13%).

In the optimum farming system, income through goat enterprise increased by 4.5 times over the existing level. The over all increase in the level of total income in small farm was only 28.7% with major portion being accounted for by goat enterprise. On marginal farm under optimal farming system, income through goat enterprise increased 10 times over the existing level. The over all increase in the level of total income was about 161% with major portion being accounted for by goat enterprise. Singh *et al.* (1990) evaluated the economics of buffaloes and crossbred cows under mixed farming systems in the semi-arid tract of Haryana and revealed that mixed farming with three crossbred cows was more profitable as compared to mixed farming with three buffaloes. Dangat *et al.* (1991) studied the employment and income pattern between dry bajra zone farming with and without milch animals and irrigated farming with and without milch animals in Maharashtra. The results showed that in the dry bajra more than twice of the male and female days were utilized in the case of farming system with livestock components as compared to the farming system without milch animals. In the case of irrigated farms less than half the male and female days were utilized in farming system without milch animals as compared with that of irrigated farms with milch animals and the total family income was Rs 18389 and Rs 11164 in the farming system with and without milch animals, respectively. The study based on data collected in 3 villages of Bagepalli taluka in Kolar district, a drought-prone region of Karnataka, indicated that 17.3% of the total gross income of small and marginal farmers was accounted from small ruminants (goat and sheep) and 19% from large ruminants. Agriculture contributed less than 50% of the total gross income, which was more or less equal to the share from animal husbandry (Table 10). Besides, when the poor farmers lose the *kharif* crop, they can survive on goat and sheep. The net returns per household from crop cultivation is Rs 3811 followed by large ruminants is Rs 1617 (Pasha, 1990). The relative economics of 1 buffalo vs 5 goat units was studied for 4 years at Ajmer in Rajasthan (Pasha, 1990). The profit per annum was Rs 1755 from 1 buffalo and Rs 1945 from 5 goats though the initial investment was less for 5 goats (Table 11).

Table 9 : Contribution of enterprises in income on small and marginal farms in various farming systems

Farmer	Activities	Existing			Optimal		
		Unit*	Farm family income	% Contribution	Unit*	Farm family income	% Contribution
Small	Crop	1.45	4013	61.9	1.45	3116	37.4
	Goat	2.0	850	13.1	8.0	4780	57.3
	Off-farm	--	1614	24.19	--	438	5.25
Marginal	Crop	0.52	1547	36.81	0.5	1788	16.2
	Goat	2.0	756	17.99	13.0	8501	77.3
	Off-farm	--	1900	45.20	--	699	6.36

*Unit in case of crop in hector and for goat in numbers.

Table 10 : Share of gross income from different sources

Source of income	Share of gross income (%)	Net returns/ Household (Rs)
Crop cultivation	41.3	3811
Large ruminants	19.0	1728
Small ruminants	17.3	1617
Hiring out of own labour	22.0	--
Others	0.4	--
Total	100.0	

Table 11 : Relative economics of 1 buffalo *vs* 5 goat units at Ajmer in Rajasthan

Particulars	One buffalo unit	Five goat unit
Number of animals	1	5
Breed	Local	Sirohi
Value (Rs)	3000	2500
Number of lactation in 4 years	2	6
Production of milk (Liters)	2500	6000
Price/Liters (Rs)	3.00	2.00
Value realized by sale (Rs)	7500	12000
Number of calves/kids born	2	42
: male	1	21
: female	1	21
Sale value of grown up calves/kids for reproduction/meat/milk (Rs)	3000	6000
Maintenance cost including feed labour *etc.* (Rs)	17520	10220
Profits for 4 years (Rs)	7020	7780
Profits per annum (Rs)	1755	1945

(Pasha, 1990).

Kuber Ram and Sharma (1991) estimated the average gross income per family per annum from different sources for the landless, marginal and small farmers as Rs 5304, Rs 11381 and Rs 20910, respectively. Out of which dairying contributed 51, 23 and 15 per cent of the total family income of the three categories of households in Western Uttar Pradesh. Singh *et al.* (1991c) compared three types of farming systems at Hissar, *viz.*, mixed farming with three crossbred cows, mixed farming with three murrah buffaloes and arable farming with or without one milch animal and found that the mixed farming with three crossbred cows gave the highest net return of about Rs.21, 000 and also generated the highest man-days of employment.

Singh *et al.*, evaluated during 1991 that the income of beneficiaries and non-beneficiaries of IRDP and found that the net income, family labour income on beneficiary's and farm business was Rs 1199.84, Rs 1569.53 and Rs 1629.53 per she-buffalo per lactation, respectively. Prabaharan and Thirunavukkarasu (1992) calculated the gross income obtained through sale of kids and adults and sale and / or household utilization of manure and milk from goat in Tamil Nadu and calculated the net returns as Rs 1200, Rs 1879 and Rs 6800 in small (1-8 goats), medium (9-16 goats) and large (17 goats and above) herds, respectively. Deoghare and Sharma (1992) estimated the net returns from crop, dairy, poultry enterprises in bullock operated and tractor operated farms of Karnal district of Haryana as Rs 1294.63 and Rs 1505.33 / hector / year, respectively. Sastry *et al.* (1993) investigated the contribution of livestock sub system to the income of rural household belonging to landless, marginal farmer, small farmer and big farmer categories of a South Indian Province. The net worth of produce Rs 6691, Rs 6172, Rs 3514 and Rs 6302 from livestock; and Rs 9827, Rs 7863, Rs 4151 and Rs 2884 from wage earning per household per year, respectively. Deoghare and Sood (1994) evaluated the income and employment potential of goat rearing in Mathura district of Uttar Pradesh. The gross income per household per year from sale of milk, goats manure and stock acceleration was calculated on landless goat breeders as Rs 3183 whereas on marginal, small, medium and large farms, it was Rs 2301, Rs 2575, Rs 2381 and Rs 2642, respectively. Tiwari *et al.* (1999) identified an ideal model in the Bastar tribal of Chhattisgarh state and found that on 1.5 ha land holding a model having 2 crossbreed cows + 15 goats + 10 poultry birds +10 ducks + fish (0.15 ha) + crop farming (1.5 ha) was the best with a net income of Rs 44911/year against an income of Rs 24093/year from arable farming system alone. A similar model was also developed by Ramarao (2005, 2006 and 2008) for the smallholder, marginal farmer and large farmers respectively, in the Chhattisgarh having different resources.

The research project "Contribution of livestock and crop enterprises to the economy of tribal farmers" was conducted in Kanke block of Ranchi district, Jharkhand. The study revealed that the average gross annual gross income from livestock was Rs 4366 per farmer. Among livestock milch animals contributed about 53.27 per cent of annual income followed by sheep and goat (30.46 per cent) and pig (16.27 per cent) as indicated in Table 12 (Singh, 2002).

Table 12 : Gross annual income from crop and livestock on farms-biennial average (Rs/farm)

Particulars	Landless	Marginal	Small	Medium	Large	Average
Crop	-	6209	13824	22209	38781	29014
Livestock	2632	2616	3394	5291	7899	34690
Poultry	458	263	295	324	376	299

Employment

Goswami and Bora (1966) stated that a person who work for 300 days may be considered to be fully employed and the figure 300 days is arrived at by assuming that one worker would get one day holiday for each week (52 days) and 13 days for sickness and other works. Bishnoi (1966) concluded that employment is a state of being engaged in productive work. Continuous engagement in such work with sufficient amount of labour put in and an adequate reward flowing from it constitutes full employment. Three hundred and twenty days or more of work in the year are taken as full employment. All adults working for a minimum of one hour per day in gainful employment are regarded as employed. Those not rendering even this much of work are taken to be unemployed. Eight hours of work or more per day constitute a full man-day for an adult male worker. Persons putting less hours of work than these are considered as unemployed. Grewal and Rangi (1980) recorded the average annual labour input per cropped hectare for the general field crops in Punjab as 138.25 man-days / hector against 457 man-days per hectare per annum for dairying. It may be noted that the per unit area labour input in general crop farming was only about 30 per cent of the labour use in dairying. Yadav and Mishra (1980) reported that the grants and subsidies have made significant impact in the generation of farm employment in Bastar district of Madhya Pradesh. The employment of the beneficiary families had increased by 26.17 per cent against 13.40 per cent for the non-beneficiaries.

Singh *et al.* (1981) calculated the total labour absorption in the dairy enterprise ranged from 224 man-days on small farms to 423 man-days on large farms, the overall average being 301 man-days. Madhava Swamy (1985) worked out the employment potential due to inclusion of subsidiary occupations such as dairying, poultry and sheep rearing to the crop enterprise farming and found that the labour utilization pattern was higher by 123, 131 and 116 in diversified farms of dairying, poultry and sheep rearing, respectively over the crop production in Karnool district of Andhra Pradesh. Satheesh *et al.* (1985) observed that crop-dairy-sericulture farming system with adequate credit and recommended technology created highest employment (905 man-days *i.e.* 90 per cent employment intensity) for group I (poorest 50 per cent farmers) and almost full employment (930 man-days, 96 per cent employment intensity) for group II (rest 50 per cent) of East Godavari district of Andhra Pradesh. Prabaharan and Thirunavukkarasu (1992) observed that goats have provided gainful employment to the herders, generating on an average about 184, 309 and 437 labour days per annum per household in small (1-8 goats), medium (9-16 goats) and large (17 goats and above) goat herds, respectively in Tamil Nadu. Deoghare (1993) recorded that the employment of family labour was highest on large size (above 10 goats) herd (113.38 days), followed by medium size (6-10 goats) herd (76.70 days). Low investment of family labour was observed on small size (2-5 goats) herd (43.88 days) of Mathura district of Uttar Pradesh. Usha *et al.* (1993) reported that the human labour absorption in various operations of livestock enterprise had positive relationship with the size of holdings. It was further noted that on an average a household spent about 123 days per annum in this enterprise.

In Mathura district of Uttar Pradesh, Deoghare and Sood (1994) studied the employment of labour in goat enterprise and found that employment was highest on large farms (83.52 days), followed by landless (81.18 days), small (77.94 days) and medium (71.17 days) categories, and low employment of labour was observed on marginal farms (70.23 days). In the study all adults working for a minimum of one hour per day in gainful employment were regarded as employed. Eight hours of work per day constitute a full labour day for an adult worker. Off–farm employment was taken as the employment that the sample households in other's farm fields for wage earning purpose. Singh (2002) studied under the research project "Contribution of livestock and crop enterprises to the economy of tribal farmers" was conducted in Kanke block of Ranchi district, Jharkhand. The study revealed that livestock created annual employment of 576 man-days, goat and sheep 145, milch animal 137 and pig 126 man-days, respectively per annum (Table 13).

Table 13 : Annual labour employment in rearing of livestock on selected farms-biennial average (days/farm)

Category of farms	Livestock activities				
	Draught animal	Milch animal	Sheep and Goat	Pig	Total
Landless	-	41	209	185	435
Marginal	153	68	140	155	516
Small	143	126	139	109	517
Medium	167	160	121	76	524
Large	210	292	116	107	725

Constraints of Integrated Farming Systems

Although the aforementioned studies have clearly shown that the system is feasible with respect to socioeconomic imperatives, actual adoption rates of integrated farming are limited and unevenly spread among farmers.

The study by Ngambeki et al. (1992) revealed that the major production constraints are animal feed shortages throughout the year, labour bottlenecks, and soil degradation. Csavas (1992) reported that in most farms studied in there was a dependency on imported feed rather than internal recycled inputs. This was concluded to be due to resource-poor farmers in general not having feedlot type systems in which to undertake livestock production. The main constraints to adoption of integrated farming systems are: 1. the long transition period that often occurs when implementing an integrated production system. This lead-in time can vary between 3 to10 years. Farmers could not forgo declines in food production and income generation over this period; 2. labour shortages, especially where the family size is small, which effectively prevented them from adopting integrated farming techniques; 3. lack of secure land rights; and 4. disincentives to adopting integrated farming resulting from government subsidies, credits for fertilizers, and herbicides. Banerjee et al. (1990) assessed the impact on allocation of the farm area to different types of crops and livestock. The study revealed that there are few opportunities for increasing farm net returns with the limited amount of capital available.

Thamrongwarangkul (2001) reported that resource-poor farmers often can not go beyond the transition period due to their need for food and for immediate economic returns to meet cash needs such as schooling, medical treatment, and loan-repayment. Contrasting this Tokrishna (1992) pointed out that a farmer who becomes successful and wants to expand the area of his integrated farm would be limited by access to adequate water supply, animal feed, and market outlets.

The other constraints are:

- Nutritional values of crop residues are generally low in digestibility and protein content. Improving intake and digestibility of crop residues by physical and chemical treatments is technically possible but not feasible for poor small farmers because they require machinery and chemicals that are expensive or not readily available.
- Crop residues are primarily soil regenerators, but too often they are either disregarded or misapplied.
- Intensive recycling can cause nutrient losses.
- If manure nutrient use efficiencies are not improved or properly applied, the import of nutrients in feeds and fertilizers will remain high, as will

the costs and energy needs for production and transportation, and the surplus loss in the environment.

- Farmers prefer to use chemical fertilizer instead of manure because it acts faster and is easier to use.
- Resource investments are required to improve intake and digestibility of crop residues.

Mixed farms are prone to use more manure than crop farms do. Manure transportation is an important factor affecting manure use.

Challenges

- Develop strategies and promote crop livestock synergies and interactions that aim to (a) integrate crops and livestock effectively with careful land use; (b) raise the productivity of specific mixed crop-livestock systems; (c) facilitate expansion of food production; and (d) simultaneously safeguard the environment with prudent and efficient use of natural resources.
- Devise measures (for instance, facilitating large-scale dissemination of biodigesters) to implement a more efficient use of biomass, reducing pressures on natural resources; and develop a sustainable livestock manure management system to control environmental losses and contaminant spreading.

Advantages

In an integrated system, livestock and crops are produced within a coordinated framework. The waste products of one component serve as a resource for the other. For example, manure is used to enhance crop production; crop residues and by-products feed the animals, supplementing often inadequate feed supplies, thus contributing to improved animal nutrition and productivity. The result of this cyclical combination is the mixed farming system, which exists in many forms and represents the largest category of livestock systems in the world in terms of animal numbers, productivity and the number of people it services.

Animals play key and multiple roles in the functioning of the farm, and not only because they provide livestock products (meat, milk, eggs, wool, hides) or can be converted into prompt cash in times of need. Animals transform plant energy into useful work: animal power is used for ploughing, transport and in activities such as milling, logging, road construction, marketing, and water lifting for irrigation. Animals also provide manure and other types of animal waste. Excreta have two crucial roles in the overall sustainability of the system:

(a) *Improving nutrient cycling:* Excreta contain several nutrients (including nitrogen, phosphorus and potassium) and organic matter, which are important for maintaining soil structure and fertility. Through its use, production is increased while the risk of soil degradation is reduced.

(b) *Providing energy:* Excreta are the basis for the production of biogas and energy for household use (e.g. cooking, lighting) or for rural industries (e.g. powering mills and water pumps). Fuel in the form of biogas or dung cakes can replace charcoal and wood.

Crop residues represent the other pillar on which the equilibrium of this system rests. They are fibrous by-products that result from the cultivation of cereals, pulses, oil plants, roots and tubers. They are a valuable, low-cost feed resource for animal production, and are consequently the major source of nutrients for livestock in developing countries.

The overall benefits of crop-livestock integration can be summarized as follows:

- Agronomic, through the retrieval and maintenance of the soil productive capacity;
- Economic, through product diversification and higher yields and quality at less cost;
- Ecological, through the reduction of crop pests (less pesticide use and better soil erosion control); and
- Social, through the reduction of rural urban migration and the creation of new job opportunities in rural areas.

This system has other specific advantages:

- It helps to improve and conserve the productive capacities of soils, with physical, chemical and biological soil recuperation. Animals play an important role in harvesting and relocating nutrients, significantly improving soil fertility and crop yields.
- It is quick, efficient and economically viable because grain crops can be produced in four to six months, and pasture formation after cropping is rapid and inexpensive.
- It helps to increase profits by reducing production costs. Poor farmers can use fertilizer from livestock operations, especially when rising petroleum prices make chemical fertilizers unaffordable.
- It results in greater soil water storage capacity, mainly because of biological aeration and the increase in the level of organic matter.

- It provides diversified income sources, guaranteeing a buffer against trade, price and climate fluctuations.

Key principles

- *Cyclic.* The farming system is essentially cyclic (organic resources - livestock - land - crops). Therefore, management decisions related to one component may affect the others.
- *Rational.* Using crop residues more rationally is an important route out of poverty. For resource-poor farmers, the correct management of crop residues, together with an optimal allocation of scarce resources, leads to sustainable production.
- *Ecologically sustainable.* Combining ecological sustainability and economic viability, the integrated livestock-farming system maintains and improves agricultural productivity while also reducing negative environmental impacts.

Recommendations

- The maintenance of an integrated crop livestock system is dependent on the availability of adequate nutrients to sustain animals and plants and to maintain soil fertility. Animal manure alone cannot meet crop requirements, even if it does contain the kind of nutrients needed. This is because of its relatively low nutrient density and the limited quantity available to small-scale farmers. Alternative sources for the nutrients need to be found.
- Growing fodder legumes and using them as a supplement to crop residue is the most practical and cost-effective method for improving the nutritional value of crop residues. This combination is also effective in reducing weight loss in animals, particularly during dry periods;
- Given their traditional knowledge and experience, local farmers are perfectly able to apply an integrated system. In practice, however, relatively few adopt this system, mainly because they have limited access to credit, technology and knowledge. The crop-pasture rotation system is complex and requires a substantial capital outlay for machinery and implements. Associations of grain and livestock producers are useful for filling these gaps and can promote the adoption of a crop livestock system;
- Veterinary services are generally unable to reach poor small farmers in remote areas. Therefore, for livestock production to be improved, more attention needs to be paid to making veterinary care accessible, particularly in terms of prevention;

- Better livestock management is needed to safeguard water. Livestock water demand includes water for drinking and for feed production and processing. Livestock also have an impact on water, contaminating it with manure and urine. All of these aspects need to be given due consideration.
- Intensification of agriculture through appropriate incorporation of small livestock has the potential to decrease the land need for agricultural production and relieve the pressure on forests.

Key Issues and Questions for Project Design

The increase in demand for livestock products presents opportunities for small farmers who can increase livestock production and benefit from related income. However, in terms of environmental impact, the growing number of livestock and the increase in livestock processing can have a negative impact on natural resources unless actions are taken to identify farming practices that are economically and ecologically sustainable. Thanks to the dynamic interaction of its various components, the highly improved integrated crop-livestock system can guarantee more sustainable production and therefore constitutes a valid new approach.

Experience in the use of this system has shown that (a) adopting sustainable management practices can improve production while preserving the environment; (b) residues, wastes and byproducts of each component serve as resources for the others; and (c) poor farmers have the traditional knowledge needed to integrate livestock and crop production, but because of their limited access to knowledge, assets and inputs, relatively few adopt an integrated system.

The challenge for development practitioners is to ensure that poor small farmers can increase the productivity of traditional farming systems, adopting an effective integrated system that produces usable biomass while conserving natural resources, and can therefore be sustainable in the long term.

Within this framework some key questions for project design are:

- How can livestock production increase to meet the growing demand for livestock products, using methods that the resource base can sustain?
- Do the strategies devised for raising productivity in integrated crop-livestock systems take into account the stage of development of the target population with respect to the nature of crop-livestock interactions?
- Do the farmers concerned have the right skills, knowledge, capital and technology to set up this system?

- Are the roles and responsibilities of men and women given sufficient consideration?
- How can additional needed nutrients be obtained? And, can the productivity of the system be increased without stressing the environment?
- Is enough good-quality feed available to sustain animals, especially during the dry season?
- Are nutrients that are relocated from grazing areas to croplands efficiently recovered?
- Are the different components of the farming system (crop, livestock and, eventually, fish) efficiently integrated?

References

Agbonlabor M.U., Aromolaran, A.B., and Aiboni, V.I. (2003). J. Sustain. Agr., 22: 51-62.

Ashby, *J.A.* 2001. Ecol. Soc., 5.

Banerjee B.N., Sarker S.C. and Maity A.K. (1990). *Indian J. Dairy Sci.,* 43: 295-301.

Bhogal, T.S., Sharma, J.S. and Arora, V.P.S. (1988). *Indian J. Dairy Sci.,* 41(1): 101-108.

Bishnoi, R.N. (1966). Indian J. of Agri. Economics. 21(1): 51-61.

Biswas, T.D. and Mukherjee, S.K. (1989). Tata McGraw-Hill Publication. *Soil Sci.*

Chaudhry, M.A. and Chaudhry, A.J. (1992). J. Rural Develop. Admin., 24(3): 18-30.

Csavas, I. (1992). Regional review on livestock-fish production systems in Asia. In: Mukherjee, T.K., Moi, P.S., Panandam, J.M., and Yang, Y.S. (Eds.), Proceedings of the FAO/IPT Workshop on integrated livestock-fish production systems, 16-20 December 1991, Institute of Advance Studies, University of Malaya, Kuala Lumpur, Malaysia.

Dalsgaard, J.P.T. and Oficial, R.T. (1997). *Agric. Syst.,* 55: 503-533.

Dangat, S.B., Sale, D.L. and Nawadkar, D.S. (1991). *Indian J. Agri. Econom.,* 46: 451-452.

Deoghare, P.R. (1993). *Indian J. Animal Sci.,* 63(1): 80-83.

Deoghare, P.R. and Sharma, B.M. (1992). *Agricultural Situation in India.* 47: 925-929.

Deoghare, P.R. and Sood, S.B. (1994). *Indian J. Anim. Sci.,* 64(3): 295-300.

Deoghare, P.R., Sharma, B.M. and Goel, S.K. (1991). *Agricultural Situation in India.* 46: 65-70.

Dillon, J., and McConnell, D.J. (1997). Farm management for Asia: A systems approach. FAO farm systems management Series 13. FAO, Rome Italy.

Edwards, P. (1997). Sustainable food production through aquaculture. Aquaculture Asia. Volume 2. School of Environment, Resources and Development, Asian Institute of Technology (AIT), Pathumthani, Thailand.

Grewal, S.S. and Rangi, P.S. (1980). *Indian J. Agri. Econ.*, 35(4): 120-125.

Jayanthi, C., Rangasamy, A., and Chinnusamy, C. (2000). *Agric. J.*, 87:411- 414.

Khatkar, R.K., Chamola, S.D. and Manocha, V. (1991). *Indian J. Agric. Econ.*, 46: 448-449.

Kuber, R. and Sharma, A.K. (1991). *Indian J . Agric. Econom.*, 46: 460-461.

Kumar, S., Pandey, R.N. and Sharma, K.K. (1985). *Indian J. Anim. Sci.* 56:126-130.

Lightfoot C., and Minnick, D.R. (1991). *J. Farming Systems Res. Ext.*, 2:11-34.

Little, D.C., and Edwards, P. (2003). Integrated livestock-fish systems. FAO, Rome, Italy.

Madhava Swamy, G. (1985). *Indian J. Agric. Econ.*, 40(3): p 333.

Mishra, R.R., Chawla, D.S. and Sundersan, D. (1978). Goats at National Dairy Research Institute, Karnal, Publication No. 159, NDRI, Karnal.

Muller, Z.O. (1980). FAO Animal Production and Health paper No. 18.

Ngambeki, D.S., Deuson, R.R., and Preckel, P.V. (1992). *Agric. Syst.* 38: 319-338.

Noble, A.D., and Ruaysoongnern, S. (2002). The role of indigenous technology and science in rehabilitating degraded light textured soils using high activity clays and bioremediation. International Water Management Institute (IWMI) and Khon Kaen University (KKU), Thailand.

Okigbo, B.N. (1995). major farming systems of the lowland savanna of SSA and the potential for improvement. In: Proceedings of the IITA/FAO workshop, Ibadan, Nigeria.

Panneerselvam, R. (1974). A study on consumption, saving and distribution of income in farm households in Pattukkottai division, Thanjavur district. M.Sc. thesis: Department of Agricultural Economics, TNAU. p 10.

Pant, J. (2002). Integrated agriculture-aquaculture systems in the context of socioeconomic transformation in NE-Thailand. PhD. Thesis. Asian Institute of Technology (AIT), Pathumthani, Thailand.

Pasha, S.A. (1990). Sustainability and viability of small and marginal farmers with reference to animal husbandry and common property resources. Paper presented at the National seminar held on October 8-10 at NIRD, Hyderabad.

Prabhaharan, R. and Thirunavukkarasu, M. (1992). Goat production in Tamil Nadu. Current status, problem and prospects. Research report / A. H. Econ. / 18. Dept of A.H. Economics, Madras Vet. College, TANUVAS. p 29.

Price, T. (2000). Cultivation our futures. Final Paper. OECD Publications No. 2. Organization for Economic Co-operation and Development.

Radhammani, S., Balasubramanian, A., Ramamoorthy, K., and Geethalakshmi, V. (2003). Agric. Rev., 24:204-210.

Ramrao W Y, Tiwari S P and Singh P (2005). Livestock Res. Rural Develop., Vol. 17, Art. #90. Retrieved October 15, 2010, from http://www.lrrd.org/lrrd17/8/ramr17090.htm

Ramrao, W. Y., Tiwari, S. P. and Singh, P. (2006) Livestock Res. Rural Develop., Vol. 18, *Article #102*. Retrieved October 15, 2010, from http://www.lrrd.org/lrrd18/7/ramr18102.htm.

Ramrao, W. Y., Tiwari, S. P., Sharma, Saraswat S., Pathak, R. and Gupta, R. (2008) Livestock Res. Rural Develop., Vol.20, Article #42. Retrieved October 15, 2010, from http://www.lrrd.org/lrrd20/3/ramr20042.htm

Saini, A.S. and Singh R.V. (1985). *Indian J. Agric. Econ.*, 40(3): 310-316.

Sardana, P.K. and Pangal, B.S. (1984). *Indian J. Dairy Sci.*, 37(3): 187-192.

Sastry, N.S.R., Bullerdieck, P. and Gall, Ch.F. (1992). *Indian J. Anim. Sci.*, 62(11): 1083-1091.

Sastry, N.S.R., Bullerdieck, P. and Gall, Ch.F. (1993). *Indian J. Anim. Sci.*, 63(2): 201-207.

Satheesh, A.V., Sharma, B.M. and Sharma V.K. (1985). *Indian J. Agric. Econ.*, 40(3): 323-329.

Schierre, J.B., Ibrahim, M.N.M. and van Keulen, H. (2002). *Agric. Ecosyst. Environ.*, 90: 139-153.

Singh A.K. and Sharma J.S. (1988). *Agric. Situation in India.*, 43(1): 17-23.

Singh, A.K., Singh, L.R. and Sharma, J.S. (1991a). *Indian J. Agric. Econ.*, 46: 459.

Singh, A.K., Singh, L.R. and Sharma, L.S. (1990). Levels of income on small and marginal farms under various farming system in mid-western region of Uttar Pradesh, Research paper No. 6376. G. B. Pant University of Agriculture and Technology, Pantnagar.

Singh, B., Bal, H.S. and Kumar, N. (1985). *Indian J. Agric. Econ.*, 40(3): 330-331.

Singh, C.B., Dhaka, J.P. and Sharma, S.P. (1981). *Indian J. Agric. Econ.*, 36(4): 14-20.

Singh, H.S. (1961). *Indian J. Agric. Econ.*, 16(1): 122-131.

Singh, K. (1987). *Indian J. Anim. Sci.*, 57(4): 317-323.

Singh, R.P. (2002). *Indian Dairyman*, 54 (5): 51-57.

Singh, R.P., Singh, J.P. and Singh, R.P. (1991). *Agric. Situation in India,* 46: 603-606.

Singh, S.N., Singh, K.P., Gupta, L.R., Kadian, V.S. and Singh, N. (1991c). *Indian J. Agric. Econ.*, 46: 468-469.

Sutton, A.L. (1985). St. Paul University, Minnesota. *Extension Bulletin* AG-FO-2613.

Talib, B.D. and Singh, H. (1961). *Indian J. Agric. Econ.*, 16(1): 155-162.

Thamrongwarangkul, A. (2001). For out Thailand. Annual report on sustainable community development for good livelihoods and environmental project. Khon Kaen University.

Tipraqsa, P. (2006). Opportunities and constraints of integrated farming system in Northeast Thailand. A case study of the Huai Nong Ian catchment, Khon Kaen Province. Ecology Development Series No. 35. University of Bonn. Cuvillier Verlag, Göttingen, Germany.

Tiwari, P.N. (1993). *J. Nuclear Agri. Biol.*, 22(1): 1-13.

Tiwari, S.P., Saxena, R.R., Nandeha, K.L., Sharma, R.B. and Rajagopal, S. (1999). *Indian J. Animal Sci.*, 69(6): 448-452.

Tokrishna, R. (1992). Integrated livestock-fish farming systems I Thailand. In: Mukherjee, T.K., Moi, P.S., Panadam, J.M., and Yang, Y.S. (Eds.). Proceedings of the FAO/IPT Workshop on Integrated Livestock-Fish Production Systems, 16- 20 December, 1991. Institute of Advanced Studies, University of Malaya, Kuala Lumpur, Malaysia.

Usha, R., Vyas, D.L. and Jodha, G.S. (1993). *Indian J. Agric. Econ.*, 48(3): 482-487.

Van Brakel, M.L., Morales, E.J., Turingruang, D., and Little D.C. (2003). Livelihood improving functions of pond based integrated agriculture and aquaculture systems. MRC Fisheries Programme (FP). Institute of Aquaculture, University of Stirling, Scotland, UK.

Yadav, H. and Mishra, C.S. (1980). *Indian J. Agric. Econ.*, 35(4): 69-73.

❑❑❑

Animal Nutrition, 2012
eds. Dr. (Mrs.) Usha R. Mehra et al., pp. 29-47
Satish Serial Publishing House e-mail : info@satishserial.com; website : www.satishserial.com

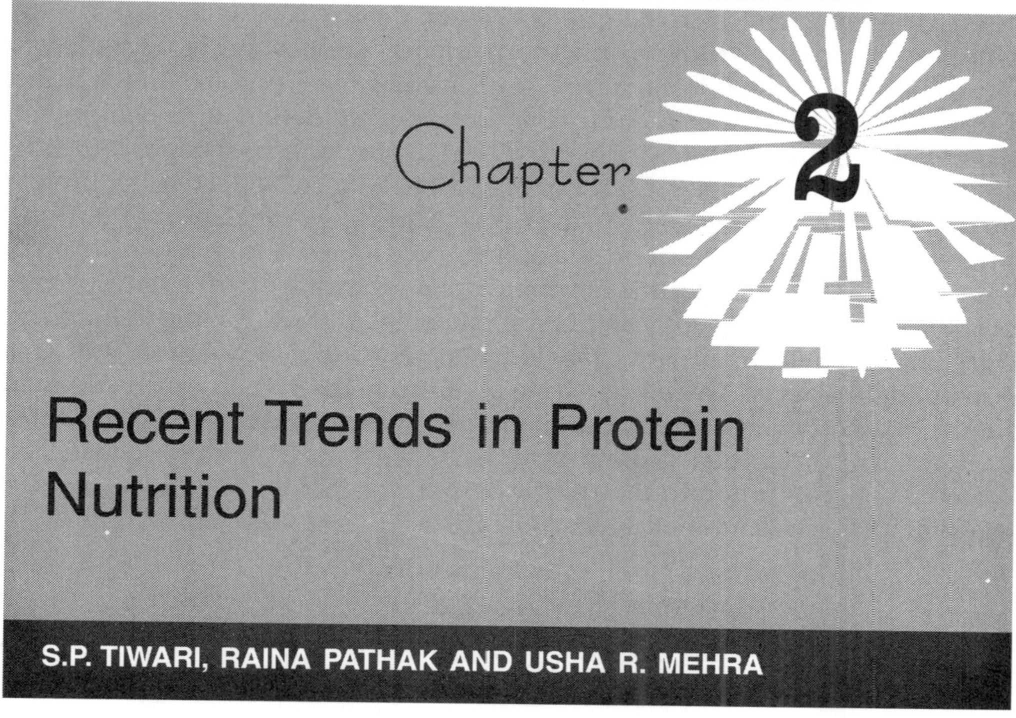

Chapter 2

Recent Trends in Protein Nutrition

S.P. TIWARI, RAINA PATHAK AND USHA R. MEHRA

Nutritional models for feeding protein to dairy cattle have evolved from basic CP (ARC, 1980) to more complex systems based on rumen-degradable (RDP) and undegradable protein (NRC, 2001). The basic structure of all the models is similar with nitrogen (N) inputs provided by dietary, recycled, and endogenous N. Dietary protein is divided into rumen-degradable and undegradable protein while RDP composed of non protein and true protein N. The Cornell Net Carbohydrate and Protein System (CNCPS) was developed to predict requirements, feed utilization, animal performance and nutrient excretion for dairy and beef cattle and sheep, using accumulated knowledge about feed composition, digestion, and metabolism in supplying nutrients to meet requirements (Fig. 1).

True protein is degraded to peptides and amino acid (AA) and eventually deaminated into ammonia N or incorporated into microbial protein. Non protein N is composed of N present in DNA, RNA, ammonia, AA, and small peptides with N from peptides, AA, and ammonia being used for microbial growth. Rumen output consists of ammonia N, undegraded protein (dietary or endogenous), and microbial protein. When dietary RDP is in excess of the amount required by ruminal microorganisms, the protein is degraded to ammonia N, absorbed, metabolized to urea in the liver, and lost in the urine. Under typical dairy cattle feeding conditions, manipulation of rumen protein degradation or the efficiency of N use (ENU) in the rumen is the most effective strategy to reduce N losses. Losses of N may be reduced by decreasing protein degradation in the rumen and (or) increasing N use by ruminal microorganisms. Microbial protein synthesis in the rumen provides the majority of protein supplied to the small intestine of ruminants, accounting for 50 to 80% of total absorbable protein. The total amount of microbial protein flowing to the small intestine depends on nutrient availability and efficiency to use these nutrients by ruminal bacteria. Therefore, N metabolism in the rumen can be divided into 2 distinct events: protein degradation, which provides N sources for bacteria, and microbial protein synthesis. Most studies have focused on ammonia concentration in the rumen despite the fact that peptides and AA are similar in concentration to ammonia.

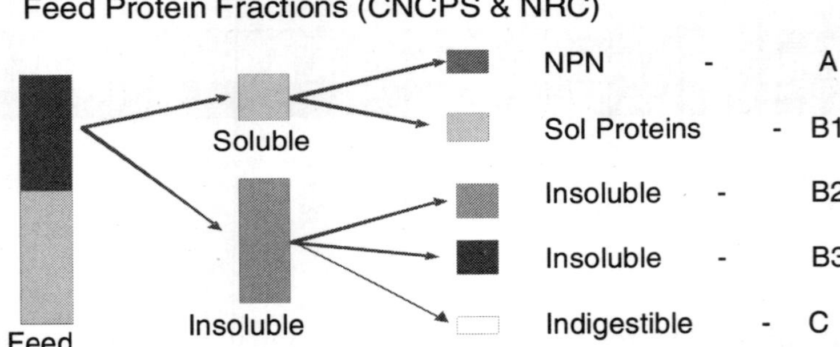

Fig. 1 :

A-Soluble in buffer (borate-phosphate)and not precipitated by tungstic acid

B1-Soluble in buffer and precipitated by tungstic acid

B2-Insoluble in buffer
= (Insoluble protein)-(protein insoluble in neutral detergent)

B3-Insoluble in buffer
= (Insoluble in neutral detergent)-(Insoluble in acid detergent)

C- Insoluble in buffer and acid detergent

Ruminal Degradation of Protein

The first step of protein degradation in the rumen involves attachment of bacteria to feed particles, followed by activity of cell-bound microbial proteases. It has been presented in Fig. 2. Approximately 70 to 80% of ruminal microorganisms attach to undigested feed particles in the rumen, and 30 to 50% of those have proteolytic activity. A large number of different microbial species form a consortium that attaches to a feed particle, acting symbiotically to degrade and ferment nutrients, including protein. Products resulting from this process are peptides and AA.

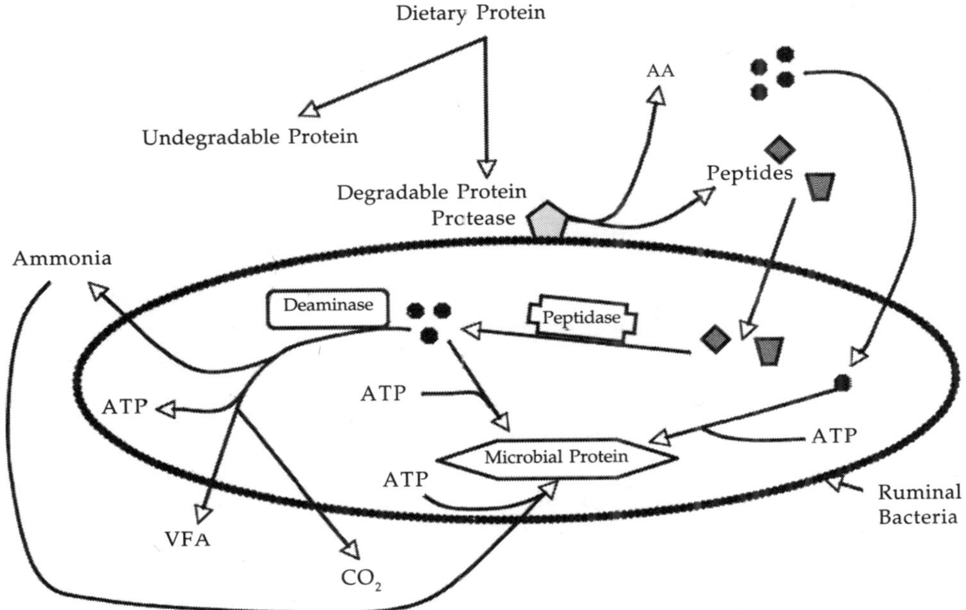

Fig. 2 : Schematic representation of protein degradation and fate of end products in the rumen.

Because the number of different bonds within a single protein is large, the synergistic action of different proteases is necessary for complete protein degradation. The rate and extent at which protein degradation occurs will depend on proteolytic activity of the ruminal microflora and the type of protein (susceptibility and accessibility of peptide bonds). Peptides and AA resulting from the extracellular rumen proteolytic activity are transported inside microbial cells. Peptides can be further degraded by peptidases into AA, and the latter can be incorporated into microbial protein or further deaminated to VFA, CO_2, and ammonia. The fate of absorbed peptides and AA once inside the microbial cell will depend on the availability of energy [carbohydrates (CHO)]. If energy is available, AA are transaminated or used directly for microbial protein synthesis. However, if energy is limiting, AA are deaminated, and their carbon skeleton will be fermented into VFA. Some ruminal bacteria lack mechanisms of AA transport from the cytoplasm to the extracellular environment, and AA absorbed in excess must be excreted from the cytoplasm as ammonia.

Most studies evaluating protein degradation in the rumen have been conducted using the *in situ* technique, which only measures protein degradation, but not the use of peptides and AA by ruminal bacteria. It was observed that peptides and AA did not accumulate after feeding proteins and suggested that proteolysis was the rate-limiting step and, therefore, key in controlling protein degradation. However, Broderick *et al.* (1991) demonstrated that rapidly degraded proteins may result in the accumulation of peptides and AA within the first 2 h after feeding, suggesting that rates of peptidolysis and deamination play an important role in the control of protein degradation. Recently, Cardozo *et al.* (2004) found in continuous culture fermenters receiving a typical dairy ration that the concentration of peptides, AA and ammonia were within the same range for up to 8 h after feeding. They reported an accumulation of AA-N at 2 and 4 h after feeding, suggesting that AA uptake could be the limiting factor of protein degradation in the rumen. Therefore, manipulation of protein degradation can be achieved not only by modulation of proteolysis, but also through changes in peptidolysis and deamination. For example, monensin reduced ammonia N concentration through the inhibition of the hyper-ammonia-producing bacteria, a small group of ruminal bacteria that are responsible for the production of most of the ammonia. Ferme *et al.* (2004) also reported that the inhibition of major ammonia-producing bacteria such as *Prevotella ruminantium* and *Prevotella bryantii* resulted in a reduction in ammonia N concentration in continuous culture fermenters of ruminal microbes. Amino acid fermenters in the rumen are as follows:

High numbers	Low numbers
Low activity	High activity
Butrivibrio fibrisolvens	*Clostridium aminophilum*
Measphaera elsdenii	*Clostridium sticklandii*
Selenomonas ruminantium	*Peptostreptococcus anaerobius*
10^9 per ml	10^7 per ml
10 to 20 Nmol NH_3/min/mg protein	300 Nmol NH_3/min/mg protein
Monensin resistant	Monensin sensitive
Ferment CHO strongly	Ferment CHO slowly or not

Continuous culture fermenters have low numbers of protozoa; however, *in vivo*, protozoa play a major role in protein degradation. The most important aspect of protozoa is their ability to engulf large molecules, protein, CHO, or even ruminal bacteria (Van Soest, 1994). In addition, protozoa play a role in regulating bacterial N turnover in the rumen, and they supply soluble protein to sustain microbial growth. Because protozoa are not able to use ammonia N a fraction of previously engulfed insoluble protein is later returned to the rumen fluid in the form of soluble protein (Dijkstra, 1994). This is one of the main reasons why defaunation decreases ammonia N concentration in the rumen (Eugene *et al.*, 2004).

Factors Affecting Ruminal Protein Degradation

The most important factors affecting microbial protein degradation include the type of protein, interactions with other nutrients (mainly CHO within the same feedstuff and within the rumen contents), and the predominant microbial population (dependent on the type of ration, ruminal passage rate, and ruminal pH).

Type of Protein

Solubility of proteins is a key factor determining their susceptibility to microbial proteases and, thus, their degradability. For example, prolamins and glutelins are insoluble and slowly degraded, but globulins are soluble and highly degradable in the rumen (Romagnolo *et al.*, 1994). However, the structure of the protein is also important. Some albumins are soluble but contain disulfide bonds, making them slowly degradable in the rumen, illustrating that factors other than solubility affect rumen degradability of proteins. The presence of bonds within and between protein chains (tertiary and quaternary structure) play an important role in determining protein degradation. For example, the acidic subunit glycinin (with strong disulfide bonds), the basic glycin, and several Leu-containing peptides in the N-terminal group in soybean meal are fairly resistant to degradation (Schwingel and Bates, 1996). In addition, specific peptide bonds are more resistant to ruminal degradation than others. For example, dipeptides formed of Lys-Pro are hydrolyzed in the rumen 5-fold slower than the dipeptide Lys-Ala, and dipeptides formed of Pro-Met are degraded 2.5-fold slower than dipeptides formed of Met-Ala. It has also been suggested that peptidases and deaminases may be regulated by end-product inhibition processes. Velle *et al.* (1997) infused increasing quantities (75, 150, 300, and 600 mmol) of different AA in the rumen and found that AA degradation decreased as the quantity infused increased.

Ruminal Dilution Rate

Protein degradation is inversely related to passage rate through the rumen. The NRC (2001) developed equations of passage rate for wet and dry forages and concentrates based on DMI, fibre content, and forage-to-concentrate ratio of the diet. Digesta passage rate of a cow consuming 18 kg of DM of a 70:30 forage-to-concentrate ration would increase from 0.049 to 0.057/h for wet forages, from 0.040 to 0.046/h for dry forages, and from 0.056 to 0.068/h for concentrates if the same cow would consume 26 kg of DM of a 40:60 forage-to-concentrate ration. With a standard ryegrass silage, alfalfa hay, and soybean meal, this increase in passage rate would result in a reduction in protein degradation of 1.2, 2.1, and 3.5 percentage units, respectively. These changes are small and represent only a modest increase in the flow of undegraded dietary protein supply to the small intestine.

Ruminal pH and Substrate

The optimal pH of rumen proteolytic enzymes ranges from 5.5 to 7. However, protein degradation is reduced at the lower end of the ruminal pH environment. Cardozo *et al.* (2002) conducted 2 dual flow continuous culture fermentation studies comparing high forage vs. high concentrate rations at pH ranging from 4.9 to 7.0 and demonstrated that protein degradation was reduced as pH decreased with both types of rations. Although amylolytic bacteria tend to be more proteolytic than cellulolytic bacteria, protein degradation was consistently lower when high-concentrate rations provided substrate to microbes, regardless of pH. In addition, a decrease in ruminal pH from 6.5 to 5.7 reduced ruminal ammonia concentration only when bacteria were obtained from cattle fed a 100% forage ration, whereas bacteria from cattle fed 90% concentrate had lower ammonia N concentration regardless of pH. These results indicate that protein degradation is affected by pH and type of ration, which may dictate the predominant type of microbial population present in the rumen. Devant *et al.* (2001) incubated soybean meal and heat-processed soybean meal in the rumen of dairy cattle fed a 60:40 forage-to-concentrate ration or in the rumen of beef cattle fed a 10:90 forage-to concentrate ration using the in situ technique. Results demonstrated that protein degradation was lower with the beef-type ration, despite the fact that pH was 6.0 in both types of animals, illustrating that the reduction of protein degradation is not only due to a pH effect, but is also related to type of substrate being fermented or the predominant microbial population induced by a particular ration.

Nutrient Interactions

The combined effect of pH and substrate on ruminal protein degradation may be explained by the resulting predominant microbial population. It is obvious that protein degradation occurs by the action of proteolytic enzymes, but there is evidence that supports the importance of other enzymatic activities on the degradation of protein. Assoumani *et al.* (1992) demonstrated that starch interferes with protein degradation. They noted that the addition of amylase increased total ruminal protein degradation of cereal grains between 6 and 20 percentage units. Positive effects of amylases on protein degradation were also demonstrated by others (Aufrere and Cartailler, 1988; Toma´nkova´ and Kopecny, 1995). Debroas and Blanchart (1993) found that NDF-bound protein was degraded by proteolytic bacteria only after microbial depolymerization of cellulose began. Kohn and Allen (1995) also reported an increase in protein degradation from 42.4 to 53.1% when cellulases were added to an *in vitro* proteolytic digestion. Similar results were obtained when forages were pretreated with cellulase before undergoing an in vitro digestion with *Streptomyces griseus* protease. Many plant proteins are trapped in a fiber matrix that needs to be degraded before proteases can gain access to proteins for degradation. Therefore, it appears that protein degradation in the rumen requires the presence of several proteolytic and non proteolytic enzymes, and the combination of several microbial and enzymatic activities are required for maximum protein degradation.

It is likely that with a high-concentrate ration, even if pH is high, starch-degrading bacteria predominate, and fiber digestion is limited by the reduced number of cellulolytic bacteria, reducing the degradation of protein. Therefore, the effect of pH and(or) the substrate being fermented may affect the predominant microbial population and modify protein degradation caused by interactions among nutrients. It could be hypothesized that reduction in cellullolytic bacteria as a consequence of low pH leads to a reduction in fibre degradation, reducing access of proteolytic bacteria to proteins, indirectly diminishing protein degradation.

Efficiency of Microbial Protein Synthesis (EMPS)

Microbial protein synthesis (MPS) in the rumen usually provides the majority of amino acids (AA) available for absorption. The total amount of microbial protein flowing to the small intestine depends on nutrient availability in the rumen and efficiency of use of these nutrients by ruminal microorganisms (Bach *et al.*, 2005; Firkins *et al.*, 2006)). In protein evaluation systems, EMPS is usually expressed on an OM basis (usually in g microbial protein per kg OM degraded). Various OM components differ in energy yield, however, and EMPS values were more statistically revealing in a number of experimental studies when expressed on a carbohydrate rather than an OM basis. In general, empirical protein evaluation systems predict MPS using a constant EMPS value. In some systems, EMPS is variable and depends on, e.g., level of feed intake, fractional passage rate or fractional degradation rate. Yet there are many mechanistic factors that affect EMPS. Mathematical equations to describe variation in microbial growth and microbial efficiency in open or closed anaerobic systems are well documented in the literature but are applied surprisingly little in empirical protein evaluation systems for ruminants. Basically, substrate consumption by microorganisms will follow enzyme kinetics represented by rectangular hyperbola, and efficiency depends upon the partitioning of substrate consumed for growth and non-growth purposes. Critical elements in these equations include the maintenance requirement and the amount of substrate required per unit growth once maintenance has been met. Usually, the goal of rumen nutrition is to maximise EMPS to use ruminal degradable N as efficiently as possible and to decrease N losses to the environment. It should be noted that substrate utilized by microbes is partitioned between fermentation end-products (mainly VFA) and microbial biomass formation. Thus, an increase in EMPS usually coincides with a decrease in VFA produced per gram of carbohydrate degraded, which reduces the supply of non-protein energy to the animal. The concept of microbial efficiency and production of biomass versus production of fermentation end-products is central to many other fermentative systems as well, but the aim in some other systems (e.g. environmental bioremediation systems like water purification) is to waste as much energy and to produce as least biomass as possible and is thus opposite to that in the rumen. Therefore, mathematical equations developed may be applicable to many fermentative situations with widely different ultimate goals.

Maintenance requirement comprises any energy or substrate necessary to the growth of the micro-organism and used in such a way that this energy or substrate is not available for biosynthesis. Thus this includes true maintenance as well as endogenous metabolism and spilling of energy or substrates. Chemostat cultures is used to estimate the maintenance requirements of mixed rumen bacteria and the value derived (0.05 g glucose/g bacterial DM per h) is applied in most mechanistic models. However, maintenance values can vary widely according to the bacterial species involved and chemical conditions in the rumen. Given the impact of maintenance requirement on microbial growth efficiency in the usual (low) range of growth rates of microbes in the rumen maintenance requirement raised from 0.05 to 0.15 g carbohydrate/g microbial DM per h), surprisingly few maintenance requirement values have been reported in literature, and clearly more data are required to improve extant mechanistic models.

Energy spilling may form a significant part of the maintenance requirement. Conceptually, energy spilling can be regarded as energy decoupling between anabolic and catabolic functions of the cell through 'futile cycles'. The term futile cycles describes the concept where the microbial cell has both an irreversible pathway for a chemical transformation process in one direction and a different and irreversible mechanism for the reverse process. If one or the other functions at a different time, metabolism is not wasteful, but if they act simultaneously, there might be no or a small net transformation and the result would be that cellular energy is dissipated, thus reducing EMPS. In the rumen, energy availability is usually the determinant most limiting microbial growth and energy spilling would be of minor importance. However, in certain situations (particularly immediately after feeding a diet high in easily degradable carbohydrates), the availability of nutrients other than energy may limit microbial growth, and spilling of energy in the excess of carbohydrate availability may occur.

In many cases, maintenance activity still remains a relatively fuzzy concept in biological terms but for prediction purposes, representation of the phenomenon seems satisfactory. Pirt (1982) proposed to account mathematically for non-growth requirements by including a constant maintenance energy term independent of the specific growth rate and a term which decreases with increase in specific growth rate. Evaluation of this representation showed good accuracy when compared with observed data, but application to predict EMPS in the rumen would require quantitative data for parameterization and these are not available. Baldwin (1995) used a different representation and adopted a Michaelis-Menten relationship in which the fermentation of carbohydrates to VFA for non-growth purposes was limited by increased availability of N sources. A similar representation can be applied for other nutrient sources that may impair the biosynthetic use of energy in carbohydrates. The pH value might also affect the apparent maintenance requirement, as *in vitro* EMPS decreases at lower pH values. A meta analysis to assess the effect of pH on EMPS was done, and found no relationship between pH and EMPS. Ruminal pH may obviously have a large impact on the degradation of OM (especially fibre). In this respect, to predict MPS in dairy cattle accurately, representation of pH affects on nutrient degradation is of greater importance than representation of pH affects on microbial maintenance requirements. Synchronisation of energy from degraded carbohydrate and various N sources will theoretically increase EMPS by proper matching of nutrients and avoidance of energy spilling, but benefits of synchronisation *in vivo* are equivocal (Firkins *et al.*, 2006). Recycling of urea-N to the rumen and temporary storage or depletion of intracellular polysaccharides will assist in overcoming instantaneous deficiencies. Overall, the practical impact of energy spilling and the need to account for it in models of rumen metabolism seems to be limited in most situations in dairy cattle nutrition.

In current protein evaluation systems, the source of N (preformed AA or peptides versus ammonia) usually does not affect MPS or EMPS. However, substrate degradation and bacterial growth have been shown to increase with addition of AA or peptides in fibrolytic and amylolytic bacteria. In various models, the theoretical improvement in EMPS when all N required is provided by AA rather than ammonia varied widely. A major part of the variation in these values can be explained by differences in the units in which EMPS is expressed (i.e. microbial protein per unit OM or per unit carbohydrates degraded). Incorporation of preformed AA or peptides directly into microbial protein, rather than synthesis of AA from ammonia and a carbon skeleton, enables more carbohydrate to be used for other purposes and consequently results in more efficient growth. Current mechanistic models include the effect of N source by representation of various N-containing substrate pools, and this representation allows for some variation in predicted EMPS.

Crude protein (CP) content of the microbial material flowing to the duodenum varies widely between 300 and 660 g/kg bacterial DM (Clark *et al.*, 1992). Although some of these differences in composition may be attributed to methodology, major variation in composition related to diet and time after feeding exists when the same techniques are used. Faster fractional microbial growth rates coincide with higher RNA and lower DNA and microbial cell wall contents. In addition high availability of carbohydrates relative to N sources gives rise to storage of polysaccharides, and N concentrations in bacteria from cows consuming slowly fermentable carbohydrates are higher than those from cows consuming rapidly fermentable carbohydrates. The stoichiometry of synthesis of microbial cell components is well established and EMPS calculated theoretically varies significantly with changes in microbial composition. Thus, actual expenditure of available OM or energy by microorganisms to synthesise protein can be very different, depending upon microbial composition. The EMPS increases upon a decrease in storage polysaccharide content (polysaccharide content from 0.2 to 0.0 g/g microbial DM) and corresponding increase in CP content (from 0.6 to 0.8 g/g microbial DM). In contrast, current protein evaluation systems usually assume a fixed total CP content of microbial DM. Moreover, individual AA composition observed in various experiments is not constant and again varies with growth rate and with microbial subpopulation. In addition, mechanistic models also do not include a representation of variation in AA composition, likely due to paucity of data. Thus, appreciation of dietary factors affecting abundance of individual groups of micro-organisms and their distinct AA compositions is desired to estimate microbial AA flow accurately. Such variation in composition led to conclude that improved procedures and data for measuring and predicting microbial AA flow to the duodenum are required to make real progress in efficient use of protein for production purposes.

Faster fractional microbial growth rates will increase EMPS by reducing the non-growth requirements. Many mathematical functions are available to estimate growth parameters (including fractional growth rate and lag time) in batch (closed) systems. In open systems, such as continuous cultures, fractional rate of passage is amongst the most important determinants of fractional microbial growth rate, as in (quasi-) steady state and when no other clearance routes of microbial matter occur, these should be equal. Whilst most empirical protein evaluation systems assume a constant EMPS, some indeed relate EMPS to rate of passage or feed intake level. The Cornell net carbohydrate and protein system and some systems derived from the gas production technique assume fractional microbial growth rate to be related to fractional degradation rate of substrate. However, although such a relationship may be valid for batch cultures, the development of models to describe microbial metabolism shows that this relationship is not directly applicable to repeatedly fed and continuous cultures (Dijkstra *et al.*, 2005) which are more representative of the *in vivo* situation. For example, Oba and Allen (2003) found *in vivo* that EMPS was negatively related to the fractional degradation rate of starch, but positively related to the fractional passage rate of starch.

It is important to note that fractional growth rate of micro-organisms is not exactly equal to fractional passage rate. Another major determinant of net growth, largely ignored in predicting EMPS, is recycling of microbial material within the rumen. The major contribution to microbial turnover is likely to be related to protozoal activities, since protozoa engulf large amounts of bacteria and since a considerable amount of protozoal biomass is recycled within the rumen. Defaunation of the rumen almost invariably increases EMPS, although MPS is not necessarily increased due to a possible simultaneous reduction in OM degradation upon defaunation. On a variety of diets, simulated recycling of microbial N in the rumen ranged from 35 to 70% whilst observed recycling, measured using isotope dilution techniques, ranged from 20 to 90%. Recycling of microbial protein wastes energy, although the VFA production may well be increased due to recycling. The released AA may be deaminated and this gives rise to further wastage of N as urea in urine.

Although recycling has a large impact on EMPS, quantitative data are very limited and mathematical. Predicting the profile of absorbed nutrients representation of recycling has not received much attention. The limited knowledge about rumen protozoal metabolism is mostly because of their dependence on live bacteria, which confounds their in vitro culture. A requirement for live bacteria appears to be manifested in particular in culture periods longer than 2 to 4 days. Moreover, a widely accepted marker to measure the protozoal fraction of microbial protein separate from the bacterial fraction is lacking. New molecular techniques such as real-time polymerase chain reaction (PCR), targeting the gene encoding 18S rDNA to quantify the amount of protozoal biomass (Sylvester *et al.*, 2004), may be promising tools to obtain more quantitative data on protozoa. Protozoal predation is usually represented by rectangular hyperbola, assuming that at low concentrations of microbes, protozoa search thoroughly to secure an adequate uptake of microbial matter, whereas at high microbial concentrations, protozoa reduce their search efforts because of satiation. On a wide range of predator species, the rectangular hyperbola has been found to provide a good description of experimental data, and this relationship was also central to the levels of predicted recycling mentioned previously. Information on preferential uptake of certain bacterial species does not reveal a consistent pattern. The engulfment of solid feed particles by protozoa is well known and this is also expected to result in engulfment of bacteria attached to these particles. On the other hand, the converse hypothesis of protection against engulfment by means of attachment, has been supported by that the observations fluid-phase, non-fibrolytic bacteria increase to a far higher extent upon defaunation than do the attached bacteria. However, it should be noted that the preference of protozoa for starch and sugars, rather than fibre, will result in a relatively higher availability of starch and sugars compared to fibre upon defaunation and hence a smaller increase in attached, fibrolytic bacteria compared to non-attached bacteria. Interestingly, Rasmussen *et al.* (2005) reported that some bacterial pathogens appear to be resistant to degradation in vacuoles of mixed rumen protozoa. Survival of several types of Salmonella in vacuoles, in particular multiresistant types, results in higher intestinal cell invasion capacity. On the other hand, toxin-producing Escherichia coli were not engulfed by or attached to mixed ciliate protozoa (Burow *et al.*, 2005). Representation of uptake and digestion of bacteria by protozoa is further complicated because of adaptive mechanisms that bacteria develop to survive protozoal predation. Adaptive mechanisms to increase the survival of bacteria under predation pressure include changing cell surface properties, modification of swimming speed, secretion of bioactive metabolites, or formation of micro-colonies (Matz and Kjelleberg, 2005). Given the large impact of microbial turnover on microbial efficiency and the small amount of experimental data, it appears that mathematical representation of selective engulfment and digestion of bacteria by protozoa may well be improved further. Quantification of microbial recycling will help to establish more accurate estimates of microbial protein yield factors to be applied in protein evaluation systems.

Finally, it is essential to note that virtually all of our present quantitative knowledge on microbial metabolism in the rumen and consequently its mathematical representation is based on culturable rumen microbial species. Recent molecular techniques indicate that understanding on the presence of various microbial species is far from complete though. For example, Edwards *et al.* (2004) showed that only 11% of the diversity of the rumen microbial ecosystem is represented by cultured isolates. Hence the information on biochemical properties used to develop mechanistic models may represent only a small fraction of the properties of the total microbial population in the rumen. Molecular techniques may give a wealth of information, but to include such findings in systems predicting the nutrient profile requires quantitative rather than qualitative data as well as close collaboration between molecular scientists and mathematical modellers on interpreting and evaluating data. Novel cultivation techniques have been described that have shown success in the isolation and cultivation of previously unculturable organisms but none of these systems is suitable for application to anaerobic ecosystems. Application of such novel cultivation approaches to the rumen ecosystem will contribute directly to increasing the understanding of microbial metabolic and fermentation processes by recovering in culture previously uncultivable organisms, and may lead to further improvements in the mechanistic representation of MPS.

Contribution of Microbial Protein to Metabolizable Protein (MP) Systems

The AA of microbial origin are well balanced with respect to requirements of absorbed AA and are assumed to be relatively constant in AA profile (NRC, 2001), although microbial subpopulations probably vary significantly in AA proportions (Rodrý´guez-Prado *et al.*, 2004) and the AA composition of bacteria could change with growth rate (Bach *et al.*, 2005). Moreover, the complementary AA in RUP must be digestible in the small intestine. Consequently, a metabolizable AA system needs further research. The NRC (2001) plotted milk protein responses against lysine and methionine supplies, calculated as percentages of MP supply. Although being a necessary format because of limitations of the data set, many subsequent users have inferred requirements of metabolizable lysine and methionine from the breakpoints in these dose-response graphs. This practice allows the metabolizable AA supply to be increased either by increasing AA flows to the duodenum or by independently decreasing the supply of MP. That is, one could conceivably increase methionine as a percentage of MP by changing dietary conditions such that MP is decreased to a greater degree than methionine is decreased, perhaps explaining some of the variability shown in the response curves (lower precision) but also potentially explaining why expected responses (accuracy) are sometimes not realized.

When expressed as a percentage of MP, the prediction of metabolizable AA requirement is even more sensitive to errors associated with MPS prediction. If MPS is under- or overpredicted, both lysine and MP supply could be under- or overestimated proportionately, and the effect on accuracy might be partially buffered. However, as the error in MPS prediction increases, making a ratio of AA: MP could compound this error and decrease precision. The requirement of RDP is calculated as microbial protein flow/0.85, and the requirement of digestible RUP is calculated after the predicted digestible microbial protein supply is subtracted from the factorial requirements for MP. Such an enormous impact of MPS calculations for both supply and requirement functions disposes the model to be susceptible to amplification of errors from using predictions for predictions and even more from using ratios. Therefore, real progress for matching supply of MP with requirements depends heavily on improved procedures for measuring and predicting microbial N flow to the duodenum (Firkins and Reynolds, 2005).

Even in more mechanistic models, improved quantification of MPS can help provide data for sensitivity analyses and other evaluations or, in some cases, by direct parameterization. Increasing dietary starch can increase both the production of protozoa and the protozoal-mediated recycling of microbial matter. Most other models either ignore protozoal-mediated recycling or consider it relatively constant. Yet, despite its potential importance for direct parameterization or for challenges of models, methods to quantify protozoal N have received little attention until recently (Sylvester *et al.*, 2005). Also, models often partition bacteria into 2 pools: those that degrade fiber, which typically attach to the particulate phase, and those that degrade nonstructural carbohydrate (**NSC**), which often are considered to be non adherent. These models often are based on the ruminal pool sizes, but such data are rarely reported, and such data might help in future meta-analyses evaluating MP systems.

Importance of Microbial Protein to Ruminants

Contribution of microbial protein to total protein requirement was determined using NRC values (2001) for a 680-kg lactating dairy cow producing 25, 35, or 45 kg/d of 4% FCM. At these three milk yields, microbial protein would contribute 51, 49 and 48%, respectively, of the total protein required by the cow when microbial synthesis in the rumen is 30 g of N/kg of organic matter truly digested (OMTD). When milk yield is 45 kg/d, the contribution of microbial protein to total protein required by the cow would increase from 32 to 63% as efficiency of microbial protein synthesis increases from 20 to 40 g of N/kg of OMTD (Table 1). Calculated contributions of microbial protein clearly depicted the importance of optimizing microbial protein synthesis in the rumen of high producing dairy cows. In addition, these calculations demonstrate that, as milk yield increases, a substantial quantity of rumen undegradable protein from protein supplements must leave the rumen to meet the protein requirement of the cow.

Contribution of microbial protein to total protein requirement was determined for a 250 kg growing beef animal (Table 2) with average daily gains (ADG) of 300, 1200 and 1700 g/day. At these three ADG, microbial protein would contribute 95, 57 and 40%, respectively, of the total protein required by the animal when microbial synthesis in the rumen is 25 g of N/kg of organic matter truly digested (OMTD). Lower efficiencies of microbial protein synthesis, ranging from 20 to 30 g N/kg OMTD, were used because beef cattle are generally less efficient, most probably due to a high population of amylolytic bacteria. Microbial protein contribution to total protein requirement demonstrated a more dramatic difference in beef cattle compared with dairy cattle. This response is probably due to the lack of increase in dry matter intake in beef cattle as ADG increases. However, in both situations, it is clear that substantial quantities of RUP from protein supplements must be incorporated into the diet of high producing ruminants.

Table 1 : Contribution of microbial protein to total protein requirement of lactating dairy cattle.[a]

Contribution of microbial protein when daily milk production (kg) equals:			
Microbial synthesis, g N/kg of OM truly digested[b]	25 (55 lb)	35 (77 lb)	45 (100 lb)
		%	
20	34	33	32
30	51	49	48
40	68	65	63

a Requirement determined using NRC (2001).
b Assumed that 55% of OM intake is truly digested in the rumen.

Table 2 : Contribution of microbial protein to total protein requirement of beef cattle (250 kg).[a]

Contribution of microbial protein when average daily gain (g/d) equals:			
Microbial synthesis, g N/kg of OM truly digested[b]	300 (0.64 lb)	1200 (2.7 lb)	1700 (3.75 lb)
		%	
20	76	46	30
25	95	57	40
30	114	69	48

[a] Requirements determined using NRC (1996).
[b] Assumed that 55% of OM intake is truly digested in the rumen.

Estimates of Rumen Un-degradable Protein

Under ideal circumstances, the ruminant nutritionist would prefer to use "book values" for RUP of various protein supplements, such as those found in the NRC (2001) publication. However, ruminal protein degradation is a complex process influenced by various factors such as solubility, protein structure, microbial proteolytic activity, microbial access to the protein and ruminal retention time of dietary protein. There is an inherent variability in reported values for RUP of feeds that is related to conditions under which experiments are conducted; however, part of the variation can also be attributed to differences in quality of protein supplements.

Intestinal Protein Digestion

Methods for Measuring Intestinal Protein Digestion

The total amount of protein available for absorption from the small intestine depends on the flow of microbial and dietary protein to the duodenum and their respective intestinal digestibility. Digestion of protein that leaves the rumen starts in the abomasum with acid-pepsin digestion and is completed in the small intestine with pancreatic and intestinal proteases. The intestinal digestion of protein supplements may differ; however, empirical data were lacking, and as a result, a constant value of 80% was used for all feeds. The main problem was the lack of reliable techniques for estimating intestinal digestion of proteins. *In vivo* estimation of intestinal protein digestion involves expensive and labor-intensive experiments and requires the use of surgically prepared animals. Apparent digestion of protein is calculated as the disappearance of CP or amino acids between the duodenum and ileum, which is subject to considerable error associated with digesta sampling, use of digesta flow rate markers, and inherent animal variation. Therefore, several alternative procedures for estimation of intestinal protein digestion in ruminants have been developed. An *in situ* mobile bag technique was devised to determine intestinal protein digestion in ruminants. A three-step procedure that combines *in situ* and *in vitro* methods was developed to estimate intestinal digestion of proteins in ruminants. Using these improved techniques, the NRC (2001) has assigned estimates of intestinal digestion to the RUP fraction of each feedstuff. More recently, McNiven *et al.* (2002) modified the three-step procedure by replacing the *in situ* step with an *in vitro* method involving a pre-incubation with a protease enzyme followed by incubations in pepsin and pancreatin. They concluded that their method could predict intestinal protein digestion of heat damaged soybeans. However, recent evaluation of this modified procedure demonstrated that estimates were not accurate among a wide variety of feedstuffs and further research is warranted to evaluate the modified procedure.

Three-step *in situ* / *in vitro* procedure

The three-step procedure was developed to: 1. closely simulate physiological conditions of ruminants, including potential effects of ruminal fermentation; 2. be rapid, reliable, and inexpensive; 3. be applicable to a wide variety of protein supplements; and 4. be accurately reflect differences in protein digestion. Dacron bags containing feed samples were suspended in the rumen for 16 h. Residue was incubated for 1 h in a 0.1 *N* HCl solution containing 1 g/L of pepsin. After incubation, pH was neutralized with 1 *N* NaOH and a pH 7.8 phosphate buffer containing 3 g/L of pancreatin was added to the solution followed by incubation at 38° C. After a 24-h incubation, a 100% (wt/vol) trichloroacetic acid solution was added to precipitate undigested proteins.

Intestinally Absorbable Dietary Protein

Intestinally absorbable dietary protein (IADP) is defined as the amount of protein from a specific feed that is available for absorption in the small intestine and is calculated as RUP multiplied by intestinal protein digestion. The IADP value provides an index of the quality of protein supplements as sources of RUP for ruminants. Because there is a large amount of variation associated with measurements of ruminal degradability and intestinal digestibility among and within protein supplements, and there seems to be no correlation between RUP and intestinal protein digestibility, the use of published values for RUP and intestinal digestion to calculate IADP is not adequate.

Estimating Microbial Protein Production-use of Purine Derivatives

External markers such as ^{15}N or ^{35}S as well as internal markers such as nucleic acids have been used to determine ruminal microbial protein production (Broderick and Merchen, 1992). However, determining digesta flow is necessary when using these markers which require cannulated animals. As a result, finding a non-invasive method to estimate microbial protein production in the rumen of cattle would be beneficial in ration formulation. In ruminants, purine derivatives (PD) are excreted in urine and milk as allantoin, uric acid, xanthine and hypoxanthine. Because of the high xanthine oxidase activity found in the blood of cattle, xanthine and hypoxanthine are converted to uric acid in blood and tissues prior to urinary excretion. Through the use of nucleic acid infusion, PD were found to originate from the catabolism of purines of both endogenous and exogenous origin. Concentrations of nucleic acids in the rumen are used to estimate MN production because nucleic acids from the diet were shown to be degraded in the rumen. As a result, most of the purines and pyrimidines found in the duodenum are assumed to originate from microbial protein production. Urinary excretion of PD such as allantoin could be a useful indicator of rumen microbial protein flow from the rumen. Since then, many researchers have used urinary and milk excretion of PD including allantoin and uric acid as a non-invasive method to predict rumen microbial protein production with varying results in different ruminants.

References

ARC (1980). The Nutrient Requirements of Ruminant Livestock. CAB International, Wallingford, UK.

Assoumani, M. B., Vedeau, F., Jacquot, L. and Sniffen, C. J. (1992). *Anim. Feed Sci. Technol.,* 39:357-368.

Aufre're, J. and Cartailler. (1988). *Annual Zootechnol.,* 37:255–270.

Bach A.S., Calsamiglia, S. and Stern, M.D. (2005). *J. Dairy Sci.,* 88 (suppl. E): E9-E21.

Baldwin R.L.(1995). In "*Modeling ruminant digestion and metabolism*". Chapman and Hall, London.

Broderick, G. A. and Merchen, N. R. (1992). *J.Dairy Sci.,* 75:2618-2632.

Broderick, G. A., Wallace, R. J and Ørskov E. R. (1991). Control of rate and extent of protein degradation. Pp.541–594. In "Physiological Aspects of Digestion and Metabolism in Ruminants" (T. Tsuda, Y. Sasaki, and R. Kawashima, editors) Academic Press, New York, NY.

Burow L.C., Gobius, K.C., Vanselow, B.A and Klieve, A.V. (2005). *Letters Appl. Microbiol.,* 40: 117-122.

Cardozo, P. W., Calsamiglia, S., Ferret, A. and Kamel, C. (2004). *J. Anim. Sci.,* 82: 3230-3236.

Cardozo, P., Calsamiglia, S. and Ferret, A. (2002). *J. Dairy Sci.,* 85(Suppl. 1):182.

Clark, J. H., Klusmeyer, T. H. and Cameron, M. A. (1992). *J. Dairy Sci.,* 75:2304–2323.

Debroas, D. and Blanchart, G. (1993). *Reprod. Nutr. Develop.,* 33: 283-288.

Devant, M., Ferret, Calsamiglia S., Casals, R. and Gasa, J. (2001). *J. Anim. Sci.,* 79:1944-1953.

Dijkstra J, Kebreab, E., Bannink, A., France, J. and Lopez, S. (2005). *Anim. Feed Sci. Technol.,* 123/124: 561-578.

Dijkstra, J. (1994). *British J. Nutr.,* 72: 679–699.

Edwards, J.E., McEwan, N.R., Travis, A. J. and Wallace, R.J. (2004). Antonie van Leeuwenhoek 86: 263-281.

Eugene, M., Archimede, H. and Sauvant, D. (2004). *Livestock Prod. Sci.,* 85: 81–97.

Ferme, D., Banjac M., Calsamiglia, S., Busquet Kamel, C. and Avgustin, G. (2004). *Folia Microbiol.,* 49: 151–155.

Firkins, J. L, Hristov, A.N., Hall, M.B., Varga, G.A. and St-Pierre, N.R. (2006). *J. Dairy Sci.,* 89 (suppl. E): E31-E51.

Firkins, J. L., and Reynolds, C. K. (2005). Whole animal nitrogen balance in cattle. pp.167–185. In "Nitrogen and Phosphorus Nutrition of Cattle and Environment" (A.N. Hristov and E. Pfeffer, editors), CAB International, Wallingford, UK.

Kohn, R. A. and Allen, M.S. (1995). *Anim. Feed Sci. Technol.*, 52: 15-28.

Matz, C. and Kjelleberg, S. (2005). *Trends Microbiol.*, 13: 302-307.

McNiven, M. A., Preslokken, E., Mydland, L. T. and Mitchell, A.W. (2002). *Anim. Feed Sci. Technol.*, 96: 1-13.

NRC (1996). Nutrient Requirements of Beef Cattle (6th revised). National Academy of Science, Washington, D.C.

NRC (2001). Nutrient Requirements of Dairy Cattle (7th revised). National Academy of Science, Washington, D.C.

Oba, M. and Allen, M.S. (2003). *J. Dairy Sci.*, 86: 195-207.

Pirt, S. J. (1982). *Arch. Microbiol.*, 133: 300-302.

Rasmussen, M.A., Carlson, S.A., Franklin, S.K., McCuddin, Z.P., Wu, M.T. and Sharma, V.K. (2005). *Infection and Immunity*, 73: 4668-4675.

Rodrý´guez-Prado, M., Calsamiglia, S. and Ferret, A. (2004). *J. Dairy Sci.*, 87: 1413–1424.

Romagnolo, L.C., Polan, C.E. and Barbeau, W.E. (1994). *J. Dairy Sci.*, 77: 1093-1099.

Schwingel, W. R. and Bates, D. B. (1996). *J. Anim. Sci.*, 74: 475-482.

Sylvester, J.T., Karnati S.K.R., Yu, Z., Morrison, M. and Firkins, J.L. (2004). *J. Nutr.*, 134: 3378-3384.

Sylvester, J. T., Karnati, S.K.R., Yu, Z., Newbold, C.J. and Firkins, J.L. (2005). *J. Dairy Sci.*, 88: 2083–2095.

Toma´nkova´, O. and Kopecny, J. (1995). *Anim. Feed Sci. Technol.*, 53: 71–80.

Van Soest, P. J. (1994). Nutritional Ecology of the Ruminant. Cornell University Press, Ithaca, NY. P. 261.

Velle, W., Sjaastad, Ø.V., Aulie, A., Grønset, D., Feigwinter, K. and Framstad, T. (1997). *J. Dairy Sci.*, 80: (7th revised). 3325-3332.

□□□

Animal Nutrition, 2012
eds. Dr. (Mrs.) Usha R. Mehra et al., pp. 49-75
Satish Serial Publishing House e-mail : info@satishserial.com; website : www.satishserial.com

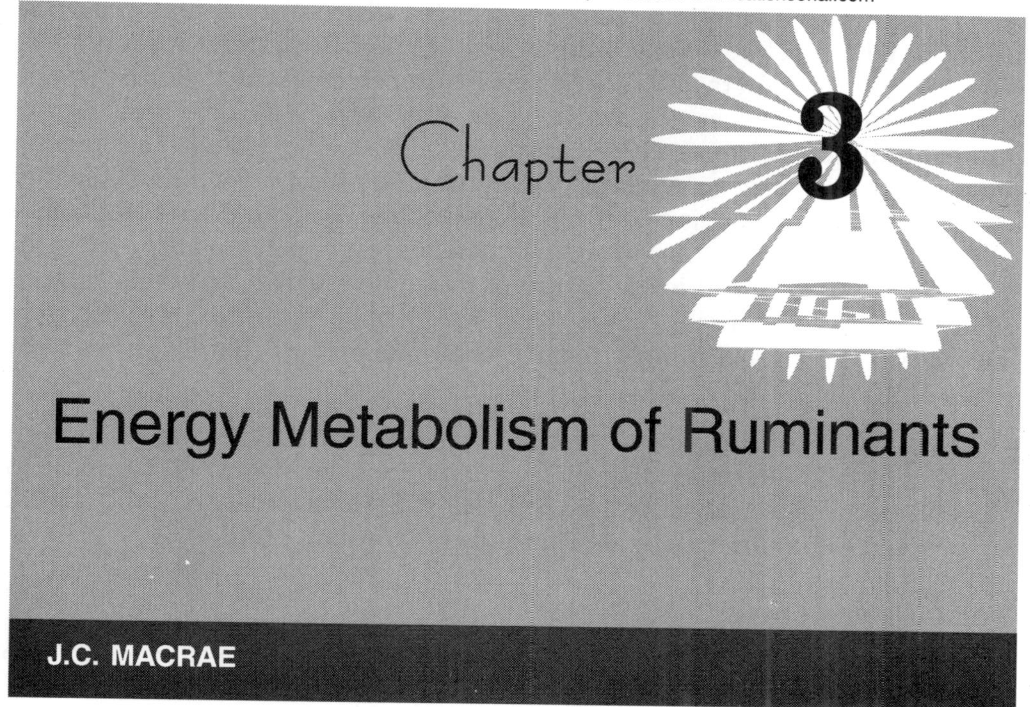

Chapter 3

Energy Metabolism of Ruminants

J.C. MACRAE

In 1965 the Agricultural Research Council proposed that the United Kingdom should replace the Starch Equivalent (SE) system of ration-formulation (Kellner, 1920) by a new system to be known as the Metabolizable Energy (ME) system. The ME system which evolved mainly from work carried out by Blaxter and his colleagues at the Hannah Research Institute in Scotland (Blaxter, 1962) differs from other systems e.g. SE system, the Scandinavian Fodder Unit system, the American Total Digestible Nutrients system in that it recognises that individual feeds cannot be thought to have a unique value characterising their ability to sustain all energy-demanding processes of the body. Instead the value of the feed depends on the ration in which it is fed, the amount of that ration fed and the physiological state of the animal which consumes it. To make the system work requires a knowledge of (i) the usable or metabolisable energy (ME) content of the ration (ii) the energy requirement of the animal for basic metabolic processes and for growth, milk production etc., and (iii) the efficiency with which the ME contained in the particular ration can be utilized to sustain basal processes and to promote the synthesis of tissue or export product.

This chapter attempts to consider selected observational and analytical findings which relate to the empiricism of the ME system; the animal's requirements for growth and lactation and the biochemical mechanisms which regulate these processes. Throughout emphasis will be given to the understanding that energy *per se* is an ill-defined entity when it comes to satisfying the needs of an animal. Although it is common to refer to the energy metabolism of animals this is very much a misnomer; animals do not metabolise energy, they metabolise the substrates (metabolites) which are absorbed from the digestive tract and it is the nature of these metabolites and their balance relative to the needs of the animals which are likely to determine the efficiency with which the animal utilizes the ME component of its diet for growth (or lactation).

Although the majority of the data presented in the chapter have been obtained in the U.K. or in other temperate regions, an effort will be made to concentrate on aspects which might have relevance to tropical and substropical regions and to the more extensive systems of livestock production.

Metabolizable energy (ME) content of rations

Classically, the study of the energy metabolism of ruminants involves a consideration of processes of energy transfer, in particular the transfer of the chemical energy contained in feedstuffs into combinations of chemical energy contained in animal products (e.g. meat, milk, wool etc.) plus work energy and heat energy.

Gross energy (GE) content of feedstuffs

The GE content of a material can be assessed as the heat liberated when the substance is combusted. There are two units of energy commonly used now-a-days, the calorie and the joule. Calorie is preferred in certain parts of the world including the U.S. and most parts of Asia, including the Indian subcontinent, whereas the Joule (the product of international volts x international amps x seconds) has been adopted as the preferred unit in Europe and Australasia.

Feedingstuffs comprise a mixture of different chemical components each with its own energy density. Thus carbohydrates on combustion liberate approximately 16.0 MJ per kg, protein 23.5 MJ/kg and fat 39.5 MJ/kg. Minerals have no energy value. The GE content of any particular feedstuff will depend on its chemical composition, especially its fat and mineral content. Column 1 of Table 1 gives the GE contents of a selection of some of the different types of feedstuffs fed in the UK and evaluated over the last 12 years by the Feedingstuffs Evaluation Unit at the Rowett Institute (FEU, 1975; 1978; 1984). Apart from materials which have a high content of sugar (e.g. sugar beet products, cassava) or oil (soyabean and groundnut meals) most of the materials have GE content between 18 to 19 MJ/kg DM (i.e. 4.3 to 4.55 kcals/g).

The GE intake of an animal can be calculated simply as:-

GE intake (MJ/d) = DM intake (kg/d) x GE content of ration (MJ/kg)

Digestible energy (de) content of feed stuffs

The GE intake says little about the amount of energy available to the animal, because a proportion of that energy will be voided as faeces and urine as well as some being eructated as methane. Of these three routes of energy loss (wastage), the energy lost in faeces is by far the largest and most variable component. The amount of GE consumed but not voided in faeces is termed **digestible energy** (DE) intake.

DE intake = GE intake - faecal energy excreted

The digestibility coefficient of a ration is calculated as:

$$\frac{\text{GE intake - Faecal energy excreted}}{\text{GE intake}}$$

Comparison of columns 1 and 2 of Table 1 will indicate that whereas the GE contents of most feedingstuffs fall within a narrow range their DE content can vary widely. Generally speaking, forages are digested less well than cereals or beans and the more mature forages are digested less well than the younger vegetative stage materials. Thus forages in general rarely have digestibility coefficients much above 0.75 and are frequently much lower than this whereas the non-forage materials seldom have coefficient below 0.80. The effect of stage of maturity of forages can be seen clearly when comparing the coefficients for vegetative stage frozen grass (> 0.70), hay (0.56-0.66) and straw (0.37-0.47).

The metabolizable energy (ME) content of feedingstuffs

The prime concern of nutritionists is to determine the proportion of any ration which is available to support the metabolic processes of the animal. As discussed already the digestibility of the diet can lead to a large but variable loss of dietary energy in the faeces. However there are other losses which also need to be taken into accout in calculating the ME value of a ration.

Some energy is excreted in urine, mainly as partially degraded nitrogen compounds. In ruminants these would comprise mainly urea, which is the end-product of amino acid degradation or ammonia absorption, creatinine, a breakdown product of muscle protein and allantoin, the non-usable moiety of microbial nucleic acids, aromatic compounds like hippuric acid and phenolic conjugates can also be important contributors to urinary energy on some diets. The energy contained in these compounds is likely to represent anywhere between 2% and 7% of the GE intake on most types of rations (FEU, 1975; 1978; 1984).

The other loss of DE which represents a wastage to the animal is the energy lost as methane, one of the end-products of microbial fermentation.

Table 1 : The gross energy (GE) content (MJ/kg DM), digestible energy (DE) coefficients and metebolzable energy (ME) contents (MJ/kg DM) of a range of feedstuffs determined in the Feedlngstuffs Evaluation Unit (FEU) at the Rowett Institute (FEU, 1975; 1978; 1984).

Feedstuffs	GE content	DE coefficients	ME content
Frozen grass	18.7-19.1	0.71-0.75	10.4-11.5
Silages lages grass	18.4-19.4	0.68-0.79	9.9-12.8
Lucerne	18.1-18.4	0.59-D.62	8.5-9.0
Maize	18.3-18.8	0.67-0.76	9.6-12.0
Dried grass			
RRI	18.2-19.5	0.67-0.78	10.4-12.4
Commercial	18.3-19.5	0.610.74	5.8-11.7
Hays	18.4-19.0	0.56-0.66	8.3-10.4
Straws	17.9-18.9	0.37-0.47	5.4-6.6
Wheats	18.1-18.5	0.80-0.94	11.7-14.8
Wheat offals	18.7-19.3	0.68-0.85	8.6-14.7
Maizes	18.7-19.1	0.81-0.95	12.5-15..5
Soya beet products	16.2-17.3	0.80-0.96	11.0-14.8
Cassavas	16.7-17.1	11:84-0.93	11.5-12.9
Sorghums	18.6-18.9	0.77-0.90	10.4-14.5
Soyabean meals	19.4-19.9	0.89-0.94	12.5-14.0
Groundnut meals	20.2-20.8	0.86-0.88	13.3-14.2

Early in *vitro* experiments (ARC, 1980) indicated microbial fermentation of carbohydrate could be represented by the stoichiometric equation:

hexose → acetate + propionate + butyrate + methane + CO_2
52 mol 68 mol 18mol 9 mol 33 mol 53 mol

However, it is now known that this is likely to vary with the nature of the hexose. In fact according to the data obtained using sheep in the Rowett

Feed Evaluation Unit the proportion of the GE lost as methane can vary enormously from as little as 2.596 of GE on certain brewery byproducts to as high as 12-13% of GE with certain concentrate feed ingstuff. Methane losses on forage type rati Jns usually represent approximately 6-8 % of the GE intake.

Faeces, urine and methane all represent wastage of dietary energy. The remainder can be reasonably assumed to be available to the animal for the support of basal metabolic processes. The proportion of the dietary energy which is available to metabolic processes is termed the Metabolisable Energy (ME) content.

ME intake = GE intake - [Faecal energy + urine energy + methane energy]

The ME content of a feed is represented as the amount of ME/kg DM. Column 3 of Table 1 indicates the range of ME contents for the various feedstuffs determined at the Rowett (FEU, 1975; 1978; 1984). It will be seen that they show a much wider between-category difference than do the GE contents.

Additivity of ME values

Two general observations from the many hundreas of trials performed in the FEU are perhaps worthy of comment. The first concerns the additivity of ME values.

In practice, diets often comprise combinations of forage with concentrates. The experimental' design adopted in the most of the trials in the Unit has involved feeding four ratios of forage: concentrate (i.e. 100:0, 80:20, 60:40 and 40:60). The ME content of each component is calculated from the least squared linear relationship relating ME value to the proportion of the constituent in the test ration. At the level of feeding used (maintenance level of intake for all rations) there has seldom been evidence of the non-linearity in these relationships. The phenomenon of non-linearity indicating interaction between dietary components and known as associative effect is seen more often at higher levels of intake and indeed there are many reports of such effects in animals given forage plus concentrate rations. On the other hand energy digestibility is perhaps less prone to being affected than other parameters. Fig. 1 illustrates data obtained many years ago in sheep given different proportions of a ration comprising hay plus barley (MacRae, 1967). It would be difficult to justify a non-linear function for the coefficients of energy digestibility whereas there is marked non-linearity with both the N and crude fibre moiety. The increase in crude fibre digestibility and the reduction in N digestibility at the intermediate incorporations of barley probably result from a change of microbial populations in the rumen (more to an amylolytic and less cellulolytic fermentation) when the ecosystem has access to the soluble carbohydrate components of barley. As a result structural carbohydrates pass out of the rumen and subsequently fermented in the hindgut. This hindgut fermentation compensates for reduced rumen fibre digestion but penalises the N digestion because the microbes draw on blood urea as a N source in the caecum colon, trapping this as bacterial protein which subsequently is excreted in the faeces. The lower N digestibility need not be detrimental to the N economy of the animal in that it probably represents only a re-routing of N excretion away from the urine and into faeces. Introduction of readily fermentable carbohydrate into the caecum of lambs has elegantly demonstrated this re-routing effect (Orskov and Food, 1969) and indeed inadequacy of N digestibility as a parameter of assessment of protein availability to ruminants has been abundantly demonstrated (ARC, 1980). In terms of the digestible energy coefficients the effects on fibre and N digestion at the intermediary points would tend to cancel each other out.

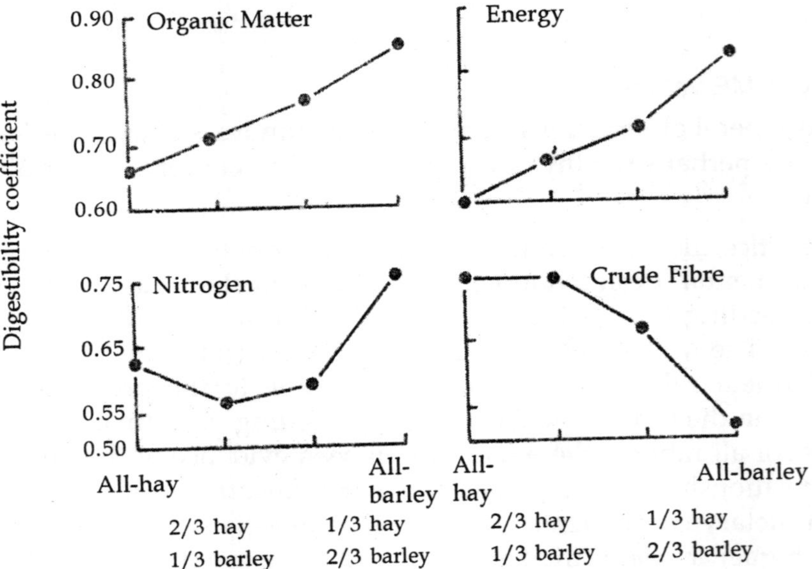

Fig. 1 : Digestibility data for sheep given rations ranging from all-hay to all-barley (data of MacRae, 1967).

The second observation worthy of comment comes from the fact that the Unit's statistical design for carrying out trials has been a "car ousel-type" procedure whereby each roughage is examined in combination with two different concentrates and likewise each concentrate is examined in combination with two different roughages. The findings have been that the ME values derived for any particular material are little affected by the other component of the mixed ration. Thus when in 1975 eight samples of dried grass were fed in combination with both wheat and barley, calculated mean ME contents (MJ/kg DM) of the grass in each mixture was 11.22 (SE 0.149) when fed with wheat, and 11.22 (SE 0.1391 when fed with barley. Similarly the mean ME content of the sixteen wheat samples when fed with the dried grass were 13.39 (SE 0.261) com. pared with 13.55 (SE 0.183) when subsequently fed with grass silage, (FEU, 1978). Likewise the ME values for the barley samples fed in combination with dried grass and grass silage were 12.89 (SE 0.183) and 12.91 (SE 0.196), respectively (FEU, 1978). Similarly when a further sixteen, samples of commercially produced dried grass, which tended to be poorer quality than the Rowett material, were fed in combination with sugar beet byproducts and maize, the mean ME contents of the dried grass were 9.95 (SE 0.417) and 9.64 (SE 0.396), respectively.

Having derived an ME intake value for a ration consideration can be given to how this ME will be utilized by the animal.

Utilization of ME - the bioenergetic approach

The classic approach to the bioenergetics of ruminants has been to consider ME intake and energy expenditure as composite entities; little consideration has been given to the different forms in which the energy is absorbed. This section will consider this classical approach in the light of recent availability of data on the energy costs of vital body processes.

The chemical energy bound up in the substrates absorbed as ME is used by the animal for a variety of processes including:

i) Maintenance of vital body functions,

ii) Building of body tissue.

iii) Production of saleable commodities (e.g. milk, wool, eggs),

iv) Production of metabolic heat generated both as an inevitable consequence of (i) above and also as a wasteful component of (ii) and (iii) above.

Animal production ofcourse represented by aspects (ii) and, (iii), and for this reason physiologists and nutritionists have performed many experiments to measure the energy retained in these processes, either directly by the comparative slaughter technique or indirectly by calorimetry. Such experiments can help distinguish between the heat losses of an animal which are the inevitable cost of vital processes and the heat loss associated with the inefficient use of absorbed nutrients.

Energy requirements of the animal

Vital processes such as protein and fatty acid synthesis, ion pumping, blood circulation and posture all require energy. Even when an animal receives no nutrient (is fasted) it still produces appreciable quantities of metabolic heat, indicating that it is drawing on body reserves to support its energy demanding basal processes.

The heat produced when an animal is fasting (in ruminants this is measured usually during the last 48 h of a 96 h fast in animals which had previously been fed at the maintenance level of intake for 3 weeks) gives an indication of the summated energy demands tor its **basal metabolic processes.** It is termed the **Fasting Metabolic Rate** (FMR) of the animal. The FMR of mature animal expressed relative to their metabolic body size (live weight 0.75) is a relatively constan't value irrespective of species (Kleiber, 1947). Table 2 gives FMRs for, a number of species ranging in size from 5 kg rabbits to 475 kg steers. In all cases the FMR is somewhere around 300 kJ/kg $W^{0.75}$. This value is usually referred to as the **interspecies mean.**

Table 2 : Fasting metabolic rates of different species.

Species	Weight (kg)	Approximate fasting metabolic rate MJ/d	KJ/kg $W^{0.75}$
Rabbit	5	1	280-300
Sheep	50	5	270
Red deer	80	8.9	330
Pig	130	10.5	270
Steer	475	34.5	340

There are systematic variations from this interspecies mean value, the FMR of mature cattle are usually slightly higher than 300 kJ/kg: $w^{0.75}$ whilst those of sheep tend to be lower than 300 kJ. Young immature animals have higher FMRs, but these tend to decline with age and/or size and/or maturity. Blaxter (1962) computed data which illustrate the decline in FMR of lambs and calves as they grow through to mature size. Table 3 gives data obtained recently at the Rowett on the FMR I. of steers grown from 100 to 345 kg (J.S. Smith, personal communication).

Table 3 : Mean fasting metabolic ratas (FMR) ± SE of growing steers. (unpublished data of J.S. Smith)

Weight of steers (kg)	(n)	FMR kJ/kg $W^{0.75}$
100	(7)	400 ± 10.9
185	(8)	370 ± 6.5
235	(4)	367 ± 12.2
345	(3)	327 ± 10.1

Over recent years nutritionists have started to study the relative energy requirements of the different basal processes. Current information on the proportional costs of protein synthesis and ion pumping was reviewed recently (MacRae and Lobley, 1986). Briefly present knowledge would indicate:

Energy Cost of Protein Synthesis

In any consideration of the energy cost of protein turnover it is important to differentiate between protein synthesis and protein deposition. The experiments of Reeds and co-workers (1980) on growing pigs provide a clear indication that an animal synthesises much more protein than it accumulates. Fig. 2 summarizes their data on the N kinetics of pigs given low, medium and high levels of a mixed cereal plus fish meal ration. From these data it can be calculated that when pigs are in zero N balance they are synthesising 212g protein/day. Synthesis of the peptide bonds is the main energy cost of protein turnover. Biochemically, it takes 4-5 mol ATP to synthesise 1 mol peptide bond, this being equivalent to approximately 4.5 kJ of energy/g protein synthcsised. Using this relationship on data from the pigs (Reeds *et al.*, 1980) and in other data from several species of mature animals fed at energy equilibrium (the maintenance level of intake) indicates that the calculated energy requirement for protein synthesis at this intake would be 60-70kJ of energy/kg $W^{0.75}$.

Calorimetric experiments would indicate the energy expenditure at this intake is relatively constant also, at approximately 420-450 kJ/kg $W^{0.75}$ (Kleiber, 1947). Thus it might appear that protein synthesis represents approximately 15% of the total energy expenditure. Limited data available for experiments where rates of protein synthesis and energy expenditure have been determined at more than one level of intake are shown in Fig. 3. These values for both pigs and cattle were slightly higher at approximately 20% of the total of heat production.

The high correlation coefficients of the relationships are perhaps surprising if the proportional costs are only in the region of 20% of total energy expenditure and it has been stressed that the values obtained for rates of protein turnover by present day techniques (i.e. use of ^{14}C leucine" to measure rates of irreversible loss and fractional oxidation of protein) provide minimal values only (MacRae and Lobley, 1986).

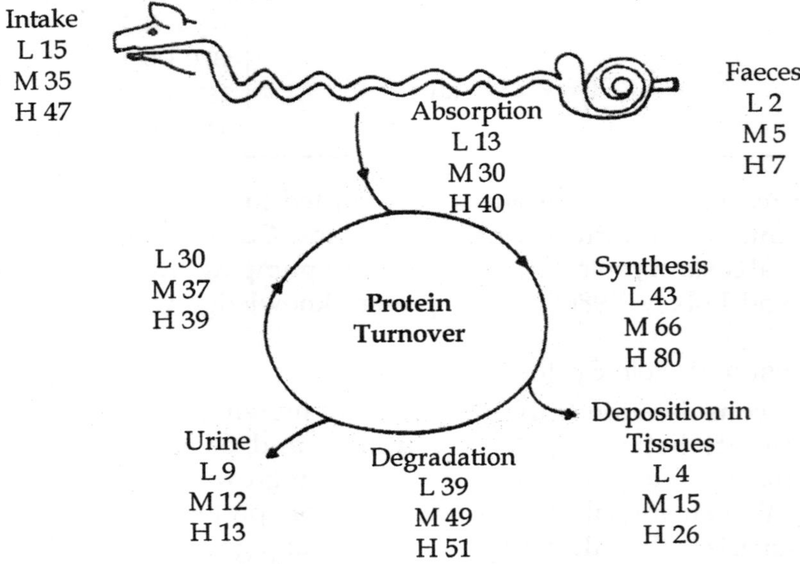

Fig. 2 : Protein turnover (g N/d) in 30 kg pigs given a mixed cereal plus fishmeal/soyabean meal ration at low, medium and high levels of intake (data of Reeds *et al.*, 1980).

Energy Cost of Ion Pumping

Despite limitations on the present techniques for measurements rates of protein synthesis, they do provide a means of obtaining estites in live animals. At present the measurement of ion pumping (Na^{+}/+ ATPase activity) across cell membranes, which is essential for the maintenance of cellular function, is restricted to in *vitro* measurements as it depends on the determination of the reduction in oxygen consumption of tissue slices and/or cells when ouabain is added to inhibit the sodium pump. The relative sensitivities of muscle and liver preparations appear to be species dependent. With ruminant tissues addition of ouabain reduces oxygen consumption by 30-40% (Gregg and Milligan, 1982) whereas with rat tissues the values are much lower (<5%) (Chinet *et al.*, 1977). Assuming that these, values are valid it sets up an intriguing possibility that ion pumping may be a major means of dissipating heat in ruminants whereas it would appear not to be in non-ruminants.

Energy Cost of Other Vital Processes

If ion pumping represents up to 40% of the total basal energy expenditure in ruminants then protein turnover plus ion-pumping together represent a minimum of 60%. At present differentiating what the remaining 40%

represents is little more than speculation, but in a recent review Reeds (Reeds *et al.*, 1985) suggested that the energy cost of fatty acid turnover may represent 10-15%, the energy cost of futile cycles may represent another 10-15% leaving perhaps the last 15% to posture, respiration, circulation secretory processes etc.

Clearly much more work is required before can give precise indications as to the true proportional energy requirement of the various vital processes.

The relationshp between energy expenditure and ME intake

The fact that the various vital body processes require energy means that even when an animal is fasted it must derive this energy from somewhere (N.B. interspecies mean FMR approximately 300 kJ/kg $W^{0.75}$). It derives this energy by mobilising' body tissues. When the animal starts to eat again the dietary ME will progressively spare this mobilisation until such time as the animal is consuming sufficient ME to maintain its various processes without the need to draw on body reserves. Beyond this point it will start to store a proportion of its ME intake as protein and/or fat. The basic relationship between ME intake and energy expenditure (heat production) is illustrated in Fig. 3.

Efficiency of Utilization of ME below Maintenance

One of the major differences between ruminants and non-ruminants is the type of absorbed nutrients which fuel metabolic processes. On most non-ruminant diets glucose derived from starch digestion in the small intestine-is the main energy-yielding nutrient. In ruminants the volatile fatty acids (VFA), acetate, propionate and butyrate, produced during microbial fermentation in the rumen and to a lesser extent the hindgut are the main fuels; on many ruminant diets absorbed VFA represent 60-70% of the total ME intake of the animal.

Experiments carried out at the Hannah Institute in Scotland in the 1950s (Blaxter, 1962) indicated that mixtures of VFAs infused into the rumen of fasted sheep can substitute for body reserves with a high degree of efficiency (0.3-0.87). Efficiency of using protein was 0.81 and of using glucose infused into the abomasum was 1.00. As ruminants absorb very little glucose, these data indicate that, if this were the only factor, the efficiency of utilization of total ME below maintenance should be in the region of 0.83-0.85. However, further energy losses as heat of fermentation and in the cost of eating reduce the net efficiency of utilization of ME below maintenance (km) to approximately 0.75. Blaxter (1962) suggested that the efficiency of utilization of ME can be calculated as:

$$km = 0.546 + 0.30 \times q$$

where q is metabolizability of ration.

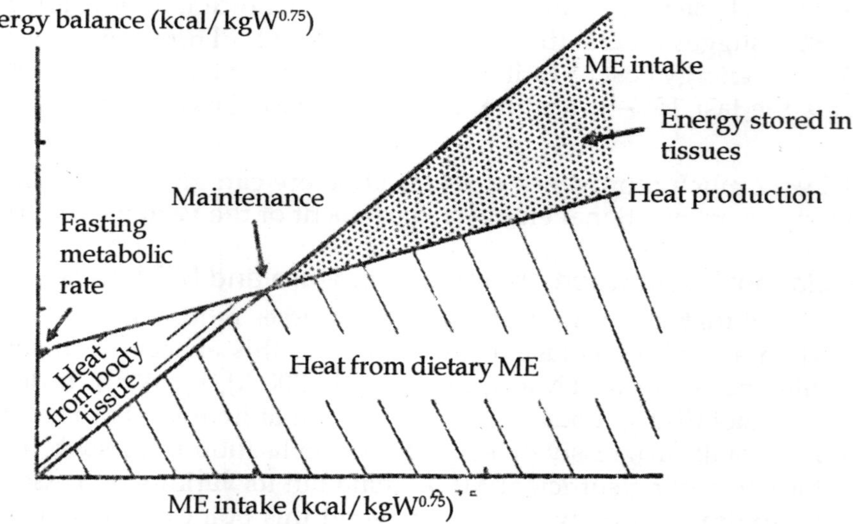

Fig. 3 : Relationship between energy balance and ME intake

Efficiency of Utilization of ME above Maintenance

As intake of ME is increased above the maintenance level of energy expenditure that ME in excess of the maintenance requirement is deposited as tissue (retained energy; E). The measurement of the efficiency of utilization of ME for tissue deposition has been the subject of many experiments. E has been obtained by two different approaches. Either it can be measured directly in experiments where animals are slaughtered at different weights and the energy content of their bodies is measured directly (i.e. **the comparative slaughter technique)** or it has been obtained indirectly from the relationship ME intake = E + heat production-by determining the heat production of the animal using respiration chambers or other means as descrIbed elsewhere in this book (see Chapter 28 by J.M. Brockway).

The latter approach has major advantages in terms of costs (1 animal can be used to determine utilization of many rations), duration of experiment (a calorimetric experiment consisting of 3-4 weeks preliminary feeding period plus 7-14 days measurement of energy intake and faeces and urine energy output, the latter 4-5 days of which might carried out in a respiration chamber for measurement of heat production and methane output, is much quicker than a 3-4 month growth period for a comparative slaughter experiment) and the fact that comparisons say between different feeds can be made on a within-animal basis.

Either way, it must be remembered that the measurement of efficiency of utilization of ME is by definition an incremental measurement and is represented more correctly as:

$\Delta E_r \div \Delta ME$ intake

Consequently, to determine the value for any particular feedstuff requires the measurements to be made atleast at two levels of intake and necessitates a large number of animals for a comparative slaughter trial.

From the many experiments that have been reported using these two techniques it is obvious that efficiency of utilization of ME above maintenance is almost invariably lower in ruminants than in non-ruminants and is particularly low on some forages. Possible reasons for the low efficiency of utilization of ME on forage rations are discussed in following section.

Overall Relationship between ME Intake and Energy Retention

The overall relationship between MEI and E is traditionally represented in a two component linear form with an inflection point at the maintenance level of intake (see Fig. 4a). This indicates that efficiency of utilization of ME is much higher below maintenance. When Blaxter and Boyne (1978) re-analysed some 80 calorimetric experiments which all included measurements of FMR they concluded that the relationship between gross energy intake (GEI) and energy expenditure was best represented by a single exponential function (see Fig. 4b). Since then there has been much discussion on the relative merits of the two representations. Whilst biologically the single exponential relationship is attractive, some experimental data tailed to show any evidence of non-linear relationship unless constrained to take in the FMR values. Hopefully, further experimentation will help to identify the more correct interpretation, but in the meantime the ME system is based on the two component linear relationship as indicated in equation 1 which assumes different but linear efficiencies of utilisation of ME below and above maintenance.

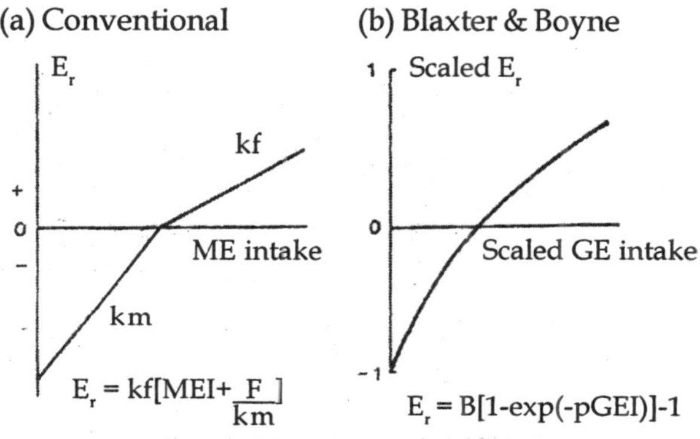

Fig. 4 : Linear aoo curvilinear representations of the relation ships between energy retention (E_r) and energy intake.

Utilization of ME - a metabolic approach

Anyone who has worked in the field of energy metabolism cannot fail to have been struck by the poor efficiency of utilization of ME in ruminants compared with non-ruminants. Fig. 5 summarises the differences and emphasises the very low efficiency that can occur with certain poor quality forages. The facts are that where mixed rations containing grain are fed, the efficiency is much higher than where forage alone is fed, and that where forage alone is fed the quality has an important bearing on efficiency. Such dietary effects occur mainly because the nature of the VFAs absorbed from the rumen has a major influence on the efficiency with which the animal can retain its MEI. Indeed inspection of Table 4 would indicate that on diets which support only poor utilization of ME (poorer quality forages) the VFAs absorbed from the rumen are predominantly acetate, whereas on diets which support better utilization of ME (i.e. mixed rations and better quality fresh pastures) there is proportionally less acetate and more propionate. The question then arises "Why should the nature of the VFA influence efficiency of utilization of ME".

Table 4 : Molar proportion of VFA in rumen of animals given various types of ration

Diet	molar proportions of VfA (%)			
	Acetate	Propionate	Butyrate	higher
Hay	70	18	11	4
grazed pasture	66	19	12	3
Hay + concentrate	60	23	14	3
ground hay + concentrate	52	31	12	6
alfalfa + steamed corn	42	41	4	7
steamed corn alone	34	46	6	14

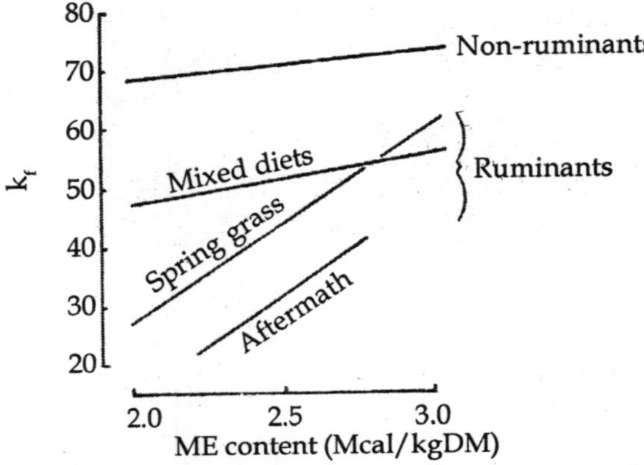

Fig. 5 : Efficiencies of utilization of ME above maintenance intake (kf) in ruminants and non-ruminants (from Webster, 1978)

Historical consideration of the relationship between nature of VFA absorbed and efficiency of utilization of ME

Earlier work at the Hannah Institute (Blaxter, 1962) seemed to indicate that a possible reason for the low efficiency of utilization of ME on forages was that ruminants cannot utilise acetic acid as efficiently as they can utilize propionic or butyric acid. Fig. 6 gives the data that suggested that efficiency of utilization of added acetate was lower than that of added propionate or butyrate. This led Blaxter (1962) to formulate a causal relationship between the amounts of acetate produced by the microbial fermentation of different diets and the efficiency of utilization of the ME of those diets.

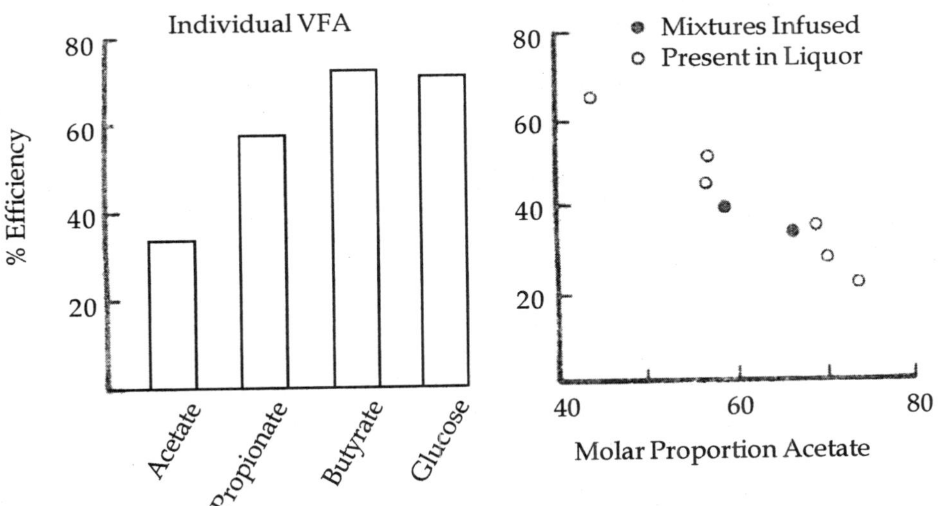

Fig. 6 : Efficiecies of utilization of individual VFAs and mixtures in sheep given a basal ration of 1 kg dried grass (data from Blaxter, 1962).

Unfortunately when this postulate was later tested in feeding trials with calves (Rook *et al.*, 1963) and lambs (Orskov and Allen, 1966) the findings cast doubts on the general applicability of the relationship. Later still experiments with lambs which were sustained entirely by infusions of mixtures of VFA into the rumen and casein into the abomasum seemed to discredit the original interpretation totally; when the VFA infusion mixture was changed from one having a molar composition of acetate 75: propionate 15: butyrate 10 to one of 45:35:20 respectively, the efficiency of utilization of ME was unchanged (approximately 60%).

Recent evidence on possible importance of glucogenic precursors in utilization of acetate

Over the last 5 years, studies carried out at the Rowett have led us to think that many of the observations reported above can be resolved if the efficiency of utilization of acetate depends on its conversion to fatty acids and then into triglycerides (MacRae and Lobley, 1982). These metabolic steps require both reducing equivalents (NADPH) and glycerol phosphate and where the provision of precursors of these co-factors is adequate - probably mainly from propionate in animals given roughage plus concentrate diets or from glycogenic amino acids in the "infusion animals" which were receiving 23% of their ME intake as casein - conversion of acetate into fatty acids can proceed and so efficiency of utilization of ME is high. On the other hand, on roughage diets where neither of these two precursors of glycolytic intermediates is particularly abundant the animal may have a problem in clearing the acetate which it absorbs and may need to catabolize the acetate via the TCA cycle with the resultant production of heat giving the lower efficiency of utilization of ME observed on forage diets.

Further indirect evidence that the provision of extra amino acids can be associated with increased efficiency of utilization of ME on rations which yield a high acetate; low propionate fermentation can be drawn from experiments conducted at the Rowett Institute using two seasonal grasses (MacRae *et al.*, 1985).

Calorimetric studies indicated that the efficiency of utilization of ME was higher for spring grass (SHG; Kf = 0.58 between maintenance M and 1.5 M) than for autumn grass harvested from the same sward (AHG; kf = 0.49). Measurements of the amounts of amino acids absorbed from the small intestine of sheep given grass at both M and 1.5 M levels of intake indicated that for each unit of extra ME available when the intake of each grass was raised above M. there was a higher net absorption of amino acids between the duodenum and the ileum for the SHG compared with AHG (29% of the extra ME from the SHG was as amino acid compared with only 13% for the AHG). When in a subesquent calorimetric experiment sheep given AHG at the same two levels of intake (M and 1.5 M) were infused with either water or casein (30 g/d) into the abomasum at both levels the infusion of casein resulted in an increased ($P<0.05$) efficiency of utilization of ME supplied from the extra AHG. Table 5 summarises these data. The extra ME fed on each. grass was approximately the same but the extra heat produced when casein was infused (1575 ± 10^3 kJ/d) was 18% lower ($P<0.025$) than when water was infused (1917 ± 103 kJ/d). This raised the calculated efficiency of utilizaiton of extra ME supplied by the grass from 0.45 to 0.57 ($P < 0.025$), i.e. to a value similar to that observed with the better quality SHG.

Table 5 : Effect of infusing casein (30 g/d) on utilization of ME in sheep given autumn harvested grass (MacRae *et al.*, 1985).

	Without	Wi th casein	Significance casein
Extra ME Intake from 1.5 M (kJ/d)	3500	3673	n.s.
Extra heat production			
from M to 1.5 M (kJ/d)	1917	1575	P 0.02
Efficiancy ([2-1] + 1)	0.45	0.57	P 0.05

Implications of the glucogenic amino acid concept on the economy of the animal

If the availability of propionate or the glucogenic amino acids can influence the efficiency of utilisation of ME if ruminants then this represents dramatic illustration of the interactions between substrates that are all too often artificially divided into the classes of energy and Protein. Direct proof of the concept is still required but there is some indirect evidence which suggests that it is worthy of further consideration. The data presented in Fig. 7 which is taken from the experiment of prskoy and colleagues (1979) where different mixtures of VFAs were infused into the rumen and casein was infused into the abomasum of mbs shows that where there was a plentiful supply of propionate the retention of N was much higher than where propionate was in scarce supply.

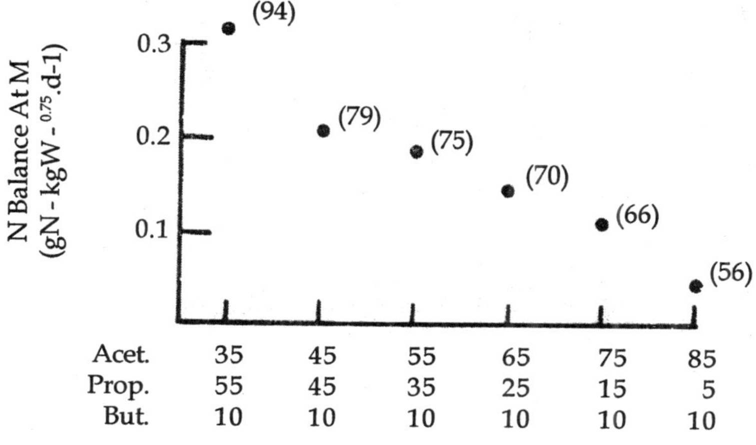

Fig. 7 : Relationship between N balance and the molar ratio of VFA infused (calculated from experiments of Orskov *et al.*, 1979).

This would seem consistent with the concept that where there is little propionate available to provide the glycogenic intermediates to help with the anabolism of acetate into triglyceride, glucogenic amino acids substitute for the propionate and so less amino acid is available for protein synthesis and subsequent protein deposition.

Two more recent studies lend support to this theory. The first (Lobley and MacRae, 1986) involved lambs given grass cubes at a 2M level of intake. When they were infused abomasally with 2 mol acetate daily, the N retention of the lambs went from approximately 5g N/d positive to approximately 3gN/d negative. The same amount of. energy infused as propionate restored N retention to positive values. The second (Girdler *et al.*, 1968) concerned lambs maintained by infusion of VFA mixtures and casein. The animals were infused with mixture containing acetate, propionate and butyrate in the molar proportions 65:25:10 plus sufficient casein to maintain N equilibrium. When the VFA ratio was then changed to 86:0:14, the animal went into negative N balance (approximately -2.4g N/d). However as increasing quantitites of glucose (26, 38 and 52 g/d) were infused abomasally with this same 86:0:14 VFA mixture the N balances progressively improved (approximately -0.4, +0.8 and + 1.5 g N/d, respectively).

The implications of such findings to the ARC protein scheme (ARC, 1980) lie in the fact that the efficiency of utilization of absorbed amino acids is assumed to be a constant value (i.e. 75%; a value obtained in one unpublished experiment conducted on 100 kg calves at the National Institute for Research in Dairying, Reading, U.K.) If the nature of the VFA absorbed from the rumen can alter the efficiency of utilization of amino acids then the protein requirement of the animal will change considerably. Fig. 8 illustrates the way in which reducing the efficiency of utilization of absorbed amino acids from 75% down to 65% would affect the requirements for undegraded dietary protein or the requirements for crude protein in a ration which had a constant degradability of 65% for a cow giving 35 kg of milk per day from an ME intake of 225 MJ/d when losing 0.5kg body weight. Reducing the efficiency by 10% units increases the requirement for UDP by 50% or alternatively increases the crude protein content of the ration from 17 to 23%.

Obviously, the question of efficiency of utilization of absorbed amino acids is a very sensitive aspect (If the ARC (1980) scheme. They set the value at a constant 75%. The updated version of the equivalent scheme used in the States, to be published later this year, adopts a 2-tier value (reminiscent of the current ME system) of 67% efficiency for maintenance and 50% for productive purposes but there would seem to be little experimental evidence for these values.

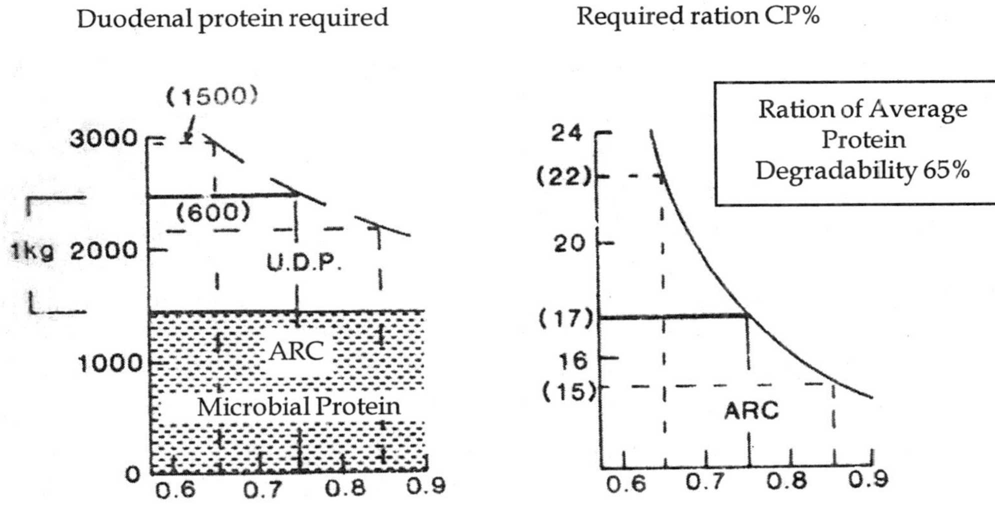

Fig. 8 : Relationship between efficiency of uiilization of amino acids and protein requirements (adapted from Oldham, 1980).

As yet there are very few published experiments from which one can obtain values for efficiency oi utilization of amino acids in ruminants. Derived data from dairy cows, lactating ewes and rapidly growing lambs all of which tend to be fed diets containing high levels of concentrates and thus generate adequate propionate the efficiency of utilisation of amino acids indicate values reasonably near to 75%. However the values for more mature and less productive animals given forages are rarely over 60%. Whether this difference is primarily due to the physiological state of the animal or to the nature of the diet fed remains to be determined. However, when forage-fed ruminants have been supplemented with cereal their N retention has increased significantly and, this might indicate that the diet and in particular, the relative amount of acetate: propionate absorbed from the rumen have considerable influence on the way the animal can utilize its absorbed amino acids.

The considerations raised in IV B and IV C need careful consideration in areas of the world where animal productivity is based on more extensive system and where forage makes up the bulk of the ration. In this respect readers might refer to two publications, the first concerned with matching livestock production systems to available resource in developing countries (Preston and Leng, 1986) and the second concerning drought feeding stratagems (Leng, 1986).

Energy requirements in lactation - the bionergetic approach

Calorimetric experiments carried out mainly in the last 25 years have provided the basis for making reasonably accurate assessments of the energy requirements of the lactating animal. These have been reviewed on a number of occasions (Flatt *et al.*, 1972; Van Es and Van der Honig, 1979) and it is not intended to discuss them here except to use the information now available on the efficiency of conversion of metabolizable energy (ME) into milk energy (k_l; 0.60-0.65) and on the maintenance requirement of lactating animals (490-530 kJ/kg$^{0.75}$) to demonstrate the simplicity of calculating energy requirements of the lactating animal from a knowledge of milk yield. Thus in a 550kg cow producing 30 1 of milk daily, with fat, protein and lactose contents of 40, 35 and 47 g/l, respectively the energy requirements can be calculated as:

1. Energy content of milk, fat	30 x 40 x 39.5	= 47400	kJ/d
protein	30 x 35 x 23.5	= 24675	"
lactose	30 x 47 x 16.5	= 23265	"
		= 95340	"
2. Efficiency of utilization of ME lactation		= 0.65	"
∴ ME requirement for milk production		= 146676	"
3. Maintenance requirement of cow		= 550$^{0.75}$x 510 = 57921	"
4. Total energy requirement		= (2) + (3) = 204597	"

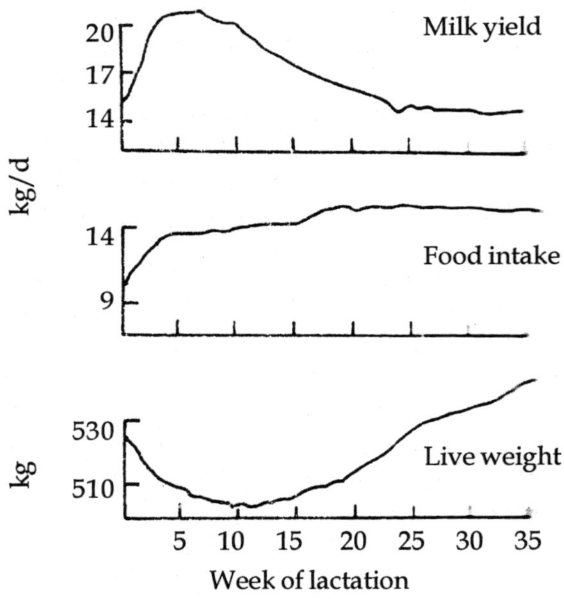

Fig. 9 : Milk yields, food intake and liveweight of 'Friesian hefters (data of Bines *et al.*, 1979).

Such calculations carried out in the first 4 weeks of lactation for high yielding dairy cows almost invariably indicate that the cow's requirements for energy are not being met by its energy intake. Typical data obtained over this period (Bines, 1979) are given in Fig. 9. Friesian heifers given a 40% roughage 60% concentrate ration during the first 2 to 3 months of lactation secrete more energy in their milk than available from their food and so a proportion of their milk production is supported by the mobilization of body tissues. It can be seen in Fig. 10 that the live weight of the heifers falls over the first 10 weeks of lactation. The loss of approximately 0.5 kg body weight per day, presumably mainly as fat (39.5 MJ/kg) would be consistent with the calculated deficit in energy intake i.e. 15-20 MJ/d. Later in the lactation cycle when milk yield had fallen away from peak output and voluntary feed intake had increased to a maximum (3 to 5 months) the animals consumed more than sufficient energy for milk and maintenance requirements and so could then replenish the body reserves used during peak lactation. A further example of this same phenomenon is given .in a recent review on the control of nutrient partition. (Bauman and Elliot, 1983).

Energy requirements in lactation – The metabolic approach

The data presented in Fig. 9 illustrate the critical nature of the balance between energy supply and demand in the first 2 to 3 months of lactation. It is generally accepted that the secretory ability of the mammary gland is determined by events which occur both before and after puberty and during pregnancy (Baldwin, 1966; Cowie *et al.*, 1980) and that the ability of animals to realise their potential for lactation depends on the availability of nutrients presented to the mammary gland. It is necessary therefore to consider what governs this supply, not just in terms of energy *per* se but in terms of specific metabolites needed for the biosynthesis of each of the milk's constituents.

Again there are many research publications and reviews which discuss milk composition (Balch, 1972; Oldham and Sutton, 1979) and the biochemical and cytological mechnisms associated with the biosynthesis of milk constituents by the mammary gland (Larson and Smith 1974; Mepham, 1983) and it is not intended to discuss these mechanisms in detail here. It is necessary however to consider the various roles of the major precursors of milk constituents and how these may interrelate when alterations in milk volume and composition are brought about by manipulation of the diet. Fig. 10 presents a simplified diagram of the main metablic pathways leading to the formulation of milk constituents.

Most of the lipid in milk (98%) is in the form of triglycerides. Approximately 50-60% of these are obtained from preformed plasma glycerides, mainly the chylomichra and low-density lipoproteins (Reaction

1), The remaining 40-50% are formed in the mammary gland from acetate and b-hydroxybutyrate (Reactions 2 & 3). Glucose is needed as a precursor of some if not most of the NADPH required for the synthesis of fatty acids as well as for the provision of glycerol-P for the subsequent esterilfication of the fatty acids. There is still some debate as to the relative contribution of the pentose cycle and the isocitrate dehydrogenase mechanism in the provision of NADPH for fatty acid synthesis in ruminant mammary tissue (Smith *et al.*, 1983). Most of the milk proteins (90 to 95%) are synthesised in the mammary gland from a free amino acid pool which is in equilibrium with that of the blood stream (Reaction 5). The remainder are taken up as preformed proteins from blood (e.g. serum albumin and immuno-globulins (Reaction 6). Milk lactose is synthesised from glucose and UDP-galactose, itself derived from glucose (Reaction 7 &8) and here there is evidence to suggest that the rate of biosynthesis of lactose is controlled by a complex mechanism at the level of the Golgi apparatus involving ex lactalbumin which exerts an nce on the enzyme galactosyltransferase.

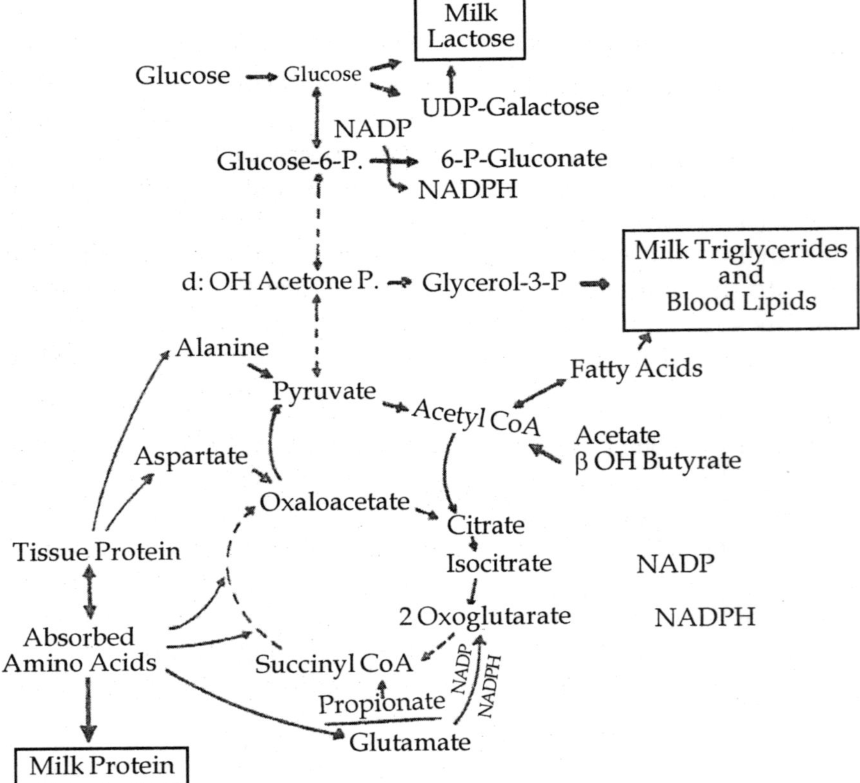

Fig. 10 : Simplified diagram of metabolic pathways involved in the biosynthesis of milk constituents.

The biosynthesis of milk therefore requires provision at the mammary gland of the correct balance of,

i) Acetate, S-hydroxybutyrate and blood lipids to produce milk lipid.

ii) Glucose or glucogenic precursors to provide milk lactose and at least some of the reducing equivalents as well as the glycer phosphate required for synthesis de novo of milk lipids.

iii) Amino acids for the synthesis of milk protein

iv) Precursors of TCA cycle intermediates to provide the enegy needed for the synthetic process.

Although the precise mechanisms are not easily documented a indication of the normal pattern of metabolite availability can be appriciated by considering why problems arise if that normal pattern is distorted.

Low milk fat syndrome

As mentioned earlier the problems with voluntary feed intake in early lactation cause the availability of energy from dietary sources to be limiting and so it is usual to maximize energy intake by providing considerable quantities of energy dense feedingstuffs, i.e. concentrate. Problems can arise with such diets in that milk fat levels may fall. At first sight this might appear to be caused by a simple alteration in the balance of nutrients being presented to the mammary gland. Such diets tend to cause a reduction in the molar ratio of acetate and increase in the molar ratio of propionate present in the rumen and this might be expected to increase the glucose and decrease the acetate which is presented to the mammary gland. However the molar ratio of the VFAs does not necessarily give a clear indication of their respective production rates. Indeed it is probable that the increased propionate:acetate molar ratios in high yielding cows in early lactation is related more to an increase in propionate production rather - than a reduction in acetate production (Bauman *et al.*, 1972).

Once high levels of propionate are absorbed they are converted to glucose in the liver. When this glucose is released into the blood stream it causes an increased insulin secretion which then partitions not only the glucose but also glycerides and acetate towards lipogenesis in adipose tissue rather than in the mammary gland (Obstvedt *et al.*, 1967). As a result the lipogenic enzymes in adipose tissue are elevated in lactating cows given high grain diets which stimulate high circulating levels of blood insulin.

This concept of insulin partitioning nutrients away from the mammary gland is by no means new. Vallance and McClymont in 1959 demonstrated a reduction in milk fat when intravenous glucose (2 kg/d for 48h) was given to lactating cows. These workers latter suggested that the low-fat syndrome might be mediated via an insulin response which would result in a reduction in the- mobilization of tissue glycerides. Indeed they reported a reduction in the plasma glyceride level in one cow whose milk fat had been reduced during an intravenous glucose infusion.

Recent studies (Sutton *et al.*, 1982) are perhaps starting to show how this insulin effect can be alleviated. Lactating Friesian cows were fed four rations containing hay plus 60, 70, 80 and 90% concentrates under two different feeding regimens, one where the animals were given hay plus concentrates twice daily at 0600 and 1630h and the other where the animal received their allocations of hay at 0600 and 1645 h but their allocation of concentrates were automatically dispensed in six equal amounts at 4h intervals. With all but the highest concentrate diet the more frequent feeding gave more milk and with a higher fat content. Cows on the 90% concentrate ration gave less milk on the more frequent feeding (21.4 versus 23 kg/d) but their milk fat content was markedly higher (29.7 versus 17.9 g/kg). Rumen samples showed a progressive decrease in the molar proportion of acetate and an increase in the molar proportion of propionate as level of concentrate was increased. There was no attempt to study the diurnal patterns of VFA production but the patterns and levels of plasma insulin were markedly different in animals given the two feeding regimens. Fig. 11 shows how 4 hourly feeding of concentrates halves plasma insulin concentrations on the 90% concentrate diet; and greatly reduced the post-feeding "spikes" of insulin presumably because propionate absorption was more evenly distributed throughout the 24h.

Supplementation at pasture

The benefits of feeding concentrate little and often could have considerable significance to the grazing animal, by allowing more of the rumen ammonia to be trapped into microbial protein. Thus grazing experiments with steers (Losada *et al.*, 1982) tend to confirm earlier findings with sheep (MacRae and Ulyatt, 1974) that ruminants given fresh pasture can wastefully absorb a considerable proportion of their dietary nitrogen as ammonia anterior to the duodenum [20-35% in sheep (MacRae and Uiyatt, 1974) 20-50% in steers (Losada *et al.*, 1982) and then excrete it in the urine as urea. If it were practicable, feeding concentrates little and often whilst the animals graze instead of say twice daily at milking time would help to even out the energy supply to the rumen. microbes and improve the efficiency with which they convert the protein of their concentrate. Supplement into microbial protein rather than absorb it as ammonia. This in itself could have a beneficial effect on milk prpduction, particularly in early lactation when the animal is in negative energy balance.

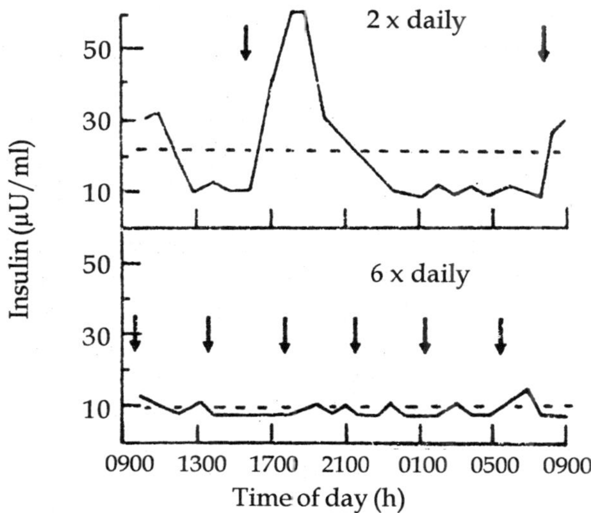

Fig. 11 : Plasma insulin levels (II U!mJ) In blood samples taken throughout a 24 h period from cows (n=4) given the concentrate part of their ration twice or six times dally (data of Sutton et al., 1982).

Conclusion

It is not possible in the space available to cover more than a few selective aspects of energy metabolism in ruminants. Other important aspects, for example the bioenergetic and metabolic aspects of pregnant animal contain their own specific problems. One of these which are also common to the lactating animal is the specific requirement for glucose. Whilst a number of misconceptions have been built up around the quantitative requirements of the ruminant for glucose the major drain for that metabolite for foetal growth and lactose production only emphasises the need to understand the inter-relationships that are becoming apparent at the metabolic level. The study of the energy: protein interactions and the relationships between specific nutrients are now starting to be considered and this departure from the classical approach of energy and protein metabolism wi11 surely gain prominence over the next few years as animal nutritionists start to demand ration formulation schemes which are more universal1y applicable than the present ones.

References

Agricultural Resaarch Council (1965). The Nutrient Requirements of Farm Uvestock No.2. Ruminants. Technical reviews and summaries. London ARC.

ARC (1980). **In:** The Nutrient Requirements of Ruminant Livestock. pp. 89, CAB, Slough.

Belch, C.C. (1972). In: Handbuch Der Tlerernahrung. VoL 2, pp. 259 (editors W. Lenkelt, K. Breirem and E. Crassmann), Verlag Paul Parey, Hamburg.

Baldwin, R.L. (1966). *J. Dairy Sci.*, 49, 1533-1542.

Bauman, D.E., DB vis, C.L. and Bucholtz, H.H. (1972). *J. Dairy Sci.*, 54, 1282-1287.

Bauman, D.E. and ElDot, J.M. (1983). In : Biochemistry of Lactation. p. 437 (editor T.B. Mepham) Elsevier: Amsterdam.

Bines, J.A. (1979). In: Feeding Strtagies for the High Yielding Dairy Cow. EAAP Publ. No.25, p. 23. (editors W.H. Brester and H. Swami). Granada Publishing Ltd.: London.

Biaxter, K.L. (1962). The Energy Metabolism of Ruminants. London: Hutchinson.

Blaxter, K.L. and Boyne, A.W. (1978). *J. Agric. Sci.*, Cambridge, 90, 47-68.

Clinet, A., Clausen, T. and Girardier, L. (1977). *J. Physiol.*, 265, 43-61.

Cowie; A. T., Forsyth, I.A. and Hart, I.C. (1980). Hormone control of lactation. Springer Verlag: Berlin.

Feedingstuffs Evaluation Unit (1984). Rowett Research Institute Feedingstuffs Evaluation Unit, fourth Report (editors F.W. Wainman, P.J. Dewey and A.W. Boyne). DAFS : Edinburgh.

FEU (1978). Rgwett Res. Inst. Feedingstuffs Evaluation Unit 2nd Report, editors F.W. Wainman, PJ.5. Dewey and A.W. Boyne. (DAFS : Edinburgh).

Flatt, W.P., Moe, P.W., Moore, L.A., Brelrem, K. and Ekern, A. (1972). In : Handbuch Der Tierernahrung, Vol., 2, p. 341. (editors W. Lenkelt, K. Brierem and E. Crasemann). Verlag Peul Parey: Hamburg.

Girdler, C.P., Thomas, P.C. and Chamberlein, P.G. (1968). *Proceedings of Nutrition Society*, 45:43A.

Gregg, V.A. and Millgan, L.P. (1982). *British J. Nutr.*, 43, 65.

Kleiber, M. (1947). *Physiological Reviews*, 27, 511-541.

Kellner, O. (1920). Die Ernahrung lier Landwirtschaftlichen Nutztier, 9th ed. Berlin: Parey.

Larson, B.L. and Smith, V.R. (1974). Lactation, A comprehensive Treatise Vol. II Biosynthesis and Secretion of Milk/Diseases, Academic Press, London.

Leng, R.A. (1986). In: Drought feeding strategies, theory and practise. Penambue aooks, Armidale, N.S.W., Australia.

Lob1ey, G.E. and MacRae, J.C. (1986). In: Proceedings of 10th Energy Metabolism Symposium, Airlie, Virginia, Sept. 1985 (In press).

Losada, H.R., Cammel, S.B., Beever, D.E. and Austin, A.R. (1982). In: Forage Protein in Ruminent Animal Production, BSAP Occasional Publ. No.6, pp. 144 (eds. D.J. Thomson, D.E. Beever and R.G. Gunn). BSAP : Thames Ditton, U.K.

MacRae, J.C. (1967). Ph.D. Thesis, University of Newcastle-upon- Tyne.

MacRae, J.C. and Lobley, G.E. (1982). *Livestock Prod. Sci.*, 9, 447-456.

MacRae, J.C. and Lobley, G.E. (1986). In : Control of Digestion and Metabolism In Ruminants. pp. 367-385 (eds. L.R. Milligan, W.L. Grovum and A. Dobson), New Jersey, Prentice-Hall.

MacRae, J.C., Smith J.S., Dewey, P.J., Brewer, A.C., Brown, D.S. and Walker, A. (1985). British J. Nutr., 54, 197-209.

MacRae, J.E. and Uiyatt, M.J. (1974). *J. Agric. Sci., Cambridge*, 82, 309-319.

McClymont, G.L. and Vallanc, S. (1962). *Proceedings of Nutrition Society*, 21, XLI.

Mapham, T.B. (1983). Biochemistry of Lactation, Elsevier, Amsterdam.

Obstvedt, J., Baldwin, R.L. and Ronning, M. (1967). *J. Dairy Sci.*, 50, 108.

Oldham, J.D. (1980). In: Proc. 3rd EAAP Symp. on Protein Metabolism and Nutrition. Vol. 3, p. 98. EAAP Publ. No.27 (Eds. H.J. Oslage and K. Rohr).

Okdham, J.D. and Sutton, J.D. (1979). In: Feeding Strategies for the High Yielding Dairy Cow, EAAP Publ. No.25, p. 114 (eds. W.H. Broster and H. Swan), Granada Publishing, London.

Orskov, E.R. and Allen, D.M. (1966). *British J. Nutr.*, 20, 509-517.

Orskov, E.R. and Food, M.H. (1969). *Proceedings of Nutrition Society*, 28, 31A-32A.

Orskov, E.R., Grubb, D.A., Smith, J.S., Webster, A.J.F. and Corrigall, W. (1979). *British J. Nutr.*, 41, 541-551.

Preston, T.R. & Leng, R.A. (1986). In: Matching Uvestock proouctlon systems to available resources. Internetlonel Uvestock Centre for Africa, Addis Abebe, Ethiopia.

Reeds, P.J., Cadenhead, A., Fuller, M.F., Lobley, G.E. and McDonald, J.D. (1980). *Bri. J. Nutri.*, 43, 445-455.

Reeds, P.J., fuller, M.F. and Nicholson, B.A. (1985). In: Substrate and energy metabolism in man. pp. 46-57 (eds. J.S. Garrow and D. Halliday), London, John Libbey.

Rock, J.A.F., Balch, C.C., Campling, R.C. and fisher, L.J. (1963). *British J. Nutr.*, 17, 399-406.

Rowett Research Institute (1975). Feedingstuffs Evaluation Unit first Report. Edinburgh: Department of Agriculture and fisheries for Scotland.

Smith, G.H., Crabtree, B. and Smith, R.A. (1983). In: Biochemistry of lactation (Mepham, T.B., ed.) Amsterdam, The Netherlends, Elsevier. p. 121-140.

Sutton, J.D., Hart, I.C. & Broster, W.H. (1982). In: Energy Metebolism of farm Animal EAAP Publ. No. 29, p. 26. (eds. A. Ekern and F. Sundstol).

Vallance, S. and McClymont, G.L. (1959). Nature 183, 466-467.

Van E.S., A.J.H. and Van der Honig, Y. (1979). In: feeding Strategies for the High Yielding Dairy Cow. EAAP Publ. No.25, p. 68. editors WoH. Broster and H. Swann. (Granada Pulr Ushing Ltd., London).

Webster, AJ.F. (1978). The Manegement and Diseases of Sheep, pp. 166-174. Slough: Commonwealth Agricultural Bureau.

□□□

Animal Nutrition, 2012
eds. Dr. (Mrs.) Usha R. Mehra et al., pp. 77-109
Satish Serial Publishing House e-mail : info@satishserial.com; website : www.satishserial.com

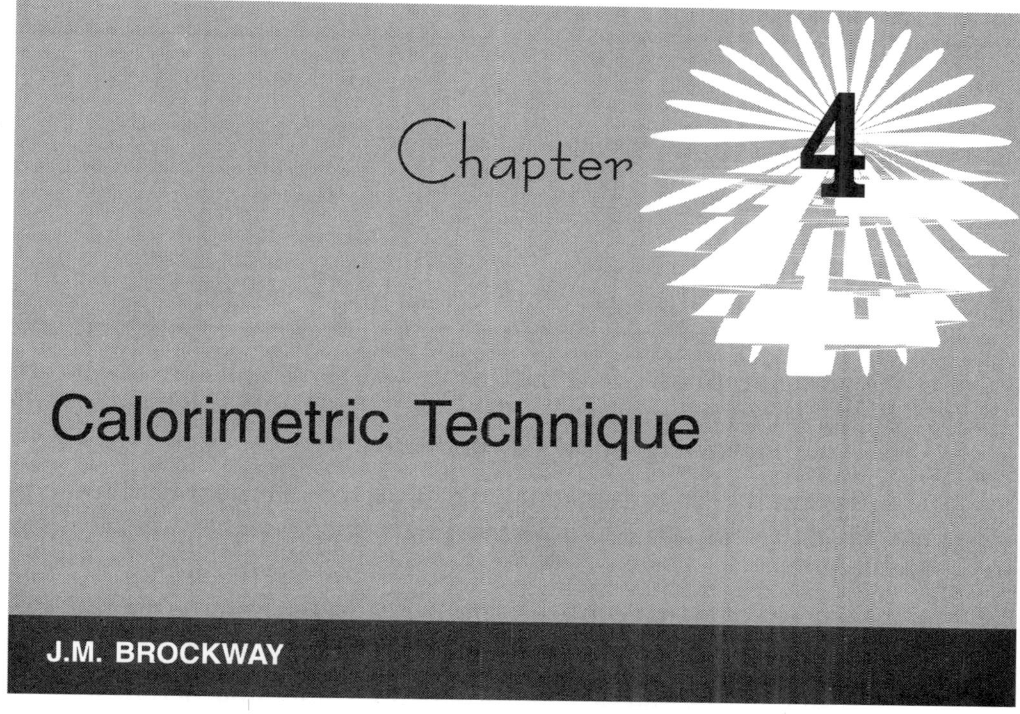

Calorimetric Technique

J.M. BROCKWAY

In the nutritional context "calorimetry" is usually understood *to* mean the measurement *of* metabolic rate; the latter term may appear under a variety of synonyms, *(or* near synonyms) such as energy expenditure, heat loss or heat production. This variable is of fundamental importance in the measurement of the energy balance *of* an animal. The difference between metabolic rate and (metabolizable) energy intake re-presents energy retention: if the algebraic sign *of* retention is positive the animal is growing or fattening - i.e. it is productive; if the sign is negative the animal is catabolizing body tissue and is in the process of starvation.

I. UNITS

To begin, it is necessary to define the units in which metabolic rate is expressed. In current scientific literature the nearest approach to a globally accepted system *of* units for the expression of physical quantities is the Systeme International d'Unites - or, as it is *more commonly* known, the "SP". The seven basic units of the, 51 are listed in Table 1.

Table 1 : SI basic units

Length	- metre	-m
Mass	- kilogram	- kg
Time	- second	- s
Electric current	- ampere	- A
Temperature	- Kelvin	- K
Luminous Intensity	- candela	-cd
Amount of substance	- mole	-mol

For the present purposes only the first three *of* these units are of concern. The **metre** (m) is defined in terms of the wavelength of the radiation of the krypton-86 atom under fully specified conditions.

The **kilogram** (kg) is a mass equal *to* that -of the International Prototype Kilogram which is kept at the International Bureau of Weights and Measures in France.

The **second** (s) is defined in terms *of* the period of radiation of the caesium-133 atom under specified conditions.

Derived units under the SI are obtained .by combining two or more of the basic units. For example, the SI unit of force is the Newton, N: it is defined as that force which when applied to a mass of kilogram for 1 second produces a velocity of 1 metre per second, or, alternatively a force of 1 newton acting upon a mass of 1 kilogram produces an acceleration of 1 metre per second per second. The newton has the dimensions, in SI units, of kg m S^{-2}. Energy is the capacity to do work; work and energy are measured in the same units, which in the SI, is the joule, J. The joule is defined as the work done when a force of 1 newton acts through a distance of 1 metre, and has the SI unit dimensions of kg m^2 s^{-2}. Power is the rate at which work is performed, and under the SI the unit of power is the **watt**, W, defined as work performed at a rate of 1 joule per second, with the dimensions kg m^2 s^{-2}.

The joule is often an inconveniently small unit of energy; for example, 1 gram of sugar, when fully oxidized yields about 18500 joules, or a sheep may have a daily energy expenditure of perhaps 7500000 joules. Such numbers are unwieldy so, at least when dealing with animals of agricultural importance, it is customary to express energy in terms of kilojoules (1000 J, or lkJ = 10 joules) or even as megajoules (1000000 J, or IMJ = 10^6 joules). The metabolic rate of the sheep would then be said to be 7.5 MJ day^{-1} or 7500 KJ day^{-1} 1. This value is equivalent to a power output of about 90 watts, i.e. about that of an average sized electric light bulb.

While metabolic rate is, strictly speaking, an expression of power it is none-the-less often more convenient to express it in term of joules per unit time (rather than as watts) in that for many purposes it is the energy balance of an animal that is under discussion, and energy intake is expressed as joules per unit time. However in cases where metabolic rate *per se* is of prime importance, as for example when evaluating the heating or air conditioning requirements for an animal house, expression of metabolic rate as watts may well is preferable.

The calorie is a unit for the measurement of energy which has been superceded by the joule; it has virtually disappeared from European scientific literature, although It may still be found in current publications: from other parts of the world. In fact, there are, or were three separately defined calories, each with slightly differing values,

These were:

1. The International Table calorie, equivalent to 4.1868 J
2. The 15°C calorie equivalent to 4.1855 J
3. The thermochemical calorie equivalent to 4.1840 J

The thermochemical calorie was probably the most used form in' nutritional work, although in many older textbooks one may still find the 15°C calorie, defined as that quantity of heat which is required to raise the temperature of I gram of pure water from 14.5°C to 15.5°C. While the difference between the thermochemical and 15°C calories may seem trifling, at less than 0.04%, it was none-the-less an occasional nuisance; it is an inconsistency that has been removed by the use of SI units. The calorie was also an inconveniently small unit, particularly when referring to man or to animals of agricultural importance, so the kilocalorie (kcal, or sometimes Calorie or Cal. = 10^3 calorie) and less commonly the megacalorie (Mcal =10^6 calorie) were used.

The other units which are required in handling data for calculation of metabolic rate are concerned with quantities of gases such as air, oxygen, carbon dioxide, methane and water vapour. The SI unit for amount of substance is the mole (mol) which is defined as the amount of the substance in question which contains as many elementary units as there are carbon atoms in 0.012 kg of pure carbon-12. Although the mole is every convenient unit for the majority or chemical or biochemical measurements and calculations, it is less so when dealing with gases, which are usually measured volumetrically. The SI derived unit for volume is the **cubic metre** (m^3) **litre** (1, formally the cubic decimeter dm^3, or 10^{-3} m^3) is probably more commonly used. The litre was originally defined as the volume occupied by 1 kg of water at its maximum density that volume differs by 28 parts in 1000000 from the current SI defined litre.

The volume occupied by a given amount of gas is, of course, dependent upon its temperature and pressure. Temperature is expressed, under SI, as "degree kelvin" (°K). The degree kelvin is defined as the fraction 1/273.15 of the thermodynamic temperature of the triple point of water. The "degree kelvin" is of the same magnitude as the "degree celsius" and the former "degree centigrade" (both °C), but whereas the kelvin scale starts at absolute zero, 0.0°K, the celsius scale's zero point is at 273.15°K. In the 51 the unit of pressure is "newton per square metre" (N m^{-2}) and is known as the pascal (Pa). When dealing with atmospheric pressures the pascal is rather too small, so the kilopascal (kPa) is used. In probably somewhat more familiar units: 100 kPa - 1 bar, 1 kPa = 10 mb or 133.322 Pa = 1 torr (= 1 mm mercury). When performing calculations involving quantities of gas expressed as volumes it is usual to convert all such volumes to conditions of standard temperature and pressure (s.t.p., dry). These standard conditions are 273.15° K and 101.325 kPa (these are the 51 unit equivalents of 0°C and 760 torr). It is recognized that many older mercury barometers are graduated, and will be read, in millimeters, or even inches of mercury; while reporting pressures in these units is to be discouraged, there is no reason why local calculations should not be made with them.

Gas volumes recorded in any calorimetric facility depart from "s.t.p., dry" conditions in temperature, pressure and humidity. The former two variables are simply dealt with by conventional "gas law" calculations, but before these can be made it is necessary to reduce the measured gas pressure by the partial pressure of the water vapour present in that gas. Water vapour pressure can be measured directly on a dew point apparatus, or by an electronic capacitance hygrometer, or more simply and cheaply by wet and dry bulb temperature sensors (thermometers, thermocouples or thermistors). Water vapour pressure is derived from wet and dry bulb temperature using any standard meteorological tables or nanograms of by use of a polynomial equation such as:

Water vapour pressure = 4.74 + 0.817W + 0.0081. W + 0.000378W - 0.5D (mm mercury)

Where W and D are wet and dry bulb temperatures, °C. Volumes of gas at s.t.p. may be easily converted to moles; e.g. 1 mole of ideal gas occupies 22.414 litres of s.t.p., or the conversion may be made on the basis of published gas densities at s.t.p., viz. oxygen 1.428 gl^{-1} carbon dioxide 1.964 g r1 and nitrogen 1.250 gl^{-1}.

II. CALORIMETRY

An idealized system for feeding farm animals can be thought of as follows

Energy expenditure + desired level of production = metabolizable energy to be supplied by food intake

Many different systems of description of the energy supplied by foods have been proposed at different times. This is not the place for discussion of these systems, but in Fig 1 the metabolizable energy/net energy system is outlined to show the pre-eminent quantitative importance of energy expenditure. In Fig. 1 the gross energy intake or the heat of combustion of the food consumed is arbitrarily set at 100 units, and the loss of energy is shown at each stage. It will be appreciated that the exact values will vary considerably under differing circumstances: those shown in Fig. 1 are presented to give the reader an idea of their relative magnitudes. Draught work can be ascribed to either activity or to production.

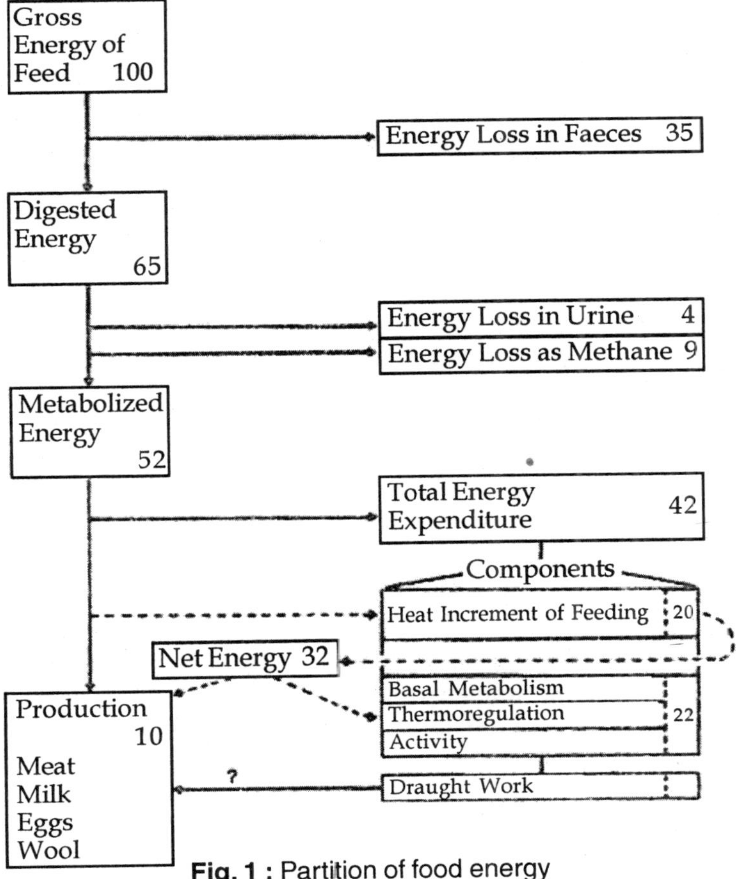

Fig. 1 : Partition of food energy

A. The Bomb Calorimeter

Although this chapter is primarily concerned with animal calorimetry it is appropriate to introduce this section with a brief account of the bomb calorimeter. This instrument is used to measure what is termed the, gross energy value, the calorific value, or the heat of combustion, of materials such as feeding stuffs, faeces or urine. The underlying principle of the bomb calorimeter is simply that the material under test is burned, in an excess of oxygen, inside the calorimeter bomb which is immersed in a known quantity of water. The heat liberated by the combustion of the test sample warms this water and can be calculated from the increase in temperature.

The calorimeter bomb is a hollow, thick-walled stainless steel Cylinder of about 300 ml capacity and fitted with a screw-on lid. The material to be tested is usually dried, and a sample of it, of about 1.0 g to 1.5 g is formed into a pellet for ease of handling. A short length of cotton thread may be included in the pellet: the free ends of this thread are wrapped around the ignition fuse wire to aid the initial stage of combustion. The sample pellet is then put into the bomb's crucible and connected to the fuse wire and ignition terminals. The bomb is closed and filled with oxygen to a pressure of about 2500 kPa; it is then placed in a can containing an accurately determined quantity of water, usually about 2 litres. The can containing the bomb and water is placed inside an outer insulating jacket. In the modern adliabatic calorimeter, this outer jacket takes the form of a temperature controlled water jacket; whose temperature exactly follows that of the water in the bomb can. Once an initial thermal stability has been obtained the test sample in the bomb is ignited electrically and the heat liberated by the burning sample warms the bomb, water and can. This rise in temperature is precisely mimicked by that of the water in the outer jacket, until a new temperature equilibrium is attained. Calculation of the heat of combustion of the test material is straightforward: the amount of heat liberated is the sum of the products' of the masses and specific heats of the bomb, can and water. In practice, from initial calibrations with material of known heat of combustion (usually benzoic acid) the products of mass and specific heat for bomb and can are expressed as their "water equivalent". As the specific heat of the stainless steel of the bomb and can is approximately one tenth of that of water, the water equivalent is approximately one tenth of their actual mass. There are minor corrections to be made to the total heat liberated. For instance, small quantities of sulphuric and nitric acids are sometimes formed in the combustion of the test material. These acids represent only partially oxidized material, so, the amount of acid found is determined by titration and from known equivalences between acids and heat a correction can be added to the heat liberated by the test sample. A further correction must be made for the energy liberated from the cotton thread used to assist ignition of the sample.

Microprocessor units are available which can be attached to the adiabatic bomb calorimeter and which can automatically monitor the rise in temperature following ignition of the sample and then calculate the calorific value with virtually no intervention on the part of the operator.

The ballistic bomb calorimeter : This instrument is considerably simpler, and less expensive, than the adiabatic calorimeter, and, inevitably, lacks some of the accuracy of the latter instrument. In the ballistic bomb calorimeter the bomb assembly is very similar to that in the adiabatic version, but there is no water, can or outer jacket. Instead the peak temperature following ignition of the sample is recorded. The ballistic peak is measured with a thermocouple and galvanometer. Calculation of calorific value is made by reference to peak temperatures obtained when differing amounts of material of known calorific value, such as benzoic acid, have been burned in the ballistic bomb.

B. Direct Calorimetry

Some of the earliest animal calorimeters resembled the bomb calorimeter in so far as the increase in temperature of a known amount of water was recorded. These early static calorimeters were only suitable for measurements on small animals over relatively short time spells. To enable longer term measurements on larger animals it became necessary to use a dynamic system in which the increase in temperature of a water flow around the animal chamber was measured. In the ideal calorimeter of this type:

Heat loss from animal = mass flow of water x specific heat of water x temperature difference of water (outlet - inlet).

A calorimeter working on these genera principle has been designed (Mount et. al. 1967) to hold several pigs at one time. In that design all heat, exchange is constrained to take place between the animals and the ventilating air flow through the chamber. Incoming air temperature is varied to give a constant outgoing temperature which matches that in the so-called "shell-space" surrounding the animal chamber. The control of incoming air temperature is achieved in a heat exchange unit through which cooled water is circulated. The amount of energy extracted from the ventilating air in the heat exchanger is estimated from comparison of the range of water temperature across the heat exchanger with the change of temperature of the same water flow across a heater of known power. The heat loss- measured in this way is the "sensible" heat loss from the animals. Sensible heat 1oss, sometimes called Newtonian heat loss, is the sum of the radiant, convective and conductive heat losses. The other route of heat loss from an animal, and the one which is of paramount importance in warm climates, is evaporative heat loss, which can take place through sweating, panting of wallowing. In the above calorimeter the magnitude of the evaporative heat loss is assessed from the differences in water vapour content between the air entering and leaving the animal chamber, and from the flow rate of that air. Water vapour pressure is measured with wet and dry bulb thermometers.

Direct calorimeters usually tend to overestimate evaporative heat loss and underestirnate sensible heat loss, although the combined figure for total heat loss may be correctly estimated. This error in partitioning between evaporative and sensible losses arises from evaporation from drinking water, from voided urine and from faeces: such evaporation takes place at the expense of part of the sensible heat loss from the animal.

Another class of direct calorimeter, is the gradient layer instrument in calorimeters of this type the temperature gradient is measured across a layer of thermal insulation between the animal (the heat source) and some from of heat sink of virtually infinite thermal capacity (usual1y a rapidly circulating constant temperature water jacket). If heat is emitted from a single point source in the centre of a spherical enclosure of uniform thermal characteristic, then, to estimate the rate of heat emission from the source, it is only necessary to measure the temperature gradient across the wall of the enclosure at one point. However, in a real situation this 3-dimensional symmetry is lacking; the heat source is an animal which is not necessarily in the centre of the enclosure, which in its turn is more likely to be rectangular box than a sphere. It then becomes necessary to measure the temperature gradient over the entire surface of the enclosure. In practice, this means that at several thousand points over the surface of the animal chamber the local temperature gradients are individually measured with thermocouples. The thermocouples are connected in series to form large but diffuse integrating thermopile whose "hot" junctions are on the animal surface of the temperature gradient material, and whose "cold" or reference, Junctions are the constant temperature water jacket surface. The temperature gradient material consists of some form of plastic sheeting which affords both thermal and electrical insula1ion between the pairs of hot and cold junctions. Because the thermocouples are connected in series their combined electro-motive force is adequate to drive a potentiometric recorder with a range of 0-9 mV, or even 0-10mV, directly, i.e. without the need for any direct current amplification.

The fact that the heat source in the chamber is an animal introduces two further complications: 1) the requirement for a ventilatory air flow, which will forcibly convict some sensible heat out of the chamber, and 2) the need to measure evaporative heat loss. These complications were dealt with in an elegant manner in a gradient layer calorimeter built for sheep and other animals up to 100 kg live weight at the Rowett Research Institute (Pullar, 1958). This calorimeter has four air conditioning units, situated two each on the inlet and outlet air flows of the animal chamber (see Fig. 2). Conditioning

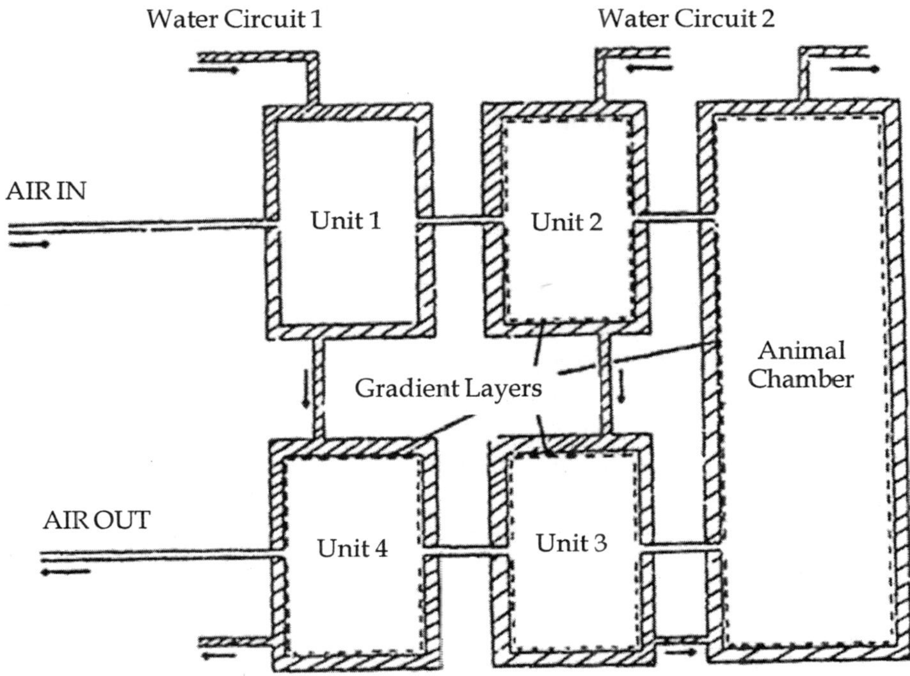

Fig. 2 : Gradiant layer Calorimeter

units 2, 3 and 4 have gradient layer between their air channels and water jackets. Units 1 and 4 are operated on the same cold water circuit (no. 1) to chill the air passing through them to a temperature which is usually in the region of 2-6°C. Units 2 and 3 are operated at the same temperature as the animal chamber (all on water circuit no. 2) which is always higher than that at units 1 and 4. Sensible heat losses as conduction, radiation and part of the total convection are detected by the gradient layers of the animal chamber; the remainder of the convective heat loss, i.e. that part swept out of the chamber by the ventilating air stream (the "forced" convection) is detected in Unit 3. Before air enters unit 1 it is humidified as needed, so that at the exit port of that unit it is saturated with water vapour at the low operating temperature of the unit. All the air conditioning units work with high efficiency to bring the air flow through them into temperature equilibrium with the water flow. The saturated air leaving Unit 1 is warmed in Unit 2 to reach the chamber operating temperature, and in the process the saturation of the air is reduced to an extent which is dependent on the relative temperatures of Units 1 and 2. Should there be no source of evaporation within the animal chamber the air will leave. Unit 3 at exactly the same degree of saturation as it left unit 2: it then passes to Unit 4 where it is cooled, to just reach full saturation again. The amount of heat transferred from water jacket to air in Unit 2 will exactly equal the amount transferred from air to water jacket in Unit 4: the voltages generated by the gradient layers in these two units will be equal and can be conncected electrically to give a net output of zero voltage. If, however, there is a source of evaporation in the animal chamber that additional 'water added to the air stream will be condensed in Unit 4 as the air stream is returned to full saturation. The additional latent heat released in the condensation will appear as an extra voltage on the gradient layer output from Unit 4; the net output voltage (Unit 4 - Unit 2) will be a function of the amount of additional water vapour added to the air stream in the animal chamber and condensed out in Unit 4. Gradient layer calorimeters thus can produce continuous output records showing total heat loss partitioned into its sensible and evaporative components. These records, if plotted on a multi-channel chart recorder require to be integrated to produce cumulative, quantitative data on heat loss. The process of integration of a chart record is conveniently carried out using a planimeter, an instrument which measures areas. The electrical signals from the gradient layer thermopiles can be handled in other ways, such as with digital counters driven by integrating motors, or by feeding the signals to a computer, either directly ("on line") or by way of some form of data logging instrumentation.

A meticulously built and operated direct gradient layer calorimeter, after careful calibration (see below), should be capable of measuring heat losses from an animal to within ± 0.5%. The **absolute** error on this type of instrument, operated under constant conditions, is fixed and independent of the heat loss being measured; conversely the relative error is reduced as the heat loss is increased.

It must always be remembered that the direct calorimeter measures heat **loss** which may be equated with heat **production,** or metabolic rate, only if no heat storage (or either algebraic sign) has occurred in the animal's 'body within .the period of calorimetric measurement. If heat storage is known to have taken place heat loss measurements can be adjusted to give a close approximate to heat production, although never with the theoretical precision with which the original heat loss measurements were made. The sort of problem that may occur involving a heat storage term can be envisaged with young growing pigs at, say, 10-20 kg live weight: these animals can change their bodyweight by ± 10% within a 24 hour period; such a change represents quite a large adjustment of the measured heat loss in order to derive metabolic rate. Apart from change in body weight, change in mean body temperature is the other major source of heat storage. Correction of storage due to change in body temperature is bound to be somewhat imprecise as it is notoriously difficult to measure mean body temperature. Deep body (core) temperature is stable and relatively easy to measure, but the so-called shell temperature (i.e. the temperature of those peripheral parts of the body that are not at core temperature) presents considerable difficulty, and even if it could be assessed accurately, there remains the problem of' the relative weightings to be given to core and shell contributions to overall mean body temperature. Fortunately the problem of heat storage due to body temperature change diminishes with time. Unlike heat storage due to weight change, which is often progressive, body temperature fluctuates about some mean, if. immeasurable, level so that, in most instances it can be ignored in any measurement of heat loss lasting more than 24 hours.

A further effect which may need to be considered in questions of heat storage is that of the heat content of ingested food and water however, except when feed of high moisture content is consumed at low temperatures the magnitude of the effect is usually small.

C. Indirect Calorimetry

Indirect calorimetry involves the calculation of metabolic rate from knowledge of respiratory exchange and nitrogen excretion. Respiratory exchange comprises oxygen consumption and carbon dioxide production, and, where appropriate, methane production. An animal's metabolic rate is assumed to arise from the oxidation of three types of physiological fuel, viz. carbohydrate, fat and protein. Within each of these classes it is considered that the materials are sufficiently, homogenous as regards chemical characteristics upon oxidation, that, for example, all carbohydrates are identical. Obviously this is not a rigorously tenable point-of-view, but the errors thus introduced are relatively small.

Before discussion of the derivation of formulae for the calculation of metabolic rate from respiratory exchange and nitrogen excretion it is necessary to consider two points: 1) the respiratory quotient, and 2) the catabolism of protein. The respiratory quotient (R.Q.) is defined as the ratio of the amount of carbon dioxide produced to that of 'oxygen consumed. Strictly speaking the R.Q. should be derived from molar quantities, but in practice, volumes are more commonly used, so:

$$\text{R.Q.} = \frac{\text{litres } CO_2 \text{ produced}}{\text{Litres } O_2 \text{ consumed}}$$

The heat of combustion of an average protein when tested in the bomb calorimeter is about 23.8 kJ g^{-1}, or 149 kJg^{-1} nitrogen content of the protein, on the assumption that the average protein contains 16% by weight of nitrogen. In the bomb calorimeter the protein is fully oxidized to water, carbon dioxide and oxides of nitrogen; in the animal the oxidation of protein is incomplete, with the formation of nitrogenous end-products such as urea or uric acid, substances which are (chemically) capable of further oxidation, and which have significant heats of combustion. The nitrogen content of urine has an average energy equivalence of about 34kJ g^{-1}. Thus the biologically available energy content of the average protein would be 149 - 34 = 115 kJ g^{-1} protein nitrogen, or approximately 18kJ g -1 protein. All the nitrogen that appears in urine is assumed, for this purpose, to be derived from 'the catabolism of protein, so that, starting with urinary nitrogen excretion it is possible to calculate the quantity of protein that was metabolized. Each gram of protein catabolized required 0.957 litre of oxygen, or 5..981 litre oxygen per gram protein nitrogen.

Table 2 : Properties of the physiological fuels

	Oxidation of 1g fuel		
	1 O_2 used	1 CO_2 produced	heat produced kJ
Carbohydrate	0.829	0.829	17.573
Fat	2.013	1.431	39.748
Protein	9.57	0.774	18.410

The simplest derivation (Brouwer, 1958) of a formula to calculate metabolic rate starts with a listing (Table2) of the relevant metabolic properties of the three types of physiological fuel, and the list of abbreviations and symbols used in the calculation are as follows:

O_2 Oxygen consumption, litre
CO_2 carbon dioxide production, litre
K carbohydrate metabolized, gram
F fat metabolized, gram
P protein metabolized, gram
N urinary nitrogen excretion, gram
H heat production, kJ

From the above table, three simple linear equations are derived which describe oxygen consumption, carbon dioxide production and heat production respectively, in terms of the quantities of carbohydrate, fat and protein metabolized

O_2 (1) = 0.829 K + 2.013 F + 0.957 P ....(1)
CO_2 (I) = 0.829 K + 1.431 F + 0.774 P ....(2)
H (kJ) = 17.573 K +39.748 F +18.410 P.................(3)

Equations (1) and (2) are solved for K and F, which values are substituted into equation (3). Following substitution the equation can be solved for H, the heat production, in terms of the amounts of oxygen consumed, carbon dioxide produced and protein metabolized:

$$H = 16.175\ O_2 + 5.022\ CO_2 - 0.957\ P \quad .... (4)$$

P is readily assessed from the amount of urinary nitrogen excreted during the experimental period: each gram of urinary nitrogen represents the catabolism of 6.25 g protein, so equation (4) can be written:

$$H = 16.175\ O_2 + 5.022\ CO_2 - 5.983\ N \quad ... (5)$$

Here, heat production is expressed in terms of the amounts of oxygen and carbon dioxide exchanged and the amount of urinary nitrogen excreted.

Equations (4) and (5) are unsuitable for use with ruminant animals as they take no account of the unoxidised fuel being lost to the animal as methane, but analogous equations can be derived whjch do take account of this energy loss. The equations are:

$$H = 16.175\ O_2 + 5.022\ CO_2 - 2.167\ CH_4 - 0.957\ P \quad ... (6)$$

$$\text{and } H = 16.175\ O_2 + 5.022\ CO_2 - 2.167\ CH_4 - 5.983\ N \quad ... (7)$$

where CH_4 is the methane production, litre.

These are the well known "Brouwer" equations, which are extensively used and which have attained world wide recognition.

The Brouwer equations are ideally suited for use with the closed circuit type of indirect calorimetry (see below) where quantities of oxygen and carbon dioxide involved are represented by the primary measurements, but in open circuit indirect calorimetry the primary measurements are of outlet volumetric flow rate and of inlet and outlet gas concentration differences. An algebraic development (McLean, 1972) of the Brouwer equation no. (7) allowed for the calculation of heat production of ruminant animals from the primary measure melts in open circuit indirect calorimetry. The Brouwer equation can be transformed from:

$$H = 16.175 O_2 + 5.022\ CO_2 - 2.167\ CH_4 - 5.983\ N \quad ... (7)$$

$$\text{to } H = Vo\ [20.464\ X + 0.732\ Y - 6.456\ Z] - 5.983\ N \quad ... (8)$$

where

Vo = outlet ventilation rate, 1 min^{-1}, from an open-circuit system

X, Y, Z = concentration differences, signs always positive, between inlet and outlet air streams for oxygen, carbon dioxide and methane respectively.

H and N are as in the Brouwer equation. In equation (8) the carbon dioxide term (0.732 Y) has less weight than in the Brouwer equation, and the error involved in omitting it altogether is not very great. The full equation (8), above, can be further manipulated to:

$$H = Vo\ [21.196\ X - 6.402\ Z] - 5.983\ N \quad \text{... (9)}$$

in which form it can be shown that it is always accurate to within t 0.8%. Equation (8) can also be reduced to terms for ventilation rate and oxygen concentration differences only:

$$H = 20.46\ Vo\ X \quad \text{... (10)}$$

in which form, it is estimated, it will be accurate to ±2% under all but severely abnormal feeding conditions. These modifications of the Brouwer formulae have made a significant contribution to the ease of calculation of open-circuit data.

D. Apparatus for Indirect Calorimetry

1. Closed Circuit Respiration Chambers

This type of apparatus consists of an animal chamber and an absorption train connected together into a closed loop, into which oxygen may be admitted. Air from the animal chamber, depleted of oxygen and enriched with carbon dioxide is circulated to the absorption train where it is first dried and then passed through an absorber for carbon dioxide, then re-dried and returned to the animal chamber. The carbon dioxide absorbent is usually a strong alkaline solution, such as sodium or potassium hydroxide. In the reaction between carbon dioxide and alkali the appropriate carbonate and water are formed e.g.

$$2\ KOH + CO_2 \rightarrow K_2\ CO_3 + H_2O$$

The absorption of carbon dioxide tends to reduce pressure within the closed circuit; this reduction in pressure is counterbalanced by the admission of oxygen through some form of demand value. The animal's carbon dioxide production is measured as the gain in weight of the carbon dioxide absorbent and its subsequent drier. Oxygen consumption is measured volumetrically as the amount of oxygen entering the system; methane accumulates within the system and is estimated as the product of the volume of the system and the concentration of methane. Fig. 3 shows the arrangement of the components in a closed circuit chamber built (Wainman and Blaxter, 1958) for studies on the energy metabolism of sheep at the Rowett Research Institute. The gas flow from the animal chamber is driven by an oil-free blower through three parallel pathways before returning to the chamber. The ratios of the gas flows in the three paths, adjusted by manually controlJed valves, give a measure of control of the humidity of the air in the animal chamber. The first of the pathways is a simple by-pass, which allows for complete control of the flow rates in other parts of the circuit; it is preferred to use this form of control rather than the more conventional throttle value as the latter may impose undue stresses upon the blowers shaft seals, whose integrity is essential to the system. That part of the gas stream not going through the by-pass is cooled in a heat exchange unit and passed through a drying tower packed with silica gel. The pre-cooling before drying is desirable in that. the capacity of silica gel for water vapour is severely reduced with increasing temperature. Other drying agents could be used - e.g. calcium chloride, but in many cases these would need to be discarded once their drying capacity is exhausted, whereas silica gel is easily re-generated in a stream of hot air (circa 150°C). After it has been dried the air stream is split once more: part returning to the animal chamber by way of a variable area flowmeter ("Rotameter") while the remainder is cooled again and directed through a further train of absorbers. The absorption train consists of a silica gel pre-drying column, a potash bubbler stage and a further silica gel drier. The potash bubbler stage consists of two large polythene bottles, each of about 15 litre capacity, connected in series, and each holding 4 litre concentrated solution of potassium hydroxide. The gas stream enters the potash solution through a diffuser which ensures that it is broken up into small bubbles to produce the maximum possible area of gas/liquid interface. In series, the pair of absorbers remove carbon dioxide with an efficiency of approximately 95%. The water produced in the reaction between the carbon dioxide and the alkali is largely carried over as vapour to be absorbed in the final drying columns of the absorption train, after which the gas stream returns to the animal chamber.

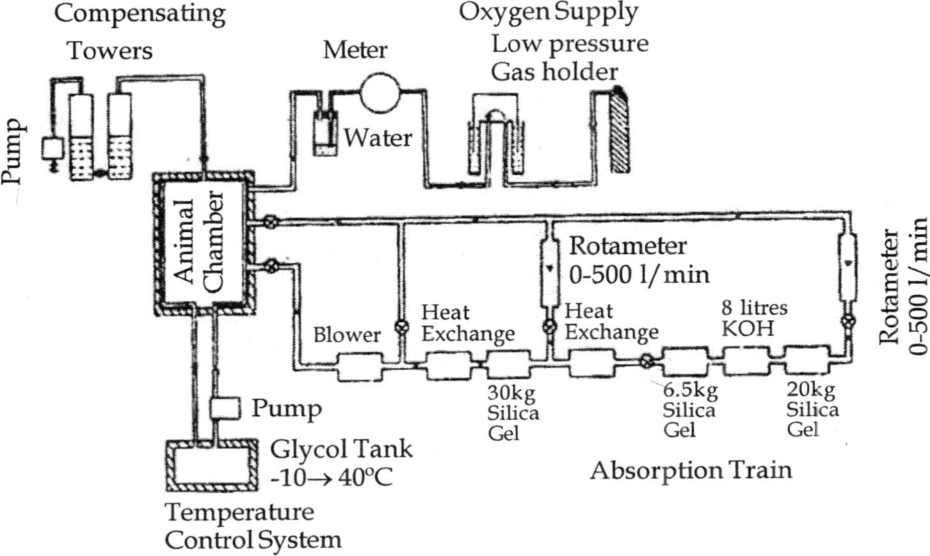

Fig. 3 : Closed circuit respiration chamber.

Oxygen is stored at high pressure in gas cylinders and automatically transferred to a low-pressure water sealed gas holder. When gas pressure in the animal chamber falls below atmospheric it is restored by the ingress of oxygen from the low pressure gas holder, through a small capacity (250 ml rev^{-1}) wet gas meter and a water sealed bubbler demand valve.

Chamber gas is sampled for analysis at the beginning and end of the each period of measurement (usually a nominal 24 hours). The analysis is necessary to estimate methane production from the sheep, which simply accumulates in the system; the analysis is also necessary so that any start/finish alteration in oxygen and carbon dioxide concentration within the chamber may be corrected for in the final calculation of heat production. These latter corrections may amount to about 5% of the primary measurements of oxygen and carbon dioxide. Two points are worth noting in connection with the methane measurements: 1) methane is reversibly adsorbed by silica gel as a function of its concentration - the quantity involved may not be very large, but the phenomenon can give rise to problems in gas analysis if silica gel is used as a drying agent, and in the c1osed- circuit chamber system it does lead to a small systematic under-estimate of methane production; 2) and potentially more serious, the accumulation of methane within the chamber after 24 hours can result in levels of up to 5% - 5.3% is the lower explosive limit for methane in air. Such high levels of methane production are rare from diets used in Western Europe, but may arise more frequently from those used in other parts of the world.

At the beginning and end of each period measurement the individual components of the absorption train are weighed. There are, in all, five absorbent containers involved in the measurement of carbon dioxide production: viz. two potash bottles and the three silica gel columns that form the final drying stage. Each item weighs between 10 kg and 20 kg and can easily be weighed to the nearest 1 gram on an electronic balance of 30 kg capacity.

The wet gas meter used for the measurement of oxygen has a totalizing counter with a resolution of 0.1 litre. The meter is used water-filled (although it could be filled with oil) and it is essential for accurate measurement that the water level be precisely maintained. The best way of achieving the required constancy of water level is to ensure that the gas passing through the meter is saturated with water vapour and that it is at the same temperature as the water in the meter. Saturation is achieved in the low pressure gas holder which is water sealed and presents a large water surface area to the oxygen stored within. Oxygen is delivered to the gas meter through a relatively long length of copper tube which allows for the establishment of thermal equilibrium between the laboratory which houses the gas meter and the oxygen in the gas line.

The animal chamber has a usable size of 1.95 x 0.60 x 1.45m (high), with a total system volume of about 2.4 m^3. The chamber can be maintained to provide environmental temperatures from –10°C to over + 40°C. The experimental animal (usually a sheep) is kept in a modified metabolism crate which can be wheeled into the chamber. Drinking water is continuously available and provision is made to feed, once or twice daily, or continuously from a conveyor belt feeder, without opening the chamber. Lighting is arranged so that diurnal patterns of light and dark can be simulated.

The compensating towers shown in Fig 3 are used to alter the volume, and hence the pressure, of the system to compensate for changes in barometric pressure during the period of measurement when the chamber is hermetically sealed from the atmosphere. This feature is necessary in that, unless the animal chamber is of very heavy construction, it is liable to deform significantly in the face of varying barometric pressure opposing constant internal pressure. For example, a closed circuit chamber with a roof area of 2 x 1m would experience a loading, on that face alone, of over 500 kg for a change of atmospheric pressure of 2.5 kPa. Such a change in atmospheric pressure can occasionally occur within a 24 hour period, and would readily buckle a chamber built of 3 mm. thick steel sheet. The compensating towers are each 0.20m internal diameter and 2.40 m tall. At the beginning of each period of measurement the water levels are equilibrated (each tower half filled), and the valve on the interconnecting pipe at the bottom of the towers is closed. If the barometric pressure rises during the course of the period of measurement, a differential pressure is imposed upon the chamber: this is counteracted by transferring water into the tower connected to the chamber thus reducing the volume and increasing the pressure in the sealed system. Should barometric pressure fall during a period of measurement the differential pressure is of the opposite sign and is counterbalanced by transferring water out of the tower connected to the chamber. The transfer of water between the towers is affected by opening the valve on the interconnecting pipe and altering the pressure in the air space above the water in the tower not connected to the chamber. The tower connected to the chamber is fitted with a full-height sight glass which is graduated to show the amounts of' water that must be transferred, in either direction, to counterbalance each 100 Pa change in barometric pressure.

Closed circuit chambers of this type have accuracy as an over whelming advantage in their favour; they are capable of affording a higher degree of precision than can be obtained from other indirect calorimetric systems although this margin of superiority is being eroded by improvements in the physical instruments used in the other systems. The error, in terms of purely physico-chemical measurement, in a closed circuit chamber can be as low as

± 1%. Over and above the physico-chemical, or 'machine' error, which is associated with any type of instrument there is the biological variability introduced by the experiment animal. The drawback of the closed -circuit apparatus is its high running cost in terms of labour, reagents and energy, although the capital cost is relatively low. Closed-circuit instruments cannot provide a minute-by minute dynamic picture of the animals metabolic rate, but this is not necessarily a disadvantage: for example, in the work of nutritional rather than physiological nature the 24 hour total heat production may of tell be all the information that is required. Calculation of results from dclsed-circuit measurements is not onerous - it is certainly well within the capabilities of logarithms, slide rule or pocket calculator.

2. The Confinement Chamber System

In its simplest form the confinement chamber may be pictured as a closed-circuit chamber without its absorption train. The animal chamber is sealed from the atmosphere and a "start" gas sample is taken for analysis, and then, after a period of time in which carbon dioxide and methane concentrations increase and that of oxygen is reduced, an "end" sample of chamber gas is collected and the chamber opened to atmosphere, ready to begin a new measurement. The duration of the period of measurement is obviously a function of the volume of the chamber, the animal's heat production, and its ability to tolerate elevated levels of carbon dioxide without distress or alteration of its metabolic rate. The first physiological effect of increasing carbon dioxide concentration in the inspired air is an increased respiration rate, which in most animals occurs at about 2 to 2.5% carbon dioxide in the inspired air. At that level of carbon dioxide the increased respiration rate gives rise to no detectable increase in metabolic rate because the incremental demand of the respiratory musculature represents only a very small proportion of the total. None-the-less most workers have come down upon the side of caution and decided that 2.0% carbon dioxide shall be their upper working limit. A rough calculation will show that a sheep with a metabolic rate of 6000kJ d^{-1} confined in a chamber of 2, capacity will reach 1.0% carbon dioxide concentration in about 2 hours, or that a cow with a daily energy expenditure of 60MJ in a 15 m^3 chamber would reach that level of carbon dioxide in less than 1 hour. It appears that with practical sized confinement chambers the measurements are unlikely to exceed 2 to. 3 hours duration; this may be considered to be an unduly short period. The solution is to make a series of successive measurements, which may be controlled manually or automatically. Once the apparatus is used with a number of cycles of operation the confinement chamber can perhaps be better pictured as a "Stopped-flow" open-circuit system in which the animal chamber is the device for the measurement of gas volumes. Such an automated confinement chamber has been described (Blaxter et al., 1972) and Fig. 8.4 shows diagramatically the principles involved in its operation.

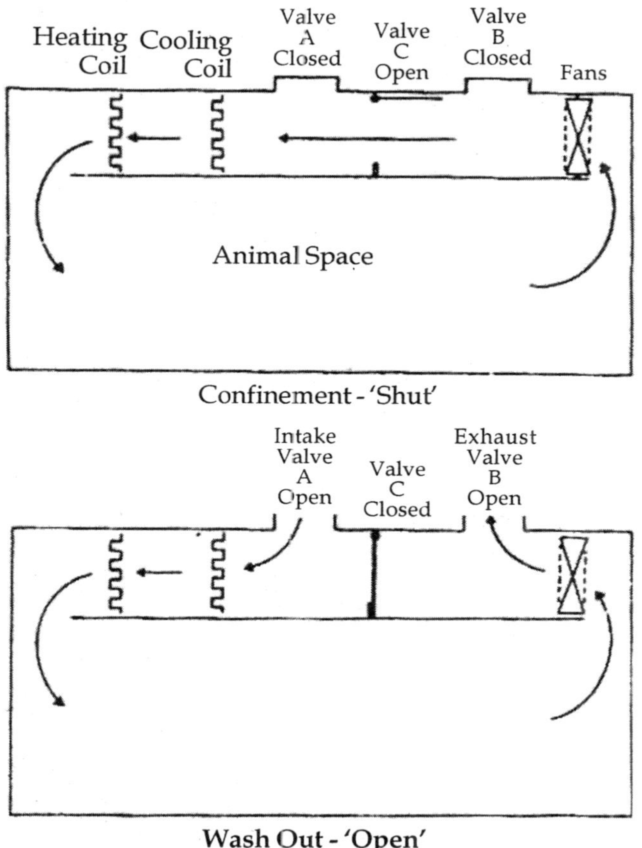

Fig. 4 : Automated confinement chamber.

During the measurement phase of the cycle of operation (confinement - "shut" in Fig. 4) the intake and exhaust valves (A and B) are closed while an internal valve (C) is open and the air within the chamber is circulated through the animal space and through a duct which contains the valves and air conditioning heat exchangers. These latter units first cool the air to condense out the water vapour produced by the animal and then re-heat it to the chamber operating temperature. At the end of the measuring phase valves A and B are automatically opened and valve C closed: The air circulation during this washout or "open" phase is inward through valve A, through the air conditioning units, through the animal space and exhausted through valve B. In this "open" phase the vitiated air accumulated during the "shut" phase is washed out, to be replaced by fresh air. Because of the presence of the respiring animal in the chamber this wash out can never be complete, but, for all practical purposes, four volumetric air changes are sufficient to produce virtually atmospheric concentrations within the chamber. This condition is achieved in 3 to 4 minutes "open" phase. The duration of the "shut" phase is minimally 30 minutes, but this can be extended to several hours if necessary when an animal of small body size and hence low absolute metabolic rate is in the chamber.

At the Rowett Research Institute two identical chambers of this type were built. Their operational cycles are run 180° out-of-phase to one another: as samples for gas analysis are required only immediately after and immediately before the "shut" phase starts and finishes, running the chambers out-of-phase allows a single set of gas analyzers to serve both chambers. Control of the operation of the chambers can be by electro-mechanical or electronic programmer or by computer. Calculation of results is not difficult, but with operational cycles of less than I hour (as is almost invariably the case with cattle) it is very tedious, and is well suited to handling by computer. Indeed, apart from the labour requirement for animal care, the total operation of these chambers in terms of control, data acquisition and calculation of results is all performed by computer.

As well as the actual animal chamber (or chambers) and the associated air conditioning equipment, a confinement system requires gas analyzers for oxygen, carbon dioxide and perhaps methane, wet and dry bulb temperature sensors, and a barometric pressure transducer. A major capital cost in any system is that of the gas analyzers: this cost can be shared between two chambers, as described above, and there is no reason why it could not be spread over four or possibly even six of them. Another major capital item is the data acquisition/recording system. It would be possible to use a multi-channel potentiometric recorder, but the extraction of the data and subsequent calculation would be very demanding of the time of a skilled technician. An intermediate stage between direct "on-line" computer recording and processing is to use some form of data logger, recording neither punched paper tape or magnetically, for subsequent processing by computer.

Confinement chambers are not as accurate as closed-circuit respiration chambers, but are capable of operating (as a physico-chemical measuring instrument) with a coefficient of variation of 1.5% to 2%.

3. Open-Circuit Respiration Chamber

Open-circuit systems are conceptually simpler than either closed circuit or confinement systems: they consist (Fig. 5) of some form of enclosure for the animal through which an airstream is drawn at a measured rate and from which a gas sample is extracted for analysis. Inevitably the practical realisation of this concept is somewhat more complicated and indeed some open-circuit systems are technologically very sophisticated (Cammell et al., 1981), but a ventilated hood system for short-term measurements can be quite simple (Brockway and McEwan, 1969), as shown in Fig. 6. The essential information that must be recorded is the same in a simple hood system as it is in the apparently more complex chamber-based apparatus.

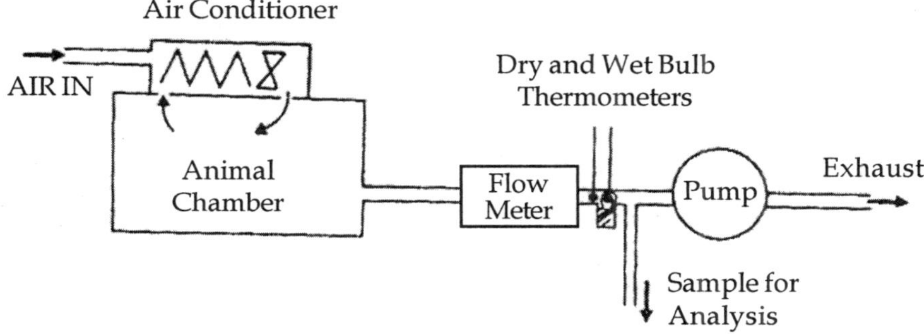

Fig. 5 : Open circuit Respiration Chamber

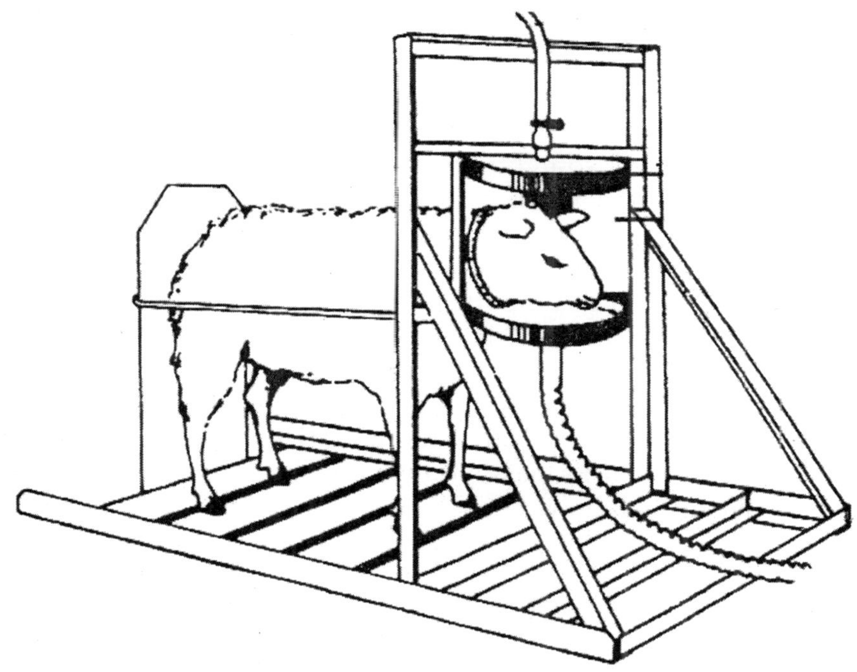

Fig. 6 : Ventilated hood

When it becomes necessary to make measurements over a period of longer than, say, 8 hours it is usually more convenient to use a respiratory chamber, which, with large animals at least, almost invariably requires some form of air conditioning, either of the incoming air, or as a recirculatory unit for the chamber air, or as shown in Fig 5. as a combination of both.

It is usual, in an open circuit system, to place the ventilation pump at the end of the circuit so that the whole system is operated under negative pressure. Any leakage is then of atmospheric air into the system and merely represents a small part of the total inlet air flow. It is essential, however, that no leak occurs between the point at which flow rate is measured and the gas analyzers. If the system were to be operated under positive pressure any outward leakage of gas would represent a loss of some of the expired air from the animal, and lead to an underestimate of heat production.

If the inlet air supply is of uncontaminated atmospheric air its composition can be assumed, but if there is any risk of contamination it is essential to measure the differences between inlet and outlet air. The other measurements that must be made are of cumulative air flow and the wet and dry bulb temperatures of the air at the flowmeter, and the absolute pressure at the outlet of the flowmeter, so that the recorded air flow can be reduced to s.t.p. Considerable savings can be made on the capital costs of gas analyzers if the simplified "Open circuit" equations (9) and (10), described previously, are used.

At their best open-circuit systems are capable of "machine" accuracies of better than ±2% coefficient of variation. The calculation of energy expenditure by this technique is very straightforward if the sample gas is collected into a suitable receiver over the whole period of the measurement, so presenting a single integrated value for gas concentration applicable to the single, cumulative value for flow. If, for any reason there is a requirement for open-circuit calculation of results other than by the simple equations (9) and (10) it is necessary to derive inlet flow rate as a parameter in the further stages of the calculation; unless the respiratory quotient is known to be 1.00, the inlet flow rate will differ from the measured outlet flow. Inlet flow is calculated from outlet flow on the assumption that the **quantity** (not concentration) or of nitrogen is unaltered in its passage through the open-circuit system. The calculation is made as follows:

Concentration of nitrogen in outlet stream =

1.00 - (conc. O_2 + conc. CO_2 + CH_4) = cNo

Volume of nitrogen leaving system = cNo x outflow s.t.p.=N

= volume of nitrogen entering system

Concentration of nitrogen in inlet air stream = 1.00 -(conc. O_2 + conc. CO_2) = cNi

Volume of nitrogen entering system = N = cNi x in-flow s.t.p.

In-flow s.t.p. = N/c Ni, or = cNo/cNi x outflow s.t.p.

The ventilated hood such as that shown in Fig. 8 may be further reduced in size to the extent that it becomes a simple oro-nasal mask. If it is considered advantageous to reduce to a mask of this type there is probably little or no benefit in ventilating the mask: instead, if the mask is fitted with separate inlet and outlet air valves the animal's own respiration is adequate to drive the system. In such a case it may be worth while to provide additional power to collect the sample of gas for analysis but this is by no means essential; respiratory gas meters have been built, primarily for use with human subjects, which utilize the movements of the components of a dry gas meter to drive a gas sample pump. A meter of this type was used for sheep (Young and Webster, 1963), in a technique where the reduction in size of the mask was carried to the extreme of incorporating the inlet/outlet valve assembly into a tracheal cannula. It is claimed that this approach allows the animal to graze normally while measurements of energy expenditure are being made, but it seems unlikely that there is much normality associated with the animal's respiratory heat exchange mechanisms under these circumstances, as the upper respiratory tract, especially the nasal cavity, serves as an important heat exchange system between inspired and expired air.

E. Gas Analysis

1. Chemical Methods

Before the introduction of gas analyzers working on physical principles, some 30-40 years ago, the only methods for gas analysis were chemically based absorption/volumetric techniques. These methods were capable of high degrees of precision but were time consuming and required the work of high skilled technicians if their potential accuracy was to be achieved. The various types of apparatus were known under the names of their originators, such as Haldane or Scholander.

The Haldane apparatus was probably the most commonly used chemical method for respiratory gas analysis (Consolazio et al., 1951). A number of variations of the original Haldane apparatus have been described, the most radical of which was the so-called Lloyd-Haldane apparatus in which the glassware was made much more compact and more easy to use, albeit at the expense of a relatively complicated multi-way glass stopcock (Lloyd, 1958). In most types of Haldane apparatus the burette had a capacity of 10 ml, although some analyzers were made with 20 ml burettes, for which an extremely high degree of precision was claimed. Carbon dioxide was absorbed in potassium hydroxide solution, while oxygen was absorbed in pyrogallol, sodium antraquinine beta sulphonate or chromous chloride. Calculation of carbon dioxide and oxygen concentrations in the sample is a straight forward expression of the volumes of these gases which were absorbed as percentages of the volume of the initial sample.

Methane can be analysed on a Haldane apparatus modified to incorporate a combustion chamber into which the remaining gas sample can be introduced, after the absorption of carbon dioxide and oxygen. In the combustion chamber the residual gas sample is mixed with an excess of air and the mixture is ignited electrically converting the methane to carbon dioxide. The carbon dioxide thus formed is analysed by a further absorption in the potassium hydroxide solution.

The scholander analyzer relies upon the same basic principles as does the Haldane, but it is a much small piece of equipment. The Scholander apparatus only requires 0.5 ml gas sample, and instead of the conventional glass burette a micrometer piston is used as the volume measuring element in this apparatus.

2. Physical Methods

Gas analyzers operating on physical principles are now common place: their capital cost is high in relation to chemical apparatus, but they do not require skilled personnel to operate them, although in the event of electronic breakdown skilled attention certainly will be required. The other advantage of physical gas analyzers is that they are generally ideally suited to, continuous or "on-line" operation.

The principles underlying physical gas analyzers are varied: thermal conductivity, paramagnestism, infra-red absorption and mass spectrometry have all been used in the analysis of the various respiratory gases. At the present time it is probable that the majority of gas analyzers for carbon dioxide and for methane are infra-red absorption instruments, and the majority of oxygen analyzers are paramagnetically based.

All gases with heteroatomic molecules (e.g. CO_2, CH_4) display absorption associated with specific vibration-rotation bands in the infrared wavelengths between approximately 2 and 15 μm. Analyzers which detect such absorption fall into two categories depending on whether they use one or two optical pathways. The earlier, and still the most sensitive, analyzers are of the so-called "Luft" pattern (see Fig. 7) and employ two beams of infra-red radiation. The two beams originating from a single source are chopped by a shutter rotating at about 6 Hz and then, with identical initial energies, pass through reference and sample cells, and thence to the detector. The detector takes the form of an electrical capacitor, and is filled with the gas which the analyzer is intended to measure. The plates of this capacitor consist of one which is perforated but rigid and one which is a continuous, but flexible diaphragm. The reference cell is a sealed unit containing none of the gas to be analysed: when the sample cell is also free of that gas the energy content of both beams of radiation remains identical when the beams impinge upon the detector. As radiation is absorbed by the gas molecules within the detector, the extent of the heating, and hence the increase in pressure, will be symmetrical on either side of the diaphragm of the capacitor thus there will be no change in the output signal to the instrument's amplifier. However, if the sample cell contains some of the gas to be analysed, energy will be absorbed in that cell, so less will reach the detector. This leads to unequal heating of the gas within the detector, and hence to unequal pressure across the diaphragm, which will deflect, altering the capacitance and signal to the amplifier.

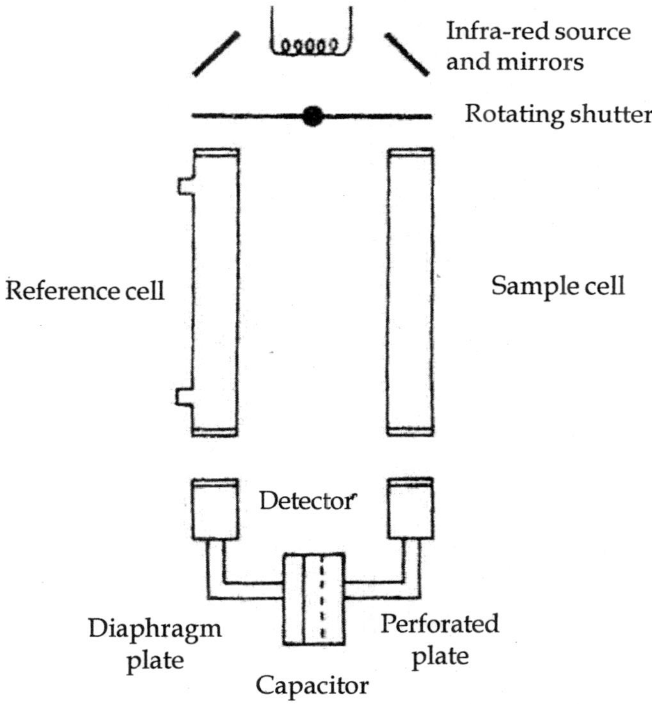

Fig. 7 : "Luft" Infra-red analyzer.

In single beam infra-red absorption analyzers optical filters modulate the beam of radiation emitted by the source, to produce a beam of, radiation of a wavelength specifically absorbed by the gas being analyzed. The detector used in this type of analyzer is a solid-state device: which directly transduces infra-red radiation into electrical energy. If various types of optical filter are mounted in a disc which rotates to change' the wavelength of the single beam of radiation the analyzer can be made to regulate its own "zero" baseline, or to allow it to be used to analyse more than one gas at a time.

The output from infra-red analyzers is essentially non-linear with concentration, but it can be linearized electronically. Analyzers with full-scale ranges as low as 0-0.1% for methane and 0-1.0% for carbon dioxide are readily available from several manufacturers. Such instruments are well suited for use in open-circuit or confinement chamber systems.

Among the gases encountered in the measurement of respiratory exchange oxygen is alone in the possession of paramagnetic properties; the other gases are all diamagnetic. The molecules of a paramagnetic gas are attracted into a magnetic field whereas those of a diamagnetic gas tend to be repelled from such a field. Use is made of the paramagnetic properties of oxygen in two types of analyzers. The more common versions are of the Pauling, or magnetodynamic type in which the analysis cell consists of a diamagnetic glass dumb-bell suspended horizontally in a strong non-uniform permanent magnetic field (Fig. 8). When a change takes place in the oxygen concentration within the analysis cell oxygen molecules *move into* or out of the magnetic field, thereby tending to displace the dumb-bell test-piece. The (horizontal) angular position of the dumb-bell is sensed optically, and any deviation from its set position is restored by an alteration of the current in the feedback coil. This current drives an electromagnetic field to oppose the forces displacing the dumb-bell. The strength of the feed-back current is a measure of the oxygen concentration of the gas in the analysis cell: this current is used to drive a local indicating meter or to provide an analogue output to some form of data logging equipment.

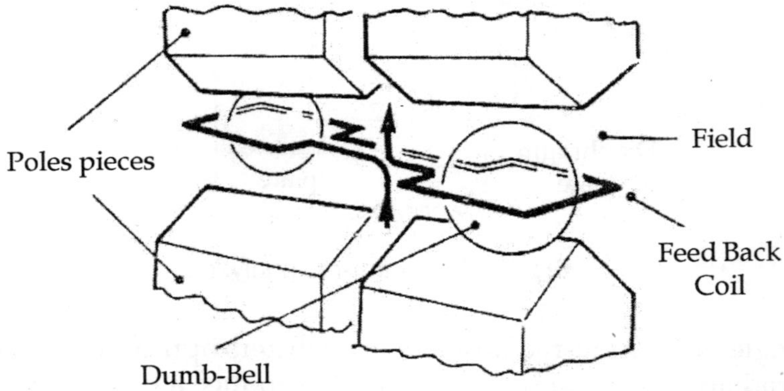

Fig. 8 : Paramagnetic oxygen analysis cell

The other version of the paramagnetic oxygen analyzer is the so-called "magnetic wind" type in which a combination of paramagnetism and thermal conductivity is used to separate and detect the oxygen present in the sample gas.

Oxygen analyzers covering the range 20-21% oxygen (which is complimentary to 0.0-1.0% for carbon dioxide) are available from a number of commercial sources. These instruments are, in reality, 0-21% analyzers with a heavily suppressed zero i.e. a stabilized electrical voltage equivalent to 0-20% oxygen is subtracted from the analyzers output signal. Although the meter is scaled in percentage oxygen the analyzer, in fact, measures the partial pressure of oxygen within the cell. Partial pressure of oxygen (pO_2) is the product of absolute pressure and fractional concentration. The suppressed zero on the oxygen analyzer renders it very sensitive to changes in absolute pressure when gas of constant oxygen content is being analyzed. Table 3 shows that a change in 4kPa in barometric pressure leads to change in pO_2 of atmospheric oxygen which is approximately the same as the change in pO_2 due to an 0.8% change in oxygen concentration at constant barometric pressure. A comparable analysis for pCO_2 world reveals that changes in absolute pressure have only very small effects compared to changes in concentration in the 0-1.0% range.

Table 3 : Effect of concentration and absolute pressure on pO_2

Oxygen concentration Barometer, kPa	0.2095 pO_2, kPa	Barometric pressure Oxygen concentration	101 kPa pO_2, kPa
101	21.1595	0.2095	21.1595
97	20.3215	0.2015	20.3515
Δ 4 kPa	Δ 0.838 kPa	Δ 0.0080	Δ 0.808 kPa

3. Estimation of Methane

The overall contribution of the methane loss to the energy balance of ruminant animal is relatively small. The Brouwer equation (no.7) shows that 1 litre of oxygen consumed makes approximately eight times more contribution to heat production than does 1 litre of methane produced, and on normal diets the volume of methane produced is only about one tenth of that of oxygen consumed, although on some types of feed methane production may be considerably greater.

In the assessment of the metabolizable energy values of diets (see Fig. 8) knowledge of methane production is necessary, but it is expensively obtained if respiration chambers must be built solely for that measurement. So various workers have tried to derive equations to predict methane production from characteristics of the diet. In what is probably the best known of these (Blaxter and Clappekton, 1965) methane production is expressed in terms of the gross energy, digestibility and feeding level of the diet:

$$CH_4 = 1.30 + 0.1120 + L (2.37 - 0.0500)$$

Where CH_4 is the methane energy loss expressed as kJ/I00 KJ gross energy intake, D is digestibility, expressed as kJ/100 kJ gross energy intake, and L is feeding level expressed as multiples of maintenance energy intake. It must be remembered that this empirical relationship describes methane production from ruminant animals fed upon materials commonly available in Western Europe: its applicability to feedstuffs from other parts of the world cannot be taken for granted.

F. Measurement of Gas Flow Rate

It is necessary to measure gas flow rates in virtually every type of system for indirect calorimetry, with the exception of the confinement chamber. When working with small animals such as rats or chickens the flow rates may be in the order of 1 1 min^{-1} or even less; with cattle they may be as high as 500 1 min^{-1}. A wide range of instruments is available, each with its own advantages and disadvantages.

I. Variable Area Flowmeter

Simplest of all flow rate instruments in the "Rotameter"- type variable area flowmeter, in which the gas flow carries a conical float up a vertical tube, usually made of glass or plastic, whose cross sectional area increases slightly with the height of the tube. These instruments are relatively inexpensive, and only provide a reading of instantaneous flow rate. At considerable extra cost they are available with automatic photo-electric scanning for float pcsition in the tube which allows for remote reading, recording and totalization of flow. Variable area flowmeters usually cover a ten-fold range of flow rate (e.g. 10-100 1 min^{-1} or 50-500 1 min^{-1}). They are generally considered to be rather inaccurate, although if all precautions are taken and, all necessary corrections applied, their usable accuracy can be upgraded appreciably.

2. Dry Gas Meter

This is the common type of gas meter used to measure supplies of domestic or industrial fuel gas, and is comparatively inexpensive. Care must be taken in use to avoid condensation of water inside the meter which is usually vulnerable to corrosion. Dry gas meters are available in a wide range of capacities and care should be taken to match meter capacity to flow rate: dry gas meters may become very inaccurate if used outside their stated range. Dry gas meters have been used in open circuit chamber systems, but they are generally considered to be insufficiently accurate for that type of work.

3. Wet Gas Meter

Wet gas meters are capable of high degrees of accuracy, provided that their upper rated flow limits are not exceeded and that the water level in the meter is accurately set, and maintained, at the datum mark. The latter constraint means that in many cases some degree of air conditioning will be needed before the gas is fed to the meter. Wet gas meters are very expensive and large capacity meters are not readily available.

In the past several laboratories constructed their own meters for use in open circuit systems for cattle, where the high required flow rate (ca 500 I min^{-1}) made it impossible to find a commercially manufactured meter. These home-made meters were generally the "mercury pump" pattern; they consist of large slow-moving pistons made gas tight with mercury seals, and they operated both as gas metering and pumping devices. The present-day large animal calorimetrician is more fortunate in that there are at least four types of instrument that can measure these high flow rates with sufficient accuracy. These are the turbine, the pressure drop, the vortex shedding and the mass flow meters.

4. Pressure Drop Flow Meter

These instruments are available in a variety of configurations, but essentially they consist of a system that measures the loss in pressure head as the gas flows past an obstruction. The obstruction may take the form of an orifice plate, a sintered or wire mesh resistance plate, or merely a narrowing (a "throat") in the pipework. The measurement of the pressure drop can be done by a variety of means ranging from a simple liquid filled manometer up to highly sophisticated electronic strain gauge or capacitance manometers. The aerodynamic behaviour of this type of flowmeter is well documented and accounts of its use and limitations may be found in standard textbooks (Ower and Pankhurst, 1966). Pressure drop flowmeters are available commercially from a number of sources they are moderately expensive but when used correctly are quite accurate enough for use in open-circuit systems.

5. Vortex Shedding Flowmeter

The vortex shedding flowmeter makes use of the phenomenon of the generation of vortices from alternate sides of the trailing edge of an obstruction to fluid flow. In practice the obstruction consists of a narrow strut mounted diametrically across a section of pipe; the vortices are detected as a modulation of the frequency of an ultrasonic beam transmitted across the pipe a short distance downstream of the strut.

Although primarily measuring linear velocity' of flow in the pipe the vortex shedding flowmeter can be obtained with a volumetric calibration. This type of flowmeter is moderately expensive, has a stable and virtually linear calibration, offers very low resistance to flow and has no moving parts. Any particular instrument covers a two-hundred-fold range of flow rates and its stability of calibration and its accuracy make it a very suitable instrument for use in open-circuit systems.

6. Mass Flowmeter

This type of instrument, more rigorously called the thermal mass flowmeter, has as its sensor element temperature detectors up and downstream of an electric heater. At zero gas flow the responses of the symmetrically placed detectors are equal, but when flow is established the downstream detector will register a higher temperature. The difference between the two temperatures is a function of the mass flow of gas past the detectors. It is the mass of gas which is measured so the flowmeter is virtually independent of the temperature or pressure of the gas flowing through. However separate calibrations must be established for gases or gas mixtures of significantly differing thermal conductivities and specific heats, although this is not a problem for open circuit indirect calorimetry; the exhaust gas from the animal chamber is sufficiently similar to air (at the same water vapour content) as regards their thermal conductivities. Over the range of flow rates required for animals of agricultural importance the mass flowmeter transducer is mounted on a by-pass tube connected to the main gas flow line. This is because the transducer itself can only deal with relatively small flow rates: no difficulty arises from this arrangement so long as the transducer and the main flow lines are kept scrupulously clean and free of any water droplets. Failure to maintain cleanliness may result in a perturbation of the ratio of flows between the transducer by-pass and the main flow pipe.

The mass flowmeter offers low resistance to flow, and the instruments calibration is highly stable and it is very accurate; it is, however, rather expensive compared to other types of flowmeter.

G. Calibrationof Calorimetric Systems

I. Direct Calorimeters

The most satisfactory way to calibrate a direct calorimeter is to generate heat electrically within the chamber. The amount of heat generated can be measured to a high degree of accuracy with a high grade wattmeter, and provided that cable of generous cross-sectional area is used, certainty is assured that all the power dissipation registered by the wattmeter is taking place inside the chamber. Depending on the nature of the heating element used nearly all the heat can be produced as, say, radiation from a high temperature source such as an electric bulb, as convection from an open-spaced resistance winding run at a temperaure well below red-heat, as conduction from an element closely applied to a surface of the chamber and well insulated on its other faces, or as evaporation from an open trough of water containing an immersion heater.

Direct calorimeters can also be calibrated by burning pure fuels such as alcohol or butane, but this method suffers from the drawback of incomplete combustion of the fuel. A small, but significant, amount of fuel escapes combustion either totally or is only partly oxidised. Most workers with experience in this method of calibration would agree that it is fairly easy to achieve 97 to 98% combustion, and very difficult to do much better.

2. Indirect Calorimeters

The calibration of apparatus for indirect calorimetry is a more complex and technically demanding task than is the case for direct calorimeters. In indirect systems the flow meter, the gas analyzers and minor items such as temperature, humidity and pressure sensors may all require separate calibration, as well as ideally, an overall calibration as an intact working system.

Flow meters can be calibrated either against a high quality wet gas meter of known accuracy, or possibly against a mass flowmeter, or they may be calibrated using weighed cylinders of compressed air. The latter process is fairly straight forward: for flow rates up to about 200 I min^{-1} one cylinder is adequate, but above that flow it is desirable to use two cylinders in parallel. For example, a cylinder containing 3,500 I air (s.t.p.), i.e. approximately 4.5. kg air, might weigh 38 kg when full; such a cylinder can be weighed to the nearest gram on a digital balance of 60 kg capacity which affords a comfortable degree of accuracy. Compressed air normally quite a low vapour content but it would be a wise precaution to check this; alternatively, compressed nitrogen could be used, which from the nature of its production will certainly have very low water vapour content.

The simplest method of calibrating a gas analyzer is to use two gas mixtures whose overall compositions approximate to those in normal use. One of these mixtures, "zero gas", is usually dry atmospheric air taken from outdoors at a point where it is free from contamination. Such air is of constant composition and presents no problems. The second gas mixture, "span" gas, should be such that it produces approximately 80% full scale deflection on the analyzer. This gas may be purchased from a commercial source, or it can be mixed on site using gas mixing pumps or blenders. In either case it is necessary to know the composition of the span gas mixture with sufficient accuracy for the purpose in hand. For closed circuit and non-ventilated hood systems there is no problem in that chemical volumetric analysis, e.g. on the Haldane apparatus can be used, but for open circuit systems the necessary accuracy can only be obtained with considerable difficulty. None-the-less, gas mixtures are very useful for checking the day-to-day stability of calibration of an analyzer: for that purpose the exact compositipn of the gas mixtures is of less importance than the stability of that composition.

Paramagnetic oxygen analyzers can be calibrated by reducing (the absolute pressure of atmaspheric air within the analysis cell. For example a reduction in the air pressure within the cell from 101 to 98 kPa brings about a reduction of 0.629.5 kPa in the partial pressure of oxygen, which is equivalent to a reduction of 0.62% in the concentration of oxygen at a constant barometric pressure of 101 kPa. Unfortunately a comparable approach cannot be employed far calibratian of the carbon dioxide to a level equivalent to say 0.75% would require the application of pressure well in excess of those which the analyzer could tolerate. For example, to increase pCO_2 in atmaspheric air by 760 Pa (equivalent to a change of 0.75% carban dioxide at Constant pressure) it is necessary to increase the absolute pressure to 26 atmospheres.

Gas analyzers can be calibrated by a gravimetric gas dilution technique (Brockway et al., 1971). In essence, this method cansists of the injection of a pure gas into an airstream at such a rate as to produce the required final concentratian of that gas. For example, if air flows through an open circuit system at an exhaust flow rate of 100 1 min^{-1}, pure carbon dioxide injected at a rate of 750 ml min^{-1} would increase carbon dioxide concentration from 0.03% to. 0.78%. To calibrate the oxygen analyzer in the open circuit system it is necessary to reduce the oxygen concentration below its atmospheric level. This can be achieved by the injection of nitrogen into the system; in this context nitrogen can be thought of as "negative oxygen". If nitrogen is added at 3.58 1 min^{-1} to the air stream, and the exhaust flow rate maintained at 100 I min^{-1}, the resultant oxygen concentratian will be 20.20% - a reduction of 0.75%. It is not possible to control volumetrically the injection rates with sufficient accuracy, but the exact amount injected can be determined gravimetrically. For example, the small cylinders often used on anesthetic machines weight less than 3 kg, and can be weighed to. 0.1 g on a suitable electronic balance. Cylinders of this size can hold enough gas to enable the calibratian process to last for 10-20 minutes.

Strictly speaking, the gravimetric calibratian procedure refers to the entire system of barometric pressure, temperature, humidity, flow rate and gas analyzer, but if the calibratian of all other instruments is already known, and appropriate correction applied in the calculation, the process can be used to calibrate the analyzer by itself.

References

Blaxter, K.L. Brockway, J.M. and Boyne, A.W. (1972). *Quart J Expl Physiol*, 57: 60-72.

Blaxter, K.L. and Clapperton, J.L. (1965). *Brit J Nut*, 19: 511-522.

Brockway, J.M., Boyne, A.W. and Gordon, J.G. (1971). *J Applied Physiol*, 31: 296-297.

Brockway, J.M. and McEwan, E.H. (1969). *Lab Practice*: 18, 552-559.

Brouwer, E. (1958). On simple formulae for calculating the heat expenditure and the quantities of carbohydrate and fat metabolized in ruminants, from data on gaseous exchange and urine-No. 1st Symposium on Energy Metabolism. Publication of European Aassociation for Animal Production, no. 8, p. 182.

Cammell, S.B., Beever, D.E., Skelton, K.V. and Spooner, M.G. (1981). *Lab Practice*, 30: 115-119.

Consolazlo, C.R. Johnson, R.E. and Marek, E. (1951). Metabolic methods. Clinical procedures in the study of metabolic functions. Henry Kimpton, London.

Llyod, B.B. 1956. Physiolo., London, 143: 5P

Mclean, J.A. (1972). *Brit J Nut*, 27: 597-600.

Mount, L.E., Holrres, C.W. Start, I.B. and Legge A.J. (1967). *J Agric Sci*, (Cambridge), 68: 47-55.

Ower, E. and Pankhurst, R.C. (1956). The Measurement of Air flow. Pergamon Press, Oxford.

Puller, J.D. (1958). Direct calorimetry of animals by the gradient layer principle. 1st Symposium on Energy Metabolism. Publication .of European Association for Animal Production, no. 8, p.95.

Wainman, F.W. and Blaxter, K.L. (1958). Developments in the design of closed-circuit respiration apparatus for animals weighing up to 70 kg 1st Symposium on Energy Metabolism. Publication of European Association for Animal Production, no. 8, p.85.

Young, B.A. and Webster, M.E.D. (1963). *Aust Agric Res*. 14: 867-873.

□□□

Animal Nutrition, 2012
eds. Dr. (Mrs.) Usha R. Mehra et al., pp. 111-134
Satish Serial Publishing House e-mail : info@satishserial.com; website : www.satishserial.com

Feeding and Nutrient Requirements of Ruminants

D.V. REDDY

A nutrient is one that aids in support of animal life. We know that the animal requires different nutrients. The metabolic changes they undergo in serving the body's various functions are also known to us. Knowledge of the quantitative needs of the body for these nutrients and of the relative value of feeds as sources of them is the basis of scientific feeding. Nutrient requirements are defined as the amounts which must be supplied in the ration to meet the needs of the normal healthy animal.

When we think of nutrient requirements, energy requirement first comes to mind because, energy supplies the driving force necessary for the maintenance of life, growth, lactation and work. However, consideration must be made also for similar requirement for protein, minerals and vitamins.

Evolution of Nutrient Requirements from Crude Biological Assays

Energy Evaluation

Crude Biological Assays

The earliest work on the nutrient requirements of ruminants was based on the practical observations in terms of crude biological assays as reported in 1810 by Albrecht Thaer in which both feed values and feed requirements were expressed in terms of 'hay'. Later in the year1884 Professor Fjord in Scandinavia came out 'barley' as the standard, where animal needs were expressed as feed units and one feed unit being equivalent to 1 kg barley. A still later version of the biological assay principle was the attempt of Max Kleiber and coworkers in 1941, who expressed nutrient needs and feed values in terms of glucose/casein equivalents.

Digestible Nutrients

In the early 19th century attempts were made to place these assays on a chemical basis. Towards this the next step in assessing nutrient requirements was taken at Weende (Gottingen) in Germany by Wilhelm Henneberg and Friedrich Stohmann in 1860s. They devised the analytical scheme for feeds and conducted numerous digestion trials. Thus, digested proximate principles came with Woolff in 1874 and later Lehmann assumed the responsibility for their continuation in 1898 as Woolff-Lehmann standard. These standards expressed as total digestible nutrients (TDN) formed the basis of Haecker's standards in the USA. They were incorporated in the standard text book published first in 1898 by W.A.Henry and then by F.B.Morrison from 1947 and TDN system was the basis of the energy requirements employed by the National Research Council (NRC) of the USA.

Net Energy (NE) Principle

A major advance was then made at Mockern in Germany by G.Kuhn in 1894 and his successor O.Kellner in 1908 and also by H.P.Armsby in 1917 at Pennsylvania State College, USA. At both the centres attempts were made to measure by calorimetry the change in energy retention following changes in diet intake. Kuhn and Kellner gave 'pure nutrients' as additions to a basal diet and measured the increase in retention. Kellner devised his feeding system, the Starch Equivalent system, by expressing values of feeds and requirements relative to the energy of starch. Armsby's experiments were mostly conducted at lower intakes of feed than Kellner's, but his conclusions were much the same. Neither Armsby nor Kellner measured the fasting metabolism.

The completeness of the net energy scheme, coupled perhaps with the cost of calorimetric work, probably inhibited progress in the next 30 years.

The work done by Armsby's successor, E.B.Forbes revealed the shortcomings of net energy scheme. By 1933, Forbes showed that the net energy of feeds varied, and the more practical studies conducted later showed that the net energy system did not work in practice.

Metabolizable Energy (ME) System

The findings of J.Barcroft and coworkers in 1944 about the significance of steam volatile fatty acids in ruminant metabolism and the increasing dissatisfaction with Kellner system led new research at Hannah Institute, UK in the 1950s. Sir Kenneth Blaxter and his coworkers undertook calorimetric work which led to the metabolizable energy system, which was adopted by the Agricultural Research Council (ARC, 1965; ARC, 1980; ARC, 1984).

Net Energy System

Net energy is most scientifically sound for expressing energy requirements and energy value of feeds. The NE value of a feed depends on whether it is used for maintenance, fattening, growth or milk production. Metabolizable energy is used with different degrees of efficiency for maintenance and body gain in non-lactating animals but is used with similar degrees of efficiency for maintenance and milk production in lactating animals. For this reason NRC (for Dairy cattle) tables (1989) gave three NE values for feeds: NE_m, NE_{gain} and $NE_{lactation}$. NE_m is the value of feeds for the maintenance of non-lactating animals (dry animals). NE_g is the NE value of feeds for the deposition of body tissue in growing males and females and mature bulls. $NE_m + NE_g$ = Total energy needs of growing cattle. In lactating animals, the NE value of feeds as well as requirements for all physiological functions is described in terms of single value as NE milk (NE_l), since energy is used with similar degrees of efficiency for maintenance and milk production.

Protein Evaluation

The system of expressing the protein requirement for ruminants and the nutrient content of feedstuffs to satisfy these requirements in terms of digestible crude protein (DCP), available protein or crude protein (CP) is inadequate and unsatisfactory. The DCP system regards the ruminant as a monogastric and takes no account of the ability of the ruminant to utilize nonprotein nitrogen (NPN). It is well known that diets containing the same amount of DCP do not necessarily support the same productivity. The DCP system does not differentiate between true protein and NPN in the diet, and it does not account for the effects of microbial activity in the rumen on the supply of protein for digestion in the small intestine.

Metabolizable protein (MP) system proposed by NRC in the USA, rumen degradable protein (RDP) and undegradable dietary protein (UDP) system proposed by ARC (1980) for the UK (The UK MP system), true protein digested in the small intestine (PDI) system of France and a similar system proposed by Germany are the new protein systems. Important features of these systems are consideration of two protein synthesizing systems, rumen microbes and ruminant tissues and linking of protein needs to available energy. ARC (1980) recognizes that dietary protein should be considered in terms of RDP and UDP. The system is fully described in the report of the Agricultural and Food Research Council (AFRC 1992) Technical Committee on Responses to Nutrients, No.9. The microbial demand for protein is stated in terms of Effective Rumen Degradable Protein (ERDP). The demand for amino acids at tissue level is quantified in terms of truly digestible protein required to be absorbed from the small intestine and designated as 'Metabolizable Protein' (MP). The NRC (1989) gave the protein requirements as rumen degradable intake protein (DIP) and undegradable intake protein (UIP).

Nutritional models for feeding protein to dairy cattle in the USA have evolved from basic CP (NRC, 1978) to more complex systems based on rumen degradable protein (RDP), rumen undegradable proteins (RUP) and intestinal digestion of RUP (NRC, 2001). The NRC (1989) recognized that intestinal digestion of protein supplements differs; however, empirical data were lacking and as a result, a constant value of 80% was used for all feeds. The main problem was the lack of reliable techniques for estimating intestinal digestion of proteins. With improved techniques, the NRC (2001) has assigned estimates of intestinal digestion to the RUP fraction of each feedstuff.

The function of dietary CP is to supply the cow with metabolizable protein (MP) as absorbed amino acids; but any extra dietary CP that does not contribute to absorbed amino acids that are used in production will be largely lost in the urine. Over-feeding protein actually appeared to suppress production. There is a cost of about 7 kcal of net energy per g of nitrogen converted to urea (NRC, 2001).

Feeding Standards

Feeding standards are statements of the amounts of nutrients required by animals. Feeding standards may be expressed in quantities of nutrients or in dietary proportions. Various units are used for feeding standards. It is obviously desirable that the units used in standards should be the same as those used in the evaluation of feeds. Different countries have evolved their own feeding standards, based on experiments conducted with farm animals in the agro-climatic conditions and economic conditions prevalent in the respective countries.

Feeding Standards for Cattle and Buffaloes

ARC / AFRC Feeding Standards

In UK a techincal committee was set up to develop the standards in 1959, by the ARC, which later known as Agricultural Food Research Council (AFRC). Between 1960 and the mid-1980s, feeding standards in the UK were drawn up by research scientists and then translated into practical manuals by extension workers of the Ministry of Agriculture, Food and Fisheries (MAFF) and associated Governmental and commercial organizations. In 1983 AFRC set up, a single organization for the UK, Technical Committee on Responses to Nutrients (TCORN) and this became responsible for both revising the standards and producing practical manuals.

NRC Feeding Standards

In USA the Committee on Animal Nutrition under the auspices of the National Academy of Sciences-NRC and US Department of Agriculture (USDA) has been publishing the Nutrient Requirements for all types of farm animals since 1945. NRC published the Recommended Nutrient Allowances from 1944 to 1964. These allowances were set higher than average determined requirements to provide a margin of safety for the simple reason that an individual's requirement for nutrients is influenced by numerous interdependent physical, environmental, social and dietary characteristics and it is not practical to determine each individual's exact needs. In 1953, the Committee on Animal Nutrition of NRC decided not to include such margins in future recommendations and thus NRC 'Nutrient Requirements' of Domestic Animal series have been issued from time to time.

The term 'requirement' implies that it is the minimum amount of a given nutrient needed to promote a given body function to the optimum in a perfectly balanced ration. After 1964 the committee considered nutrient requirements to represent values sufficient to promote maintenance, optimum production and prevention of all symptoms of deficiency. The NRC 1989 for Dairy Cattle has been designed to meet the needs of those individual animals that have higher than average requirements for essential nutrients and not those that have merely average requirements. Thus, the requirement values are higher than average and in this respect, provide a margin of safety for animals whose requirements are average or below average.

Indian Feeding Standards

K.C.Sen in 1956 came up with the first Indian standards for dairy cattle based on mid-Morrison values of 1954. The Western data, on which the Morrison standard is based, pertains to the animals which are larger in body size, body weight and are superior in their productive performance. The Indian cattle are smaller in size, lower in body weight, low in production and are adapted to the adverse climatic and low input farming / poor feeding conditions. So lot of work has been done in India in ICAR Institutes and the State Agricultural / Veterinary Universities to determine the energy and protein requirements (primarily) for Indian Cattle, buffaloes, sheep and goats. Thereafter, these were revised by S.N.Ray in 1964 and later Ray and Ranjhan (1978) based on the research findings of Indian studies. The ICAR published the first report on the nutrient requirements of livestock and poultry in 1985. The second revised edition has been brought out in 1998 under the authorship of Dr. S.K. Ranjhan.

Requirements for Maintenance: Energy

Maintenance can be defined as that state in which there is neither gain nor loss of a nutrient by the body. Maintenance requirements are estimates of the amounts of nutrients needed to achieve such equilibrium states. The energy requirement for maintenance is the minimum amount needed to keep the animal in energy equilibrium. Energy requirements are best determined by measurement of energy expenditure. Energy requirement in dry animals for maintenance are low (61 to 104 Kcal / $W^{0.75}$) whereas in lactating animals it is high (113 to 160 Kcal / $W^{0.75}$). Since in the case of milch cows basal metabolic rate (BMR) is higher than the dry animals (Brody, 1945), the maintenance requirements are higher (10-15%) in the milch animals. Energy requirements for maintenance are calculated using 122 Kcal of ME/$W^{0.75}$ for cattle and buffaloes.

Requirements for Maintenance: Protein

The amount of protein (N x 6.25) lost in the urine and faeces of animals, and additional losses, such as hair, skin, and hooves represent the amount of protein required for maintenance. The estimation of maintenance requirements for protein as compared with that of energy is more complicated because of the following reasons. Protein may also be used as a source of energy in case of energy shortage. An excessive supply of protein results in deamination of protein and utilization of the resulting N-free-substances as a source of energy, since deposition of protein in reserve tissue of mature animals is limited.

Protein requirement for maintenance has been determined using factorial method and later regression model. The requirement of 2.84 g/$W^{0.75}$ is used for calculating the DCP requirement for maintenance. NPN compounds such as urea can be used to replace about 30% of the protein requirements of the dairy cattle and buffaloes after the rumen functions are established. Easily available carbohydrates should be incorporated in diets whenever urea is fed.

Requirements for Growth

With the exception of the humans, the growth curves of many animals are quite similar (Brody, 1945). Typical growth curves are sigmoid in shape, showing that gains are faster in young animals than in older animals. Composition of the gains of growing animals changes as they become older and larger. The water, protein, and ash content of the gain declines steadily, while the fat increases from 20% in excess of 50% of the gain. Because of these variables, the assessment of requirements for growth is complicated. In feeding standards for growing animals, requirements of both protein and energy for maintenance and growth are combined to give a single figure against the body weight.

Requirements of Milk Production

Energy requirements for milk production are based on the composition of the milk, its yield and the efficiency of conversion of dietary energy into milk energy. Generally, the energy requirement increases with fat content of milk. Milk secretion represents a direct loss of protein to the animal body which needs to be replaced. Estimates of the efficiency of utilization of digestible protein for milk production vary from 60 to 70%; hence one kg FCM with 35 g of protein need 50 to 55 g digestible protein in the diet.

Requirements of Reproduction

At the initiation of pregnancy, the nutrient requirements of the breeding male per unit size above maintenance may be nearly comparable to those of the breeding female. Thereafter, however, the nutritional needs of the pregnant female enhance. It has been reported that the deposition of energy is moderate during the first two-thirds of gestation and materially increases during the last one-third of the gestation. Further the heat increment of pregnancy, which is primarily due to the increase in the metabolism of the maternal tissue, accounts for more than three-quarters of the energy used throughout gestation; hence the additional requirement for energy above maintenance increases materially during the last trimester of gestation. The requirement for protein during gestation closely parallel to that of energy.

Requirement for Vitamins and Minerals

The requirements for vitamins can logically be divided into two categories: the fat soluble vitamins and water soluble vitamins. The fat soluble vitamins are required for the maintenance of tissue and bone, whereas the B vitamins play roles in metabolism as enzyme cofactors and their requirement increase in parallel with that of energy and protein.

The dietary requirement for minerals depends on animal factors and the bioavailability of the minerals which differs among the feedstuffs and diets. Requirements for calcium and phosphorus are fairly well established because of their greater occurrence in the body and greater role to play in the body. Calcium and phosphorus make up the bulk of milk ash and hence the two minerals have received the most attention in relation to lactation. The minerals of major concern in the reproduction are calcium, phosphorus and iron. The requirements for calcium and phosphorus for milk production can be calculated from the following: one kg of FCM contain about 1.3 g of Ca and 1.0 g of P. If the dietary Ca and P are used with an efficiency of approximately 60%, about 2.2 g of Ca and 1.6 g of P are required per kg of FCM.

Use of Maintenance Requirement Values in Practice

Although there are situations under which farm animals are fed for maintenance only, for the most part they are fed primarily for productive purposes. Here maintenance values serve as basic figures to which additions are made in accordance with number of calvings, milk production, gestation, etc. to calculate the total requirements of nutrients and formulate a ration.

Research Work on Nutrient Requirements of Buffaloes

Buffaloes are of two types, namely riverine and swamp. Riverine buffaloes (chromosomes 2n=50) account for the majority of buffaloes present in India, while swamp buffaloes (chromosomes 2n=48) are localized in North eastern parts of India.

In India, Dr S K Ranjhan and his coworkers at IVRI, Izatnagar and Dr V D Mudgal and his coworkers at NDRI, Karnal did great amount of research on nutrient requirements of buffaloes although many animal nutrition research workers from State Agricultural/Veterinary Universities did contribute substantially. Feeding standards recommended by Sen et al. (1978) are being followed for dairy cattle and buffaloes. Kearl (1982) also has published the requirement for buffaloes. Digestible protein (DCP) requirement for maintenance is 2.84 g per kg metabolic body size (Ranjhan and Pathak, 1979) while Kearl (1982) used a value of 2.54 g.

Nutrient Requirements of Cattle and Buffaloes

Taking 122 Kcal of ME and 2.84 g of DCP per unit metabolic body size, the maintenance requirements were calculated for Zebu cattle, buffaloes and crossbred animals (Table 1). The requirements for TDN and DCP have been calculated per kg of milk production taking 1188 Kcal of ME per kg of 4% fat-corrected milk (FCM) and 132 g digestible nitrogen for 100 g of milk nitrogen (Table 2). In case of feeding heavy milk yielders with high planes of nutrition there is depression, in the digestibility of the feed. To compensate for depression 3% extra feed may be given for each 10 litres of milk produced above 20 kg.

During the last trimester (last two months with a gradual increase for a month) of gestation an additional amount of 90 to 130 g of DCP and 1.0 kg to 1.1 kg TDN have to be provided to cattle and buffaloes of 350 kg to 500 kg (Table 1) body weight. During the pregnancy nutrients are required for the development of foetus and membranes. During the last 60 days, weight of

Table 1 : Daily Nutrient Requirements for Maintenance, Pregnancy and Lactation for Cattle and Buffaloes (Ranjhan, 1998).

Live weight, kg	Dry feed, kg	DCP, g	ME, Mcal	TDN, kg	Ca, g	P, g	Carotene, mg	Vitamin A, 1000 IU
1	2	3	4	5	6	7	8	9
Maintenance of Mature Cows/Buffaloes*								
200	3.5	150	6.0	1.7	8	7	21	9
250	4.0	170	7.2	2.0	10	9	26	11
300	4.5	200	8.4	2.4	12	10	32	13
350	5.0	230	9.4	2.7	14	11	37	15
400	5.5	250	10.8	3.0	17	13	42	17
450	6.0	280	12.4	3.4	18	14	48	19
500	6.5	300	13.2	3.7	20	15	53	21
550	7.0	330	14.4	4.0	21	16	58	23
600	7.5	350	15.5	4.2	22	17	64	26
650	8.0	370	16.2	4.5	23	18	69	28
700	8.5	390	17.3	4.8	25	19	74	30
750	9.0	410	18.0	5.0	26	20	79	32
800	9.5	430	19.1	5.3	27	21	85	34
Maintenance and Pregnancy (last 2 months of gestation)								
250	4.9	270	10.8	3.0	14	12	51	21
300	5.6	290	12.4	3.4	16	14	56	25
350	6.4	320	13.2	3.7	21	16	67	27
400	7.2	350	14.1	4.0	23	18	76	30
450	7.9	400	15.9	4.4	26	20	86	34
500	8.6	430	17.3	4.8	29	22	95	38
550	9.3	465	18.8	5.2	31	24	105	42
600	10.0	500	20.2	5.6	34	26	114	46
650	10.6	530	21.6	6.0	36	28	124	50
700	11.3	550	22.7	6.3	39	30	133	53
750	12.0	600	24.2	6.7	42	32	143	57
800	12.6	630	25.6	7.1	44	34	152	61

* During the first and second lactation, in order to allow the growth of the lactating cows / buffaloes, add about 20 and 10 per cent of the maintenance allowance.

the pregnant animal increases by about 25 to 35 kg depending upon the breed and their condition. Besides the requirement for foetal growth and uterus, nutrients are also deposited in reserve that may be utilized for milk production in early lactation. The nutrient requirements for growing calves (Tables 3, 4 and 5) working animals (Table 6) and breeding bulls (Table 7) are presented.

Table 2 : Nutrient Requirements per kg of milk Production (Ranjhan, 1998).

Fat, %	DCP, g	ME, Mcal	TDN, kg	Ca, g	P, g
3.0	40	0.97	0.270	2.5	1.8
4.0	45	1.13	0.315	2.7	2.0
5.0	51	1.28	0.370	2.9	2.2
6.0	57	1.36	0.410	3.1	2.4
7.0	63	1.54	0.460	3.3	2.6
8.0	69	1.80	0.510	3.5	2.8
9.0	75	2.06	0.500	3.7	3.0
10.0	81	2.16	0.600	3.9	3.2
11.0	85	2.34	0.650	4.1	3.4

Table 3 : Nutrient requirements of pre-ruminant cattle- and buffalo-calves (Ranjhan, 1972)

Age, day	Live weight, kg	Daily gain, g	DCP, g	TDN, kg	ME, Mcal	Ca, g	P, g	Vitamin A, 1000 IU	Vitamin D, IU
Birth to 15	25	200	80	0.40	1.5	2.5	1.5	1.5	200
16 to 30	30	300	90	0.50	1.7	3.0	2.0	1.5	250
31 to 60	40	300	125	0.80	2.4	3.5	2.5	1.7	250
61 to 90	50	350	150	1.00	3.6	4.0	3.8	2.0	300

Feeding of Ruminants

In India, the nutritive values of feedstuffs and nutrient requirements have been widely expressed in terms of DCP, TDN and ME. However, protein fractions such as RDP and UDP values for certain feedstuffs are also available. In addition to the several commercial feed manufacturers, National Dairy Development Board, Anand has been promoting the manufacturing and supply of 'bypass protein' feeds to the dairy farmers.

Table 4 : Nutrient requirements for growing cattle-calves (Ranjhan, 1998)*

Live weight, kg	Growth rate, g	DM, kg	DCP, g	TDN, kg	ME, Mcal	Ca, g	P, g	Carotene, mg	Vitamin A, 1000 IU
70	550	2.1	255	1.4	5.0	8	6	7	3
	600	2.3	260	1.5	5.4	8	6	7	3
80	550	2.4	260	1.5	5.4	9	7	7	3
	600	2.5	270	1.6	5.8	9	7	8	3
100	550	2.8	270	2.1	7.6	10	8	10	3
	600	3.0	280	2.2	7.9	10	8	10	3
120	550	3.2	280	2.3	8.3	14	11	11	4
	600	3.7	290	2.4	8.6	14	11	11	4
140	550	3.7	290	2.5	9.0	14	11	16	6
	600	4.2	300	2.6	9.4	14	11	16	6
160	550	4.2	300	2.7	9.7	15	12	16	6
	600	4.7	320	2.8	10.1	15	12	16	6
180	550	4.7	310	2.9	10.4	15	12	18	8
	600	5.2	320	3.0	10.8	15	12	18	8
200	550	5.2	320	3.1	11.2	16	13	22	9
	600	5.7	330	3.2	11.5	16	13	22	9
220	550	5.7	330	3.3	11.9	18	14	24	10
	600	6.2	340	3.4	12.2	18	14	24	10
240	550	6.2	340	3.5	12.6	20	16	28	12
	600	6.7	350	3.6	13.0	20	16	28	12
260	550	6.7	350	3.7	13.3	20	16	30	13
	600	7.2	360	3.8	13.7	20	16	30	13

* Calcium, phosphorus, carotene and vitamin A are from NRC (1989)

Ranjhan and Kiran Singh (1993) compared and analysed the various feeding standards such as NRC (1989), ARC (1980), Sen et al (1978) and ICAR (1985) and found no large difference in the requirements for large ruminants for both maintenance and production. Considering the livestock productivity from Indian farmers, say for example, milk production which is by and large "production by masses", we should not lose sight of the feed resources available and socio-economic situation of the farmers. Farmers mostly depend on crop residues such as straws and stovers, natural grasses, tree foliages and limited quantities of byproducts of concentrates from milling of grains and oilseeds.

Table 5 : Nutrient requirements for growing buffalo-calves (Ranjhan, 1998)*

Live weight, kg	Growth rate, g	DM, kg	DCP, g	TDN, kg	ME, Mcal	Ca, g	P, g	Carotene, mg	Vitamin A, 1000 IU
70	450	2.0	156	1.3	4.7	8	6	7	3
	550	2.1	168	1.5	5.4	8	6	7	3
80	450	2.2	177	1.4	5.0	9	7	7	3
	550	2.3	183	1.6	5.7	9	7	8	3
100	450	2.7	198	1.7	6.1	10	8	10	3
	550	2.8	210	1.8	6.5	10	8	10	3
120	450	3.1	264	1.9	6.8	14	11	11	4
	550	3.2	276	2.1	7.6	14	11	11	4
140	450	3.6	279	2.2	7.9	14	11	16	6
	550	3.7	291	2.2	7.9	14	11	16	6
160	450	4.1	288	2.5	9.0	15	12	16	6
	550	4.2	300	2.6	9.4	15	12	16	6
180	450	4.6	300	2.7	9.9	15	12	18	8
	550	4.7	316	2.8	10.1	15	12	18	8
200	450	5.1	312	2.9	10.4	16	13	22	9
	550	5.2	329	3.1	11.2	16	13	22	9
220	450	5.6	345	3.1	11.2	18	14	24	10
	550	6.2	357	3.2	11.5	18	14	24	10
240	450	6.1	375	3.3	11.9	20	16	28	12
	550	6.2	390	3.4	12.2	20	16	28	12
260	450	6.2	410	3.5	12.6	20	16	30	13
	550	6.5	420	3.6	12.8	20	16	30	13

* Calcium, phosphorus, carotene and vitamin A are from NRC (1989)

Strategic Supplementation of Critical Nutrients

Dr R.A.Leng challenged the description of crop residues as being of low quality and preferred to relate to them as imbalanced forages. Strategic supplementation of critical nutrients (Reddy, 1989) ably utilizing the inherent potential in ruminant mode of digestion has the potential to sustainably feed the fabulous ruminant population exploiting their genetic potential for economic milk and meat production. While practising so, the latest advances made in ruminant nutrition need to be put to use in formulating rations.

Table 6 : Nutrient Requirements for Working Bullocks and Buffaloes (Sen, Ray and Ranjhan, 1978)

Live weight, kg	Normal work*				Heavy work**			
	DM, kg	DCP, kg	TDN, kg	ME, Mcal	DM, kg	DCP, kg	TDN, kg	ME, Mcal
200	4.00	0.24	2.0	7.2	5.0	0.25	2.7	9.5
300	5.80	0.33	3.1	11.4	7.0	0.42	4.0	14.4
400	7.60	0.45	4.0	14.4	9.8	0.57	4.8	17.3
500	9.40	0.56	4.9	18.0	11.2	0.71	6.4	23.0
600	11.2	0.66	5.8	20.8	13.40	0.82	8.0	28.8

* 6 hrs of carting or 4 hrs of ploughing
**8 hrs of carting or 6 hrs of ploughing

Table 7 : Nutrient Requirements of Breeding Bulls (Sen, Ray and Ranjhan, 1978).

Live weight, kg	DCP, kg	TDN, kg	ME, Mcal	Ca, g	P, g	Carotene, mg	Vitamin A, 1000 IU
400	380	3.6	13.0	18	13	40	16
500	450	4.5	16.2	20	15	53	21
600	530	5.4	19.4	22	17	64	26

Amino acids are supplied to the duodenum of ruminants by microbial protein synthesized in the rumen, undegraded dietary protein and endogenous protein. Stern and Hoover (1979) reviewed the literature and reported that approximately 30 g (values ranged from 10 to 50 g) of nitrogen was synthesized per kilogram of organic matter (OM) digested in the rumen. AFRC (1992) used 32 g microbial nitrogen per kg apparently digested OM in the rumen. Microbial protein usually accounts for a substantial portion of the total amino acids entering the small intestine. Hence, the goal of the ruminant nutritionist should be to maximize efficiency of microbial protein synthesis (EMPS) as well as to maximize microbial CP (MCP) flow. The total amount of microbial protein flowing to the small intestine depends on nutrient availability and efficiency of utilization of these nutrients by ruminal bacteria.

NRC (2001) model prioritize to meet the RDP requirement first, since microbial protein accounts for most of the dairy cow's MP, followed by supplying matching ruminal fermentative energy. Matching ruminal energy fermentation with RDP will be effective for improving N efficiency, regardless of dietary protein degradability. Microbial nitrogen yield in the rumen is taken as 1.34 g per MJ fermentable ME or 8.38 g MCP per MJ. Ruminal acidosis and associated metabolic problems limit the amount of readily fermented carbohydrate that may be fed to produce MP from microbial growth. There are likely "optimal" levels of dietary concentrate (Table 8) and forage that will support maximal ruminal protein synthesis and milk production.

Table 8 : Recommended minimum concentrations (% of DM) of total and forage NDF and maximum concentrations (% of DM) of NFC for diets of lactating cows when the diet is fed as a total mixed ration, the forage (being alfalfa or corn silage predominantly) has adequate particle size, and ground maize is the predominant starch source.

Minimum forage NDF	Minimum dietary NDF	Maximum dietary NFC	Minimum dietary ADF
19[a]	25[a]	44[a]	17[a]
18	27	42	18
17	29	40	19
16	31	38	20
15	33	36	21

[a]Diets that contain less fibre (forage NDF, total NDF or total ADF) than these minimum values and more NFC (non-fibre carbohydrates) than 44 % should not be fed (NRC, 2001).

"Optimal" Levels of Dietary Concentrate and Forage and Physically Effective NDF

High-concentrate diets for high-yielding dairy cows must contain sufficient physically effective fibre (i.e., fibre that stimulates rumination, saliva production, and rumen buffering) to prevent ruminal dysfermentation and subacute ruminal acidosis (SARA). The concept of physically effective fibre was created to amalgamate the chemical characteristics and particle size of forages, and to quantify its value to rumen function (Mertens, 2000). Physically effective NDF (peNDF) is related to the physical characteristics of NDF (primarily particle size) that affect chewing activity and the biphasic nature of ruminal contents. The NRC (2001) does not give requirements for peNDF due to lack of a standardized, validated method for measuring effective fiber in feeds and to establish requirements for effective fibre. NRC (2001) gave an average effective value of NDF from nonforage sources (e.g., soyhulls, beet pulp, maize gluten feed, and grains) as 50% of that for NDF from forage based on the published reports.

Urban livestock production caters the needs of urban population for milk and milk products. In urban dairies concentrate feeds may account over 70% of the ration, especially in case of high yielding cows/buffaloes, which can lead to acidosis, depressed butterfat content of the milk, etc. In those cases, it is necessary to provide a minimum quantity of fibre (33% NDF) in the total DM provided to the animal. If a ration consists of a concentrate mixture of about 14% NDF, the minimum amount of roughage DM that is to be provided is 25% if the roughage contains 70% NDF, e.g. rice straw, wheat straw and finger millet straw or 30% if the roughage contains 60% NDF, e.g. maize and sorghum stover or 39% if the roughage contains 50% NDF, e.g. lucerne, berseem and cowpea.

Cornell Net Carbohydrate and Protein System (CNCPS)

Nutritionists formulate cattle rations as per the nutritional recommendations which often contained significant "safety factors" because nutritional requirements and availabilities for all types of cattle, feeds and environmental or management conditions are at variance. The extra nutrients contained in these safety factors to ensure that nutrient requirements were met often increased nutrient excretion and contributed to adverse effects on water and air quality. The Cornell Net Carbohydrate and Protein System (CNCPS) is a mathematical model to evaluate diet and animal performance that was developed from basic principles of rumen function, microbial growth, feed digestion, passage and animal physiology.

The most widely used and sophisticated multi-chemical approach for quantifying N fractions in feedstuffs is the protein fractionation scheme used in the CNCPS (Sniffen *et al.*, 1992). The CNCPS partitions CP into 5 fractions: **A** (NPN; soluble in borate-phosphate buffer), **B1** (rapidly degraded true protein), **B2** (moderately degraded true protein and large peptides), **B3** (slowly degraded true protein) and **C** (undegraded true protein). The protein content of the diet has soluble intake protein (SIP), degradable intake protein (DIP) and undegraded intake protein (UIP). SIP is the fraction of feed protein that is rapidly degraded in the rumen. SIP is referred to as the A fraction. DIP is the fraction of feed protein that can be degraded in the rumen and this includes fractions A, B1, B2 and B3. UIP is the portion of feed protein that is not degraded in the rumen and remains intact as it passes to the lower tract. It includes available UIP as the B3 fraction and unavailable UIP as the C fraction.

Although microbial protein alone may be adequate for low producing ruminants, it can be inadequate for supporting higher levels of growth, wool or milk production. As animal production increases, additional protein must be provided from dietary protein that leaves the rumen undegraded to meet the animal's protein requirement. The use of high rumen undegradable proteins

(RUP) in diets fed to ruminants with high protein requirements can improve the amino acid supply to the animal provided that enough degradable protein is included in the diet to maximize microbial protein. When formulating diets for ruminants, various criteria can be used to select the protein supplement including palatability, ruminal protein degradability, protein quality, intestinal absorption of amino acids, cost per unit of protein, availability and consistency of product, and impact on animal performance. Similarly, the relevant information is looked for while selecting energy and other feeds.

Tree Foliage as a Source of Available UIP

Tree foliage could be considered promising and interesting sources for incorporation into ruminant diets. The B3 values for *Acacia auriculiformis*, cashewnut, *Gliricidia sepium*, jack, *Sesbania grandiflora*, subabul and yellow gold mohur leaves, respectively, were 4.81, 3.13, 6.12, 4.56, 7.90, 4.94 and 4.81% (Reddy and Elanchezhian, 2008). Among the tree leaves studied, *Sesbania grandiflora* had highest amount of slowly rumen-degraded protein followed by gliricidia, subabul, acacia, yellow gold mohur, jack and cashew.

Table 9 : Nutritive value (%) of common feedstuffs (on as fed basis)

Feedstuffs	DM	DCP	TDN	Ca	P
Rice straw	90	0.00	44.0	0.5	0.12
Bund grass (grasses naturally grown on farm bunds during crop farming)	25	1.5	15.0	0.07	0.04
Green grass (Hybrid napier / Para / Guinea)	25	1.0	16.0	0.11	0.05
Leguminous green fodder (Berseem / Lucerne / cowpea)	15	2.5	12.0	0.3	0.05
Agathi (*Sesbania grandiflora*) green foliage	35	6.0*	22.0	0.6	0.07
Subabul (*Leucaena leucocephala*) green foliage	30	6.9*	22.0	0.6	0.07
Groundnut cake	90	42.0	71.0	0.2	0.7
Gingelly cake	90	38.0	78.0	2.0	0.8
Rice bran (deoiled)	90	6.0	66.0	0.08	1.5
Wheat bran	90	10.0	68.0	0.1	0.8
Gram husk	90	0.5	55.0		
Tapioca flour	90	2.0	64.0		

* Crude protein; DCP 3.0 to 3.5%.

Table 10 : Requirement of a 400 kg cow / buffalo giving 8 or 10 kg milk.

Particulars	DCP	TDN	Ca	P
	----Kg------			
Maintenance	0.25	3.00	0.017	0.013
Milk production per kg (4% BF)	0.045	0.315	0.0027	0.002
8 Kg milk production	0.36	2.52	0.0216	0.016
10 Kg milk production	0.45	3.15	0.027	0.02
Total for 8 kg milk production	**0.61**	**5.52**	**0.0386**	**0.029**
Total for 10 kg milk production	**0.70**	**6.15**	**0.044**	**0.033**

Table 11 : Requirement of a 350 kg cow / buffalo giving 6 or 7 kg milk.

Particulars	DCP	TDN	Ca	P
	----Kg------			
Maintenance	0.230	2.7	0.014	0.011
Milk production per kg (4% BF)	0.045	0.315	0.0027	0.002
6 Kg milk production	0.27	1.89	0.0162	0.012
7 Kg milk production	0.315	2.205	0.0189	0.014
Total for 6 kg milk production	**0.50**	**4.59**	**0.0302**	**0.023**
Total for 7 kg milk production	**0.545**	**4.905**	**0.0329**	**0.025**

Formulating Rations using the Feedstuffs Readily Available with the Farmer

Several rations (Table 12) have been formulated using roughages such as bund grass (green), rice straw, *Sesbania grandiflora* or subabul green foliage and concentrates such as oilseed cakes, brans, husks or tapioca thippi for cows / buffaloes producing 6 to 10 kg milk.

1. Ration for a cow / buffalo of 350 kg producing 6 kg milk

Particulars	RM*	DM	DCP	TDN	Ca	P
		----Kg----				
Requirement		8.75	0.50	4.59	0.0302	0.023
From roughages						
Bund grass	8.0	2.0	0.12	1.2	0.0056	0.0032
Rice straw	5.0	4.5	0.0	2.2	0.025	0.006
Total		6.5	0.12	3.4	0.0306	0.0092
Nutrients to be supplied from concentrates (DCP 15.2% TDN 47.6%)	2.5	2.25	0.38	1.19	Met; but straw has oxalate also	0.0138

*RM=Raw material

Percentage Composition of the concentrate mixture

Feedstuffs	Kg	DCP, kg	TDN, kg
Groundnut cake	26.1	10.96	18.53
Wheat bran	40.9	4.09	27.81
Gram husk	30.0	0.15	16.50
Mineral mixture	2.0	-	-
Salt	1.0	-	-
Total	100.0	15.2	62.84

Composition of the concentrate mixture, 2.5kg

Feedstuffs	Kg	DCP, kg	TDN, kg
Groundnut cake	0.653	0.274	0.464
Wheat bran	1.03	0.103	0.7
Gram husk	0.75	0.004	0.415
Mineral mixture	0.05	-	-
Salt	0.025	-	-
Total		**0.381**	**1.579**

2. Ration for a cow / buffalo of 350 kg producing 7 kg milk: ration 1

Particulars	RM	DM	DCP	TDN	Ca	P
	---------	---------	Kg---------	---------	---------	
Requirement		8.75	0.545	4.905	0.0329	0.025
From roughages						
Agathi (*Sesbania grandiflora*) green foliage	2.0	0.7	0.12	0.44	0.012	0.0014
Bund grass	8.0	2.0	0.12	1.2	0.0056	0.0032
Rice straw	3.5	3.15	0.0	1.54	0.0175	0.0042
Total		5.85	0.24	3.18	0.0351	0.0088
Nutrients to be supplied from concentrates (DCP 9.53% TDN 53.91 %)	3.2	2.90	0.305	1.725	Met	0.0162

Percentage Composition of the concentrate mixture

Feedstuffs	Kg	DCP, kg	TDN, kg
Groundnut cake	13.04	5.48	9.26
Wheat bran	21.96	2.20	14.93
Rice bran (deoiled)	21.96	1.32	14.49
Gram husk	30.00	0.15	16.50
Mineral mixture	2.0	-	-
Salt	1.0	-	-
Total		9.15	55.18

Composition of the concentrate mixture, 3.2 kg

Feedstuffs	Kg	DCP, kg	TDN, kg
Groundnut cake	0.417	0.175	0.296
Wheat bran	0.703	0.070	0.478
Gram husk	0.96	0.005	0.55
Deoiled rice bran	0.703	0.042	0.464
Tapioca flour	0.32	0.0006	0.205
Mineral mixture	0.05	-	-
Salt	0.025	-	-
Total		0.2926	1.993

3. Ration for a cow / buffalo of 350 kg producing 7 kg milk: ration 2

Particulars	RM	DM	DCP	TDN	Ca	P
		Kg				
Requirement		8.75	0.545	4.905	0.0329	0.025
From roughages						
Agathi (*Sesbania grandiflora*) green foliage	4.0	1.4	0.24	0.88	0.024	0.0028
Bund grass	6.0	1.5	0.09	0.9	0.0042	0.0024
Rice straw	4.0	3.6	0.0	1.76	0.002	0.0048
Total		6.5	0.33	3.54	0.0302	0.01
Nutrients to be supplied from concentrates (DCP 8.6% TDN 54.6%)	2.5	2.25	0.215	1.365	0.0027	0.015

Percentage Composition of the concentrate mixture

Feedstuffs	Kg	DCP, kg	TDN, kg
Groundnut cake	10.4	4.37	7.38
Wheat bran	23.3	2.33	15.84
Deoiled rice bran	23.3	1.40	15.38
Gram husk	30.0	0.15	16.50
Tapioca flour	10.0	0.20	6.40
Mineral mixture	2.0	-	-
Salt	1.0	-	-
Total		8.45	61.50

Composition of the concentrate mixture, 2.5kg

Feedstuffs	Kg	DCP, kg	TDN, kg
Groundnut cake	0.26	0.109	0.185
Wheat bran	0.583	0.058	0.396
Gram husk	0.75	0.004	0.415
Deoiled rice bran	0.583	0.035	0.385
Tapioca flour	0.25	0.0005	0.16
Mineral mixture	0.05	-	-
Salt	0.025	-	-
Total		0.2065	1.541

4. Ration for a cow / buffalo of 400 kg producing 8 kg milk

Particulars	RM	DM	DCP	TDN	Ca	P
			Kg			
Requirement		10.0	0.61	5.52	0.0386	0.029
From roughages						
Rice straw	7.0	6.3	0.0	3.08	0.035	0.0084
Total						
Nutrients to be supplied from concentrates (DCP 14.88% TDN 64.5%)	4.1	3.7	0.61	2.44	0.0036	0.0206

Percentage Composition of the concentrate mixture

Feedstuffs	Kg	DCP, kg	TDN, kg
Groundnut cake	25.0	10.5	17.75
Wheat bran	26.0	2.6	17.68
Deoiled rice bran	26.0	1.56	17.16
Gram husk	10.0	0.05	5.50
Tapioca flour	10.0	0.20	6.40
Mineral mixture	2.0	-	-
Salt	1.0	-	-
Total		14.91	64.49

Composition of the concentrate mixture, 4.1 kg

Feedstuffs	Kg	DCP, kg	TDN, kg
Groundnut cake	1.025	0.431	0.728
Wheat bran	1.066	0.107	0.725
Gram husk	0.41	0.002	0.226
Deoiled rice bran	1.066	0.064	0.704
Tapioca flour	0.41	0.0008	0.262
Mineral mixture	0.080	-	-
Salt	0.050	-	-
Total		0.605	2.645

5. Ration for a cow / buffalo of 400 kg producing 10 kg milk

Particulars	RM	DM	DCP	TDN	Ca	P
		Kg				
Requirement		10.0	0.70	6.15	0.044	0.033
From roughages						
Rice straw	6.5	5.85	0.0	2.86	0.0235	0.0078
Total						
Nutrients to be supplied from concentrates (DCP 15.22% TDN 66.0%)	4.6	4.15	0.7	3.29	0.0206	0.0252

Percentage Composition of the concentrate mixture

Feedstuffs	Kg	DCP, kg	TDN, kg
Groundnut cake	12.84	5.39	9.12
Gingelly cake	12.84	4.88	10.02
Wheat bran	30.66	3.07	20.85
Deoiled rice bran	30.66	1.84	23.91
Gram husk	10.0	0.05	5.50
Mineral mixture	2.0	-	-
Salt	1.0	-	-
Total		15.23	69.40

Table 12 : Daily rations consisting of roughages and concentrate ingredients for Cows / buffaloes

Particulars	Rati on 1	Rati on 2	Rati on 3	Rati on 4	Rati on 5	Rati on 6	Rati on 7	Rati on 8	Rati on 9	Rati on 10
	350 kg; 6 kg milk production		**350 kg; 7 kg milk production**			**400 kg; 8 kg milk production**			**400 kg; 10 kg milk production**	
Roughages, kg										
Bund grass, green	8.0	-	8.0	6.0	6.0	-	9.0	9.0	-	9.0
Sesbania / subabul green foliage	-	5.0	2.0	4.0	4.0	-	-	4.0	-	-
Rice straw	5.0	5.0	3.5	4.0	4.0	7.0	5.0	4.0	6.5	5.0
Concentrates, g										
Groundnut cake	650	400	420	260	250	1000	750	450	600	550
Gingelly cake	-	-	-	-	-	-	-	-	600	550
Wheat bran	1000	2000	700	600	600	1000	1000	1000	1400	1000
Deoiled rice bran	-	-	700	600	600	1000	1000	1000	1400	1000
Gram husk	750	1000	1000	750	750	500	450	500	500	1000
Tapioca thippi	-	-	250	250	250	500	450	500	-	-
Mineral mixture	50	50	50	50	50	80	80	80	100	100
Salt	25	25	25	25	25	50	50	50	50	50

Composition of the concentrate mixture, 4.6 kg

Feedstuffs	Kg	DCP, kg	TDN, kg
Groundnut cake	0.591	0.248	0.420
Gingelly cake	0.591	0.225	0.461
Wheat bran	1.41	0.141	0.959
Gram husk	0.46	0.002	0.253
Deoiled rice bran	1.41	0.085	0.931
Mineral mixture	0.100	-	-
Salt	0.050	-	-
Total		0.701	3.024

References

AFRC, (1992). Technical Committee on Responses to Nutrients, Report No 9, Nutritive requirements of ruminant animals: protein. *Nutr. Abstr. Revi.*, Series B 62, 787-835.

Agricultural Research Council (1965). The Nutrient Requirement of farm livestock No.2. Ruminants. London, UK.

Agricultural Research Council (1980). The Nutrient Requirement of ruminant livestock Technical Review by an ARC Working Party, Commonwealth Agriculture Bereau, Farmham Royal, UK.

Agricultural Research Council (1984). The Nutrient Requirement of ruminant livestock Supplement No. 1. Slough, UK; Commonwealth Agriculture Bereaux.

Brody, S. (1945). Bioenergetics of Growth. New York: Reinhold.

Community. Published by Pudoc, Wageningen, Netherlands. Pp 308.

ICAR (1985). Nutrient Requirements of Livestock and Poultry. Indian Council of Agricultural Research, New Delhi.

Kearl, L.C. (1982). Nutrient requirements of ruminants in developing countries. Utah State University, Logan, USA, International Feedstuffs Institute.

Mertens, D.R. (2000). *Feedstuffs*, 10: 11–14.

National Research Council (1978). Nutrient Requirements of Dairy Cattle. 5th revised edition, National Academy Press. Washington, D. C., USA.

National Research Council (1989). Nutrient requirements of diary cattle. 6th revised edition. Update. National Academy Press. Washington, D. C., USA.

National Research Council (2001). Nutrient Requirements of Dairy Cattle. 7th revised edition, National Academy Press. Washington, D. C., USA., and New World Camelids, National Academy Press. Washington, D. C., USA.

Prasad Anjaneya Reddy, D.V. and Murthy, A.S.N. (1983). *J. Nuc. Agric. Biol.*, 12:29-32.

Ranjhan, S.K. (1972). Animal Nutrition and Feeding Practices, Vikas Publication, New Delhi.

Ranjhan, S.K. and Singh Kiran (1983). Nutrient requirements, feeding standards and feeding of ruminants and their relevance to Indian conditions. In: Feeding of Ruminants on Fibrous Crop Residues Kiran Singh and J.B.Schiere (Eds) Proceedings of an international workshop held at the NDRI, Karnal, February 4-8, 1991. pp 117-130.

Ranjhan, S.K. and Pathak N.N. (1979). Management and feeding of buffaloes. 1st edn. Vikas Pub House Pvt Ltd, New Delhi

Reddy, D.V. (1989). "Response to supplementation of critical nutrients in buffaloes fed with diets based on ammoniated wheat straw". Ph D Thesis IVRI Deemed University, Izatnagar

Reddy, D.V. (2001). Development of straw based practical diets for buffaloes using catalytic level of supplements. Review papers of the X Animal Nutrition conference on "Emerging Nutritional Technologies for Sustainable Animal Production and Environmental Protection" held at National Dairy Research Institute, Karnal during 9-11 November, 2001, pp.60-69.

Reddy, D.V. and Elanchezhian, N. (2008). Evaluation of tropical tree leaves as ruminant feedstuff based on cell contents, cell wall fractions and polyphenolic compounds. Livestock Research for Rural Development 20, *Article #70.* Retrieved from http://www.cipav.org.co/lrrd/lrrd20/5/redd20077.htm

Sen, K.C., Ray, S.N. and Ranjhan, S.K. (1978). Chemical Composition of Cattle Feeds and Feeding of Farm Animals. ICAR, New Delhi.

Sniffen, C.J., Van Soest, P.J., Fox, D.G. , O'Conner, J.D. and Russell, J.B. (1992). *J. Anim. Sci.,* 70: 3562-3577 http://www.animal-science.org/cgi/reprint/70/11/3562

Stern, M.D. and Woover, W.H. (1979). *J. Anim. Sci.,* 75: 2256-2276.

□□□

Animal Nutrition, 2012
eds. Dr. (Mrs.) Usha R. Mehra et al., pp. 135-161
Satish Serial Publishing House e-mail : info@satishserial.com; website : www.satishserial.com

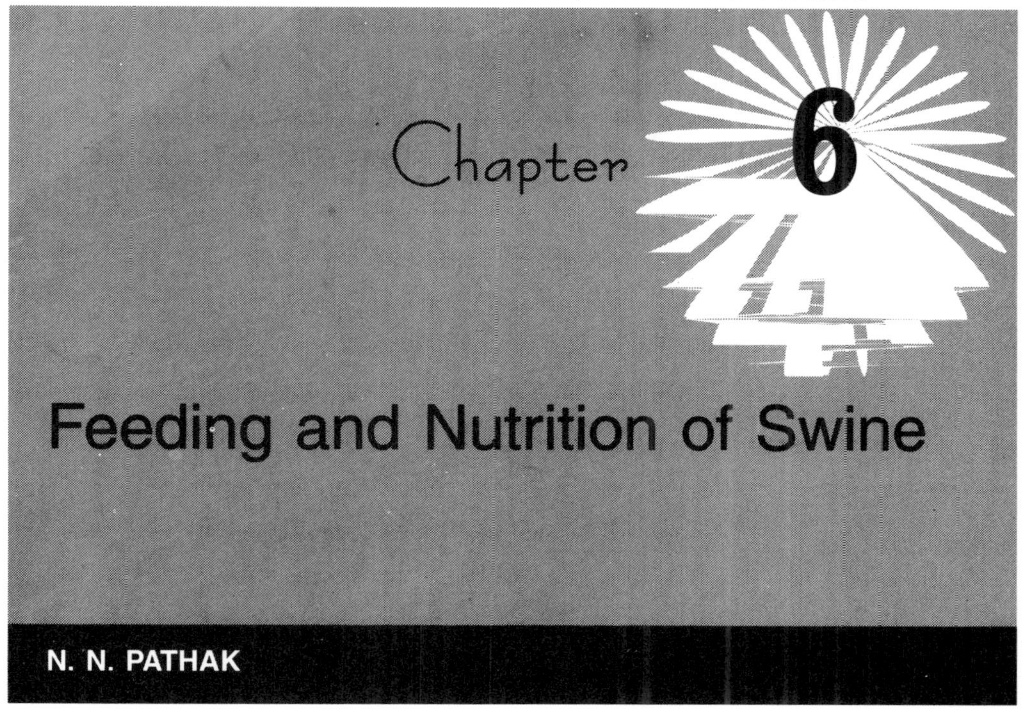

Chapter 6

Feeding and Nutrition of Swine

N. N. PATHAK

Being simple stomached animal of low feed intake capacity but very high growth rate and prolificacy, pigs require nutrient rich feeds for the supply of their nutritional requirements for optimum performance. During the past half century swine husbandry for pork production is gradually emerging from the traditional scavenging system to semi-intensive and intensive system. Alongwith the continuous increase in human population and importance of animal proteins in the diet, the demand of proteinous foods of animal origin is also increasing. At the present level of growth in the production of various proteinous foods of animal origin it may be possible to cope up with the demand from the products of one or two species. There is also demand of variety of products. Therefore, for the production of wholesome pork, it is becoming necessary to rear pig according to scientific management and feeding systems. The other reasons for intensive pig production is the shrinkage of resources for scavenging.

Feeds for Pigs

The pigs are simple stomached animals with little scope of utilization of fibrous herbages. The nutritional requirements of pigs are quite high due to higher growth rate and prolificacy. Therefore, pig diets are prepared from the energy and protein rich feeds. While selecting proteinous feeds the content of essential amino acids are also taken into consideration. The feeds of pigs are derived from the following sources.

Cereal Grains

Yellow maize is considered the feed of choice for the pigs, but all edible cereal grains may be used in various proportion for compounding the diets for different categories of pigs. Sorghum, pearl millet (bajra), barley, wheat, oats, rice and minor millets are the common conventional sources of dietary energy for pigs.

Leguminous Seeds

These are good sources of energy and protein and may be used for the feeding of pigs. However, most of the leguminous seeds require treatment before feeding for the inactivation of antinutritonal factors present in most of the feeds.

Oil Seeds

These are richer sources of protein and energy but seldom used for the feeding of livestock. However, shortings are used for feeding.

Extraction Products

The residue or byproducts of cereal grains, pulses and oil seeds are extensively used for the feeding of pigs and other farm animals.

Brans

Wheat bran, rice bran and deoiled rice polish are the common byproducts available from the milling of wheat and rice.

Pulses Milling Byproducts (Dal Chunnies)

These include hulls, embryos and fine broken cotyledons obtained by separation after milling the pulses. Although these byproducts are good sources of protein and minerals but less popular for the feeding of pigs due to high fibre content. The common dal chunnies marketed in India are gram chunni, moong chunni, masoor chuni, urad chunni and arhar (toor) chunni.

Oilseed Cakes

Most of the oilseed cakes are rich sources of protein and used as protein supplements for balancing the cereal based diets. Although three types of oilseed cakes, i.e. ghani pressed (traditional old system of oil extraction), expeller pressed and solvent extracted cakes are produced, but due to increasing demand of vegetable oils in human dietary the solvent extraction process has prevailed over the other two methods. Average oil content may be 7-10%, 5-6% and less than 1% in the ghani pressed, expeller pressed and solvent extracted oil seed cakes. The reduction in oil content has reduced the energy value but increased the protein content and keeping quality of the cakes. The various oil seed cakes used for the feeding of pigs are soybean cake, groundnut cake, mustard/rape seed cake, linseed cake, sesame cake, cotton seed cake, sunflower cake, safflower cake and coconut cake.

Sources of Animal Protein

Almost all foods of plant origin are deficient in several essential amino acids which are present in adequate quantity in the animal tissues. Therefore, small amount of proteinous foods of animal origin are incorporated in the compounded diets of pigs for balancing the nutritional requirements of otherwise deficient essential amino acids in the grain based diets. The common sources of animal protein are fish meal, meat meal and dried skim milk powder, and less known feeds are liver residue, silkworm pupa meal, frog trash meal and blood meat etc.

Miscellaneous Feeds

The other conventional feeds incorporated in the diets of pigs are grain shortings, maize gluten meal, tapioca waste meal, yeast, sugarcane molasses and brewers grain etc.

Tubers and Roots

In certain areas extensive cultivation of several succulent roots and tubers is quite common, and the shortings and often roots and tubes (when available at cheaper rate) are used for the feeding of swine. These crops are rich in digestible carbohydrates and also provide some protein, minerals and vitamins. The common root crops are carrot, turnip and beet root. The common tubers are potatoes, sweet potatoes and tapioca.

Some of the roots and tubers contain antinutritional factors like cyanogenic glucosides in the tapioca tubers. Boiling tubers for some time destroys the cyanogenic glucosides. Potatoes are rich sources of starch and also contain 9 to 12 per cent crude protein in dry matter. The antinutritonal and harmful substances are present in young tubers.

Sprouting tubers and greenish tubers contain chaconine and solanidine. Feeding of raw potatoes causes the occurrence of gastroenteritis which may be fatal on the feeding. The potatoes should be properly cooked before feeding the swine.

The tubers of sweet potatoes do not contain any harmful substance. The tubers are harder than the potatoes due to higher dry matter content. Crude protein content is very low but energy content is high.

Average chemical composition of some common roots and tubers is presented in Table 1 on dry matter basis.

Table 1 : Average chemical composition of some common roots and tubers fed to pigs (% in DM)

Feeds	Dry matter	Organic matter	Crude Protein	Crude fibre	Ether extract	Ash
Carrot	11	96	11	10	0.9	4
Beet root	20	97	5	5	1.8	3
Potatoes	20	96	10	4	0.9	4
Sweet potatoes	32	97	4	4	0.8	3
Tapioca	36	97	3	4	0.8	3
Turnip	9	92	12	11	0.8	8

Forages

Succulent leafy fodder may be fed for the partial supply of protein, vitamins and minerals. Feeding of small amount of leafy forages improves the appearance of pigs.

Non-Conventional Feeds

Due to short supply of conventional feeds different kinds of weed seeds, kernels, fruits and extraction residues have been identified for the feeding of livestock during the past half contury. These are minor oil seed cakes, fruits and vegetable processing wastes, sugar mill byproducts, forest products, aquatic plants, animal wastes, marine animal byproducts and others.

Most of the non-conventional feeds are poor sources of nutrients either due to low digestibility or due to harmful effects of antinutritional factors. Available information about the chemical composition and nutritive value of the some of the non-conventional feeds are provided in the following order:

1. *Minor oil seeds and cakes*: These are deoiled salseed meal, mahua seed, neem seed cake, rubber seed cake, nahar seed cake and bijada cake. Tannin is a common antinutritional factor in almost all these feeds. There are also feed specific antinutritonal factors in many of these feeds.

2. *Fruits and vegetable processing wastes*: The fruits and vegetable processing wastes suitable for the feeding of pigs are mango seed kernel, pine apple bran, rejected banana, residue of ripen jackfruit, jackfruit seeds, apple pomace, tomato pomace and citrus fruit pulp etc.
3. Sugar mill byproducts are molasses, press mud and yeast sludge.
4. *Forest products*: These are ripen fruits of mahua, flowers of mahua, ripen fruits of wild fig, gular, peepal, bargad etc.
5. Aquatic plants include lemna, azolla, hydrilla, spirulina, pistia and water hyacinth etc. These are fed in small quantity because energy content is quite low in most of the aquatic plants.
6. Marine animal byproducts include fish waste, frog trash and prawn wastes.
7. Animal byproducts include meals prepared from fallen animals, slaughter house byproducts and wastes etc.
8. Miscellaneous byproducts include Brewers grains, date stone, tamarind seeds, silk worm pupa meal and sago processing residues etc.

Non conventional feeds are used in small quantity. Necessary processing is done for the removal or inactivation of antinutritional and harmful factors. Too many non conventional feeds are not included together. For the better utilization of non conventional feeds pelleting should be done. Sugar cane molasses is used for masking the unpleasant taste and increasing the palatability of diets containing non-conventional feeds.

Nutritional Constituents of Swine Diet

Like feeds of any other simple stomached mammalian species the diets of swine include sources of carbohydrates, proteins, lipids, minerals and vitamins. The carbohydrates and lipids are the main sources of energy and protein metabolism is diverted for energy supply only when diets are deficient in energy or pigs are starving due to clinical reasons.

Carbohydrates

Since pigs are unable to utilize large amount of fibrous carbohydrates they are provided starch and other digestible carbohydrates for providing greater proportion of energy requirement. In the diet of suckling piglets, lactose available in sow's milk is the main source of highly digestible carbohydrate. On introduction of solid feeds, grains and their byproducts are the main sources of dietary energy. Lactose fermentation in the gastrointestinal tract of the young pigs produces acidic environment due to production of lactic acid which promotes the absorption of calcium, phosphorus and other minerals. The utilization of sucrose and starch is quite less in the young piglets. It is preferred to incorporate lactose in the milk replacers and pre-starter (creep) rations of piglets weaned at 4-5 weeks of age and also for the feeding of orphaned piglets and those from the agalactic sows.

The fibre digestion potential of pigs of all age group is very low due to lack of adequate amount of fibre digesting enzymes like cellulase and hemicellulase. These enzymes are synthesized by the gastroenteric microorganisms which are very few in the large intestine of pigs. The energy contribution of dietary fibres for body functions is very little and crude fibre content should not exceed 10 per cent even in the diets of adult pigs.

The carbohydrates are very sensitive component of the diets of very young nursing piglets. Inadequate supply of milk in large litters may cause hypoglycemia due to deficiency of lactose supply. Thus, special care is required in the supplementary feeding of baby pigs and diets for such piglets should contain sufficient quantity of lactose or dried milk powder or milk of other mammalian species.

High fibre diets some times fed during scarcity conditions results in the partial energy starvation. This causes lowered growth rate, craving for food, unthriftiness and poor carcass quality.

Lipids

These include different fats and oils and are condensed sources of energy capable of supplying about 2.25 times more metabolizable energy when compared to carbohydrates and proteins. The most important roles of lipids in the swine nutrition are the absorption and metabolism of fat soluble vitamins A,D, E and K, and the supply of essential fatty acids i.e. linoleic and arachidonic acids. For optimum performance swine diets should contain more than 2 per cent fat in the diets on dry matter basis.

A deficiency of fat in the diet causes occurrence of fat soluble vitamin deficiency symptoms and the symptoms of essential fatty acid deficiency. The common fatty acid deficiency symptoms in growing pigs are dullness, dry and rough coat, characteristic scaly dandruff like skin. If diet is not corrected, the condition progresses and characterized by deposition of brownish pasty exudate around the ears, axillary space and under the flanks finally resulting in the erosion and necrosis of the skin and tail. The growth is slow and sexual development specially in males is impaired.

Proteins

Being simple stomached animal pigs are unable to synthesize several amino acids essential for the normal physiological functions like growth and reproduction. These amino acids are called essential or indispensable amino acids. Among the nine essential amino acids i.e. histidine, isoleucine, leucine, lysine, methionine, phenylalanine, threonine, tryptophan and valine, three amino acids-lysine, tryptophan and threonine have been identified as critical amino acids for the cereal based diets. Arginine is not essential in the diets of pigs.

The deficiency of protein and more specifically the amino acids results in retarded growth, rough body coat, anaemia and lowered resistance against the infectious diseases. The other signs are hypoproteinaemia, delayed healing of wounds and infertility.

Minerals

Common feedstuffs of natural and cultivated sources absorb a large number of minerals and many of these minerals are absorbed in the body from feeds but all are not essential for the animals. So far seven major and six trace elements were recognized essential for the normal functions upto middle of the previous century. Later on four more trace elements were found essential. After 1970 few more trace elements have been identified to contribute in the body functions but detail metabolic role is yet to be concluded. The minerals required less than 100 mg per kg dry matter of the diet are delineated as micro, minor or trace elements.

The seven macro minerals are calcium, phosphorus, potassium, sodium, sulphur, chlorine and magnesium in descending order of concentration in the body of animals. The trace elements are iron, zinc, copper, iodine, manganese and cobalt in which molybdenum, selenium, chromium and fluorine were added during the third quarter of the twentieth century. The role of some more trace elements like arsenic, boron, lead, lithium, nickel, silicon, tin (stanus) and vanadium has been observed in later studies but detail functions in different species of farm animals are still in progress and may take some more time.

Calcium (Ca)

Calcium is the main mineral element in the body and almost 99 per cent is used for the development of skeletal system. The remaining one percent is distributed in the cells and tissue fluid pools. The other functions of calcium are the coagulation of blood, transmission of nerve impulses, muscle contraction and in various enzyme systems. Blood calcium is present in plasma and optimum level of plasma is maintained by mobilization of calcium from the long bones in conditions of dietary deficiency. In the body of animals metabolism of calcium is dependent on the calcium : phosphorus ratio and the supply of vitamin D. The minerals in bones are not fixed permanently and exchange of calcium between the bones and other tissues is a continuous process and it is also regulated by the action of parathyroid hormone in addition to routine function of controlling absorption through the intestine.

Phosphorus (P)

It is another main constituent of skeletal system and about 80 per cent of body phosphorus is the component of bones and teeth. The absorption and utilization in the body depends on the Ca:P ratio and the availability of vitamin D. The phosphorus is also a constituent of phospholipids, phosphoproteins, nucleic acids and blood cells. The important functions of phosphorus in the body other than the bone development are the active role in energy metabolism.

Magnesium (Mg)

It is third mineral constituent of bone alongwith calcium and phosphorus, and more than 70 per cent of magnesium is present in the skeletal system. The magnesium is an important activator of the several enzyme systems in the body and contributes significantly in the metabolism of carbohydrates and lipids. The other important functions are the cellular respiration and energy metabolism.

Potassium (K), Sodium (Na) and Chloride (Cl)

Potassium, sodium and chlorine alongwith biocarbonates are responsible for the maintenance of acid-base equilibrium and osmotic pressure of the body fluids. These are usually present in ionic form. The potassium is cellular cation and sodium is cation in extracellular fluid systems and soft tissues. These are responsible for the excitability of nerves and muscles. The potassium is associated with carbohydrate metabolism and sodium plays an active role in the absorption of sugars and amino acids from the digestive system. The chlorine is coworker of sodium and potassium in the maintenance of acid-base equilibrium and osmotic pressure of the tissues. Chlorine is essential for the synthesis of hydrochloric acid in the gastric juice. Feeds contain adequate amount of potassium and supply of sodium and chlorine is made by supplementation of common salt. However, it should be limited to about 1 per cent of dry matter in the diets and should not exceed 2 per cent otherwise salt poisoning may occur.

Sulphur (S)

Utilization of inorganic sulphur is quite less in pigs but some studies have shown the sparing effect of sulphur containing amino acids to certain extent on the supplementation of organic sulphate.

Trace/Micro/Minor Elements

Iron (Fe)

Although required in minute quantity of less than 30 mg per kg dry matter of the diets, iron is one of the most important elements for the survival. Greater proportion of iron in the body is present in the blood as a component of haemoglobin in the red blood cells and transferrin in the blood serum. Excess iron in the body is stored in the form of ferritin in liver, kidneys, spleen and bone marrow. The another storage compound in the body is haemosiderin. Iron is either constituent or activator in the many enzyme systems in the body.

The main functions of iron are the transportation of oxygen to each living cell and collection of carbon dioxide from cells to lungs for expulsion in the expired air, transportation of electrons through the oxidation reduction function and various enzymes required in energy metabolism and other activities.

Copper (Cu)

Copper is essential for the formation of haemoglobin (Hb) although it is not a constituent of Hb. It is also present in some other enzymes like ceruloplasmin required for the liberation of cellular iron into the plasma. Copper is also present in other blood proteins like erythrocuprein. As a component of cytochrome oxidase enzyme it is involved in oxidative phosphorylation in energy metabolism. It is also a constituent of many pigments and distributed in all cells but liver is the seat of copper storage. Tolerance of copper in pigs is quite high and excess has growth stimulation effects.

Cobalt (Co)

Cobalt is required for the synthesis of vitamin B_{12} by the gut microorganisms. The quantity of vitamin B_{12} (Cyanocobalamin) produced by the enteric microorganisms of pigs is not sufficient to meet the requirements and supplementation is necessary for optimum production.

Iodine (I)

It is essential for the synthesis of triiodothyronine and tetraiodothyronine or thyroxine by the thyroid gland. Supply of amino acid tyrosine is required for the synthesis of thyroid hormones. The element is required in very small quantity and present distributed in the body, but concentration is higher in the thyroid gland. These hormones increase body functions and stimulate basal metabolism, better utilization of nutrients, improved growth and better utilization of oxygen in the body.

Manganese (Mn)

Very minute amount of manganese is required in the diet. Greater proportion of manganese is present in the bones, kidneys, pancreas, liver and pituitary glands. It is activator for several enzymes. Lameness is a sign of manganese deficiency in pigs. This is also associated with glucose metabolism and blood coagulation property of vitamin K.

Zinc (Zn)

Zinc is another important trace element in the diets of pigs. It is distributed in almost all cells of the body and bones are the organ of storage for surplus zinc in the body. The zinc content is more in skin, body coat and skeletal system. Zinc is also constituent of many enzymes and activator of some other enzyme systems. It is required for growth, development of immunity, secretion of hormones and maintenance of electrolyte balance.

Selenium (Se)

Normally diets provide adequate amount of selenium and high levels are toxic. Selenium may replace part of the vitamin E requirement. The requirement of selenium is about 0.1 mg/kg dry matter of the diet.

Vitamins

Both fat soluble vitamins A,D,E and K and some of the water soluble vitamins of b-complex group are essential for the normal functions of pigs. The pigs are capable to synthesize adequate amount of vitamin C from glucose metabolism and dietary supplementation is not required. Among the b-complex group only thiamine, riboflavin, niacin, pantothenic acid, pyridoxine, choline and cyanacobalamine (B_{12}) are dietary essential for the pigs. They do not require supplementation of inositol, biotine, para amino berozoic acid (PABA) and folic acid.

Vitamin A

Pigs are capable of converting cryptoxanthine and carotenes into vitamin A activity. Green herbages are the good source of carotenes. The main functions of vitamin A are the maintenance of optimum growth, visual functions, integrity of epithelial cells and immunity. Liver is the main site of storage of vitamin A and can maintain supply for few months on the feeding of deficient diet. Fish liver oil, viz., shark liver oil and cod liver oil are good sources of vitamin A.

Vitamin D

It is a sunshine vitamin and problems of deficiency in Indian conditions may be only due to intake of some antivitamin D factor. The two natural precursors of vitamin D are the cholicalciferol (D_3) and ergocalciferol (D_2); the former is much potent than the later. The vitamin is essential for the metabolism of calcium and phosphorus for skeletal development. The important functions of vitamin D are the synthesis of calcium and phosphorus binding proteins for bone formation; absorption, mobilization and retention of bone forming mineral elements and maintenance of the functions of immunogenic cells.

Vitamin E

It is a very effective anti-oxidant for the fats and fat soluble vitamins. The various functions of vitamin E is to reduce the production of harmful free radicals from the oxidation of unsaturated fatty acids, synthesis of phospholipids in cell membranes, enhancement of resistance against infections and regulation of oxidation reduction reactions. It may meet part of the requirements of selenium for the protection of phospholipids of cell membranes.

Vitamin K

It is required for the formation of prothrombin and other factors necessary for the clotting of blood. Small amount of vitamin K is present in cereal grains and oil cakes. The animal products, liver and fish meal are the good sources and used in the diets of pigs.

Thiamine (Vitamin B_1)

It is found in the form of thiamin pyrophosphate in animals. The vitamin is highly water soluble and disintegrates in neutral solution. The thiamin pyrophosphate is a coenzyme named cocarboxylase, which is associated with the oxidative carboxylation of pyruvate in the tricarboxylic acid cycle for energy metabolism. It is important for the synthesis of nucleic acids through pentose phosphate pathway. The thiamine is essential for the integration and functions of cell membrane of nerve tissue. It is also involved in the synthesis of acetyl choline and fatty acids.

Cereal grains and their byproducts are good sources of thiamine. The other rich sources are brewers's yeast, liver, kidney, egg yolk and meat.

Riboflavin (B_2)

This is a crystalline compound of low solubility in water. The vitamin is heat stable but easily decomposes on exposure to light. Most of the common feeds are deficient in riboflavin. The important functions are the energy generation from the metabolism of organic constituents i. e. glycogen, glucose, lipids and proteins. It is a component of several enzyme systems in the form of flavin mononucleotide (FMN) and flavin adenine dinucleotide (FAD). The various flavoproteins are resposibe for the transport of hydrogen and electrons in oxidation reduction reactions in the body.

The vitamin is found in all green herbages, yeast, liver and fermented milk. Food grains contain very little amount of riboflavin.

Niacin/Nicotinamide

This vitamin is active in the amide form. The vitamin is highly stable and most affected by acids, alkales, oxidizing agents and heat. This vitamin is an active component of coenzymes, nicotinamide adenine dinucleotide (NAD) and nicotinamide adenine dinucletotide phosphate (NADP) involved in the release of energy from carbohydrates, fats and proteins in the tissue.

Common sources of vitamin are proteinous feeds like liver, yeast, groundnut cake, sunflower cake and feeds supplying higher amount of tryptophan. The vitamin complexed in cereal grains are not easily available to the pigs. However, animals are capable of synthesizing nicotinamide from tryptophan. Therefore, adequate supply of tryptophan should be assured in the diet.

Pantothenic Acid

It is an amide pantoic acid and alanine. The vitamin is a component of coenzyme A. The common feeds are mostly deficient and supplementation is required. It is destroyed by moist heat and loss of its potency is quite high due to pelleting and moist cooking.

The important functions are in the form of coenzymes A and acetyl carrier protein. Antibody production is improved. The coenzyme A is involved in the oxidation of fatty acids for supply of energy and acetyl carrier protein is required for the synthesis of fatty acids. Pantothenic acid is also essential for the synthesis of acetyl choline which is the chemical transmitter at the nerve synapses. It is also associated with the biosynthesis of citric acid and haemoglobin.

The common sources of vitamin are cereal by products, brans, germs, oil seed cakes and sugarcane molasses.

Pyridoxine (B_6)

The vitamin is present in three interconvertible forms of pyridoxol, pyridoxal and pyridoxamine in the tissues. The pyridoxol (Pyridoxine) is more stable than the other two forms (aldehyde and amine).

The various functions of vitamin B6 are the catabolism and synthesis of amino acids, synthesis of biogenic amines, production of energy from the metabolism of carbohydrates, proteins and fats in tricarboxylic acid cycle. The vitamin is involved in a large number of enzymes. It is associated with transportation of amino acids into the body from the intestinal contents.

The common sources are herbages, pulses, cereal grain, yeast, liver and milk in different forms.

Choline

It is produced in liver and absorbs large amount of water. The vitamin is heat tolerant and not destroyed by pelletting, cooking and extrusion. However, it decreases the potency of other vitamins in mixture. The requirement of choline increases with the increase in protein and fat content in diets.

The vitamin is a structural component of cells and phospholipids, and required for the maturation of cartilage matrix of bones. It plays an important role in fat metabolism.

The cereal grains and their by products, green leaves, eggs and yeast are rich sources of choline.

Vitamin B_{12} (Cyanocobalamin)

The synthesis of vitamin B12 by enteric microorganism in pigs is negligible and supplementation is necessary for optimum production. Cobalt is an essential constituent of vitamin B_{12}. Its potency is most affected by minerals in premixed and by pelleting of compounded feeds.

For absorption from the gut the vitamin is found to need a specific glycoprotein called intrinsic factor. The intrinsic factor is secreted by the gastric mucosa. It is a coenzyme in many enzyme systems. It is required for the biosynthesis of methionine, choline and folacin. It is associated with the synthesis of methyl group, and purine, pyrimidine and proteins. The sources of vitamin B_{12} are only animal and fish products. It is not found in any feeds of plant origin.

Feed Additives

Some organic and inorganic substances are used in small quantity in the diets of pigs for (i) the stimulation of growth, (ii) improvement of feed utilization efficiency and (iii) protection of animals from subclinical infectious diseases. In recent past some herbal products have also been incorporated in the list of feed additives. These are mostly used for lean meat production.

These feed additives may be placed under different categories on the basis of their chemical nature, action on the tissues, protection from diseases, improvement of performance and production of desired quality of pork.

Antibiotics

Some of the antibiotics used in small quantity for the improvement of performance are oxytetracycline, chlorotetracycline, zinc *bacitracin*, flavomycin, virginiamycin, lincomycin and avilamycin etc. However, use of antibiotics as a growth promoter is being discouraged and in many countries their use as feed additives has been banned due to (a) possibility of adverse effects of antibiotic residue in pork on the health of consumer and (b) the development of antibiotic resistant pathogens hazardous for human health.

Antioxidants

These are mixed in high fat diets for preventing oxidative changes (rancidity) because (a) rancidity decreases palatability of feeds, (b) lowers the availability of nutrients, and (c) reduces the activity of fat soluble vitamins A, D, E and also biotin. Besides being important nutrients vitamin E and C, and selenium are good antioxidants. Some of the synthetic antioxidants are the butylated hydroxyl anisole (BHA), butylated hydroxyl toluene (BHT) and ethoxyquin.

Copper sulphate

The tolerance for copper in pigs is very high (about 250mg/kg dry matter of diet) and it has growth promoting effect. Although greater proportion of dietary copper is excreted in faeces but in the digestive system it improves the availability of nutrients by changing the microbial environment. This results in better growth and feed utilization efficiency. Now it is not used in many countries.

Probiotics (Direct-fed microorganisms, DFM)

The direct-fed microbes include Aspergillus oryzae, Bifidobacterium bifidinum, some species of lactobacillus (*L. acidophilus, L. bulgaricus, L. casei* and *L. plantarum*), some species of streptococci (Streptococcus diacetylactis, Str. faecium, and Str. lactis), and several strains of Saccharomyces cerevisiae. These probiotics multiply at a fast rate and suppress the growth of harmful microorganisms in the digestive tract. Thus, releases the stress resulting in improved performance.

Arsenicals

Earlier some arsenic compounds like phenyl arsenic acid, parahydroxy phenyl arsenic acid and 3 –nitro-4-hydroxyphenyl arsenic acid were used at a very low level (0.05 to 0.02 per cent of the dry feed) increased growth (Carpenter, 1951) but the effect was non consistent (Hanson *et al.*, 1951). Now it is not used in the diets of pigs in many countries.

Hormones

Thyroidectomy and feeding of goiterogenic compounds like thiouracil favour faster fattening and better feed utilization efficiency in the later part of the finishing period. However, with the increase in the demand for lean meat, use of goitrogens is not favoured.

Growth stimulating effect of oestrogens has been utilized for better finishing and feed utilization efficiency. However, uncontrolled feeding of some forages containing oestrongenic activity may be harmful.

Measures of Protein and Energy System

Since pigs are simple stomached animals, the formulation of their diets requires special consideration of protein quality and availability of essential amino acids and energy besides balancing for minerals and vitamins.

Ideal Protein System

The diets of pigs reared in intensive system contain greater proportion of grains and oilseed cakes supplemented with small amount of proteinous feeds of animal origin for balancing the limiting amino acids. Although crude protein system is quite satisfactory but does not provide precise information about the content of essential amino acids. Of late, a modification of chemical score has been evolved on the basis of the amino acid pattern of a reference tissue of the pig muscles. This has been defined as "ideal protein". The values of essential amino acids in reference to ideal protein suggested by Agricultural Research Council of the commonwealth Agricultural Bureau (1981) are presented in Table 2. These values are used for the determination of the quantity of limiting amino acid (s) from the protein for balancing the diets.

Table 2 : Balance of amino acids (g/kg) in ideal proteinous feeds recommended by ARC (1981).

Amino acid	Amount (g/kg)	Amino acid	Amount (g/kg)
Lysine	70	Isolencine	38
Leucine	70	Methionine	35
Phenylalanine	67	Histidine	23
Valine	49	Tryptophan	10
Threonine	42	Non essential AA	596

Note : In this score the amount of methionine and phenylalanine should not be less than half of the recommended value as the part of methionine can be replaced by cystine and part of phenylalanine by nonessential tyrosine.

The concept of ideal protein envisages the supply of correct rations of essential amino acids in balance with the availability of non-essential amino acids so that excess protein is not fed. In this system there is no scope of feeding excess of any amino acid. This may be harmful in some cases. Therefore, supply of any essential amino acid should not be allowed to exceed 20 per cent of reference value. The reference values of amino acids in the diets for growth, pregnancy, lactation and maintenance will be different in the reference protein. This concept still requires more exercise for optimization. Therefore, in practical diet formulation the supply of total protein and essential amino acids in the true proportions should be assured.

Energy System for Pigs

The various systems for depicting the energy content in the diets of pigs are the classical old system of total digestible nutrients (TDN) and later evolved systems of digestible energy (DE) and metabolizable energy (ME). Since grains and oil cakes are the common constituents of swine diets, there is less scope of significant deviation in the ratio of DE and ME due to dietary levels of less digestible fibrous feeds. For most of the common feeds of pigs the ME value is about 96 per cent of the DE value. However, in case of brood adult sows and mature boars the value may reduce to 90 per cent as sufficient quantity of succulent greens are fed for satiety. Therefore, any of the three systems may be used for the formulation of diets for the feeding of pigs.

Feeding Standards for Pigs

In most of the countries feeding standards suggested by National Research Council (NRC) of USA or Agriculture Research Council (ARC) of UK are followed. In India, Bureau of Indian Standards has also suggested a standard for the feeding of pigs. However, this standard is less precise than the earlier two standards, and needs more exercises for the development of a precise feeding standard for pigs. The three feeding standards are summarized as follows:

Feeding of Neonatal Piglets

Feeding piglets in early life upto 5 weeks of age requires some special consideration in the selection of feed ingredients for the formulation of pre-starter or creep rations due to the following reasons:

- The sow's (mother's) milk is deficient in iron and body reserve in most of the piglets is inadequate to meet the demand for erythropoiesis in early life.
- The activity of salivary amylase is meager in the first week of life. It shows a little increase during the second and third week of life and then

again declines. The salivary amylase activity, therefore, has little significance in starch digestion.

- Despite the presence of peptic and parietal cells in gastric glands there is significant proteolytic activity in gastric juice upto second week of life. However, it has a significant merit in helping the absorption of immunoglobulin present in the colostrum.
- The pancreatic secretion contains nominal activities of amylase, lipase, trypsin and chymotrypsin upto 3, 2, 4 and 2 weeks of life respectively (Corring *et al.*, 1978).
- The brush border of the cells of small intestine contains six types of carbohydrases, viz. lactase, trehalase, sucrase, two types of maltase and isomaltase. However, activity of lactase is maximum at birth and then starts decreasing gradually. The activities of sucrase, isomaltase and two types of maltase start during second to third week of life but that of trehalase upto 5th weeks of life (Kidder and Manners, 1980).
- Transport of sodium (Na) ion across the intestine decreases sharply after the intake of colostrum but simultaneously increases across the colon mucosa. This happens due to damage of the cells of small intestine due to pinocytosis of the colostral antibodies.

Therefore, it is important to consider the supply of iron and digestible carbohydrate (Lactose followed by sucrose, and maltose). The scope of starch utilization in considerable amount is only after 5 weeks of age. Indeed, some amounts of starchy grains are used in prestarter diets for the development of microbial digestion in the large intestines.

Feeding of Adult Pigs

With the increase in the age the pattern of digestion in the pigs particularly that of carbohydrates is almost reversed. The digestion of lactose comes down to only about 15 per cent of the initial by 5 weeks of age while that of sucrose becomes more than 200 times and maltose more than 80 times of the initial at birth.

In natural habitat pig is an omnivorous animal but domestication has made it almost herbivorous although fibre handling capacity is low. This change in food habits has favoured considerable development of microbial digestion in the large intestines. The microbial digestion starts in the stomach itself and traces of volatile fatty acids (VFA) may be observed in the stomach and small intestine but considerable amount is produced only in the caecum and colon. (Arganzio and Southworth, 1975). The pigs reared on scavenging and ranges consume different types of roots, tubers and tender leafy plants, and also aquatic plants like azolla, lemna and water hyacinth etc.

Formulations of Compounded Diets for Different Classes of Pigs

The various diets will include prestarter, starter, grower, finisher and diets for pregnant and lactating gilts and sows, and breeding boars.

Pre-Starter Diets

Special care is taken for the supply of iron and lactose. A pre starter diet is introduced in the second week of life and fed up to 4th week of life. A few examples are presented in Table 3.

Table 3 : Composition of pre-starter diets (%).

Ingredients	1	2	3
Dried skim milk	40.0	30.0	40
Ground maize	30.0	30.0	30
Ground soyabean cake	10.0	10.0	-
Groundnut cake	-	10.0	10.0
Fish meal	8.0	8.0	10.0
Molasses	10.0	10.0	8.0
Mineral mixture	1.5	1.5	1.5
Common salt	0.5	0.5	0.5
Vitamin premix	as per manufactures recommendations		

NB : 1. Brewers's yeast may be used @ 1 per each. Other probiotics may also be used.
2. If hygienic condition is not satisfactory antibiotics may be supplemented.

Starter Diets

These are fed from 5th week to weaning at 6 to 8 weeks of age. By this age carbohydrate and protein utilizing enzymes are secreted in adequate quantity. The piglets are now capable of digesting starch, sugars and proteins efficiently due to which lactose rich ingredient like skim milk powder can be safely replaced by an energy rich cereal like maize, wheat, sorghum and rice etc. A few examples of starter diets are presented in Table 4.

Creep Ration

The high protein-high energy balanced diets fed inside the creep to suckling piglets are known as creep rations. These include both pre-starter and starter diets fed upto weaning. The name creep ration has been derived from structure allowing the entrance and exit of piglets but preventing the dam. The structure is called creep. An example of creep ration worked out by Pathak and Raujhan (1972) is given in Table 5.

Table 4 : Composition of starter diets (%).

Ingredients	1	2	3	4
Ground maize	68	38	30	-
Ground wheat	-	30	20	50
Ground barley	-	-	18	18
Skim milk powder	10	-	-	-
Fish meat	-	10	10	10
Soybean cake	20	-	-	20
Groundnut cake	-	20	20	-
Mineral mixture	1.5	1.5	1.5	1.5
Common salt	0.5	0.5	0.5	0.5
Vitamin premix	as per manufactures recommendations			

Note : Probiotics and antimicrobials may be used as per the requirements.

Table 5 : Composition of creep ration

Ingredients	Amount (%)
Fine ground yellow maize	40.0
Skim milk powder	10.0
Groundnut cake	10.0
Sesame cake	10.0
Wheat bran	10.0
Molasses	10.0
Fish meal	10.0
	per 100 kg
Brewers yeast	6.0
Mineral mixture	2.0
Common salt	1.5
Vitamin premix	As per manufactures recommendations

Note : 1. Total fat should be more than 2% and preferably 5 per cent.
2. Maize may be replaced upto 25 percent with ground wheat, dehusked barley, pearl millet, broker rice.
3. Groundnut cake can be replaced with soyabean cake.

Growers Diets

In Indian conditions three different types of grower diets are used for the growing pigs reared under intensive system. These are (A) cereal based diets, (B) grainless diets and (C) grower diets containing non-conventional feeds.

Cereal Based Grower Diets

These diets contain about 18 per cent protein balanced for essential amino acids and 3200-3300 Kcal digestible energy (DE). A few examples are presented in Table 6.

Table 6 : Per cent composition of cereal based grower diets

Ingredients	1	2	3	4
Crushed maize	60.0	60.0	50.0	40.0
Crushed groundnut cake	20.0	20.0	20.0	20.0
Wheat bran	-	10.0	10.0	15.0
Fish meal	8.5	8.0	8.0	8.0
Molasses	10.0	-	10.0	15.0
Mineral mixture	1.5	1.5	1.5	1.5
Common salt	0.5	0.5	0.5	0.5
Vitamin premix				

Note : 1. About half of maize may be replaced with crushed wheat, white sorghum or broken rice.
2. Groundnut cake may be replaced with soyabean cake but only 25 per cent by mustard rapeseed cake.
3. Deoiled rice bran may be incorporated upto 10 per cent in place of wheat bran.

Grainless Diets for Growers

The main ingredient of these diets is wheat bran and various formulations contain about 17 per cent crude protein and 2900 kcal DE. A few examples are given in Table 7.

Table 7 : Percent composition of grainless diets for growing pigs

Ingredients	1	2	3	4
Wheat bran	60.0	40.0	85.0	70.0
Deoiled rice bran	-	20.0	-	-
Ground nut cake	15.0	15.0	7.0	7.0
Fish meal/meat meal	8.0	8.0	6.0	6.0
Molasses	15.0	15.0	-	15.0
Mineral mixture	1.5	1.5	1.5	1.5
Common salt	0.5	0.5	0.5	0.5
Vitamin premix	As per recommendation			

NB : Incorporation of deoiled rice bran at higher level (more than 50%) may result in retarded growth

Grower Diets Containing Non-Conventional Feeds

A few non conventional feeds like deoiled sal seed meal, detoxified mahua seed cake and treated neem seed cake may be incorporated upto 10 per cent level. However, diets should be adjusted for balancing. Only one non-conventional feed should be used at a time.

Finisher Diets

The eating capacity of pigs increases considerably by the terminal stage of growing period. Therefore, pigs are able to compensate energy requirement by increasing intake of a low energy diet (Pathak and Ranjhan, 1973, Bhar *et al.*, 2000). Like grower diets, finisher diets are also (A) cereal based, (B) grainless and (C) containing non conventional feeds.

Cereal Based Finisher Diets

The protein level of diets for feeding during finishing period is reduced to about 14 per cent to meet the requirements during 35 to 90 kg body weight in fast growing breeds (Table 8).

Table 8 : Per cent composition of cereal based grower diets

Ingredients	1	2	3	4
Crushed maize	60.0	65.0	45.0	35.0
Deoiled GN cake	10.0	10.0	10.0	7.0
Wheat bran	13.0	13.0	25.0	50.0
Fish meal	5.0	5.0	5.0	6.0
Molasses	10.0	5.0	13.0	-
Mineral mixture	1.5	1.5	1.5	1.5
Common salt	0.5	0.5	0.5	0.5
Vitamin premix	As per recommendation			

Note: Almost half of the maize may be replaced with wheat, dehusked barley, sorghum and about 25-30 per cent with pearl millet and minor millets.
2. Deoiled groundnut cake can be replaced with soyabean cake and upto 50 per cent with sesame cake, linseed cake, cotton seed cake or mustard cake etc.

Grainless Finisher Diets

The replacement of cereal grains with wheat straw brings down the DE value from 3250 to 2900 kcal per kg. However, energy intake is compensated by higher intake (Ranjhan *et al.*, 1972; Bhar *et al.*, 2000). Incorporation of deoiled rice bran in place of wheat bran causes drastic reduction in palatability and pigs are unable to perform. A few examples of palatable grainless finisher diets are presented in Table 9.

Table 9 : Percent composition of grainless finisher diets

Ingredients	1	2	3	4
Wheat bran	61.0	71.0	83.0	92.0
Deoiled rice bran	15.0	10.0	-	-
Molasses	15.0	10.0	7.5	-
Fish meal	7.0	7.0	7.5	6.0
Mineral mixture	1.5	1.5	1.5	1.5
Common salt	0.5	0.5	0.5	0.5
Vitamins premix	As per manufacturers guide			

Finisher Diets Containing Non Conventional Feeds

Non conventional feeds like deoiled salseed meal, mangoseed kernel cake and treated neem seed cake can be incorporated from 10 to 30 per cent without much decrease in palatability. However, growth rate is reduced and pigs take significantly longer period for finishing. Total cereal replacement by salseed meal from a diet containing 40 per cent maize has been demonstrated (Pathak and Ranjhan, 1973).

Diets for Pregnant Gilts and Sows

Pregnant gilts and sows of more than 100 kg body weight require 2.5 and 2.0 kg dry feed per day respectively when diets contain 13-14 per cent CP and 3250 kcal per kg DE. Requirement of gilts is higher than the sow for supporting growth of relatively younger animals. Finisher diets are equally suitable for the pregnant sows and gilts. However, use of mustard cake, linseed cake and raw soyabean meal should be avoided. The amount of grainless diets should be increased to 3.0 and 2.5 kg daily for pregnant gilts and sows respectively.

Diets of Lactating Sows

The diets of lactating (nursing) sows should contain about 15-16 per cent CP and 3200-3300 kcal DE per kg air dry feed. The first farrowed sows and mature sows are offered 2.5 and 2.0 kg feed daily alongwith additional amount of 0.2 kg per piglet suckling the dam. However, total diet should not be less than 3 kg daily.

A few examples of diets for nursing sows are given in Table 10. Adult females are able to tolerate up to 10 per cent crude fibre in the diets provided balancing is done for the supply of nutrients.

Table 10 : Percent composition of diets for lactating sows

Ingredients	1	2	3	4
Crushed maize	60.0	50.0	40.0	30.0
Wheat bran	20.0	21.0	27.0	53.0
Groundnut cake	10.0	9.0	8.0	7.0
Fish meal	8.0	8.0	8.0	8.0
Molasses	-	10.0	15.0	20.0
Mineral mixture	1.5	1.5	1.5	1.5
Common salt	0.5	0.5	0.5	0.5
Vitamins premix				

Note: 1. Maize can be replaced with all edible cereal grains. In case of barley wheat bran should also be replaced.
2. Other conventional cakes except those containing goitrogens may be fed.

Feeding Pigs on Scavenging

Even today it is the most popular system of pig production in India and many other countries. The scavenging system of pig production is almost zero input method for feeding. The system is highly variable and influenced by region, foods of humans, cropping systems, availability of natural grassland, forest cover and proportion of fruits and seeds producing trees in the agro-forestry plantation, area under seasonal and perennial water sources and types of aquatic herbages, food grain, fruits and vegetable markets, Dhabas, halwai shops, road side small restaurants, snack huts and tea huts etc. It is also affected by urban, periurban and rural habitats.

The scavenging system of pig production has been referred frequently in the litratures, but precise information are not available. On the strong recommendations of the author scavenging system of hog raising was included in the technical programmes of the All India Coordinated Project on Pig in its annual workshop at Veterinary College, Tirupathi in 1980. Some sporadic studies were conducted at 2 or 3 centers but nothing substantial could be contributed. Indeed the system is continuing and in all ill designed economic management putting almost one-fourth of population of various levels of under feeding, intermittent starvation and malnutrition the scavenging system of pig production will continue for quite some time.

A few systems of pig feeding on scavenging have been described briefly (Pathak and Ranjhan, 1988; Pathak and Kamra, 1989). There is no quantitative information and only qualitative aspects have been given.

Scavenging in Urban Areas

Free roaming pigs can be frequently seen in almost all urban locale starting from small towns to old habitation of even metropolitan cities except at some rare places where pig rearing in urban area has been banned.

The families associated with pig rearing live in small clusters of mostly small houses with some enclosure with shade for herding pigs in the night. All age group of pigs including nursing sows with two weeks old litter are let loose early in the morning before sun rise. The groups of pigs start roaming in search of edible garbage in lanes, streets and vicinity of sweets shops, milk processing shops, restaurants and hotels etc. This is followed by visit to fruits and vegetable markets and then to grain markets. Most of the animals retire beneath a shade for 6-7 hours from 10 or 11 a.m. and again come out for scavenging between 4 to 7 pm in different seasons being early in winter and late in the summer. In evening most of the pigs return to their respective shades for night or may wait for the next day.

The garbage available for feeding is highly variable and may include household residues, sweet shop residues, hotel wastes, spoiled and damaged fruits, roots, tubers and vegetables, pomace from fruit juice vendor, animal excreta, slaughter house byproducts and all such wastes thrown at the garbage collection places or elsewhere.

Scavenging in Peri-Urban Areas

The system is more or less similar to urban areas but in many regions even today plenty of night soil voided early in the morning nearby the locality is consumed by the scavenging pigs. The availability of fruits and vegetable wastes is less but other herbages are available. At many places in periurban areas seasonal water ditches and pits provide edible and nutritious aquatic plants and their succulent roots and tubers etc.

Scavenging in Rural Areas

It is highly variable and crop dependent. One of the major sources of nutrients supply is the night soil. This is supplemented with flowers (mahua flower), wild fruits, nuts, seeds, kernels, roots, tubers, herbages and aquatic plants.

In sugar cane growing areas finishing pigs are herded near the jaggery making plants, crushers and sugar mills. The pigs are offered *ad libitum* amount of scum and molasses to supplement pasturing.

In some states of north-east region, West Bengal, Orissa, Jharkhand and Chhattishgarh some nomadic tribes roam in limited area. Some families camp for short time near human habitats and then move. The camping duration ranges from 15 days to 30 days depending on the availability of food resources for their pigs.

In coastal areas coconut waste, fish trash, roots, berries and herbages are the foods for scavenging pigs.

Metabolic and Nutritional Deficiency Diseases

Several metabolic and nutritional deficiency diseases may be encountered during pig raising. The causes of metabolic diseases are mostly physiological disturbances, whereas deficiency diseases are caused by either low supply of nutrients or interference of other nutrients reducing the availability. Some of the conditions encountered in pig production are described briefly.

Hypoglycemia of Neonatal Piglets

This condition is observed in piglets of low birth weight either due to premature birth or due to very large litter size. The occurrence is higher in winter season due to higher demand of heat production to keep the body warm. The first week of life require special care because stored energy in the form of liver glycogen and fat is quite low at birth and metabolism of glycogen and fat (gluconeogenesis) fails to meet the energy requirement for vital functions in the body.

Diseases Caused by Vitamin Deficiency

The common symptoms of deficiency diseases caused by hypovitaminosis are presented in Table 11.

Table 11: Diseases caused by deficiency of vitamins

Vitamins	Deficiency diseases/symptoms
Vitamin A	• Appearance of signs of nerve degeneration like inability to stand properly, incoordination, muscular spasms and staggering gait. • Xerophthalmia or complete blindness on prolonged deficiency • Prolonged deficiency during pregnancy results in birth of weak, deformed or dead litter. • Loss of appetite, slow growth and decreased resistance against pathogenic infections.

Contd...

Vitamin D	Impaired metabolism of calcium and phosphorus leading to rickets in young and osteomalacia in adults.
Vitamin E	• Nutritional myopathy or muscular dystrophy • Cardiac dysfunction often leading to cardiac failure
Riboflavin	Loss of appetite, poor growth, vomiting, dermatitis, crooked legs, stiffness in joints and ocular disorders.
Niacin	Anorexia, poor growth, enteritis, vomiting and dermatitis.
Pyridoxine	Inappetance, slow growth, anaemia, weakness and convulsions
Pantothenic acid	Diarrhoea, poor growth, scaly skin, alopecia and goose stepping is characteristic sign
Biotin	Alopecia, dry and scaly skin, lowered feed intake, poor growth and reproductive disorders in sows
Choline	Fatty infiltration of liver, retarded growth
Vitamin B_{12}	Slow growth, weakness and incoordination in young piglets; dermatitis, loss of appetite, rough coat and weakness in growing-finishing pigs.

Diseases Caused by Mineral Deficiency

Common disorders caused by the deficiency of various dietary essential minerals are presented in Table 12.

Table 12 : Disorders caused by mineral deficiency

Minerals	Deficiency disorders
Calcium and phosphorus	1. Rickets in young and slow growth 2. Osteomalacia in aged 3. Reproductive disorders in sows
Sodium	1. Reduced growth 2. Impaired utilization of energy and protein
Chlorine	1. Alkalosis
Iron	Anaemia, piglet anaemia
Iodine	Goitre, alopecia, birth of hairless litter, stillbirth
Copper	Anaemia, slow growth, skeletal deformity in youngs, scour etc.
Manganese	Poor growth, skeletal deformities, ataxia, lameness, and reproductive insufficiency leading to failure in prolonged deficiency
Zinc	Loss of appetite, poor growth, decreased feed conversion efficiency and dermatitis (Parakeratosis)
Selenium	Mulbery heart disease, hepatic necrosis, hepatosis dietetica causing death.

References

ARC (1981). Agricultural Research Council. Commonwealth Agricultural Bureau.

Argenwzio, R.A. and Southworth, M. (1975). *Am. J. Physiol.*, 228: 454-460.

Bhar, R, Pathak, N.N. and Paul, S. (2000). *Asian-Aust. J. Anim. Sci.*, 13: 1429-1432.

Carpenter, L.E. (1951). *Arch Biochem. and Biophys.*, 32: 181-186.

Corring,T., Aumaitre, A. and Durand, G. (1978). *Pancreas and pancreative enzymes. Nutrition and Metabolism*, 22:231-243.

Hanson, L.E.1953. *59th Annual Report Nebrraska Agril exp st.*, pp.60-61.

Kidder, D.E and Manners, M.J. (1980). *Brit. J. Nutri.*, 43:141-153.

NRC(1988). *Nutrient requirements of pigs*. National Research Council, Washington,D.C.

Pathak, N.N. and Kamra,D.N.(1989). In "Livestock Feeding in Tropics". Cosmo Publications, New Delhi.

Pathak, N.N. and Ranjhan, S.K. (1972). *Indian J. Anim. Sci.*, 32: 1048-1052.

Pathak, N.N. and Ranjhan, S.K. (1973). *Ind. J. of Anim. Sci.*, 43: 424-428.

Pathak, N.N and Ranjhan, S.K. (1988). Shookar poshan. Indian council of Agricultural Research.Krishi Anusandhan Bhavan-I, Pusa, New Delhi.

□□□

Animal Nutrition, 2012
eds. Dr. (Mrs.) Usha R. Mehra et al., pp. 163-184
Satish Serial Publishing House e-mail : info@satishserial.com; website : www.satishserial.com

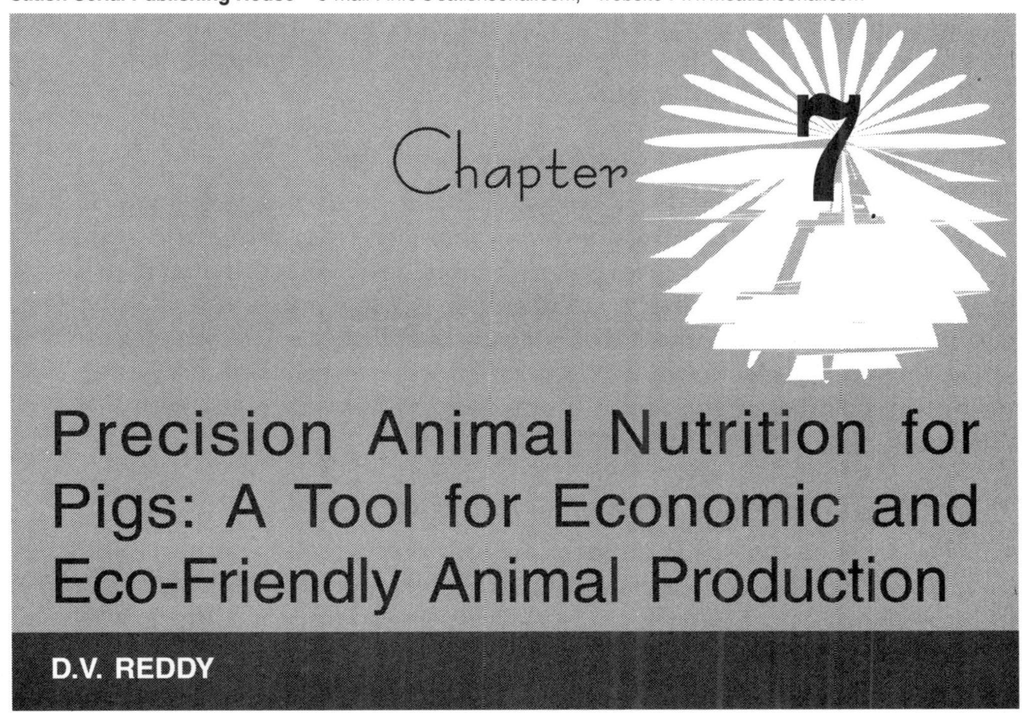

Precision Animal Nutrition for Pigs: A Tool for Economic and Eco-Friendly Animal Production

D.V. REDDY

One of the main objectives of raising livestock and poultry is to produce unadulterated wholesome animal products to the consumers as a profitable enterprise with least contribution to climate change. Precision animal nutrition (PAN) is defined as providing the animal with the feed that precisely meet its nutritional requirements for optimum productive efficiency to produce better quality animal products, and to contribute cleaner environment and thereby ensure profitability (Reddy and Krishna, 2009).

Economic Growth and Demand for Livestock Products

Economic activity has remained dynamic in the developing countries. Indian economy has experienced an accelerated growth of 9% in the recent years till global meltdown in the later part of 2008. As income grows the people are likely to consume more animal products with their diets. There is demand for a variety of animal products. Further, it is impossible to cope with the demand from only poultry, sheep or goats. Hence, pork production deserves encouragement following the precision animal nutrition practices.

The consumer led demand for animal products (Delgado *et al.*, 1999) is defining a new world order for feed characterized by low global grain and oilseed reserves, and high feed demand.

Effect of Stress on Animal Productivity

There are a multitude of stressors in swine production such as high temperature, over crowding, immune challenge, handling and transport. Selection of animals for improved growth rate and feed conversion efficiency is associated with a number of undesirable consequences and the increased susceptibility to environmental changes is one of them. The adverse effect of stress includes high mortality, decreased feed consumption and poor body weight gain. Minimizing stress to animals improves weight gain and feed efficiency (FAO 1999; LPES 2005).

Tools to Achieve Precision Animal Nutrition

The tools to achieve PAN include more precise ration formulation based on nutritional value of each batch of ingredients, proper weighing and mixing of ingredients, use of nutricines feed additives and improved feed processing techniques, implementing phase feeding and split-sex feeding. PAN seems to be the only way to improve the productivity of animals in developing countries by effective utilization of available feed resources with the aim of maximizing the animals' response to nutrients. It is generally agreed that the more feed an animal consumes each day, the greater will be the opportunity for increasing its daily production, which is dependent upon improving the digestibility.

Precise Ration Formulation

Nutrient allowances vary according to three factors, namely, live weight, gender and reproductive state. Nutrient requirements are influenced by many dietary and environmental factors and hence, modification of the allowances needs updating periodically. Factors that influence nutrient requirements include potential for lean tissue growth, propensity for fat deposition, metabolic efficiency of nutrient utilization, demands created by the environmental temperature to maintain thermal homeostasis, metabolic costs of immunological responses, expenditures associated with voluntary activity and nutrient needs of reproductive functions such as foetal development and milk production.

For ease of formulation, it is a common practice to express requirements on the basis of concentration, usually as a percent. It is then assumed that sufficient feed will be consumed to provide the absolute quantity of each nutrient needed each day. However, the demand for metabolizable energy (ME) is influenced by environmental temperature. The quantity of feed consumed is again dependent on the energy density of the diet. Addition of fat increases energy density, while addition of fibre or high-moisture feedstuffs dilutes energy concentration. Hence, nutrient to calorie ratio assumes importance. When expressed as a percentage of the diet, amino acid requirements are higher for maximal leanness than for maximal gain, higher for gilts than for barrows, decrease with age and increase with caloric density of the diet. Amino acid requirements are affected by protein level in the diet and are related to the pig's daily rate of protein accretion (Easter et al., 1996). To support optimum growth and reproduction, vitamins and minerals do play significant role. Many mineral interactions also exist. Hence, precise ration formulation should take care of these valid points.

Nutritional Manipulation for better Pork Products

The objective of pig production is to produce lean, tasty and inexpensive pork products. The body composition of pigs depends on their genetic background, sex and live weight at slaughter, apart from the more influential nutrition. Production of lean and uniform carcasses requires diets optimized for essential nutrients in relation to energy.

Live Weight and Muscle Formation

Daily body protein formation increased up to 40 to 60 kg live weight, which got plateau from 60 up to 120 kg and then decreased towards zero. Daily body fat formation increases almost linearly with increasing body weight. Daily formation of subcutaneous fat exceeds that of muscle between 90 and 100 kg live weight (Just, 1984).

Live Weight and Feed Efficiency

Feed conversion to weight gain is depressed at higher body weights usually because subcutaneous fat contains 7 to 8 Mcal of energy/kg while muscle has only 2 to 2.5 Mcal of energy/kg. The daily gain is reduced also because the fat partly replaces water. Deposition of 1 g fat increases the live weight by 0.5 to 0.7 g, whereas deposition of 1 g protein usually increases daily gain by 2 to 4 g (Just *et al.*, 1982).

Sex and Protein Deposition

Female pigs (gilts) contain more muscle, protein and water in the carcasses than do barrows (male castrates). The percentage of protein decreased and the percentage of fat increased with increasing carcass weight in both sexes (Just, 1984). An optimum rate of protein formation occurs only if the animal's daily intakes of essential nutrients and energy are sufficient.

Feeding Intensity and Body Composition

Just *et al.* (1983b) studied the effect of different feeding intensities below the feeding standards (100, 94, 88, 82, 76 and 70 %) on the chemical composition of pigs. The percentages of dry matter (DM) in empty body and of fat in empty body DM decreased with decreasing feeding intensities, whereas the percentages of protein in empty body DM and physically dissected muscle increased as the level of feeding intensity decreased.

Protein Level and Nutrient Utilization

The study on effect of excess crude protein (CP) in the diets of pigs (the levels tested being 13, 16, 20, 23, 27 and 29% of DM) on their efficiency (Just, 1982a) revealed that increasing levels of CP improved the digestibility of protein and energy. However, the amount and utilization of metabolizable energy were decreased as dietary CP levels increased due to the direct loss of energy in the urine (1.2 kcal/g catabolized CP) and indirect loss energy as heat (1.6 kcal/g catabolized CP). Pigs do not have a requirement for protein as such but they do require a certain amount of digestible amino acids. Therefore, the value of any protein source depends primarily on its digestibility and amino acid composition.

Fibre Level and Body Composition

Increasing the dietary crude fibre levels (varying from 3, 4, 7, 10, 13 to 16% from cereal grains) obviously resulted in varying dietary energy concentrations (from 2.16 to 3.77 Mcal ME/kg DM). The digestive tract contents or gut fill increased 0.4 kg/percentage unit increase in dietary fibre. The pigs fed on the low density diet consumed 1.8 times as much dietary DM as compared to those fed the high density diet to obtain identical live weights through the growth period from 20 to 90 kg (Just, 1982c). With increasing level of crude fibre in the diets, the percentage of muscle in the carcass increased while the percentage of subcutaneous fat decreased.

Fat Level and Body Composition

Inclusion of animal fat in the diets of pigs (varying levels of 4, 8, 12, 16, 20 and 24% of DM) increased the net energy by 1.2 kcal/g digestible crude fat (Just, 1982b). The results of dissection of the carcass indicated that the percentage of muscle decreased and the percentage of subcutaneous fat increased with increasing levels of dietary crude fat. In contrast to the fibrous part of the diets, crude fat is mainly absorbed in the small intestine, which contributes to the positive effect on energy utilization (Just *et al.*, 1983a,b).

Body Composition Studies of Pigs

Changes in body composition can occur while growth rate remains unaltered. Accurate measurements of changes in body composition and the energy content of live animals are key to understanding the response to the intake of nutrients. Body composition analysis is fundamental for the evaluation of growth modifiers in animal research, for genetic selection in animal production, and for carcass grading in value-based marketing. Classically, measurements have been done by direct or indirect calorimetry, comparative slaughter, or dilution techniques (McDonald *et al.,* 2002).

Slaughtering technique and chemical analysis is the 'gold standard' technique for measurement of body composition, but is destructive, time consuming and expensive. The use of dilution technique for the measurement of body water had been investigated in several species and tritiated water (TOH) was employed in the measurement of body water in living pigs (Kay *et al.,* 1966; Reddy and Prasad, 1983). Results of the study revealed that prediction of body composition from the regression equations was quite precise at 35 kg but not at 65 kg body weight (Reddy and Prasad, 1983).

Body Composition of Gains during Grower Phase and Finisher Phase

The body composition of piglets (n=3) fed a standard diet (NRC 1973; 18% CP and 3.5 Mcal DE/kg) determined using tritiated water as well as direct slaughter method served as the basis to study the effect of energy: protein ratios on the gain of protein and fat by pigs (n=4) at 35 kg body weight (Reddy and Prasad, 1985). The net energy gain (NEg) values of the experimental grower diets were determined by dividing the NE deposited with the amount of daily DM consumed. The NEg values for the four grower diets were 0.80, 0.79, 0.59 and 0.82 Mcal/kg, respectively. It was concluded that grower diet with 18% CP-3.3 Mcal DE/kg was about equivalent to diet with 16% CP-3.0 Mcal DE/kg and superior to other diets.

The composition of gains during 35-65 kg was estimated from the body compositions at 35 kg and 65 kg body weight. Gain in water was more in pigs fed 14% CP-3.0 Mcal DE/kg diet or 16% CP-3.3 Mcal DE/kg diet than those fed 14% CP-3.3 Mcal DE/kg diet. Higher amount of fat was laid down in pigs fed 14% CP-3.3 Mcal DE/kg diet than those fed 14% CP-3.0 Mcal DE/kg (Reddy and Prasad, 1985).

Conjugated Linoleic Acid as Nutrient Repartitioning Agent

Deposition of lean muscle is favoured to obtain better feed efficiency and faster live weight gains. Dugan *et al.* (1997) reported that feeding a 2% conjugated linoleic acid (CLA) diet to finisher pigs resulted in a repartitioning effect of carcass fat to lean. Their subsequent research showed that feeding diets containing CLA increased intramuscular fat levels, but did not improve palatability (Dugan *et al.*, 1999). Joo *et al.* (2002) demonstrated that CLA concentration in pork depended on the level of CLA in diet. Lipid oxidation was inhibited with increased CLA in meat. Thus, dietary CLA could not only offer beneficial effects on human health but also improved pork quality.

Importance of Energy Protein Ratios in Large White Yorkshire (LWY) Pigs

Feed accounts for the major cost of pig enterprise. Hence feeding of pigs for economic production should be based on feed intake, nutrient content of the diet and efficiency of nutrient utilization. Optimum energy protein ratio is of paramount importance for pig rearing to be a profitable enterprise. LWY pigs are acclimatized to the agro-climatic conditions of India. Rations containing 10% less energy than the NRC recommendations proved most effective for the LWY pigs in terms of feed efficiency and economy of feed conversion in view of the tropical climate of India (Rao *et al.*, 1978).

Seshi Reddy *et al.* (1982) conducted two experiments, one at 3 x 3 factorial at 3 levels of protein and energy and another at 3 levels of energy with 18% CP and the results revealed that LWY pigs required 18% CP and 3.3 Mcal digestible energy (DE)/kg diet, which worked out to be an optimum of 17 to 19 calories of DE per g of protein for growing LWY pigs from 20 to 35 kg body weight. Systematic studies had been undertaken to have a holistic view (Reddy, 1981). Two 2 x 2 factorial experiments were conducted with growing (20 to 35 kg) and finishing (35 to 65 kg) LWY barrows to determine optimum energy: protein ratios and to predict their body composition by using tritiated water dilution technique.

In experiment I, 40 barrows (randomly allotted to four groups of ten each) were fed on diets supplying 16 % CP (on fresh basis) with 3.0 or 3.3 and 18 % CP with 3.0 or 3.3 Mcal DE/kg (Reddy and Prasad, 1985). The average daily gain (ADG) and daily feed consumption decreased by about 8 and 10 % respectively, as the level of energy was increased. Energy had a significant effect on feed consumption. Feed efficiency and cost/kg gain of pigs fed 16% CP with 3.0 Mcal DE/kg and 18% CP with 3.3 Mcal DE/kg were superior to other diets. Level of energy significantly influenced digestibility of DM, CP, ether extract (EE) and nitrogen free extract (NFE). Energy: protein ratios did not affect nitrogen retention. The % loin+ham was higher in pigs fed 18% CP with 3.3 Mcal DE/kg than those fed on other diets. The optimum energy: protein ratio for grower pigs was found to be 182 to 185 kilocalories percentage units.

In experiment II, 24 barrows of experiment I were shifted to finisher diets supplying 14% CP with 3.0 or 3.3 and 16% CP with 3.0 or 3.3 Mcal DE/kg

(Reddy and Prasad, 1985). Energy density and energy x protein interaction influenced feed consumption, which was 15% lower in pigs fed 16% CP and 3.3 Mcal DE/kg diet than those fed 16% CP and 3.0 Mcal DE/kg diet. The ADG decreased by about 7% as the level of energy in the diets was increased. Feed efficiency and cost/kg gain of diet that supplies 14% CP with 3.0 Mcal DE/kg was superior to other diets. The level of energy significantly influenced N retention. Level of protein had a significant effect on dressing percentage. Energy, protein and E x P interaction influenced loin eye area, which was significantly higher in pigs fed 14% CP with 3.0 Mcal DE/kg diet than in pigs fed other diets. The body fat content in pigs fed 14% CP-3.3 Mcal DE/kg diet was higher than those fed 14% CP-3.0 Mcal DE/kg diet. The optimum energy: protein ratios for finisher pigs were 204 to 213 kilocalories percentage units, respectively.

Importance of Energy Protein Ratios in Desi Pigs

Forty-eight weaned native/desi pigs were used to investigate the effects of four diets viz. 16% CP with 3.0 or 2.7 Mcal DE/kg and 14% CP with 3.0 or 2.7 Mcal DE/kg in a 2 x 2 factorial design on the performance, utilization of nutrients and nitrogen balance (Reddy *et al.*, 1986a). The average daily gain, daily feed consumed and efficiency of feed utilization were significantly lower in pigs fed 14% CP and 2.7 Mcal DE/kg diet than in those fed other diets. Feed efficiency and cost/kg gain of 16% CP with 3.0 Mcal DE/kg diet were superior to those of 16% CP-2.7 Mcal DE/kg or 14% CP-3.0 Mcal DE/kg. Energy, protein and E x P interaction influenced ADG, daily feed consumed and feed efficiency. Energy density had a significant effect on faecal N excretion and total N excretion. For growing desi pigs (14 to 45 kg BW) a diet with 16% CP and 3.0 Mcal DE/kg diet was found to be superior to other diets.

Development of Economic Rations

Conventional feedstuffs like maize, groundnut cake, soybean meal and fishmeal are given top priority in formulating pig diets. A key task for nutritionists is to achieve cost optimization of feed formulation. The ever-increasing cost of these ingredients coupled with short supply has necessitated the search for utilization of alternative/unconventional/low cost feed ingredients. There is a global boom in the use of byproducts from non-food crop production as well as human food processing in animal feeding. Towards this several experiments have been conducted by replacing maize with rice polish and molasses (Krishna Rao and Prasad, 1980), tamarind seed and molasses (Thomas and Prasad, 1983; Reddy *et al.*, 1986b), variga grain (*Panicum milaceum*) (Seshi Reddy *et al.*, 1984), bagasse and molasses in 9:1 ratio (Reddy *et al.*, 1985), tamarind seed or rice polish (Reddy *et al.*, 1986b).

Krishna Rao and Prasad (1980) reported that partial replacement of maize with zinc-supplemented rice polish diet was superior to the maize diet. Molasses could safely be added at 10% level and replacing wheat bran by rice bran did not offer any advantage. Maize could not be completely replaced with variga, although 50% replacement could be beneficial (Seshi Reddy *et al.,* 1984). Twenty parts of maize could be replaced with bagasse and molasses mixture without any adverse effect on economy of feed conversion (Reddy *et al.,* 1985). Maize could be completely replaced with 30% tamarind seed and 10% molasses for economic pig rearing (Thomas and Prasad, 1983; Reddy *et al.,* 1986b). Replacing maize partially with 20% rice polish and 10% molasses appeared to be better than complete replacement of maize with 30% rice polish and 15% molasses (Thomas and Prasad, 1983).

Efforts of complete replacement of maize with bajra, groundnut cake with deoiled sunflower cake, wheat bran with deoiled rice bran, fishmeal with synthetic amino acids-lysine and methionine did not yield favourable results (Srinivasa Rao *et al.,* 1992). Studies of Karunakar Rao *et al.* (2005) indicated that replacement of bajra with tamarind seed kernel in grower diets or along with tapioca waste in finisher diets resulted in poor performance in pigs.

Use of Local Resources

Preston and Leng (1987) have suggested that one way to achieve sustainable animal production systems is to match them with the available local resources. Preston (2006) has suggested that the leaves from shrubs such as cassava and mulberry and from vegetables such as sweet potato and cocoyam, together with water plants such as duckweed and water spinach, can be used successfully in diets for pigs, replacing at least half the protein usually supplied as soybean meal and fishmeal.

Constraints in Utilization of Local Feed Resources and Dietary Tools to Overcome them

Locally available feed resources/byproducts and some cereal grains have high fibre, low protein and energy contents. When they are included at high levels, they may decrease the digestibility of energy (Just *et al.,* 1983a) and other dietary components (Len *et al.,* 2007) and result in low performance. Like other non-ruminants, pigs do not secrete endoenzymes that degrade cell wall and nonstarch polysaccharides (NSP) found in feedstuffs in various concentrations (Bach Knudsen, 1997).

Diet formulation based on CP is inefficient since the digestibility of CP in different feedstuffs varies from the negative to almost 100%, which is influenced by several factors that include dietary concentrations of crude fibre,

CP, presence of protease inhibitors, tannins, etc., processing methods used, heat treatment employed, age and weight of pigs. The utilization of digestible protein (amino acids) depends mainly on its amino acid composition, if the requirements of the pigs for other nutrients and energy are fulfilled.

Supplementation of Amino Acids

Swine diets may be deficient in one or more amino acids and this can limit growth rate of pigs and resistance to disease. Simply adding more protein to the diet may increase the absolute amounts of these limiting amino acids but will not provide an optimum mix of amino acids and may increase intestinal disorders. Much of the additional protein may be "wasted" because it contains excess amounts of more common amino acids. Therefore, supplements of the limiting amino acids have been added to diets to improve performance of pigs (Thomke and Elwinger, 1998). Addition of supplementary protein or synthetic amino acids is also of importance, since 60-75% of the pig's total dietary protein is supplied through cereal grains and their byproducts (Eggum *et al.*, 1990). Sharda and Yadav (1981) reported that supplementation of 14% CP diet with 0.1% lysine improved the performance of pigs and brought it at par with those fed 18% CP in the diets.

Supplementation of a barley-wheat-soybean diet containing 13.5% CP with the amino acids lysine, methionine and threonine resulted in a higher growth rate and feed conversion ratio in growing pigs than feeding an unsupplemented diet containing 15.8% CP (Askbrant *et al.*, 1994). Addition of threonine to a maize, soybean, rapeseed and cottonseed meal diet increased weight gain and feed conversion in growing pigs and also improved immune function (Kemme *et al.*, 1999). In another experiment with finishing pigs that fed a low protein corn-soybean diet, addition of individual amino acids did not improve growth (Smith *et al.*, 1999).

Supplementation of Enzymes

Commercial application of enzymes focused on removing the antinutritional effects of NSPs present primarily in viscous grains (wheat, rye, barley or triticale), nonviscous cereal grains (sorghum, maize) and other feedstuffs, increasing utilization of phytate P and also to alleviate environmental pollution; and improving the digestibility of vegetable proteins. The NSPs, proteins, phytic acid and various minerals are present as complex compounds in the cell walls of plants. Nutrients bound to NSP or phytate are released by NSP degrading enzymes or phytases so that the digestibility of the protein and of various minerals (Ca, Mg, Zn, etc.) can be improved as a concomitant effect.

In monogastric animals, enzymes such as proteases, amylases, lipases are produced and there is a need to supplement them in young animals (newly weaned piglets may produce inadequate amounts of certain enzymes) and in adults (when fed on certain feeds) to further their digestive capacity. Bedford and Schulze (1998) reviewed the currently available enzymes used as feed supplements and prospects for further developments of enzymes such as glycanases (carbohydrate degrading enzymes) as alternatives to in-feed antibiotics for the improved production performance.

Highly Digestible Feedstuffs to Improve Feed Efficiency

New sources of highly digestible feedstuffs are being developed through classical breeding techniques or genetic modification to improve feed efficiency. Low-phytate maize and low-stachyose soybean are examples under this group. Phosphorus (P) availability in classical feed maize and soybean is low for pigs as P is usually bound in a phytate molecule and phytase enzyme is lacking in the digestive system of pigs. The use of low-phytate genotypes reduces the levels of mineral P to be supplemented in the diet and reduces P excretion by 25 to 35% (FAO 1999; Sutton *et al.,* 2001).

Improvements in Feed Processing Technology

Particle size of feed has been emphasized since it could significantly improve feed efficiency and reduce the N level in the faeces. Particle size of 700 microns is recommended for swine feeds. Data from studies at Kansas State University over decades indicated that the mean size of maize particles need to be 600 microns or less, since 1-1.5% improvement in feed efficiency was reported for every 100-micron reduction from 1200 microns down to 400 microns. However, a feed using finely ground wheat may give rise to stomach ulcers. Hence, although a very fine feed structure promotes the best pig performance one should be cautious on the risk of ulcers and eventual consequences. Pelleting improves feed efficiency by 8.5%.

Split-sex Feeding and Phase Feeding

In precision animal nutrition it becomes important to feed the animal with diets that are formulated to match its nutrient requirement, as an animal's nutrient requirement changes with age, sex, and growth potential. Examples of this are split-sex feeding and phase feeding. Differences in nutrient requirements among gilts, barrows, and possibly boars are taken into consideration in case of split-sex feeding. Barrows typically have a higher feed intake capacity without a larger potential for lean gain, and thus diets should be fed with somewhat less protein.

Phase feeding refers to feeding programmes that match the animal's nutrient requirement since nutrient needs change with the animal's age/size. To minimize nutrient waste, the animal's diet should thus be changed continuously to match its requirements. Feeding programme of pigs during growing-finishing phase needs to be divided into several phases and multi-phase feeding reduces feed costs as well as nitrogen excretion. Economics and convenience drive implementation of such nutrient refinement programmes even into adult productive life stages.

Use of Antibiotics in Animals

Antibiotics are used largely for three purposes in animals: therapeutic use to treat sick animals, prophylactic use to prevent infection in animals and as growth promoters to improve feed utilization and production. Antibiotic growth promoters (AGPs) directly depress microbial growth in the gastrointestinal tract.

The Swann Committee (Swann, 1969) concluded that there was probably a hazard to human health from feeding subtherapeutic levels of antibiotics to food-producing animals. In response to the report, a number of countries including UK, European countries and Australia removed penicillin and tetracyclines from the approved list. Interestingly, the USA did not respond to this because the Food and Drug Administration (FDA) was unable to demonstrate a threat to public health (Feinman, 1998).

Antimicrobial resistance has become a global health problem (animal and human). Consequently, the World Health Organization (WHO) called for a ban on the practice of giving healthy animals antibiotics as growth promoters (FAO, 2003).

Potential Alternatives to In-feed Antibiotics

Nutricines (Adams, 1999) are components of food which are considered for their beneficial effect upon health rather than their direct contribution to nutrition. Nutricines provide the crucial link between health and nutrition. Nutricines play important roles in delaying the onset of diseases, controlling microbial spoilage of food, improving the digestion of food and helping the absorption of nutrients from the gastrointestinal tract. Examples include antioxidants, nondigestible carbohydrates (NDC), natural acids, enzymes, lecithins. Let us go through the various important alternatives to in-feed antibiotics.

Antimicrobial Peptides

As alternatives to antibiotics, antimicrobial peptides (AMPs) are of interest. Endogenous antimicrobial peptides play an important role in innate immunity.

More than 12 antimicrobial peptides have been detected in pigs. Most of these compounds kill bacteria by disrupting cell membranes, and it is believed that bacteria may be slower to develop resistance to these compounds. A recent comprehensive review of porcine antimicrobial peptides was presented by Zhang (2000). But some bacterial pathogens have developed their own form of resistance to the AMPs.

Much attention has been paid to physiological functions of non-nutritive components in the seaweeds and to immune activities of their extracts, which were reported to be non-toxic cellular and humoral immune agent, and their main components were lectins (Shan *et al.,* 1999).

Immune Modulators

These are the immunologically active compounds that affect the working of the immune system and may enhance resistance to disease. These substances include mainly antibodies in the form of colostrum from the sow vaccinated for a particular disease or antibodies from products such as spray-dried plasma, freeze-dried eggs containing pig related antibodies and possibly some whey protein products, cytokines. Some or all of the growth-promoting effects of subtherapeutic antibiotics in feeds may result from their action against sub-clinical infections or competitive intestinal bacteria. Therefore, it has been suggested that addition of antibodies or other immunoactive compounds to feed may accomplish the same purpose.

Conjugated Linoleic Acid as Immunomodulator

Conjugated linoleic acid has immunomodulating effects and appears to be a promising immunologic activator in young pigs that have not yet developed a more specific immune response repertoire. Dietary CLA isomers are excreted in colostrum and milk and are available to the suckling piglets (Bee, 2000). Corino *et al.,* (2002) reported that dietary CLA enhanced serum IgG and lysozyme production in weaned piglets fed CLA for 4 weeks. Subsequent work (Bontempo *et al.,* 2004) revealed that dietary supplementation of 0.5% CLA to sows during late gestation and lactation increased the IgG level of colostrum and also affected its fatty acid composition and increased the serum IgG and lysozyme levels. Dietary supplementation of 0.5% CLA to postweaning piglets also increased serum IgG level.

Zinc Oxide

It is well documented that supplementation of 2500~3000 mg/kg of dietary zinc oxide for piglets in a period of 1~2 weeks after weaning resulted in increased feed intake, increased growth rate and reduced the occurrence of diarrhoea. Feng *et al.*, (2006) reviewed the work done on possible mechanisms of zinc oxide in piglets.

Organic Acids

AGPs directly depress microbial growth in the gastrointestinal tract (GIT). Hence, research workers looked for products that would reduce intestinal microbial growth. Though GIT is inside the animal body, the lumen of the GIT is outside the body of the animal. The GIT provides a complete interface between the animal and its environment. The first line of defence, therefore, is to prevent harmful bacteria from entering the intestines by the oral route. Acidic conditions in the stomach are achieved by the secretion of hydrochloric acid to form a powerful antimicrobial barrier. In the newly weaned piglets, this mechanism can be inadequately developed due to insufficient production of hydrochloric acid and pancreatic enzymes.

The need for feed acidification led to revisiting the organic acids, which have been known for their feed preservation. A particular scientific interest is now paid to the antimicrobial potency of various carboxylic acids and of short chain fatty acids and their salts. Addition of organic acids offers opportunity to lower the diet's acid-binding capacity and increases gastric acidity (Reddy, 2006). These acidifiers can be administered individually or as a mix (to broaden a spectrum of antimicrobial potency) via feeds or drinking water. There is a general consensus on the efficacy of organic acids as the best alternative to antibiotic growth promoters, though the mode of action of particular organic acids and salts is not uniform (Mroz, 2005).

Essential Oils / Plant Extracts

Essential oils (EO) or plant extracts can be used as appetite stimulant, aroma, stimulant of saliva production, gastric and pancreatic juices production enhancer and antioxidant. However, the antibacterial property of essential oils is the most widely studied area as alternative to AGPs, and the inhibitory properties of 50 essential oils against 25 different bacteria have been reported. Oils that contain phenolic structures have stronger antimicrobial properties than oils without phenolic structures (Dorman and Deans, 2000).

The mode of action of essential oils may be related to changes in lipid solubility at the surface of the bacteria. Lambert *et al.* (2001) reported that essential oils impaired the functioning of a variety of enzyme systems, mainly involved in energy production and structural components synthesis, thus disintegrate the outer membrane of *E. coli* and *S. typhimurium*, and thus inactivate these pathogens. Mode of action was also through leakage of ions, ATP, nucleic acids and amino acids. Essential oils have a limited effect as a replacement of antibiotic growth promoters but they can act in synergy with organic acids both for their growth promoting effect and prevention of specific intestinal diseases.

Garlic Preparation

Number of natural substances and herbal extracts are looked on as a candidate for potential alternatives. It appeared far easier to include it as a full dose mixture constituent than crushed cloves of fresh garlic. Powder from lyophilized garlic cloves additive, especially in 5 or 10 g/kg mixture, may constitute a recommended dietary component for raising piglets up to 56 days of life (Grela and Klebaniuk, 2007). Dietary supplementation of garlic improved body weight gain, decreased piglet losses as well as triglycerides and total cholesterol concentration in blood plasma. Cullen *et al.* (2005) used garlic powder at 1g or 10g/kg mixture while Grela and Semeniuk (2006) supplemented 2g/kg mixture in grower-finisher pigs.

Prebiotics, Probiotics and Synbiotics

The bacteriostatic approach need to be supported by modification to the diet so that reduced amount of substrate is available to the intestinal microflora. This is possible only either by using highly digestible feed ingredients or by the addition of enzymes to less digestible ingredients. But in case of piglet starter diets wherein highly digestible carbohydrates are used, there may be a shift to protein fermentation in the hindgut by being 'carbohydrate' deficient. Excess protein fermentation in large intestine leads to increased ammonia concentration in colon and predisposes early-weaned piglets to diarrhoea (Dong *et al.*, 1996). The addition of selected fermentable carbohydrates has been shown to increase bacterial diversity and lead to more rapid stabilization of the microbial community (Konstantinov *et al.*, 2003) in newly weaned piglets. Such non-digestible oligosaccharides (NDOs) are found in feedstuffs such as barley, wheat, sugarbeet pulp, soybean hulls, alfalfa meal, etc. and are referred to as prebiotics.

Prebiotics have been used to induce the colonization of probiotic bacteria such as lactobacilli and bifidobacteria, considered to be beneficial for the host. Stimulation of the Lactobacillus population has their potential effect on gut function and health (Stewart, 1997), apart from their possible antagonistic activities towards other bacteria (Henriksson *et al.*, 1995). Due to the potential synergy between probiotics and prebiotics, foods containing a combination of these ingredients are often referred to as synbiotics (Collins and Gibson, 1999).

Glutamine

In stressful conditions, intestinal permeability increases allowing bacteria to enter the bloodstream, thus causing infection (Adjei *et al.*, 1994), and glutamine has been shown to decrease the incidence of infection in surgery and trauma patients (Andrews and Griffiths, 2002). Feeding glutamine at1% to broiler chicks improved growth performance and may stimulate development of the gastrointestinal tract and humoral immune response (Bartell and Batal, 2007). However, Kitt *et al.* (2002) did not observe improvements in weight gain in swine.

Nucleotides

Dietary nucleotides may potentially act as an alternative to antibiotics. The need for nucleotides is elevated during periods of rapid growth, during periods of stress, and in immunocompromised animals (Kulkarni *et al.*, 1994). In chicks and piglets (especially newly weaned pigs) all of these factors are present and hence, it can be expected that they have a high requirement for nucleotides. Nucleic acids found in many feed and food ingredients are protected by specific binding proteins, which allow only about 30 percent of them to become nutritionally available. But purified nucleotides can provide growing animals and fish with their precise dietary requirements (Hoffmann, 2007). In studies with pigs it has been demonstrated that dietary nucleotides reduce oxidative stress caused by high concentrations of polyunsaturated fatty acids in the diet (Salobir *et al.*, 2005). RNA/nucleotides are the building blocks for life and involved in diverse cellular processes. They facilitate immune response by supporting the crucial proliferation of cells involved in cellular and humoral defence mechanisms. They are regarded as an ideal management tool to control and diminish stress, improve performance, and modulate diseases in livestock (Hoffmann, 2007).

Yu *et al.* (2002) reported that a combination of a dietary supplement of glutamine and nucleotides improved feed intake, intestinal villus height, and serum IgG concentrations in pigs challenged with a lipopolysaccharide injection. Nucleotide supplementation also increased lymphocyte stimulation to phytohaemagglutinin and concanavalin-A challenges in weanling pigs by 50% and 30%, respectively (Zomborsky-Kovacs *et al.*, 1998). Results of these studies suggest that dietary sources of nucleotides/nucleosides play a role in developing, maintaining, and enhancing the immune system.

Intensive Animal Production and Environmental Pollution

The challenge for nutritionists is to formulate rations that continue to improve production levels while simultaneously minimizing environmental impacts associated with excreta. This can be achieved by optimizing nutrient availability by better adjusting and synchronizing nutrients and mineral inputs to the animals requirements, which reduce the quantity of manure excreted per unit of feed and per unit of product.

Mineral Pollution and Mitigation Strategies

A review of balance data for pigs fed commercial feedstuffs indicated the following approximate utilization values as percent of intake: 30 to 55 for nitrogen, 30 to 50 for calcium, 20 to 50 for phosphorus, 5 to 20 for potassium, 10 to 25 for sodium, 15 to 30 for magnesium, 5 to 30 for copper, 5 to 30 for zinc, 5 to 10 for manganese and 5 to 30 for iron (Kornegay and Harper, 1997). Peet-Schwering and Hartog, (2000) reported that sows, weaned pigs and finishing pigs excrete 76, 46 and 67% of the nitrogen consumed and 75, 38 and 63% of the phosphorus consumed, respectively.

Proper mineral nutrition controls animal wastes. In Switzerland the mean content of copper and zinc in pig manures decreased considerably between 1990 and 1995 (by 28% for copper, 17% for zinc), which demonstrated the effectiveness of limiting heavy metals in animal feed to required levels (Menzi and Kessler, 1998). In case of bioavailability of mineral elements, chemical form and degree of solubility can have a profound effect on utilization of supplemental sources. Using organic forms of copper, iron, manganese, selenium and zinc in pig diets reduced the level of heavy metals added to the ration and significantly reduced the excretion levels without depressing growth or feed efficiency (Sutton *et al.*, 2001; LPES, 2005). Substances stimulating their absorption (for example, dietary citric acid in case of zinc) may also be applied as feed additives.

The use of phytase has been shown to improve P digestibility in pig diet by 30 to 50% and P excretion can be lowered by 20 to 30%. Multi-phase feeding can reduce the P excretion by about 15% (Peet-Schwering and Hartog, 2000).

Nutritional Interventions to Reduce Nitrogen Excretion

Diet acidification promotes a more effective digestion of protein, since the conversion of pepsinogen to pepsin is inhibited by increase of pH above 4. Nutrient repartitioners (porcine somatotropin (pST) and β-agonists) or chromium supplement improve N deposition in growing pigs by reducing the urinary N excretion.

A more efficient intermediary metabolism will reduce N excretion in urine whereas a reduction in losses from gastrointestinal (GI) tract will reduce excretion both in faeces and in urine. These are possible through precision nutritional management. The nitrogen losses in intermediary metabolism can be reduced by following the concept of 'ideal' protein for monogastric animals. Lenis and Schutte (1990) reported that the protein content of a typical swine ration could be reduced by three percentage points (e.g., from 16% to 13%) replacing, for example, soybean meal with synthetic amino acids and maize without negative effects on animal performance. Such a reduction could exert a large impact on N excretion in manure. Schutte *et al.* (1993) determined that for each percentage point that N is reduced in the feed, N excretion is reduced by 10%.

Synthetic amino acids help to enhance the digestibility of amino acid (nitrogen), and nitrogen excretion could be reduced significantly. Small amounts of synthetic amino acids (0.1-0.3%) could spare dietary protein by 2-3% (Han *et al.*, 1998). Nitrogen excretion can drop by 30% where synthetic amino acids are used to compensate for a lower dietary level of crude protein.

Feeds are prepared based on measurement of N or CP of feedstuffs and chemical composition of which is variable. For example, CP content of maize varies from 8-11%, lysine content 1.8-2.0%, while a coefficient of variation of 16% has been found for starch digestibility in maize. Nitrogen, however, correlates poorly with the available amino acid content of feedstuffs (Van Kempen and Simmins, 1997). Hence feed manufacturers are inclined to produce feed with a higher degree of variation than desirable for precision nutrition. van Kempen and Simmins (1997) calculated that reducing the variation by using more appropriate quality control measures (e.g., analyzing each batch of feedstuff and formulating feeds) would result in a 13% to 27% reduction in N excretion.

Nutritional Interventions to Reduce Ammonia Emission

Ammonia originates predominantly from urea and is relatively stable in urine. The rate at which ammonia is emitted is dependent on many factors like mixing of urine with faeces, urea content, pH of urine and/or manure, temperature, airflow, etc. Ammonia emission can be reduced by precision nutrition. Cahn (1998) studied the effect of three protein levels in the diet (16.5, 14.5 and 12.5%) on the ammonia emission of finishing pigs. It was concluded that for every percent decrease in dietary crude protein the ammonia emission was reduced by 10.0 -12.5%.

Ammonia emission can also be reduced by decreasing the pH of urine and/or manure and reducing the pH of the urine seems to be a better proposition. Lowering the pH will result in a conversion of NH_3 (volatile) to NH_4 + and therefore, a lowered ammonia emission (Cahn, 1998). Mroz et al., (1996) demonstrated that by replacing $CaCO_3$ (limestone) in the diet with $CaSO_4$ (gypsum), $CaCl_2$ (calcium chloride), or calcium benzoate (not yet an approved feed ingredient), ammonia emission could be reduced by 30%, 33%, and 54%, respectively. The drop in urinary pH for $CaSO_4$ and $CaCl_2$ was approximately 1.3 units, while the drop in pH was 2.2 units for calcium benzoate. Brok *et al.* (1997) showed that using benzoic acid for this purpose actually improved feed conversion (from 2.92 to 2.83) while decreasing ammonia emission by 40%. Improving the feed conversion ratio is another important way to reduce the nitrogen and ammonia emission. van Kempen (2001) used adipic acid at 1% in the diet to reduce urinary pH and thus ammonia emission. Adipic acid being a flavour enhancer, it may increase the feed intake in nursery pigs.

Alum and aluminium chloride were also found to reduce swine manure pH significantly (Smith et al., 1999). In their further studies, Smith et al., (2004) observed that dietary manipulation with phytase and application of aluminium chloride (0.75% vol:vol of final manure volume) are promising management practices for the reduction of ammonia from swine farms.

Kirchgessner et al., (1994) showed that some of the nitrogen excretion was shifted from urea in urine to bacterial protein in faeces when more fermentable non-starch polysaccharides (NSPs) (e.g. sugarbeet pulp, soybean hulls, alfalfa meal) were included in the diet. A supply of fermentable organic matter to the microbes of the large intestine induced a secretion of urea from the blood (Low, 1985) and microbial growth. As a result, some N excretion shifts from urine to faeces (Mroz et al., 1996). Microbial protein goes into the manure and is less likely to release ammonia than the N in the urine. Canh (1998) investigated the effect of four different dietary NSP levels on the partitioning of N excretion. The pigs fed the diets with the highest NSP content excreted less nitrogen in the urine and more in the faeces than pigs fed diets with the lowest NSP in the diets. The ammonia emission decreased with increasing levels of NSP in the diet.

References

Adams, C.A. (1999). Nottingham University Press. Nottingham, U.K.

Adjei, A.A., Matsumoto, Y., Oku, T., Hiroi, Y., Yamamoto, S. (1994). *Nutrition Research,* 14:1591-1599.

Andrews, F.J. Griffiths, R.D., (2002). *Br. J. Nutr.,* S1, 38.

Askbrant, S., Hakansson, J., Andersson, K., Svensson, C., Malmlof, K. (1994). *Swedish J. Agrl. Res.,* 24: 115118.

Bartell, S.M. and Batal, A.B. (2007). *Poultry Sci.,* 86:1940-1947.

Bach Knudsen, K.F. (1997). *Anim. Feed Sci. Technol.,* 67: 315-338.

Bedford, M.R., Schulze, H. (1998). *Nutr. Res. Rev.,* 78: 89-102.

Bee, G., (2000). *J. Nutr.* 130: 2292-2298.

Bontempo, V., Sciannimanico, D., Pastorelli, G., Rossi, R., Rosi, F., Corino, C. (2004). *J. Nutr.,* 134: 817-824.

Brok, G.M., den; Hendriks, Vrielink, J.G.L., Peet-Schwering, M.G.M., Van der, C.M.C., (1997). Cited by Peet-Schwering, C.M.C. Van der, Hartog, L.A.den, 2000. Nutr. Abstr. Rev. Series, B 70: 912-917.

Cahn, T.T., (1998). Ammonia emission from excreta of growing pigs as affected by dietary composition, Ph D Thesis, Agricultural University Wageningen, The Netherlands, pp.163.

Collins, M.D. and Gibson, G.R. (1999). *Am.J. Clin. Nutr.,* 69: 1052S-1057S.

Corino, C., Bontempo, V., Sciannimanico, D. (2002). *Can. J. Anim. Sci.,* 82: 115-117.

Cullen, S.P., Monahan, F.J., Callan, J.J., OíDoherty, J.V. (2005). *Irish J. Agrl. Food Res.,* 44: 57-67.

Delgado, C., Rosegrant, M., Steinfeld, H., Ehui, S., Courbois, C. (1999). The Next Food Revolution. Food, Agriculture and the Environment Discussion Paper 28. International Food Policy Research Institute, Washington D C.

Dong, G.Z., Zhou, A.G., Yang, F., Chen, K.R., Wang, K.Y., Dao, D.M. (1996). *Acta Veterinaria et Zootechnica Sinica,* 27: 293-302.

Dorman, H.J.D., Deans, S.G. (2000). *J. Appl. Microbiol.,* 88: 308316.

Dugan, M.E.R., Aalhus, J.L., Jeremiah, L.E., Kramer, J.K.G., Schaefer, A.L. (1999). *Can. J. Anim. Sci.,* 79: 45-51.

Dugan, M.E.R., Aalhus, J.L., Schaefer, A.L., Kramer, J.K.G. (1997). *Can. J. Anim. Sci.,* 77: 723-725.

Easter, R.A., Ellis, M., Hollis, G.R., Baker, D.H. (1996). Dietary nutrient allawances for swine. In: 1996 Feedstuffs Reference Issue 68 (30): 38-44.

Eggum, B.O., Jorgensen, H., Danielsen, L. (1990). *Nutr. Abstr. Rev.,* 61: 4073.

F.A.O. (1999). Livestock Environment Toolbox, Livestock Environment Development (LEAD) Initiative, Rome. [Available at www.virtualcentre.org/en/dec/toolbox/homepage.html].

F.A.O. (2003). World Agriculture: Towards 2015/2030. An FAO perspective. Editied by J Bruisnsma, Rome and London, Earthscan.

Feinman, S.E. (1998). *American Society for Microbiology News,* 64: 24-30.

Feng, Z.K., Ou, D.Y., Li, X.L., Wang, F.L., Li, D.F. (2006). Possible mechanisms of zinc oxide for piglets. In: XIIth AAAP Animal Science Congress 2006, held at BUSAN, KOREA September 18-22, 2006.

Grela, E.R. and Klebaniuk, R. (2007). *Medycyna Wet.,* 63: 792-795.

Grela, E.R. and Semeniuk, V. (2006). *Anim. Sci.,* 10: 32-33S.

Han, In. K., Cho, W.T., Kim, J.W. (1998). The role of synthetic amino acids in animal production. In: Proceedings Symposium Series 1 of 8th World Conference on Animal Production held at Seoul, Korea during June 28 - July 4 1998. pp 92-109.

Henriksson, A., André, L., Conway, P. (1995). *FEMS Microbiol Ecol.,* 16: 55-60.

Hoffmann, K. (2007). The use of nucleotides in animal feed, Part 3. *Feed Mix,* 15: 36-38.

Joo, S.T., Lee, J.L., Ha, Y.L., Park, G.B. (2002). *J. Anim. Sci.*, 80: 108-112.

Just, A. (1984). *J. Anim. Sci.*, 58: 740-752.

Just, A. (1982a). *Livest. Prod. Sci.*, 9: 349-360.

Just, A.(1982b). *Livest. Prod. Sci.*, 9: 501-509.

Just, A. (1982c). *Livest. Prod. Sci.*, 9: 569-580.

Just, A., Fernandez, J.A., Jorgensen, H. (1982). In: Laplade, J. P.; Corring, T.; Rerat, A. (Eds) Digestive Physiology in the Pig. *Les Colloques de L'INRA* 12: 207-215.

Just, A., Fernandez, J.A., Jorgensen, H. (1983a). *Livest. Prod. Sci.*, 10: 171-186.

Just, A., Jorgensen, H., Fernandez, J.A. (1983b). *Livest. Prod. Sci.*, 10: 487-506.

Karunakar Rao, M., Ravi, A., Rao, Z.P., Reddy, D.V., Reddy, R.R. (2005). *Indian J. Ani. Nutr.*, 22: 97-101.

Kay, M., Jones, A.S., Smart, R. (1966). *Br.J. Nutr.*, 20: 439-448.

Kemme, P.A., Jongbloed, A.W., Mroz, Z., Kogut, J., Beynen, A.C. (1999). *Livest. Prod. Sci.*, 8, 107-117.

Kirchgessner, M., Kreuzer, M., Machmueller, A., Roth-Maier, D.A. (1994). *Anim. Feed Sci. Technol.*, 46: 293-306.

Kitt, S.J., Miller, P.S., Lewis, A.J., Fischer, R.L. (2002). Effects of glutamine on growth performance and small intestine villus height in weaning pigs. *In:* Nebraska Swine Report, Univ in Nebraska Swine Report, Univ. Nebraska, Linedn.

Konstantinov, S.R., Zhu, W.Y., Williams Barbara, A., Tamminga, S., Vos, W.M.de, Akkermans, A.D.L. (2003). *Ecol.*, 43, 225-235.

Kornegay, E.T., Harper, A.F. (1997). *The Professional Animal Scientist*, 13: 99-111.

Krishna Rao and K., Prasad, D.A. (1980). *Indian J. Anim. Sci.*, 50: 63-67.

Kulkarni, A.D., Rudolph, F.B., Van Buren, C.T. (1994). *J. Nutr.*, 124: 1422-1446.

Lambert, R.J.W., Skandamis, P.N., Coote, P.J., Nychas, G-J.E. (2001). *J. Appl. Microbiol.*, 91: 453-462.

Len, N.T., Lindberg, J.E., Ogle, B. (2007). *J. Anim. Physiol. Anim. Nutr.*, 91: 297-303.

Lenis, N.P., Schutte, and J.B. (1990). Amino acid supply of piglets and graw-finish pigs in relation to nitrogen excretion. *In :* Manure Issues : Nutritional solutions for pigs and poultry A.W. Jongbloed and J. Coppodse, ed. Service Agricultural Research, Wageningen. The Netherlands, pp. 78-79.

Low, A.G. (1985). Recent Advances in Animal Nutrition, Butterworths, London. pp. 87.

L.P.E.S.(2005). Livestock and Poultry Environmental Stewardship Curriculum: A national educational programme [Available at http://www.lpes.org/Lessons/Lesson01/1_Environmental_Stewardship.html]

McDonald, P., Edwards, R.A., Greenhalgh, J.F.D., Morgan, C.A. (2002). Animal Nutrition. 6th edn. Prentice Hall, London, U.K.

Menzi, H., Kessler, J. (1998). In: Proceedings of the International Conference of the FAO ESCORENA Network on Recycling of Agricultural, Municipal and Industrial Residues in Agriculture, Rennes, France. 26-29, May 1998.

Mroz, Z. (2005). *Adv. Pork Prod.,* 16: 169-182.

Mroz, Z., Jongbloed, A.W., Vreman, D., Canh, T.T., Diepen, J., Th., M. Van, Kemme, P.A., Kogut, J., Aarnink, A.J.A. (1996). Lelystad, The Netherlands, pp. 58.

N.R.C. (1973). Nutrient Requirements of Domestic Animals. No. 2. Nutrient Requirements of Swine, National Research Council, Washington, D C.

Peet-Schwering, C.M.C. van der, Hartog, L.A. den (2000). *Nutr. Abstr. Rev. Series* B, 70: 912-917.

Preston, T.R. (2006). Forages as protein sources for pigs in the tropics. Workshop-seminar "Forages for Pigs and Rabbits" MEJARN-CelAgrid, Phenom Penh, Cambodia, 22-24 August, 2006, Article #2 Retrieved, from http: // www.makrn.org/proprof/preston.htm

Preston, T.R., Leng, R.A. (1987). Matching Ruminant Production Systems with available resources in the Tropics and Sub-tropics. Penambul Books, Armidale.

Rao, R.M., Khan, M.Y., Ranjhan, S.K. (1978). *Indian J. Anim. Sci.,* 48: 123-125.

Reddy, D.V. (1981). MVSc thesis submitted to Andhra Pradesh Agricultural University, Hyderabad, AP, India.

Reddy, D.V. (2006). In: Compendium for ICAR sponsored Summer School on "Recent advances in the feed additives for production of residue free livestock/poultry products" held at Department of Animal Nutrition, Madras Veterinary College (Tamil Nadu Veterinary and Animal Sciences University), Chennai, India, from 17-08-2006 to 06-09-2006, pp 57-63.

Reddy, D.V. and Krishna, N. (2009). Livestock Research for Rural Development. Volume 21, Article #36. Retrieved March 11, 2009, from http://www.lrrd.org/lrrd21/3/redd21036.htm

Reddy, D.V., Prasad, D.A. (1983). *J. Nuclear Agri. Biol.,* 12: 4-7.

Reddy, D.V., Prasad, D.A. (1985). *Indian J. Anim. Sci.,* 55: 468-476.

Reddy, D.V., Prasad, D.A., Charyulu, E.K., Reddy, M.R.N., Audeyya, P. (1985). *Cheiron,* 14: 1-7.

Reddy, D.V., Prasad, D.A., Charyulu, E.K., Audeyya, P., Reddy, M.R.N. (1986a). *Indian J. Anim. Sci.,* 56: 105-109.

Reddy, D.V., Prasad, D.A., Reddy, B.S., Charyulu, E.K., (1986b). *Indian J. Anim. Sci.,* 56: 1094-98.

Salobir, J., Rezar, V., Pajk, T., Levart, A. (2005). *Animal Sci.,* 81: 135-140.

Schutte, J.B., Jong, J.de, Van Kempen, G.J.M. (1993). In: Verstegen, M. W. A.; den Hartog, L.A.; van Kempen, G. J. M.; Metz, J. H.M. (ed) Nitrogen Flow in Pig Production and Environmental Consequences. Pudoc Scienfitic Publishers, Wageningen, The Netherlands. pp 259-263.

Seshi Reddy, B., Reddy, D.V., Prasad, D.A. (1984). *Indian J. Anim. Nutr.*, 1: 24-26.

Seshi Reddy, B., Prasad, D.A., Sreeramamurthy, A. (1982). *Indian J. Anim. Sci.*, 52: 236-240.

Shan, B.E., Yoshida, Y., Kuroda, E., Yamashita, U. (1999). *Int. J. Immunopharmacology*, 21: 59-70.

Sharda, D. P., Yadav, K.R. (1981). *Haryana Agricultural University J. Res.*, XI: 311-314.

Smith, D.R., Moore, Jr. P.A., Haggard, B.E., Maxwe, C.V., Daniel, T.C., Van Devander, K., Davis, M.E. (2004). *J. Anim. Sci.*, 82: 605-611.

Smith, J.W., O'Quinn, P.R., Goodband, R.D., Tokach, M.D., Nelssen, J.L. (1999). *J. Appl. Anim. Res.*, 15: 116.

Sreenivasa Rao, T., Reddy, R.R., Rao, Z.P., Reddy, D.V. (1992). *Cheiron*, 21: 147- 152.

Stewart, C.S. (1997). Microorganisms in hindgut fermentors. In: Mackie, R.I.; White, B.A.; Isaacson, R.E. (ed). Gastrointestinal Microbiology, Chapman and Hall, New York, pp 142-186.

Sutton, A., Applegate, T., Hankins, S., Hill, B., Sholly, D., Allee, G., Greene, W., Kohn, R., Meyer, D., Powers, W., van Kempen, T. (2001). Manipulation of animal diets to affect manure production composition and odours: state of the science, In: Rice, J.M.; Caldwell, D.F.; Humenik, F.J. (ed) Animal Agriculture and the Environment: National Center For Manure and Animal Waste Management White Papers. St. Joseph, Michigan, USA, Published by the American Society of Agricultural and Biological Engineers. pp 377-408.

Swann, M. M. (1969). Use of Antibiotics in Animal Husbandry and Veterinary Medicine. UK Joint Committee Report London: H M Stationery Office.

Thomas, C.P., Prasad, D.A. (1983). *Indian J. Anim. Sci.*, 53: 738-742.

Thomke, S., Elwinger, K. (1998). *Ann Zootech.*, 4: 245271.

Van Kempen,and T.A.T.G. (2001). *J. Anim. Sci.*, 79: 2412-2417.

Van Kempen, T., and Simmins, P.H. (1997). Dietary adipic acid reduces ammonia emission from swine excreta. *J. Appl. Poultry Res.*, 6: 471477.

Yu, I.T., Wu, J.F., Yang, P.C., Liu, C.Y., Lee, D.N., Yen, H.T. (2002). *Animal Sci.*, 75: 379-385.

Zhang, G.L., Ross, C.R., Blecha, F. (2000). *Vet. Res.*, 31: 277296.

Zomborsky-Kovacs, M., Tuboly, S., Biro, H., Bardos, L., Soos, P., Toth, A., Tornyos, G. (1998). *J. Anim. Feed Sci.*, 7: 245-251.

❑❑❑

Animal Nutrition, 2012
eds. Dr. (Mrs.) Usha R. Mehra et al., pp. 185-208
Satish Serial Publishing House e-mail : info@satishserial.com; website : www.satishserial.com

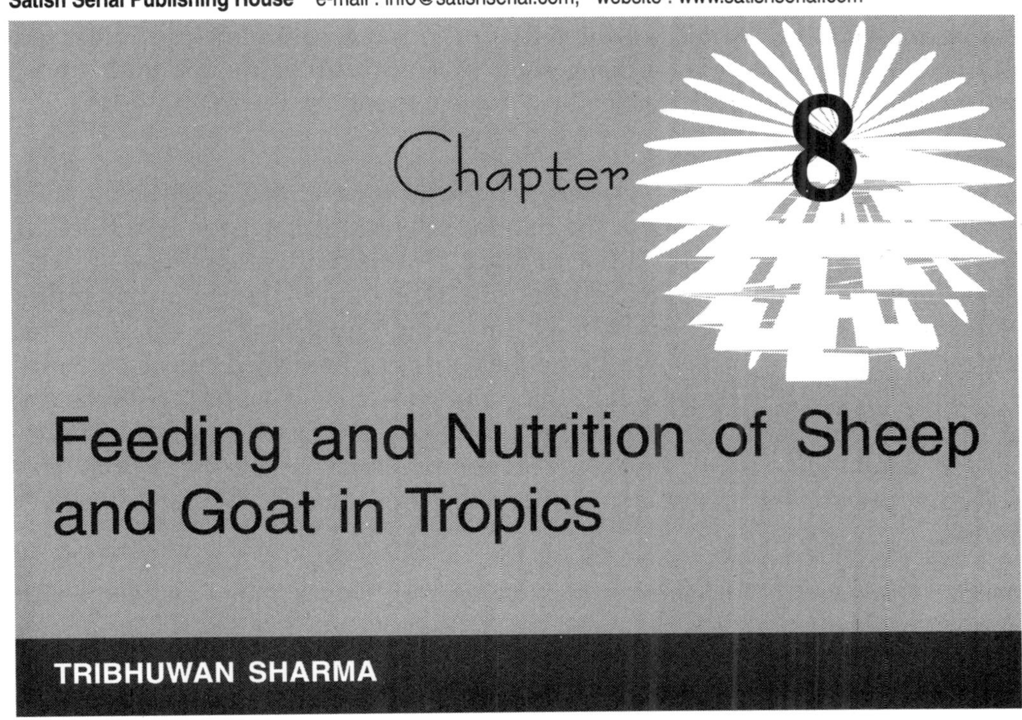

Chapter 8

Feeding and Nutrition of Sheep and Goat in Tropics

TRIBHUWAN SHARMA

The developing countries have about 55% of sheep and 95% of the goat population. The developed countries, on the other hand, have about 45% sheep and only 5% of goats. Presently there are about 53, 105 and 263 goats against 100 sheep in the world, Asia and India, respectively.

The sheep and goat are important livestock species in tropics. They play vital role in the livelihood security of small and marginal farmers and landless labourers throughout the tropics in arid and semiarid region. They are reared under most extensive and migratory system and predominate in the ecologically poor zones. The gravity of situation can be judged from the fact that India with only 2.30% of the land area of the world is maintaining nearly 16.6% of world human population and about 20.0% of livestock, subjecting available resources to great biotic pressure. Therefore, maintaining large flocks of sheep and goats under extensive system is facing difficulties and rearing of these two species under semi-intensive system is acquiring place. This changing scenario need serious review of present small ruminant production systems followed by the farmers of different ecological zones and defining of strategies and approaches for improvement. Studies have shown that improvement can be achieved in overall productivity of the small ruminants through feed and fodder resource development, their efficient utilization and nutritional interventions bring out better feeding management for sheep and goat.

Feeding Behaviour

The goats are basically browsers and spend more time for browsing than grazing but keeping in view of the habitat of goats, it has been described as browser, grazer and an animal that readily consumes both grasses and browse. Goats have also been identified as opportunist feeders as they adopt their diet according to forage class availability and forage quality (Papachristou and Nastist, 1993). Being top down grazers they start to eat seed heads of top of the canopy and progressively take the forage down. In general, goats are not meaningful competitor with grazing species i.e. sheep and cattle provided browse availability is not limited. The comparative feeding behaviour and digestive physiology in goats and sheep are presented in tabular form here under.

Table 1 : Comparative Feeding Behaviour and Digestive Physiology in Goats and Sheep (Devendra, 1989)

	Characteristics	Goats	Sheep
1	Activity	Bipedal stance and walk longer distances	Walk shorter distances
2	Feeding pattern	Browser, more selective	Grazer, less selective
3	Browse and tree leaves	Relished	Less relished
4	Variety in feeds	Preference greater	Preference lesser
5	Taste sensation	More discerning	Less discerning
6	Salivary secretion Rate	Greater	Moderate
7	Recycling of urea in saliva	Greater	Lesser
8	DMI for meat	3% of BW	3% of BW
	DMI for lactation	4-6% of BW	3% of BW
9	Digestive efficiency With coarse roughages	Higher	Less efficient
10	Retention time	Longer	Shorter
11	Water intake/Unit DMI	Lower	Higher
12	Rumen ammonia concentration	Higher	Lower
13	Water economy	More efficient	Less efficient
14	Water turnover rate	Lower	Higher
15	Nature of faeces	Less Water	Relatively higher
16	Nature of Urine	More concentrated	Less concentrated

The digestion in sheep, goats and cattle is similar when on moderate to high quality forage. But with regards to utilization of cell wall rich and nitrogen poor forages goats are more efficient than sheep. Goats retain the feed for longer time in gastro-intestinal tract and have a higher concentration of cellulolytic bacteria in rumen. The recycling of blood urea is also comparatively better in goats than sheep and other large ruminants. In adverse condition goats consumes less water.

Anatomical Feature of Sheep and Goats

Herbivores that have broad and flat muzzle have a lesser ability to feed selectively then species with narrow months and incurred incisors arcades (Shinde and Sankhayan, 2006). Sheep have a muzzle with a split upper lip and they can pick up tiny blades of herbage which are inaccessible to bigger animals and thus have a special ability to survive on natural grasses, herbs, legumes, weeds and shrubs, from an exploited range lands (Dumont, 1997). Goats, known to prefer browse on various pastures have shown evidences that they have a flexible and opportunistic grazing behaviour enable them to adapt to various range conditions. Goats have characteristic bipedal stance, give them advantage in consumption of several tree species and overhead portion of shrub species. Goats manipulate bipedal stance behaviour according to the availability of tree foliage from grazing lands (Bhatta *et al.*, 2001).

Small Ruminant Production Systems

A number of small ruminant production systems are in practice varying from country to country and region to region with in a country. In tropics, the rearing of sheep and goats are under both migratory and sedentary system. The sedentary system includes stall feeding following cut and carry system, semi intensive feeding or an extensive management system. Where as, migratory system include long distance migration or transhumance. The production system adopted in an area primarily depends on availability of wasteland and surrounding forest cover as well as market prospects. On account of these aforesaid factors about 70-80% of sheep flocks are reared under migratory system in the India. The migratory system is still most effective and practical system for small ruminants rearing in arid area because of topography, scarce vegetation and socio-economic status of farmers besides, low and erratic rainfall and recurrent drought. The sheep under migration get access to new and wide variety of vegetation, rich in vitamins, minerals and other nutrients help them to meet the requirement. In past the migration and environment were complementary to each other but now a days due to technological advancement and climatic changes this functional relationship has undergone changes and have narrowed down the migratory routes.

Over exploitation of natural resources as a result of increasing biotic pressure is throughout the tropics. The existing grazing pressure in arid India is very high i.e. 1 to 4 ACU/ha, against normal 0.2-0.5 ACU/ha (Beniwal and Singh, 2005a). Studies carried out indicate, that from Rajasthan state alone, 0.5 million sheep are in permanent migration and are not brought to their homestate at any time. About 1.0 million small ruminants from western districts of Rajasthan migrate for 6-9 months to near by states starting migration between October to February and return at onset of monsoon. Goat flocks are normally non-migrating except in case of mixed flocks.

Under the constraints of extremely degraded rangelands and shrinking of grazing lands, the targeted production never seems to be achievable. Thus, semi intensive system i.e. free range grazing /browsing plus supplementation devised to take care of limitations of extensive system seems to be the most viable proposition for sustainable small ruminant production in tropics. Further, this system is particularly more suitable for goats to perform well. The total confinement and stall feeding of goats sound good but has been observed to be detrimental many a times.

The intensive feeding system to be adopted in tropics is of two categories-

- Complete stall feeding on cultivated forage or complete feed or crop residues.
- Grazing/browsing on silvi pasture or on good grass pastures.

Stall feeding is of practical importance in areas abundantly supplied with crop residues and agro-industrial by products. In goats it is preferred for milk and meat production in urban and semi-Urban areas. In case of sheep stall feeding is not common, however weaned lambs could be raised on cultivated fodder or on complete feed. Lambs rearing on complete feed comprising of roughage (tree leaves, grasses, legumes) and concentrate (maize, barley grains, oil cakes, bran etc.) in ratio of 60: 40, 50: 50 and 60: 40 have good option for meat production. Kids after weaning at 3 months of age and fed on feed lot ration attained bodyweight of 25 Kg at 6 months with dressing yield of 48-51% and feed efficiency 10-12% (Singh and Sahu, 1997). Intensive feeding of kids have been reported to improve dressing yield and fat content but reduced bone and lean content compared to semi-intensive system. A growth rate of 150 and 170 g daily during 3-6 months of age with feed efficiency of 12-15% have be recorded in native and crossbred lambs kept on ration, containing concentrate and roughage in 50:50 ratio.

Feeds Fodder Resources and their Nutritive Value

In tropics, sheep & goat are numerically important farm animals. The climate is mostly characterized by long dry summers with mean temperature rising several degrees above mammalian body temperatures followed by low winter temperatures. Further due to late erratic and short spell of rains and soil conditions, the natural potential of range and pasture lands falls far short to meet the nutritional requirements of animals. There is marked variation in respect of availability of feed resources and its nutritive value among years and seasons. The natural range/grazing lands have been over exploited and are dominated by extremely poor and mostly annual grasses and shrubby vegetation. Even then during monsoon natural grasslands have an important place among the forage resources for sheep and goats. The grazing land support adapted native vegetation with variable proportions, comprising of predominately annual and perennial grasses, legumes, forbs and woody perennials used as forage by sheep and goats. The top feeds in arid and semi arid area particularly classed as crisis fodder for livestock. In general, they form an integral part of feed for sheep and goats in the regions, during lean periods when grazing material is scare and its nutritive value is very low. The fodder trees are the potential source of feed. About 60% of total feed available comes from these sources for sheep and goats (Beniwal and Singhal, 2005b). Most of the tree leaves contain high crude protein. *Prosopis cineraria* is an important fodder tree in arid and semi arid region, which grows even on cultivated fields without any determent to associated ground cover. The leaves contain about 15% crude protein and its average yield is 58.7 Kg per tree on complete lopping (Beniwal and Singh, 2005a). *Tecomela undulata Salvadora oleoides, Albizzia labbek, Ziziphus spp. Clophasperum mopaen, Alianthus excelsa,* etc. are important top feed plants of arid and semi arid region contribute biomass for sustainable sheep and goat production.

In areas where sheep and goats are important domesticated species, to take care of the lean periods silvi pastures having trees and shrubs adapted well to the region in association with pasture grasses and legumes have been observed to be most effective land use system,. This system helps to overcome scarcity of fodder during lean periods (Nov. to June). Silvi pasture system provides quality forage for larger span of year (Shankar and Gupta,1992). It has biomass yield between 20-25 q/ha adequate to maintain 6 sheep/goat round the year. In arid and semi arid areas, despite most judicial use of resources migration during summer months is common.

Grazing Behaviour

Feed resource availability both qualitatively and quantitatively, climatic conditions and physiological stage of animals influence the grazing behaviour. In lambs as the milk supply from dam decreases the grazing time increases. There is an increase of grazing time with age up to the age of 3 yrs as per study recorded in Marino sheep, due to change in number of bits per minute and amount of feed per bite. Pregnancy has not been recorded to increase grazing time but during lactation there is 7-12% increase in grazing time

(Arnold, 1975). Thin sheep eat more than fat sheep by increasing the rate of eating. Shorn sheep in cold climate consumed feed at faster rate and reduced the grazing time than unshorn sheep. In goats, the grazing behaviour changes from morning to evening. In first hours of the day, they utilize less time for grazing but visit different sites to explore the most grazing places (Solanki, 1994). Sheep and goat follow rhythmic periodicity in grazing pattern; graze actively during morning and evening hours. Forage quality particularly fibre content of forage influence the feed utilization pattern rumination rate (Chew/bolus) in sheep increased from 62-67 with decreased mastication rate from 69-63 due to increase in fibre content of diet (Shinde, 1997). In goats mastication rate was not influenced by fibre content of diet. It was noticed to be species specific rather than dependence on fibre content of diet. Rumination rate was noticed to be 45 chew/minute in monsoon when diet comprised of 68% shrubs and 32% grass and forbs, further, the rate increased to 72 chew per minute when shifted to sole diet of shrubs in winter and summer. Regurgitation rate is influenced by high moisture content. In a study, it was noted to be 1.44 bolus/min in monsoon which decreased in winter and summer to 1.11 and 1.08 with maturing of vegetation (Bhatta *et al.*, 2001).

Diet Selection

Several workers have studied the nutrient selectivity by sheep while grazing in the rangelands. It was found that selection of CP by sheep from grazing land when compared with its availability in grazing land was 1:35:1 during monsoon and 1:78:1 during winter and 2:25:1 during summer. It is also observed that goat select diet rich in protein and low in fibre by virtue of their opportunistic behaviour and movement. (Bhatta *et al*, 2001). In case of goats even when grasses are available in all seasons in range land, consume grasses only in monsoon period (24% of their diet) and avoid grasses in other season, on account of their maturity and age. The goat's diet contained 76% shrub during monsoon and almost 100% during winter and summer season. Browse species of plants are most preferred component of the goat diets (Ramirez *et al* 1990, Mallado *et al* 1991). In a study goats consumed 81% shrub, 9% grasses and 10% forbs species under forced grazing system on desert grassland. A better understanding of dietary preference of sheep & goats on arid and semiarid range lands help in improving the animal production. The decision of grazing by herbivorous is generally dictated by their will to maximize the energy balance. Sheep has definite motivation for their selection because of nutritional wisdom and to match nutrient intake with nutrient requirements. Sheep and goat unlike other animals are hedyphagic (They select food at minimum cost of unpleasant, olfactory and other sensation) and euphagic (They select food which provide them optimal nutrition and avoiding toxicities). Sheep select plant species not only for nutrition but also for flavour. The choice is determined by the response of chemical stimuli received through the sense of small, taste and touch and the selection is influenced by sugars, organic acids, tannin and alkaloids, presence in plant species. Some of the information on preference of forage species and nutrient by sheep and goat while grazing freely in range land has been collected at CSWRI (Table 2).

Table 2 : Preference indices for forage species and nutrients by sheep and goats

Forage species	Season				Dietary nutrients		
	Monsoon	Winter	Summer		Monsoon	Winter	Summer
			Sheep				
Vernonia cineraria	0.68	0.25		CP	1.19	2.12	3.00
Cenchrus catharticus	1.02	1.86		NDF	0.99	0.77	0.85
Eleusine aegyptiaca	0.62	0.92		ADF	0.99	0.95	0.76
Crotolaria burhia	0.43	0.28		Cellulose	0.98	0.84	0.73
Eleusine indica	1.06	0.46		H. Cellulose	0.97	0.50	1.61
Indigifera cordifolia	0.69	-		ADL	1.90	2.20	0.81
Cyanodon dactylon	0.55	0.60		GE	0.93	1.03	1.05
			Goats				
Grasses and Forbs							
Crotalaria burhia	3.85	-	-	CP	1.35	1.78	2.25
Phaseolus tribulus	2.89	-	-	NDF	0.93	0.86	0.65
Melilotus indica	0.72	-	-	ADF	0.89	0.86	0.56
Sorghum halepense	14.88	-	-	Cellulose	0.64	0.79	1.03
Shrub and trees				H. Cellulose	1.05	0.86	1.24
Acacia senegal	0.45	0.49	0.42	ADL	2.00	1.68	0.66
Acacia tortillas	-	-	0.82	-	-	-	-
Bauhinia recemosa	6.85	-	-	-	-	-	-
Cocculus pendulus	1.70	1.39	2.30	-	-	-	-
Dicrostachys nutans	1.17	2.56	-	-	-	-	-
Gymnosporia spinosa	2.76	2.54	-	-	-	-	-
Prosopis cineraria	0.79	1.42	0.65	-	-	-	-
Zyziphus mauritiana	6.63	3.16	-	-	-	-	-

Source : Shinde and Sankhyan (2006), Bhatta *et al.* (2001)

Nutrient Requirements of Sheep

The adult weight (30-40 Kg) and growth rate of Indian breeds of sheep in comparison to many foreign sheep breeds (70 Kg) is much lower. Besides, the genetic make up; inadequate nutrition is major factor for low growth rate and body weight. Under adequate feeding conditions, the crossbred have proved superior to native sheep in terms of body weight gain, feed efficiency and wool yield. Proper nutritional management is essential to exploit the full genetic potential. The Nutrient requirements for sheep available are NRC (1985), AFRC (1993), ICAR (1998) and Kearl (1982).

Energy

Energy deficiency or in sufficiency is likely the most common nutritional problem affecting performance of sheep. Energy deficiency causes slowing of growth, loss of weight, reproductive disorder, lowered production and increased mortality depending upon the severity of deficiency.

Maintenance

The energy requirement for maintenance is the amount to be consumed daily to maintain constant weight. It is the amount of ME resulting in zero change in body energy and products.

In the ARC (1980) system, the energy value of feeds is expressed in terms of ME. In 1993 a full description of the modified system was prepared by the Agricultural and Food Research Council (AFRC) and published by CAB. For sheep, the equation for predicting the maintenance requirement (as net energy) for ewes and wethers is

$$0.226\ (W/1.08)^{0.75} + 0.007\ W$$

Rams require 15% more energy for maintenance. As per ICAR the maintenance energy values reported are 93 KCal/Kg $W^{0.75}$ (ICAR, 1998) which is equivalent to 27.3 g TDN/Kg $W^{0.75}$.

Growth

Energy requirement for growth reflect the deposition of lipids, protein and water. The sheep data examined by ARC (1980) suggested large effects of sex on the energy value of gains, only small effects of breed and no effect of rate of gain.

The equation derived for sexes were

Male : Evg = 2.5 + 0.35 W

Female : Evg = 4.4 + 0.35 W

Where, Evg = energy value of live weight gain (MJ/Kg)

W = live weight in KG

Thus, predict the energy content of live weight gain of 30 Kg lambs. For example 13.0 MJ/Kg for males and 15.6 MJ/Kg for females.

Lactation

Lactation requirements are pertinent to first and second month of lactation there after in 3rd month, the requirement may be reduced by 25% due to short lactation period in sheep. The lactation requirement in first two months is twice the maintenance requirement (ICAR 1998). The ME requirement per Kg Milk is almost similar in sheep, goat and cattle and ranges between 1100 to 1300 KCal/Kg of 4% FCM. For every additional Kg of Milk produced add 1250 K cal ME (Kearl 1982).

The Energy value of ewe's milk as per AFRC (1993) is

$$EV_L \text{ (MJ/Kg)} = 0.0328\,F + 0.0025D + 2.2$$

Where F = Fat Content (g/Kg)
D = Day of Lactation

In general when information on composition is not available, a value of 4.6 MJ/Kg may be assumed.

Pregnancy

Pregnant ewes during the last 6 weeks of pregnancy should be provided with 50 % more nutrients than the maintenance needs.

As per NRC the maintenance requirement may be multiplied by 1.5 for single lamb and 2 for twin lambs, to derive the pregnancy requirement to be given during last 6 weeks of pregnancy.

Protein

The protein requirements are expressed as digestible protein (ICAR, 1985, Kearl, 1982), Crude protein (NRC, 1985) and metaboliazable protein (AFRC, 1993). For formulating diets, digestible protein values have been converted to total protein (Kearl, 1982) using the equation.

$$Y = 1.115\,X + 3.82$$

Where X = DP (% of DM)
Y = TP (% of DM)

Quality of protein is also important as protein synthesized in rumen do not meet with qualitative requirement of sheep for maximum production. The sulphur containing amino acid, methionine is prime limiting amino acid in microbial protein required by sheep for both growth of wool and weight gain followed by lysine and threonine.

Maintenance

The average digestible protein value of 1.72g/kg $W^{0.75}$ was proposed by Kearl (1982), which was translated to 18.5 g DP/Mcal ME for maintenance only. ICAR (1998) suggest protein requirement for maintenance of Indian sheep to be 2.73 g DCP/Kg $W^{0.75}$. The requirement of Metabolizable protein given by AFRC (1993) for maintenance in sheep is 2.19 g/Kg $W^{0.75}$.

Growth

NRC (1975) suggested the digestible protein requirement of sheep weighing between 29-35 Kg to be 24 g/M cal ME. It was used by Kearl (1982) ,to calculate DP requirement of sheep for maintenance, growth and early lactation. In AFRC (1993) feeding standards for estimating protein requirement, the protein content of live weight gain is added to the endogenous losses as well as deposition of protein in fleece i.e. if a 20 Kg lamb growing at the rate of 0.2 Kg/d is estimated to have endogenous losses of nitrogen equivalent to 21 g protein/d and suppose its live weight gains are estimated to be 140 g protein/Kg and 6 g of protein is stored per day in fleece.

The net protein requirement will be

$$21.0 + (0.2 \times 140) + 6 = 55g/d.$$

To calculate the requirement for MP, each of the net energy requirements must be divided by the appropriate efficiency factor. For Maintenance the factor is 1.0, for live weight gain 0.59, and for wool growth 0.26.

Therefore, the metabolizable crude protein (MCP) is

$$21 + 28.0/0.59 + 6.0/0.26 = 92\ g/d$$

Lactation

The lactation requirement for first two months in ewes producing 1 or 2 Kg milk per day is suggested to be a ratio of 30 g DP/M cal. ME. In last four months the DP requirements are reduced to 27 g DP/ M cal. ME.

Nutrient Requirements of Goats

Nutrient requirements of goats for different physiological stages have been suggestd by NRC (1981), Kearl (1982), AFRC (1993) and ICAR (1998). The dry matter intake (DMI) varies according to the energy density of diet and the physical character of roughages included in diet. The intake of dry matter suggested by NRC (1981) and ICAR (1998) have been given in tables of feeding standards.

Energy

Energy requirements are affected by age, growth, body size, pregnancy and lactation as well as environment, voluntary activity and stress.

Table 3 : Daily Nutrient Requirements of Sheep*

Category	Physiological Activity	Body Weight (kg)	kg	DMI ADG (g)	% of live ut.	Diet Density (Mcal/k)	ME (Mcal)	TDN (kg)	TP (g)	DP (g)	Ca (g)	P (g)
Ewes and Lambs	Maintenance, Growth, Non-	-	0	0.93	2.3	1.6	1.48	0.41	75	36	5.7	3.1
	lactating	40.0										
	ewes		50	1.10	2.8	2.0	2.16	0.6	100	52	5.7	3.1
	and first 15 weeks of gestation		100	1.19	3.0	2.4	2.85	0.7	121	68	5.9	3.2
Ewes	Last six weeks of gestation or last eight											
Ewes Rams	weeks of lactation	40.0	100	1.48	3.7	2.65	3.9	1.08	174	105	4.0	3.8
	First eight weeks of lactation											
	maintenance	40.0	(-)10	1.67	4.2	2.0	3.37	0.93	176	101	10.4	7.4
	and growth	40.0	110	1.43	3.6	2.15	3.07	0.85	137	74	6.3	3.5

*Adapted from Kearl (1982); 1 kg TDN = 3.62 Mcal ME

Maintenance requirement during last trimester = 171% of maintenance

Grazing

(1) open range: Add 25% of nutrient requirements

(2) Harsh conditions with long distances to water: Add 50% of requirements

(3) Sparse vegetation, mountainous country: Add 75% of requirements

Maintenance

ME requirement for maintenance in goats have been suggested to be 101.38 K cal ME/kg $W^{0.75}$ by NRC (1981). ICAR (1998) has given a value of 30.0 g TDN/kg $W^{0.75}$ for maintenance of goats. AFRC (1993) suggested considerable variation in fasting metabolism of lactating goats and arrived at 75.3 Kcal/kg $W^{0.75}$ per day. The value should be increased by 10% for goats kept in door, 20% for grazing at low lands and 30% for grazing at hills.

Growth

The ME requirements for growth has been suggested to be 7.25 Kcal/g gain (NRC, 1981) at all body weight and activity.

Table 4 : Daily Nutrient Requirements of Sheep*

Category	Physiological Activity	Body Weight (kg)	Weight Change/ day(g)	kg	DMI % of live weight	TDN (kg)	DE (Mcal)	ME (Mcal)	CP (g)	Ca (g)	P (g)
	Maintenance	50	1.0	1.0	2.0	0.55	2.4	2.0	95	2.0	1.8
Ewes	Flushing - 2										
	weeks pre		100	1.6	3.2	0.94	4.1	3.4	150	5.3	2.6
Ewes	breeding	50									
	Non-										
	Lactating and		30	1.2	2.4	0.67	3.0	2.4	112	2.9	2.1
	first 15										
Ewes	Last four	50									
	Weeks of										
	gestation-										
Ewes	expected	50.0	180	1.6	3.2	0.94	4.1	3.4	175	5.9	4.8
	first six to										
	eight weeks	50.0	(-)25	2.1	4.2	1.36	6.0	4.9	304	8.9	6.1
	of lactation										
Ewes	suckling										
Ewe lambs	-	40.0	182	1.4	3.5	0.91	4.0	3.3	176	5.9	2.6
Ram lambs	-	40.0	330	1.8	4.5	1.1	5.0	4.1	243	7.8	3.7
Lambs	Finishing 4 – 7 months old	40.0	275	1.6	4.0	1.2	5.4	4.4	185	6.6	3.3
Lambs	Early weaned	40.0	345	1.5	3.8	1.2	5.1	4.2	202	7.7	3.9

*NRC (1985); 1 kg TDN = 4.4 Mcal DE; ME = 82 % DE

Pregnancy

In last two months of pregnancy, the ME requirement has been suggested to be 177 K cal/kg $W^{0.75}$ (NRC, 1981) and 182 K cal/W kg. $^{0.75}$ (ICAR, 1998).

Lactation

NRC (1981) used a value of 1246.12 K cal ME/kg of FCM for a fat range of 2.5 to 6.0%. For each 0.5% change in fat % from 4%, an addition or subtraction of 16.28 K cal ME has been suggested. ICAR (1998) has suggested 30 g TDN/kg $W^{0.75}$ for lactating goats as requirement.

Protein

Proteins are of vital importance for growth, maintenance, reproduction and milk production. The protein requirements for various physiological processes are detailed here under.

Table 5 : Feeding Standards for Sheep*

Category	Physiological Activity	Body Weight (kg)	ADG (g)	Days from conception	DMI (kg)	ME (MJ)	MP (g)
				98	1.2	7.9	72
				112	1.2	8.8	76
Ewes	Pregnant with single lamb	55.0		126	1.2	9.9	82
				140	1.2	11.3	89
				Weeks of lactation			
Ewes	Lactating ewes Kept outdoors with single lamb (qm = 0.625)	55.0	-	1-4	1.5	16.7	154
			-	5-8	1.7	15.8	148
			-	9-12	1.6	13.2	120
			0	-	0.46	3.4	21.0
Female Lambs	Growth (qm = 0.55 metabolizability)	20.0	50		0.46	4.5	45.0
			100	-	0.46	3.9	21.0
			0	-	0.46	3.9	21.0
Male Lambs	Growth (qm = 0.55 metabolizability)	20.0	50		0.46	4.8	47.0
			100	-	0.46	5.8	61.0

*AFRC, 1993

Table 6 : Daily Nutrient Requirements of Sheep*

Physiological Activity	Body Weight (kg)	ADG (g)	DMI g	DMI % of live wt.	TDN (kg)	ME (Mcal)	DCP (g)	Ca (g)	P (g)
Maintenance			964	2.4	434	1.56	48	1.9	1.3
Pregnancy			1590	4.0	827	2.98	115	5.2	3.7
	40.0								
Lactation		-	1750	4.4	945	3.41	135	8.7	5.8
Wool production		-	1230	3.1	555	2.0	67	2.5	1.6
		50.0	600.0	3.0	360	1.08	55	3.0	2.0
	20.0								
Growth		100	680.0	3.4	410	1.44	63	3.4	2.3

*ICAR (1998)

Maintenance

Digestible protein requirement for maintenance of goats has been suggested to be 2.82 and 3.0 g/kg $W^{0.75}$ by NRC (1981) and ICAR, (1998). As per AFRC (1993) the net requirement of nitrogen for maintenance is amount needed to replace the EUN, part of MFN and loss of N in hair and scurf. The total is referred as basal endogenous nitrogen (BEN) and is 0.35g/kg $W^{0.75}$ per day or 2.19 g/kg $W^{0.75}$ per day of metabolizable protein. The metabolizable protein is considered to be used for maintenance with an efficiency of 1.0.

Growth

NRC (1981) has given an average value of 0.195 g DP equal to 0.284 g TP/g gain in goats.

Pregnancy

ICAR (1998) has given a value of 5.53 g DP/kg $W^{0.75}$ as pregnancy requirement of does in body weights between 15 to 60 kg. Where as, requirement has been suggested to be, 4.79g DM or 6.97 g TP/kg $W^{0.75}$ by NRC (1981) for pregnancy.

Lactation

ICAR (1998) has suggested the lactation requirements of does to be 45g DP/kg of 4% FCM, whereas, NRC (1981) recommendation is 57.2g DP or 81.71 g TP/kg milk with 4.86% fat.

The daily nutrient requirement suggested by NRC (1981), Kearl (1982) and ICAR (1998) for sheep and goat have been given in table form.

Feeding of Sheep (Under Organized Management)

Feeding of pre weaning lambs

Pre weaning lambs require special attention for harvesting desired economic return in active phase of growth. The newborn should be fed colostrum as early as possible. The biological significance of colostrum feeding is lost if it is delayed. The lambs may be maintained with their dams till one week after birth to avoid mis mothering and to facilitate effective consumption of colostrum. In this period the lambs are allowed free suckling. A minimum of 3-4 suckling must be ensured. In developed countries the lambs are initiated to milk replacer as early as possible to boost their nutrient intake to support higher rate of gain but it is not the practice in developing and under developed countries.

Table 7 : Daily Nutrient Requirements of Goats*

Physiological Activity	Body Weight (kg)	ADG (g)	Energy				Crude Protein			
			TDN (g)	DE (Mcal)	ME (Mcal)	NE (Mcal)	TP	DP	Ca (g)	P (g)
Maintenance only (includes stable feeding conditions, minimal activity and early pregnancy	40	-	448	1.98	1.61	0.91	63	43	2.0	1.4
Maintenance plus Low activity (=25% increment, intensive Management, tropical range and early Pregnancy	40	-	560	2.47	2.02	1.14	77	54	3	2.1
Maintenance plus Medium activity (=50% increment, Semiarid range land, slightly hilly pastures and early pregnancy	40	-	672	2.97	2.42	1.36	93	64	4	2.8
Maintenance plus high activity (=75% increment, Arid range land, sparse vegetation, mountainous pastures and early pregnancy	40	-	784	3.46	2.82	1.59	108	75	4	2.8
Additional requirements for Late pregnancy for all goat sizes	-	-	397	1.74	1.42	0.8	82	57	2	1.4
	-	50	100	0.44	0.36	0.2	14	10	1	0.7
Additional requirements for growth for all goat sizes	-	100	200	0.88	0.72	0.4	28	20	1	0.7
	-	150	300	1.32	1.08	0.6	42	30	2	1.4
Additional requirements for milk production (per kg) at 4% fat content in milk	-	-	346	1.53	1.25	0.7	72	51	3.0	2.1

* NRC (1981)

Table 8 : Daily Nutrient Requirements of Goats*

Physiological Activity	Body Weight (kg)	ADG (g)	DMI kg	DMI % of live	Diet Density (Mcal/kg)	ME (Mcal)	TDN (kg)	TP (g)	DP (g)	Ca (g)	P (g)
Maintenance,		0	0.91	2.2	1.8	1.65	0.46	70	48	25	1.9
growth, Early	40.0										
Lactation		50	0.98	2.4	2.05	2.00	0.55	80	58	3.1	2.4
		100	1.04	2.5	2.30	2.34	0.65	99	67	3.8	2.9
Last six Weeks of Gestation or Last eight weeks of Lactation	40.0	120	1.21	3.0	2.5	3.05	0.84	129	115	4.0	2.8
First ten weeks of lactation	40.0	(-) 20	1.9	4.8	2.0	3.79	1.05	160	121	5.0	3.5
Milk production (per kg FCM) 4.0 % fat	-	-	-	-	-	1.25	346	75	51	3.0	2.1

*Adopted from Kearl (1982)

DMI = 76.3 / kg $W^{0.75}$

20 % was added to the ME requirement for first kidding goats (20 to 25 kg weight)

10% was added to the ME requirement for second kidding goats (30 kg weight)

Table 9 : Daily Nutrient Requirements of Goats*

Physiological Activity	Body Weight (kg)	ADG (g)	DMI kg	DMI % of live wt.	TDN (kg)	ME (Mcal)	DCP (g)	Ca (g)	P (g)
Maintenance		-	1040	2.6	500	1.79	48	2.6	1.5
Pregnancy		-	1460	3.6	802	2.89	88	4.4	2.9
Lactation	40.0								
Yield, 0.5 kg		-	1245	3.1	673	2.43	70	6.2	4.1
Yield, 1 kg		-	1565	3.9	845	3.05	93	7.8	5.2
		50.0	640.0	3.2	385	1.39	39	3.3	2.2
Growth	20.0								
		100	790.0	3.9	475	1.71	49	4.1	2.7

* ICAR (1998)

The lamb starts nibbling in third week. The nibbling is not with the objective of providing dry matter intake but it helps in early rumen development. After 15 days the lambs are offered *ad lib* creep mixture of high energy and protein content (DCP 16 % and TDN 60 %) and free choice green fodder. This practice is in use at CSWRI. The lambs after 1 month are let out for grazing on mixed pasture in cooler parts of the day. The concentrate offered to the lambs raised for mutton production may preferably be given in early hours, before they go out for grazing.

In pre weaning phase lambs derive nutrients mainly from dam's milk and thus in pre weaning growth the milk yield of dams have significant effect. Milk yield in ewes of western India have been recorded to be 300-400 ml/day (Riyazuddin *et al.* 1998). While in flocks under organized management Singh and Singh (1987) have recorded 643 ml milk/day. The efficiency of milk utilization for growth has been reported to vary from 17 to over 30% (Sharma, 1998). The nutrition of lactating ewe to optimize milk yield could be considered as key to affect the pre weaning growth. Twins and Triplets also effect growth rate of lambs as growth rate is faster in single as compared to twins and triplets and could be ascribed to competition in milk consumption and lower birth weight. However, if both lambs survive the pooled weight is mostly higher, than single. The lambs, which are heavier at birth grow fast and attain higher weaning weight. At farmers field the native and crossbred have been reported to achieve 74 and 68g ADG, respectively (Kausuish *et. al.*,1990). While under organized feeding management with *ad lib* concentrate and free suckling, pre weaning growth rate of 172 and 168g ADG in male and female lambs have been achieved in mutton synthetic and malpura breeds (Arora *et al.*, 1986).

An average daily gain of 140 g with feed conversion ratio of 1:3.4 recorded by Santra and Karim (1999) on feeding *ad lib* creep mixture & free suckling could be considered optimum under semi arid environment.

Table 10 : Feeding Schedule for a Kid from Birth to 90 Days

Age of Kids	Dam's milk or cow milk	Creep Feed (g)	Forage, green /day (g)
1-3 days	Colostrum 300 ml, 3 feedings	-	-
4-14days	350 ml, 3 feedings	-	-
15-30 days	350 ml, 3 feedings	A little	A little
31-60 days	400 ml, 2 feedings	100-150	Free choice
61-90 days	200 ml, 2 feedings	200-250	Free choice

Weaning

Weaning is a transitional phase of growth and influence post weaning growth response which is very crucial for economic returns. The lambs are generally weaned at 3 months.

In pre weaning period lambs constantly receive maternal care and suddenly are devoid off. On account of separation lambs are nervous and gradually adjust to change. A weight loss has been observed immediately after weaning. Studies have shown that lambs require two weeks time to regain the weight loss due to weaning stress (Karim, 2004). Further, the well-fed lambs were recorded to loose more weight. Report have shown that weaning at 90 days followed by intensive feeding for 90 days to attain desired finishing weight of 30 kg at 6th month in lambs raised for mutton deposited high carcass fat even exceeding 20% with low feed conversion efficiency. Thus to improve feed conversion efficiency, reduce carcass fat% and to improve economic returns the weaning age was suggested to reduce from 90 to 60 days (Karim, 2004).

Feeding of post weaning lambs

Post weaning period in sheep is an active phase of growth and very critical for mutton production. In developed countries this phase is used for fattening ensuring an ADG of 250-300 g/day, where as, in tropics in this period, the ADG is much lower. In India it averages between 40-70 g. This low gain in due to poor plan of nutrition and suggests scope of maximization through nutrition interventions. Supplementations with grazing have been found to be very effective in improving finishing weight. Supplementation of concentrate in limited amount of 1.5-2.0% of body weight, in addition to free grazing could provide finishing weight of 25-30 kg at six months of age (Shinde *et al.*, 2008). A growth study, Kheri weaners maintained on extensive, semi-intensive and intensive (R:C, 40:60) system of feeding indicated that the finish lambs at 6 months of age attained 22.7, 30.3 and 28.6 kg weight providing ADG of 70, 175 and 136 g with cost of feed input kg gain Rs. Nil, 36.62 and 38.91, respectively. The lambs further continued upto 9 months from 6 months on free grazing with *ad lib* concentrate supplementation and attained 36.2, 42.7 and 37.6 kg weight providing ADG of 137, 134 and 131 g having higher cost of concentrate input/kg gain in semi intensive, then in extensive and intensive feeding. It was observed from the study that under organized feeding, cost was uneconomical at 6-9 months age.

Faster gain in intensively fed lambs was associated with higher carcass fat content even exceeding 20%. Thus it is advisable to reduce weaning age from 90 to 60 days. The 60 days weaner lambs under intensive feeding has

160 and 151 g ADG and 16 and 12% feed efficiencies in Malpura and Sandi lambs. While the 90 days weaner lambs of some breed had 139 and 146 g ADG with 16 and 14% feed efficiency (Karim and Arora, 1997). Intensive feeding on 50:50 RC based complete feed attained 33.5 kg finishing weight with 11% feed efficiency at six months of age (Shinde *et al.*, 1995). Such series of studies suggested that the desirable finishing weight can be achieved by least cost ration formulation utilizing conventional roughage sources, tree leaves and energy and protein supplemented complete feed in intensive feeding system.

Nutrition for Wool Production

Plane of nutrition plays important role in the production of wool both quantitatively and qualitatively. Nutrient availability relative to maintenance affects wool production. Improved pasture sustain higher wool yield. Winter pastures are more efficient for wool growth then spring pastures. Pastures in high rainfall area are less efficient than pastures in low rainfall area. Seasonal variation in pasture quality affect wool growth but it can be overcome by appropriate supplementation. Robertson *et al.* (2000) noticed that production of sound wool on maintenance feed, compared to restrictive feed reduced staple length. Nutrient availability in terms of energy, protein and minerals require special attention for wool production. Unless sufficient energy is provided to the animal, wool production is seriously affected. Protein accretion as wool is more affected by energy intake than protein intake. Different levels of energy and protein significantly influence wool growth efficiency, fat content and wool fibre diameter (Moghadam *et al.*, 2000).

Although wool is composed mainly of protein but the level of protein required in the diet is not very high. Addition of protein beyond 11% had no extra advantage on fleece weight. Feeding good quality legume fodder can easily meet protein requirement for wool production. Keratin in wool contains high proportion of sulphur containing amino acids and sulphur in wool is found in the form of dithio linkage, that gives strength to wool fibre. Sulphur content of wool of different breed varies between 2.16-3.10% and in different grades of wool between 1.44 (very coarse wool) - 3.30 (very fine wool). Presence of high concentration of sulphur containing amino acids in the sheep diet is therefore very important, 0.2% sulphur in feed is considered sufficient to meet requirements (Choudhary, 1979). Copper is also directly associated with wool quality. It acts as a catalyst for oxidation of thio groups to dithio links in keratinization process. It also contributes towards crimps in wool. The deficiency leads to upset in keratinization, steely wool condition develops. The desirable level of copper in blood is 100 ppm. A 0.001% copper in the diet is adequate to meet the requirements. Zinc, Cobalt and iron deficiency have also been reported to affect wool production due to shading of wool. Wool is sensitive to Zinc, intake above 17 ppm depresses wool growth (White and Martin, 1988).

Over and above these, vitamin A deficiency appears to cause excessive keratinization of follicular epithelium which blocks the opening of follicle and prevent wool growth. As such, the wool production is not affected directly by B-complex vitamins as they are assured from rumen microflora. Supplementation of Flavomycin with appropriate availability of sulphur containing amino acids increases wool growth by 14.5% (Murray *et al.*, 1992). But no beneficial effect of hormonal growth promoters and urea as NPN on wool growth has been appreciably noticed.

Feeding of Goats (Under Organized Management)

Feeding under intensive system is basically dependent upon the knowledge of nutrient requirements and nutritive value of feed offered. Forages (green/ dry) available in large quantities at relatively low cost could be able to meet the maintenance and production requirement only upto certain level depending upon quality. The higher production requirements can be met by concentrate supplies adjusting energy, protein, minerals and vitamin needs.

Feeding of kids

Colostrum and milk are the essential feeds for neonatal kids. Colostrum should be fed *ad lib* to all kids as soon as possible after birth to provide immunity and positive energy balance. The effectiveness of transfer of immunoglobulin from colostrum to plasma is a function of antibody concentration in the colostrum, level of intake and time to consumption after birth (Norman, 1987) 20-28 days after birth kids may loose ability to absorb immunoglobulin from colostrum. Though evidences are available, that ability may stay longer in starved kids (Havervoll *et al.*, 1991). Total intake of colostrum per day for first 2-3 days should be about 280 ml for small kids weighing 3.5-4.5 kg. Cow colostrum could also be effectively utilized in kids and can be given @100 ml per kg live weight. Both under and over feeding of milk is harmful to the health as well as growth of kids. Larger volume may be divided into multiple small volumes. Kids may be switched to three and two times per day feeding by third week of age. However, multiple small feedings are good to reduce incidences of bloat and scour.

Early consumption of forage and concentrate must be encouraged as it is essential for the early development of rumen. The forage should be provided to the kids as per their choice in plenty. Natural milk feeding is very common in goats. Milk replacer is used to save milk for sale, for feeding of multiple births and to reduce milk feeding. A milk replacer/substitute having 24% CP may be used effectively for early growing kids. Early weaning may check the post weaning growth, therefore, to take care of weaning shock the goats may be given good quality concentrate mixture for the provision of adequate nutrients.

Feeding ot Post Weaning Kids

The daily dry matter intake (DMI) of goats may vary from 2.0 to 5.8 % of their body weight. High intake in young, growing and high lactating goats is to satisfy the comparatively higher need of nutrients. For optimum growth the kids must be maintained on intensive or semi intensive feeding. They should be provided good quality roughage, energy and protein supplements. Cereal grains constitute the major parts of concentrate mixture of growing goats. Deficiency of energy significantly affects growth. High energy concentrate may be formulated but concentrate mixture rich in starch has to be avoided in 5-7 months of female kids to prevent excess fattening effect negatively milk production in first lactation. Concentration of protein in diet is also equally important. Inclusion of by pass protein results in higher growth rate and better feed conversion efficiency. NPN has also been found effective (MBA *et al.*, 1974). In order to have optimum production, feeding of concentrate to goats is essential but ration with high proportion of concentrate (more than 75% of DMI in dairy animals and more than 85% in grower kids) may cause acidosis. Two to six months period is considered as active growth period. Therefore, balanced feeding during this period is very important for getting maximum returns. About 500 g green fodder, 200 g dry fodder and 250-300 g concentrate per day in association with grazing may meet the nutrient requirement of kids from 2 to 6 months of age and 250-300 g of concentrate mixture (as per body weight) in addition to grazing can provide adequate nutrient for kids from 6 to 12 months of age.

Feeding of Goats for Maintenance, Production and Reproduction

Goat and adult non breeding bucks require maintenance diet only. Supplementation of 2.0-2.5 kg green leguminous fodder, 250-350 g of dry fodder and 100 g of concentrate mixture with grazing can meet out with requirements.

In rainy season, it is advisable to give 150-200 g of concentrate mixture, 400-500 g of dry fodder to the goats to avoid incidences of diarrhoea on account of consumption of high moisture green fodder from grazing. 100 and 150 g/day/goat concentrate mixture for small and large breeds over and above the maintenance requirement are required to attain adequate body size for breeding. 400 g/day/goat concentrate mixture for small and large breed may be given for per kg milk produced. Level of protein and energy in diet of lactating goats is very important for milk production. Even 15% low energy of their total energy requirement reduces milk production with in 24-48 hr. (Moranod Fehr and Sauvant, 1978).

For pregnancy requirements concentrate mixture may be supplemented @ 400 g/d/animal in late pregnancy (last 5-6 weeks) to meet the requirement of rapid growth of faetus. Low plane of nutrition at this stage can cause pregnancy toxaemia. Breeding bucks may be given good quality green fodder to meet maintenance requirement and 400 g (smaller breed) and 500 g (larger breed) concentrate mixture per day per animal during active breeding season (Choudhary, 2004).

Feeding for Chevon Production

Several studies have been conducted on indigenous and crossbred kids under *ad lib* feeding on concentrate including barley, maize grain, oilcakes, wheat and rice bran, molasses etc. and roughages including leaves, cultivated grasses and legumes in the ratio of 40:60, 50:50 and 60:40. The male kids weaned at 2-3 months and raised on feed lot system attained slaughter weight of 25Kg at 5 to 6 months age with dressing percentage of 48 to 51%. The kids under semi intensive system required less feed for per Kg gain than under intensive system but the dressing percentage is superior under intensive system (Singh and Sahu, 1997). The total confinent and complete feeding of goats in stall has been noticed to be detrimental many a times.

The literature in totality reveals that an improvement can be achieved both in finishing weights and carcass quality through intensive feeding of male kids. To ensure a weaning weight of 14 to 15 kg, male kids may be provided *ad lib* suckling, creep ration and green/dry leguminous fodder during pre weaning period and completely weaned at 60 days of age. These weaners then be feed *ad lib* on complete feed consisting of 50% roughage and 50% concentrate, under stall, till attain 25-30 kg finishing weight in about 6-7 months of age. Alternatively the kids may be allowed to graze on available pasture and supplemented with concentrate mixture @ 1.5 to 2% of body weight till they achieve finishing weight.

References

AFRC (1993). *CAB*. International, Walling Ford, UK.

Arnold, G.W. (1975). *Aust. Agri. Res.*, 26: 1017-1024.

ARC. (1980). The Nutrient Requirements of Livestock. *CAB, Farnham Royal, U.K.*

Arora, A.L., Prassad, V.S.S., Gupta, D.C., Mark, A., Mehta, B.S., Srivastava, C.P., Satish Kumar and Mahajan, J.M. (1986). AICRP on Sheep breeding for mutton, Annual Report, CSWRI, Avikanagar.

Beniwal, R.K. and Singh, J.P. (2005a). In: Seminar on "Augmentation of Livestock Production Using Newer Technologies" March 11-12, College of Veterinary and Animal Science, Bikaner.

Beniwal, R.K. and Singh, J.P. (2005b). In: National Seminar on "Conservation, Processing and Utilization of Monsoon Herbage for Augmenting Animal Production" December 17-18, Regional Research Station, CAZRI, Bikaner, pp. 67-74.

Bhatta, R., Sankhyan, S. K. and Shinde, A.K. (2001). *Indian J. Anim. Sci.*, 71: 62-65.

Choudhary, U.B. (2004). National seminar on "Opportunities And Challenges In Nutrition And Feeding Management of Sheep, Goat and Rabbit for sustainable Production" pp. 60-66.

Chaudhary, B.R. (1979). Effect of feed and feed additives on sulpher content of wool and its yield in different breeds of sheep. Ph.D. Thesis, University of Udaipur, Rajasthan.

Dumont, B. (1997). *Ann. Zootech.*, 46: 105-116.

Havervall, O., M. hadjipanayiotou., M.R. sanzsampelayo, Z. Nitsan and P.Schmidely (1991). In: Goat Nutrition. Ed. P. morand- Fehr, Pudoc wageningen.

ICAR. (1985). *Nutrient Requirements of Livestock and Poultry in India.* ICAR, New Delhi.

ICAR. (1998). *Nutrient Requirements of Livestock and Poultry,* New Delhi.

Karim, S.A. (2004). Nutrition and feeding management of sheep for mutton production. National seminar on "Opportunities and Challenges in Nutrition and Feeding Management of Sheep, Goat and Rabbit for Sustainable Production. pp-88-99

Karim, S.A. and Arora, A.L. (1997). *Indian J Anim. Sci.*, 6: 536-537.

Kearl, L.C. (1982). *Nutrient Requirements of Ruminants in Developing Countries.* International Feedstuffs Institute, Utah State University, Logan, Utah, USA.

Kaushish, S.K., Rawat, P.S. and Sharma, S.C. (1990). World Rev. Anim. Prod., 25: 44-46.

Mallado, M., Foote, R.H., Rodriquez, A. and Zarate, P. (1991). *Small Rumi. Res.*, 6: 141-150.

MBA, A.U., Akinsoyinu, A.O. and Olubajo, F.O. (1974). *Nigerian J. Anim. Prod.*, 1:209-216.

Moghadam, R.A., khorshidi, K.J. and Nikghah, A. (2000). Pajouhesh-va-Sazandgi, 46: 114-117.

Morand-Fehr P.and Savant D. (1978). *Livst. Prod. Sci.*, 5: 203-213.

Murray, P.J., Winslow, S.G. and Rowe, J.B. (1992). *Aust. J. agric. Res.*, 43(2): 367-377.

Norrman, N.E. (1987). Ramfolk for kalvens halsa. A Kuelt from lantbruks university 360 husdjur, pp. 60.

NRC. (1975). *Nutrient Requirement of Sheep,* Washington D.C.

NRC (1981). *National Academy Press Washington, D.C.*

NRC (1985). *Nutrient Requirement of Sheep,* 6th revised ed. National Academy Press, Washington, D.C.

Papachristou, T.G. and Nastist, A.S. (1993). *Range Manage*, 46: 220-226.

Ramirez, R.G., Rodriquez, A.., Flores, A., Carlos, J.L. and Carcia, J.G. (1990). *Small Rumin. Res.*, 3: 97-107.

Riyazuddin, Karim, S.A. and Rawat, P.S. (1998). Golden Jubilee on Sheep, Goat and Rabbit Production and Utilization, 24-26 April, Jaipur. pp. 139-143.

Robertson, S.M., Roberds, G.E. and Wolfe, E.C. (2000). *Aust. J. Agric. Res.*, 51(1): 125-132.

Santra, A.K. and Karim, S.A. (1999). *Small Rumin. Res.*, 33: 131-136.

Sharma, V. (1998). Influence of pre weaning nutrition on post weaning gain of lambs. Ph.D. Thesis Submitted to Chaudhry Charan Singh University, Meerut, India.

Shankar, V. and Gupta, J.N. (1992). *In: Restoration of Degraded Lands:* Concepts and Strategies (Ed. J.S. Singh). Rastogi Publications, Meerut, India. pp. 115-155.

Shinde, A.K. (1997). Seasonal changes in energy metabolism of grazing sheep, Ph.D. thesis submitted to Jawahar lal Nehru Krishi Viswa Vidhyalaya, Jabalpur, Madhya Pradesh.

Shinde, A.K., Karim, S.A., Patnayak, B.C. and Mann, J.S. (1997). *Small Rumin. Res.*, 26: 119-122.

Shinde, A.K. and S ankhyan, S.K. (2006). Monsoon herbage, their preference and nutritive value in sheep and goats. National Seminar on Conservation and Utilization of Monsoon Herbage for Augmenting Animal production. p 112-119.

Shinde,A.K.,Bhatt,R.S., Nassimuddin,M and Karim,S.A.(2008). *Ind. J. Small Rumin.* 14(1): 71-76.

Shinde, A.K., karim, S.A., Singh, N.P. and Patnayak, B.C. (1995). *Indian J. Anim. Sci.*, 65(7): 830-833.

Singh, N.P. and Sahu, B.B. (1997). *Indian J. Anim. Sci.*, 67(1):87-89.

Singh, N.P. and Singh, M. (1987). *Indian J. Anim. Sci.*, 57: 986-990.

Solanki, G.S.1994. Feeding habits and grazing behavior of goats in semi-arid region of India. *Small Rumin. Res.*, 14: 39-43.

Singh, N.P. and Sahu, B.B. (1997). Chevon production in three goat breeds under two feeding systems. Lead Paper. Proceedings of the Golden Jubilee Seminar on Sheep, Goat and Rabbit Production and Utilization held at CSWRI, jaipur on April 24-26, 1998.

White, C.E. and Martin, G.B. (1988). *Proc. Nutr. Soc. Aust.*, 13:86.

□□□

Animal Nutrition, 2012
eds. Dr. (Mrs.) Usha R. Mehra et al., pp. 209-219
Satish Serial Publishing House e-mail : info@satishserial.com; website : www.satishserial.com

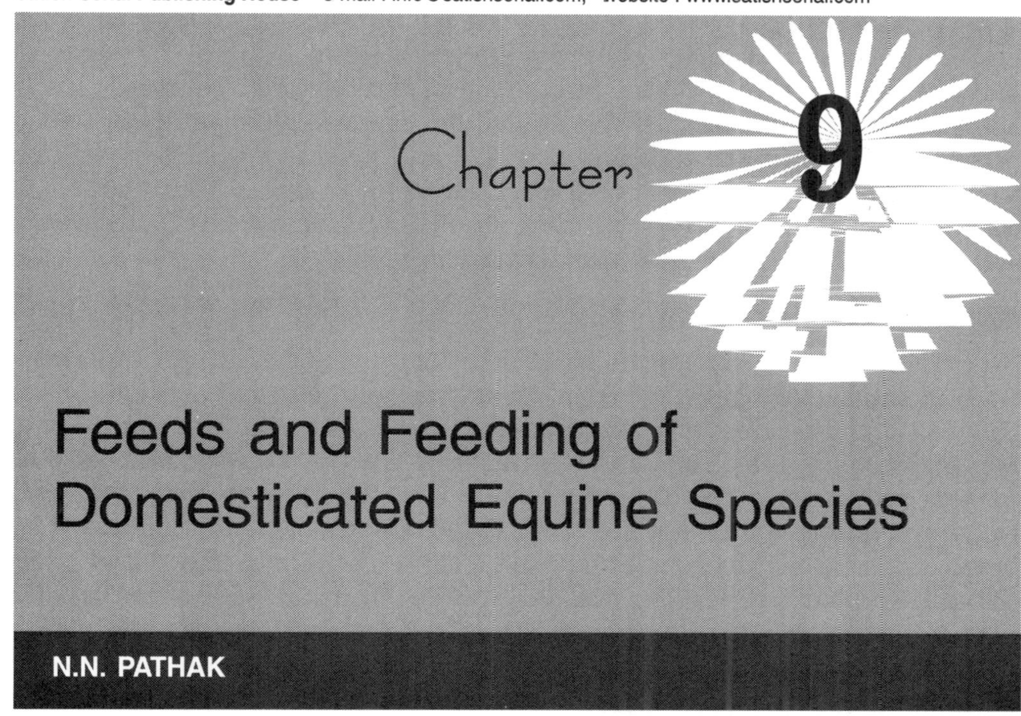

Chapter 9

Feeds and Feeding of Domesticated Equine Species

N.N. PATHAK

The use of domesticated equine species has declined due to increase in the mechanical, electrical and oil energy driven transportation facilities. However in difficult terrains of uneven hilly areas, river basins and other such areas so far not invaded by other facilities they are still very useful. The two main domesticated equine species are horses and donkeys (asses) and very useful sterile hybrid, i.e. mules and jennets are produced from the inter breeding of the two. The utility of different kinds of equines has been listed as follows :

Type of equine	Preferential uses
Horses	Race, riding, different forces, games and pulling carts
Ponies	Pulling carts, pack animal, riding and games
Mule/Jennets	Pack animal, pulling carts, riding and ploughing arable land.
Donkey/Ass	Pack animal, pulling cart, ploughing arable land and riding.

Despite various services provided by different equine species, there is lack of serious attempts on the development of scientific feeding and only a few sporadic studies have been conducted on the nutrition of equines in India. Feeding of gram to horses is an age old practice in India and instead of reasonable advancement in the feed selection and feeding of horses in many horse breeding countries, it is still difficult to convince the majority of Indian people that gram is not a dietary essential and horses can perform well on feeding of a balanced diet devoid of gram. Some empirical formulations of diets are made at the private breeding studs of race horses but these remain secret so it is difficult to make their scientific evaluation.

Feeds for Equine Species

Various equine species are natural herbivorous animals which perform well on satisfactory grass cover in grazing system. However, situation has changed and pastures for grazing are not available except in the hilly and mountaineous regions. Thus, stall feeding has become a necessity for the equine owners and under such changed situation it is important to know the feeds eaten by various equine species. They eat almost all feeds that are eaten by other domestic herbivorous animals like cattle, buffaloes, sheep and goats (Barsaul and Talapatra, 1979, Raut *et al.*, 1987). All equine species are capable of growing on natural pastures covered with satisfactory biomass and to satisfy their nutritional requirements they often resort to selective feeding. In comparison to cattle and sheep the horses are capable to maintain grass intake even at a low sward height (Mesochina *et al.*, 2000).

Various kinds of feeds required by equines are as usual concentrates and roughages as presented :

A. Concentrates

For the feeding of equines grains containing low level of soluble carbohydrates should be selected preferably to avoid acidosis (Budras *et al.*, 2001). The concentrates fed to equines may be further identified into –

(i) *Protein rich feeds* : These are oil cakes, *i.e.* linseed cake, soyabean meal, groundnut cake, mustard cake and sesame cake. However, some precautions are required in the use of various oilseed cakes in view of the presence of some anti-nutritional factors.

(ii) *Energy rich feeds* : All cereal grains are rich in energy content. However, oats and barley also contain high amount of fibrous fractions due to which these two are preferred for the feeding of equines.

(iii) *Feeds moderate in protein and energy* : These are leguminous seeds. Gram is a highly valuable and preferred feed of horses but it should not be considered essential. Even today it is believed by many horse owners that horses can not perform well without the feeding of gram which is not true.

(iv) *Feeds rich in protein and energy content* : These are oil seeds like soyabean, linseed, safflower seed and sun flower seed. Use of linseed tea is quite popular for improving the lusture of body coat.

(v) *Milling byproducts* : These include wheat bran, rice bran and dal chunnies including seed coat.

(vi) *Other feeds* : Some of the feed ingredients specially the condiments are used in small quantity for improving the appetite of animals.

B. Roughages

Almost all roughages eaten by bovines are also eaten by equine but in Indian territory Bermuda grass (dub) is considered to be forage of choice among the natural herbages. All kinds of equine species grazing on scrub and fallow lands graze dub very closely avoiding other naturally growing herbages. Various roughages fed to equines on stalls are classified as (i) dry roughages and (ii) green forages.

(i) *Dry roughages* : These include wheat straw, barley straw, oat straw and chaffed stovers of sorghum and pearl millet. Paddy straw and straws of minor millets are generally not liked by the equines and they feed on these straws only when other fodders are not available. Leguminous straws comprising of empty pods and leaves are liked by all equine species. These are straws of gram, moong, urad, moth and arhar etc.

(ii) *Green forages* : These are proteinous leguminous and similar forages like berseem, lucerne, white clover (in Himalayan region), cowpea, moong, moth and sengi etc. Voluntary intake of lucerne is satisfactory only at flowring stage and that of cowpea at flowering to immature pod formation (Raut *et al.,* 1987).

Feeding of oats from emergence of heads to dough stage of growth is most suitable and liked by horses. Other common cultivated fodders like maize, sorghum, pearl millet, teosinte (Euchlaend mexicana) and grasses like guinea grass, green panic, blue panic, themeda, para grass and many others growing in plains of India are eaten by the horses. Hay of mature natural grasses from central plateau are baled and supplied to studs for the feeding of horses and dairy animals.

In the high rain fall areas of north-eastern states some natural aquatic and semi-aquatic grasses like dal, uridal, ulu, aruna and arali etc. alongwith small quantity of water hyacinth are also fed to horses after mixing with chaffed paddy straw or chaffed dried stalk of maize because straws of wheat, barley and oats are generally not produced in the region.

Digestibility of Nutrients of Some Common Cultivated Fodder

Few Indian values of common cultivated fodder determined by Raut *et al.* (1987) in horses are presented in Table 1.

Table 1 : Digestibility coefficients of dry matter and proximate constituants of common fodders.

Attributes	Oats hay	Green maize	Green sudan	Green Baru	Berseem	Lucerne
Maturity	Flowering	Milk	Milk	Vegetative	9 week	Flowering
CP % in DM	9	9	9.5	9	23	19
CF % in DM	32	28	33	35	18	30
Digestibility coefficients						
DM	58	60	43	45	57	57
CP	62	66	50	59	73	75
CF	51	58	31	43	52	52
EE	33	26	43	37	28	28
NFE	63	68	54	52	75	66

Forage quality including their fibrous fractions, level of feeding and species of equines may have significant effect on the digestibility of feed (Pearson *et al.*, 2001). Voluntary dry matter intake of alfalfa hay has been found to be higher than the oats straw on *ad libitum* feeding, but when the supply of these feeds was restricted to only 70%, the digestibility of alfalfa increased whereas that of oats straw decreased. The decrease in later case was probably due to lack of scope for the selective feeding of more digestible parts. On voluntary feeding, intake of nutrients is mostly higher in horses. On comparison dry matter intake per unit of body size is less in donkeys than the ponies but digestibilities of dry matter, gross energy and fibrous fractions are higher.

Comparison of Digestibility of Feeds in Horses and Cattle

Both horses and cattle are herbivorous animals but there is difference in the anatomy and structure of their digestive tracts. The horses possess post stomach fermentation system whereas in cattle it is pre-stomach and in addition cattle also recycle feeds several times by rumination. Due to this digestibility of most of the nutrients is higher in cattle than the horses (Table 2).

From the perusal of digestibility values shown in Table 2 it is apparent that digestion ability of nutrients of coarse roughages like straws is very low in horses than the cattle but difference becomes much less in the digestibility of green and succulent fodders which almost turns to be equal for most of the nutrients of grains. The digestibility of lipids is always much less in horses than the cattle and there is need of exploratory studies for finding the reasons of low digestibility of lipids in horses in comparison to cattle.

Table 2 : Comparison of digestibility coefficients of organic nutrients between horses and cattle.

Attributes	Animal species	Wheat straw	Meadow hay	Oat grain	Maize grain
CF % in DM		41	22	10	2
Digestibility coefficients					
OM	Horses	21	58	69	89
	Cattle	41	67	70	90
CP	Horses	2	63	80	76
	Cattle	4	65	86	72
EE	Horses	-	22	71	61
	Cattle	31	57	80	89
CF	Horses	18	40	29	40
	Cattle	50	63	28	58
NFC	Horses	28	65	75	92
	Cattle	71	68	76	95

Factors Affecting Nutritional Requirements of Equines

The various factors affecting the nutritional requirements of the equines may be grouped into the following order.

1. Animal factor

The physiological state of animals has significant influence on the nutritional requirements being lowest for maintenance. Additional nutrition is required to be fed for all kinds of production and other functions. The various animal factors may be listed as fallow :

a. Maintenance of adult animals

b. Growth
  (i) During suckling phase
  (ii) During growth phase
  (iii) During terminal growth phase

c. Pregnancy – particularly during last 90 days.

d. Lactation
  (i) Early 3 months
  (ii) Terminal 3 months (3-6 months)

e. Activities
   (i) Slow
   (ii) Light
   (iii) Medium
   (iv) Heavy
   (v) Strenuous

f. *Species difference* : Digestibilities of energy providing fractions like dry matter, gross energy and fibre are generally higher in donkeys than the horses (Pearson *et al.*, 2001), due to which feed requirement of donkeys is less than the horses.

2. Feed factors

The palatability of feeds, their chemical composition and digestibility are the factors used for the determination of feeding value. The feedstuffs available and used for the feeding of equines may be classified as follows :

a) *Low quality feeds*: These are dry crop residues containing less than 5% crude protein (CP) and 45% total digestible nutrients (TDN) on dry matter (DM) basis.

b) *Medium quality feeds*: These are cereal fodder, grasses and hay containing 5-7% (CP) and 50-55% TDN on DM basis.

c) *Good quality feeds*: These are highly palatable and nutritious feeds containing more than 8% CP and more than 56% TDN on DM basis.

d) The availability of dietary energy is lower in fibrous feeds due to loss of energy used in the fermentation of such feeds. This results in the lower metabolizale energy (ME) value of fibrous feeds in comparison to less fibrous feeds of similar chemical composition except intake is utilized to meet the requirement of increased breathing rate in hot season and for maintaining body temperature in winter season.

4. Nutritional Requirement

The requirements of dry matter (DM), crude protein (CP) digestible crude protein (DCP), total digestible nutrients (TDN) and digestible energy (DE) have been calculated on the basis of per kg metabolic body size (kg$W^{0.75}$) from the values of NRC (1978) for different categories of horses and are presented in Table 3. For the supply of these nutrients their content in the diets of horses has been shown in Table 4.

There is wide difference in the energy requirement of horses for different works and exercises (Hintz *et al.*, 1971). The mean DE requirement per hour per kg body weight (Kcal/h/kg BW) for working horses has been presented in Table 5.

Table 3 : Feed and nutrients requirement of different categories of horses (from NRC, 1979).

Physiological state	Requirement per kg $W^{0.75}$				
	DM (g)	CP (g)	DCP (g)	TDN (g)	DE (kcal)
Adults, maintenance	70-72	6-7	3-3.5	35	155
Last 90 days gestation	70-72	7-8	3.4-5	40	175
Lactation, first 3 months	95-100	13-14	8-8.5	60	275
3-6 months	90-95	10-12	6-6.5	54	235
Nursing foals (upto 3 months)	95-105	17-19	12-14	70	310
Nursing creep (3-6 months)	85-90	13-14	8-9	60	260
Growing period					
6-12 months	75-80	9-10	5-6	50	220
12-18 months	70-75	7-8	4-5	42	185
18-24 months	65-70	6-7	3-4	38	168

Table 4 : Nutrients content in complete diets of different categories of horses on dry matter (DM) basis.

Physical class	Requirement per kg $W^{0.75}$					
	CP (%)	DCP (%)	TDN (%)	Ca (%)	P (%)	DE (Mcal/kg)
Adults, maintenance	8-9	3.5-4	50	2.20	0.30	0.20
Pregnant, last 90 days	10-11	5-5.5	57	2.50	0.50	0.35
Early lactation (upto 3 months)	13-14	8-9	64	2.80	0.50	0.35
Late lactation (3-6 months)	11-12	6-7	59	2.60	0.45	0.30
Growing period						
Upto 3 month	17-19	14-16	74	3.25	0.85	0.60
3-6 months	15-16	10-11	70	3.10	0.85	0.60
6-12 months	12-13	7-8	64	2.80	0.70	0.50
12-18 months	10-11	5.5-6	60	2.65	0.45	0.30
18-24 months	9-10	4.5-5.5	59	2.60	0.45	0.30
Working adult horses						
Light work	8-9	3.5	57	2.50		
Moderate work	8-9	3.5-4	66	2.90		
Strenuous work	8-9	3.5-4	70	3.10		

Table 5 : DE requirement of working horses.

Work done	DE (Kcal/h/kg)
Slow walking	0.5
Light (Slow trot, some canter)	5.1
Medium (Fast trot, canter)	12.5
Heavy Canter, gallop, jump)	24.0
Strenuous	39.0

Requirement of essential minerals and vitamins are not included in the tables although they are very important constituents of the balanced diets. For common purpose it has become customary to mix about 2 percent complex mineral mixture and 1 percent common salt (preferably rock salt) in the concentrate mixtures. Besides this mineral licks are also provided to horses at the organized farms for free choice consumption.

While balancing the diets care should be taken for the adequate supply of calcium, phosphorus and common salt among major elements, and trace elements like iron, zinc, manganese, copper, cobalt, iodine and selenium. Wheat bran and rice bran are the good source of phosphorus and most of the micro minerals. However, presence of phytic acid reduces the bio-availability of the many minerals.

Special precaution is required in the selection of good quality mineral mixture containing tolerance level of harmful and toxic minerals like lead, fluorine, selenium, cadmium and copper.

Feeding Schedule of Equines

The feeding schedule of equines depends on several factors like type of horse, utility of the animal, availability of feeds and physiological state of the animal. Common feeding schedule at an organized farm may be as per Table 6.

Table 6 : Feeding schedule of equines.

Category	Grazing	Roughage at stall	Concentrate mixture	Activities
1.	+	-	-	Idle and early gestation
2.	+	-	+	Draught, lactation, late gestation
3.	+	+	+	While pastures are depleted or scarce
4.	-	+	+	Training, show and race
5.	-	Complete	Ration	Horses kept for pleasure riding in cities

N.B. Complex salt and mineral mixture and fresh drinking water should be available for free choice consumption.

Colostrum feeding is very important and foals should be allowed suckling as early as possible and within 36 h of foaling. Weaning is done at 5-6 months of suckling and during this period small quantity of supplements should be offered at short intervals (Sehu, 2001).

Composition of Diets and Feed Intake Capacity for Equines

Like the diets of any herbivorous farm animal, the diets of the equines are also made of roughages and concentrate in different ratios. The ratio of roughages and concentrate in the diets depends on several factors like.

1. Feeding value of feeds-this includes voluntary feed intake and nutritive value.
2. Nutritional requirements of the animal. Which depends on physiological states like growth, gestation, lactation, activities and maintenance as well as condition of the animal.

The composition of diets and average feed intake capacity i.e. dry matter intake (DM) of horses at various physiological states are presented in Table 7.

Table 7 : Average composition of diets and DMI in horses for various stages.

Physiological state	Feed DM as % b.wt.		Ratio in DM		DMI/100 kg bodyweight
	Roughage	Concentrate	Roughage	Concentrate	
Nursing foal, 3 months	Negligible	1.0-1.5	0.20	80-100	2.5-3.5
Foal, 3-6 months	0.5-1.0	1.5-3.0	20-40	60-80	2.0-3.5
Foal, 6-12 months	1.0-1.5	1.0-2.5	30-40	60-70	2.0-3.0
12-18 months	1.0-1.5	1.0-2.0	40-50	50-60	2.0-3.0
18-24 months	1.0-1.5	1.0-1.5	50-60	40-50	2.0-2.5
2 years of age	1.0-1.5	1.0-1.5	50-60	40-50	2.0-2.5
2 years (race horse)	0.75-1.0	1.25-1.5	30-40	60-70	2.0-2.5
Draught horses					
Light work	1.5-2.0	0.5-1.0	60-70	30-40	1.5-2.5
Medium work	1.0-2.0	1.0-1.5	40-50	50-60	1.75-2.5
Heavy work	1.0-1.5	1.5-2.0	30-40	60-70	2.0-2.5
Adult horses					
Maintenance	1.5-2.0	0.0-1.0	80-100	0-20	1.5-2.0
Last 90 days of pregnancy	1.0-1.5	0.5-1.0	60-70	30-40	1.5-2.5
Early lactation	1.0-2.0	1.0-2.0	40-50	50-60	2.0-3.0
Late lactation	1.0-2.0	0.5-1.5	60-70	30-40	2.0-2.5

Water Requirement

Water requirement of an animal generally depends on the following factors

1. The type of animal
2. Age of the animal
3. Physiological state of the animal
4. Intensity of physical work
5. Physical and chemical composition of the diet
6. Climatic conditions and housing

There is relationship between feed intake and water requirement of the animals provided other factors are more or less unchanged. Asses can withstand higher dehydration than the horses and Somalian asses may survive even upto 30 per cent dehydration loss in the body weight. They regain this loss within 2 to 5 minutes of drinking about equal quantity of water. There is significant fall in feed intake at about 15 per cent loss in body weight due to dehydration and complete cessation of feed intake may occur after 22 percent loss due to acute dehydration. Ass can withstand feed and water deprivation upto 48 hours even in summer season. This is partly due to capacious caecum and colon where digesta are retained for the microbial fermentation for the supply of energy to the horse (Pathak and Kamra, 1983).

A fall in the water content of body upto 10 per cent in horses may cause physiological disturbance and beyond 20 per cent may be fatal. Rehydration of animals along with the supply of electrolyte is essential to provide protection against fatigue, muscular weakness and fall in feed intake. In addition to drinking water, animals also receive considerable amount of metabolic water produced during the metabolism of carbohydrate, fat and protein at the rate of 107, 60 and 40 ml per 100 g of substrate respectively.

Normal water requirement of an adult horse is 2 to 3 litres per kg of feed intake and it mostly depends on the dry matter content in the feed. Water requirement of animals increases under the following conditions.

1. Rise in ambient temperature beyond 25°C in temperate and 30°C in tropical climate.
2. Occurrence of diarrohea
3. Lactation
4. Extent of exercise.

Nutrition of Race Horses

Limited information is available on the actual feeding practices of race horses with the R.V.C. Stud owners keep their systems of feeding secret.

However, for satisfactory performance the balanced diet of a race horse should be less bulky and rich in instantly available energy. The roughage part of the diet should be made of highly digestible fodder.

References

Barsaul, C.S. and Talapatra, S.K. (1970). *Ind. Vet. J.*, 47: 508-512.

Budras, K.D., Scheible, K., Patan, B., Streich, W.J. and Kim, K. (2001). *J. Vet. Sci.*, 2: 1-7 (France).

Hintz, H.F., Robert, S.J., Sabin, S. and Schryver, H.F. (1971). *J. Anim. Sci.*, 32: 100-102.

Mesochina, P., Peyraud, J.L., Duncan, P., Micol, D. and Trillaud-Geyl, C. (2000). *Annales deZootechnie*, 49: 505.

NRC (1978). Nutrient Requirement of the Horse. National Research Council, National Academy of Science, Washington, D.C.

Pathak, N.N. (1989). Equine feeding in Advanced Animal Nutrition (ed. U.B., Singh) Indo Vision Publishers, Ghaziabad.

Pathak, N.N. and Kamra, D.N. (1989). Equine feeding, pp. 144-155 in Text Book of Livestock Feeding in Tropic. Cosmo Pub. New Delhi.

Pearson, R.A., Archibald, R.F. and Muirhead, R.H. (2001). *Br. J. Nutr.*, 85: 599-606.

Raut, B., Ranjhan, S.K. and Pathak, N.N. (1987). *Ind. J. Nutr.*, 4: 114-119.

Sehu, A. (2000). Nutr. Abst. Rev., 71B 84.

□□□

Animal Nutrition, 2012
eds. Dr. (Mrs.) Usha R. Mehra et al., pp. 221-258
Satish Serial Publishing House e-mail : info@satishserial.com; website : www.satishserial.com

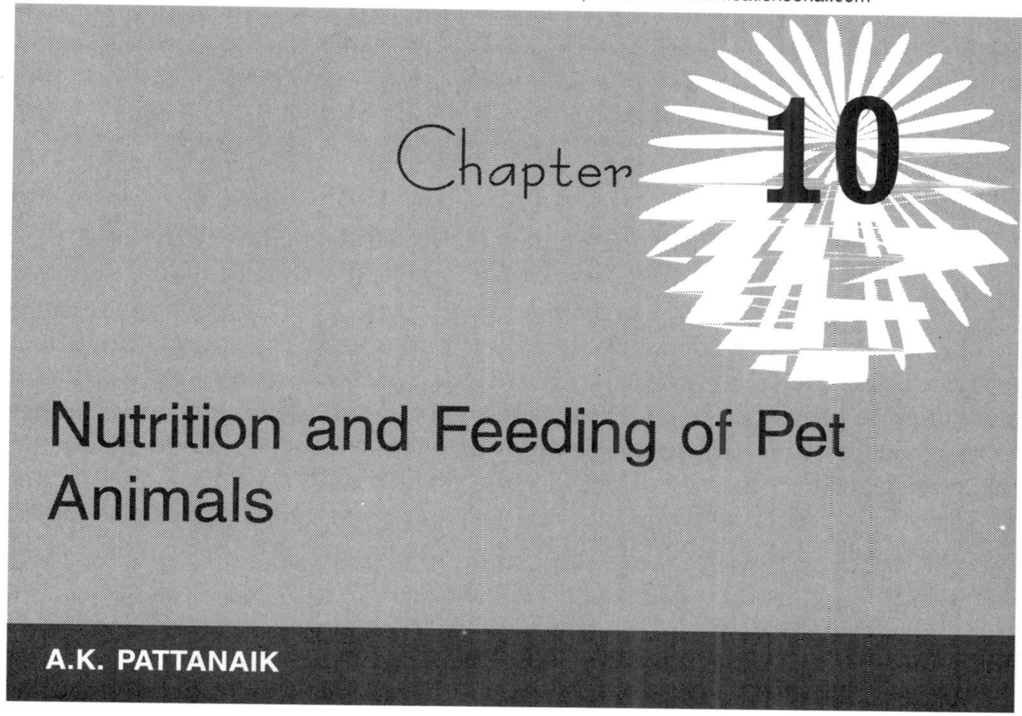

Chapter 10

Nutrition and Feeding of Pet Animals

A.K. PATTANAIK

Companion animals, namely dogs and cats, present unique challenges to the fields of veterinary medicine and nutritional science. In addition to inherent metabolic idiosyncrasies, their nutrition and care are based on promoting lifelong health, not on production traits (*e.g.* average daily gain, feed efficiency) as it often is in livestock species. The pet's behavior, happiness, health, longevity and overall well-being are inextricably intertwined with its nutrition. As such, the correct balance of nutrients is crucial to maintain health and a long and happy life for pets.

The philosophy and objective of companion animal nutrition differ from that of production animals. Farm animal nutrition focuses on providing maximum production at the lowest cost; while maintaining appropriate standards of care, trade-offs are made on the basis of economics rather than emotion. Nutritional needs are strongly influenced by the animal's life stage; life stages of concern for production animals include growth, maintenance, and reproduction. For companion animals, these life stages also apply, although maintenance describes a much longer span of a pet's life stage. In addition to life stage, lifestyle is quite different between production and companion animals. It is also quite variable between individual pets. Production animals tend to live under conditions that are similar for a particular production function, such that their level of exercise, exposure to the elements, life style and general husbandry are similar. Pets, on the other hand, can vary widely in life style. In general, the majority of dogs are house pets but there are others who hunt or work for a living.

The importance of pet nutrition has increased dramatically over the past twenty years. In the past pets were often subjected to scraps and leftover food, which has changed to a great extent. Pet owners are increasingly turning to manufactured pet foods, which they perceive to be more nutritious. Although majority of dog owners in the western countries enjoy the convenience, economic freedom and reliability of commercially produced pet foods, some owners still prefer homemade diets for their pets. In India, the situation regarding the use of pet foods is reverse with a vast majority of pet owners relying on homemade diets to rear their pet dogs. The present chapter aims to highlight the nutrition and feeding management of pets with special focus on dogs.

Importance of Pets

There is a growing body of evidence that pets can improve the health of their owners. Many scientific studies have over the period proved the fact that pet ownership is a key to heart health, social support, and long life. It is commonly assumed that owning a pet provides older residents in the community with health benefits in terms of improved physical health and psychological well-being. It has also been reported that pet owners are lower on neuroticism and higher on extraversion compared with those without pets (Parslow *et al.*, 2005). The advantages out of the relationship between pets and health encompass therapeutic, physiological, psychological and psychosocial benefits. Pet ownership has been found to be positively associated with some forms of social contact and interaction, and with perceptions of neighbourhood friendliness; social capital is another potential mechanism by which pets exert an influence on human health (Wood *et al.*, 2005). In a more specific study, Hemsworth and Pizer (2006) suggested that even immune-compromised patients should be able to continue to enjoy the significant benefits of pet ownership with proper consideration to the overall benefits of the human-animal bond and with proper handling and husbandry. Scientific studies have proved that dogs have a number of positive effects on human health and well-being. There are specific studies showing benefits of owning a pet in terms of improvements in cardiac health, anxiety, hypertension and even restoration of normal lipid profile. Recognition to this fact has lead to companion dogs being used systematically in "animal assisted therapy" in various institutions and hospitals, both as specific treatment of a medical condition and to improve well-being in certain groups of patients. Although the reasons for the positive effects of dogs on human health are not clearly identified, the attachment between people and their pets the human-animal bond seems to have important physiological and psychological effects. Additionally, companion dogs have been shown to increase physical activity and social contact, which may also influence human health.

Idiosyncrasies of Dog and Cat Nutrition

Based on their gastrointestinal system, both cats and dogs should be classified as carnivores. Historically dogs have been considered omnivores because of their scavenger hunting adaptations, but cats are considered as true carnivores. Although both cats and dogs belong to the order Carnivora, significant nutritional metabolic, behavioural and dietary differences exist between the two species. These differences include the cat's unique energy and glucose metabolism; many investigations showed that cats are unable to metabolize sugars in large quantities (Kienzle, 1993, 1994b; Washizu *et al.*, 1999). The cat's unique physiologic status involves higher protein requirement, typical need for dietary taurine and arachidonic acid, and sensitivity to deficiency of arginine, requirement for pre-formed vitamin A and inability to convert tryptophan to niacin. Many of these metabolic compulsions entail a requirement for animal tissues in diet of cats. Further, in general, cats are considered to exhibit decreased apparent nutrient digestibility than their canine counterparts.

Nutritional Requirements

Nutrient requirement is the quantity of a nutrient that must be supplied to an animal in order to satisfy its metabolic needs. It reflects the minimum average level of intake of a given nutrient which, over time, is sufficient to maintain the desired biochemical or physiological functions. Numerous factors influence the nutritional requirements of pets including age, physiological growth status, physical condition (influenced by sexual status), activity and lifestyle, health condition, size of the dog and, its breed.

The extremely heterogeneous anatomical and physiological attributes of different breeds of dogs makes breed as one of the most important factor while working out the nutritional requirements. For example, it is extremely difficult to visualize that nutritional requirements for a Yorkshire puppy, which multiplies its birth weight by a factor of 20 over just 8 months, could be the same and a Mastiff puppy, which multiplies its birth weight by 100 times in 18 to 24 months before reaching its adult size (Pibot, 2007). Many of the important factors that determine the nutritional requirements are, in turn, influenced strongly by the breed of the animal, for example, digestive capacities, type of skin and coat, pathological risks and life expectancy etc. The colic transit time represents 80 to 90% of the total transit time; it takes over 40 hours in the Great Dane, compared to less than 24 hours in a Toy Poodle (Hernot *et al.*, 2006). Small breeds are often fussy, need highly palatable diet to be fed *ad libitum,* whereas medium, large and giant breed dogs are usually willing to consume less palatable diets and need to be fed in a portion-controlled manner. The digestive tract constitutes 7% of the body weight in case of smaller breed vis-à-vis 2.7% in case of larger breed dogs. Small and medium breed dogs age slower, and need to be changed to senior diet at 7 years of age compared to 5 and 6 years, respectively, in case of giant and large breed dogs. Small breed dogs need a calorie dense diet because a higher energy requirement per unit body weight as compared to larger breed dogs. Larger breed dogs are susceptible to high Ca intake and skeletal disorders due to rapid growth rate whereas small breed dogs meet Ca requirements at lower Ca : ME ratio, and hence less prone to skeletal disorders. Skin and hair renewal can represent up to 35% of an adult dog's daily protein requirement (Scott *et al.*, 2001). Even with dogs of similar body weight, wide variations in maintenance energy requirements are observed between different breeds. For example, the Great Dane, which requires around 50% more calories than one would expect simply on the basis of its body weight (Kienzle and Rainbird, 1991; Blum *et al.*, 1992), attributable both to its shorter hair, and muscular body mass. The collective nutritional approach has therefore been progressively transformed, and nutritional requirements are arrived at first of all taking size into account, followed by the breed of the animal.

There are two sources of published information that provide nutrient requirement information for dogs and cats. The National Research Council (NRC) compiles lists of minimum requirements while the Association of American Feed Control Officials (AAFCO) has developed standards of practical nutrient profiles of dogs and cat foods based on commonly used ingredients. In its latest edition, NRC (2006) has listed the nutrient requirements data as minimal requirement (MR, minimal concentration of bioavailable nutrient that will support a defined physiological state), adequate intake (AI) and recommended allowance (RA, concentration or amount of a nutrient in a diet formulated to support a given physiological state) besides safe upper limit. The RA is based on MR and includes a safety factor for nutrients with uncertain bioavailability. A complied data on nutrient requirement of dogs is listed in Table 1.

As energy density determines the food intake in dogs and cats, it is highly essential that the diets are properly balanced so that requirements for all other nutrients are met at the same time that energy needs are satisfied. It is for this very reason, it becomes more appropriate to express levels of nutrients in the food in terms of ME concentrations rather than in terms of percentages on weight basis. The nutrient requirements tables by NRC (2006) provide nutrient allowances in "units/kg DM", "units/1000 kcal ME" and "units/kg $BW^{0.75}$". The "units/kg DM" data assume an energy density of 4.0 kcal ME/g DM; hence in order to convert "units/100g DM" to "units/1000 kcal ME" the data needs to be multiplied by a factor 2.5. However, for foods with energy densities different from 4.0 kcal ME/g DM, the recommendations should be corrected for energy density.

Table 1 : Nutrient requirements of dogs at various physiological stages.

Nutrient	Unit	NRC (2006)†			AAFCO (1994)‡	
		Post-weaning growth	Adult maint-enance	Late gestation and peak lactation	Growth and repro-duction	Adult maint-enance
Crude protein	%	-	10.0	20.0	22.0	18.0
4-14 weeks	%	22.5	-	-	-	-
> 14 weeks	%	17.5	-	-	-	-
Total fat	%	8.5	5.5	8.5	8.0	5.0
Linoleic acid	%	1.3	1.1	1.3	1.0	1.0
α-Linoleic acid	%	0.8	0.44	0.8	-	-
Arachidonic acid	%	0.3	-	-	-	-
EPA and DHA$	%	0.5	0.44	0.5	-	-
Minerals						
Calcium	%	1.2	0.4	0.8	1.0	0.6
Phosphorus	%	1.0	0.3	0.5	0.8	0.5
Magnesium	%	0.04	0.06	0.06	0.04	0.04
Sodium	%	0.22	0.08	0.20	0.3	0.06
Potassium	%	0.44	0.04	0.36	0.6	0.6
Chloride	%	0.29	0.12	0.30	0.45	0.09
Iron	mg/kg	88	30	70	80.0	80.0
Copper	mg/kg	11	6	12.4	7.3	7.3
Zinc	mg/kg	100	60	96	120.0	120.0
Manganese	mg/kg	5.6	4.8	7.2	5.0	5.0
Selenium	mg/kg	0.35	0.35	0.35	0.11	0.11
Iodine	mg/kg	0.88	0.88	0.88	1.5	1.5
Vitamins						
Vitamin A	IU/kg	5050	5050	5050	5,000.0	5,000.0
Vitamin D	IU/kg	552	552	552	500.0	500.0

contd.....

Vitamin E	IU/kg	30	30	30	50.0	50.0
Vitamin K	mg/kg	1.64	1.63	1.6	-	-
Thiamin	mg/kg	1.38	2.25	2.25	1.0	1.0
Riboflavin	mg/kg	5.25	5.25	5.3	2.2	2.2
Pyridoxine	mg/kg	1.5	1.5	1.5	1.0	1.0
Niacin	mg/kg	17.0	17.0	17	11.4	11.4
Pantothenic acid	mg/kg	15.0	15	15	10.0	10.0
Cobalamin	mg/kg	0.035	0.035	0.035	0.022	0.022
Folic acid	mg/kg	0.27	0.27	0.27	0.18	0.18
Choline	mg/kg	1700	1700	1700	1200.0	1200.0

† Recommended allowance at a presumed caloric density of 4.0 kcal ME/g DM
‡ Minimum levels at a presumed energy density of 3.5 kcal ME/g DM
$ Eicosapentanoic acid and Docesahectanotic acid

Energy

The daily energy requirement is the sum of the energy that is required for resting metabolic rate, voluntary muscular activity, meal-induced thermo-genesis besides adaptive thermo-genesis i.e. maintenance of body temperature when exposed to adverse weather conditions. Because of its critical importance, energy is always the first requirement to be met by the diet. The daily energy requirement of dog depends upon the amount of energy that the body expends each day. Very little research has been done in dogs on the internal signals that affect food intake. Information available is based on data collected from laboratory animals. The most common internal signals include (i) gastric distention, (ii) physiological response to signal sound and smell, and (iii) changes in plasma concentration of specific nutrients, hormones and peptides. The external stimuli, on the other hand, include (i) food availability, (ii) diet palatability, (iii) food composition texture and (iv) timing and size of meals (Case *et al.*, 1995).

Metabolizable energy (ME) is the preferred unit of energy for calculating the requirements in pets. The energy density (ME value) of food is of utter importance in pet animals. It is the principal factor that determines the quantity of food that an animal eats and therefore has a direct bearing on the amount of all other essential nutrients that it ingests. The energy density of any diet must be high enough to allow the pet to consume a sufficient amount (volume) of food to meet its energy demand.

The dog is unique in the sense that it has the widest range of normal adult bodyweight (in relative terms) within any single species. Three power functions have been proposed by various workers to arrive at the ME requirement in case of dogs. The allometric equation ME req = K x kg $W^{0.67}$

provides an accurate estimate of daily maintenance ME requirements for different sizes of adult dogs experiencing different activity levels; the value for K ranges between 130-300, but specifically 132 for inactive, 145 for active, 200 for very active, and 300 for endurance performance (Case *et al.*, 1995). There are two other equations suggested to be used for estimating ME in adult dogs: (i) ME = 100 x kg $W^{0.88}$, although it provides a reasonable estimate of the daily energy requirement of active dogs weighing between 1 to 60 kg, studies have shown that this equation may overestimate the energy requirement of adult dogs that have low to normal activity levels; (ii) ME = 132 x kg $W^{0.75}$, it provides a good estimate of the energy requirement for small and medium size breeds during maintenance (NRC, 1974). However, this equation may underestimate the energy needs of some of the larger breeds of dogs. In its latest recommendations, NRC (2006) has expressed ME requirements for adult maintenance as 130 x $BW^{0.75}$ using factor 0.75 for dogs with the K value ranging between 95 for inactive pets to 200 for young adult and active pets. The factor for average active kennel dogs has been suggested as 130. For cats, it has used two factors i.e., 0.67 and 0.4, the later for maintenance requirements of cats with body condition score >5.0).

Regardless which of the three equations is used to predict energy needs, the resulting number should be used only as a starting point to determine the daily energy requirement of a particular animal. ME requirement is influenced by many factors other than breed (or body size), including stages of the life cycle, environment, level of activity (exercise), metabolic status and nutritional status (malnutrition vs. obesity). Variability in BW of individual dogs and the environmental condition may result in a requirement that is up to 25% greater or less than the predicted value. The energy requirement predicted from 130 x $BW^{0.75}$ is for maintenance but there are stages of life that result in increased energy needs like growth, gestation, lactation, period of strenuous physical work and exposure to extreme environmental conditions.

After weaning, growing puppies require approximately 2 times the energy intake per unit of body weight as adult dogs of the same weight. This amount should be reduced to 1.6 times and 1.2 times of the maintenance level once a puppy reaches 40 and 80 percent of adult weight, respectively (NRC, 1985). The age at which a puppy will attain these proportions of adult weight will vary with the adult size of dog; in general, large breeds of dogs mature more slowly than the small breeds. The rate of growth in the early stages is very rapid and, in general, most breeds of dog will attain 50% of their mature adult weight at around 5 to 6 months of age.

Energy needs increase substantially for bitches during gestation and lactation. During the first 3 or 4 weeks it remains the same as maintenance but thereafter it starts increasing and becomes around 1.25-1.5 times the normal maintenance requirement by the end of gestation period (Rowsos, 1981). Lactation is one of the most energy demanding stages of life for an animal; depending upon the size of the litter, energy needs of the females during lactation can increase as much as 3 times the normal maintenance requirement. Both physical work and environmental stress can cause increased energy needs in dogs. Short bouts of intense physical exercise may cause only a small increase in energy needs, but a regular program of prolonged exercise may cause increased needs of up to 2-4 times the maintenance levels (NRC, 1985). In cold conditions, depending upon the severity, there can be an increase of 1.2-1.8 times of the normal maintenance needs in dogs (Blaza, 1982).

NRC (2006) in its latest recommendations has come out with specific equations to arrive at the ME requirements for various stages of life cycle, which are given below:

- Growing puppies after weaning: ME (kcal) = Maintenance requirement x 3.2 x $[e^{(-0.87p)} - 0.1]$
- Where: $p = BW_a / BW_m$; BW_a = actual body weight at the time of evaluation (kg); BW_m = expected mature body weight (kg); e = base of natural log = 2.718
- Bitches in late gestation: ME (kcal) = Maintenance requirement + [26 kcal x kg BW]
- Lactating bitches: ME (kcal) = Maintenance requirement + [BW x (24*n* + 12*m*) x L]

  where: *n* = number of puppies between 1 and 4; *m* = number of puppies between 5 and 8 (<5 puppies, *m* = 0); L = correction factor for stage of lactation; week 1, 0.75; week 2, 0.95; week 3, 1.1; and week 4, 1.2.

Fats

Fats are important component of pet animal's diet as a concentrated source of energy. More importantly, they supply the essential fatty acids (EFAs), which serve important structural functions in cell membranes EFAs are needed for various inflammatory and immune responses besides being essential for synthesis of eicosanoids such as prostaglandin and leukotrienes which are important regulators of cell functions. They are also vital for maintaining normal skin structure and function. Dietary fats generally improve palatability and add an acceptable texture to foods. They also serve as carriers for fat-soluble vitamins. Dogs require a minimum of 8% (growth and reproduction) or 5% (maintenance) dietary fat, on a dry-matter basis, at least 1% of which must be available as linoleic acid. In its latest edition, NRC (2006) has come up with minimal levels of requirements for arachidoxic acid, licesapentinoic acid (EPA) and docesahexaenoic acid (DHA) as well. Dogs fed foods containing normal levels of protein tolerate very high levels of fat (e.g. sled dogs). However, very high fat foods with very low protein content have been linked with adverse effects in dogs (Lindsay *et al.,* 1948).

Dogs and cats are unable to synthesize linoleic acid making it dietary essential in both species. Additionally, cats exhibit low Δ-6 desaturase activity and cannot meet their physiologic requirement for arachidonic acid through biotransformation from linoleic acid, especially for maintenance of normal pregnancy and neonatal growth and maintenance. Consequently, both linoleic acid and arachidonic acid are considered essential nutrients for cats. Of the (n-6) polyunsaturated acids (PUFA), linoleic acid is involved in the maintenance of the cutaneous water permeability barrier, and arachidonic acid regulates epidermal proliferation via prostaglandin E_2. The long chain PUFAs, arachidonic acid, and in particular DHA are known to support correct neural and visual development in mammalian species. Recent research data demonstrate the importance of dietary lipid sources, in particular DHA, on neurological function in terms of trainability (Kelley *et al.,* 2005). DHA is the preferred substrate for retinal uptake in early development when the demand for DHA is greatest. Arachidonic acid is also important for neural development. Supplementation with α-linolenic acid and linoleic acid during gestation and lactation is an ineffective means of increasing the milk content of DHA and which are often adequate respectively arachidonic acid, for neonatal nutritional needs. It is thus preferable to have small amounts of DHA and/or EPA, as well as arachidonic acid in foods for growth and reproduction (Bauer *et al.,* 2004, 2006; Heinemann and Bauer, 2006). Dietary deficiencies of EFAs are uncommon but may occasionally occur in dogs and cats that are fed poor quality, low fat dry foods or inappropriately formulated home-prepared diets. EFAs should constitute at least 2% of the daily caloric intake to prevent deficiencies. The percentage of linoleic acid in adiet varies greatly depending on the fat source. Safflower oil and corn oil constitute good sources of linoleic acid whereas fish oil is a concentrated source for arachidonic acid.

Although there is increasing evidence of beneficial effects of omega-3 fatty acids, the current information is insufficient to recommend a specific level of omega-3 fatty acids for adult dogs (NRC, 2006). The effects of omega-3 fatty acids depend on the level as well as on the ratio of omega-6 to omega-3 fatty acids. Very high levels of long chain omega-3 fatty acids can decrease cellular immunity, particularly in the presence of a low level of omega-6 fatty acids (Wander *et al.,* 1997; Hall *et al.,* 1999).

Carbohydrates

Carbohydrates are one of the most important dietary factors in a dog food supplying energy as well as the physical characteristics allowing for effective processing-manufacturing. Being an excellent source of energy, carbohydrates should be provided adequately in the diets so that protein will not be used for energy and can be used instead for growth and tissue repair. However, carbohydrate is not an essential component of the puppy's diet, provided that sufficient protein is available for glucose synthesis. Similarly, while carbohydrates are physiologically essential, it is not an indispensable component of the diet of gestating/lactating bitches. In fact, it has been shown that lactating bitches fed a carbohydrate-free diet required 30 percent dietary protein compared to 16 percent when fed a diet containing carbohydrate (Kienzle and Meyer, 1989). Nonetheless, carbohydrates form an useful and economical source of energy in the dog's diet. Fibers are the kinds of carbohydrates that modify the mix of the bacterial population in the small intestine, which can help manage optimal gastro-intestinal health. For dogs and cats to obtain the most benefit from fiber, the fiber source must be moderately fermentable. Fiber sources that have low fermentability (e.g. cellulose) result in poor development and less surface area of the intestinal mucosa. Conversely, highly fermentable fibers can produce gases and by-products that can lead to flatulence and excess mucus. Moderately fermentable fibers—including beet pulp, which is commonly used in both dog and cat foods—are the best, as they promote a healthy gut while avoiding the undesirable side effects. Other examples of moderately fermentable fibers include brans (of corn, rice and wheat) and wheat middlings. Foods that are high in fiber are not good for dogs and cats with high energy requirements, such as those who are young and growing.

Protein

Protein in the diets is required for both essential as well as non-essential amino acids that the animal need for maintenance, growth, gestation and lactation. Like fats, protein content also contributes to palatability and acceptability of food in pets. As for most other animals, dogs and cats also need 10 essential amino acids viz. arginine, histidine, isoleucine, leucine, lysine, methionine, phenylalanine, threonine, tryptophan and valine. Cats have a higher dietary protein requirement than most other species including dog, because the obligatory endogenous nitrogen loss in cats is nearly twice that of dogs. The endogenous urinary nitrogen excretion, when fed a protein-free diet, is 360 mg per kg $W^{0.75}$ per day compared to 210 mg per kg $W^{0.75}$ per day in case of dogs (Hendriks *et al.*, 1997).

Dietary factors, which affect a dog's protein requirement, include (a) protein quality and amino acid composition, (b) protein digestibility, and (c) energy density of diet. Besides, it is also affected by other extraneous factors including the animal's activity level, physiological state and prior nutritional status. An animal's protein requirement varies inversely with the digestion of the protein source, and with its ability to provide all of the essential amino acids in their correct quantity and proportion. Dogs require a minimum of 22 or 18% good quality protein, on a dry-matter basis, for growth and reproduction, and maintenance, respectively. The higher the quality of protein fed, the lower the % total protein needed in the diet. Highly digestibic protein results in free amino acids and smaller peptides that are poorly antigenic and therefore reduces the risk of protein-related food allergy. Common protein sources for dogs include oil meals, eggs, dairy products, muscle or organ meats etc. The arginine requirement increases with increased protein content owing to its role as an intermediate in the urea cycle. Therefore, for every gram of crude protein above the stated values, an additional 0.01g of arginine is required (NRC, 2006).

Minerals

As per available experimental evidence dogs and cats essentially require some 12 minerals i.e. six each as macro minerals (Ca, P, Mg, Na, K and Cl) and micro minerals (Fe, Cu, Zn, Mn, I and Se). Several others are assumed to be essential, due to evidence of their need in other species, and are normally present in sufficient amounts in food.

Minerals serve many physiological functions in animals. It includes rigidity to skeleton and teeth, nervous impulse transmission and muscle contraction, acid-base balance, essential components of cellular structure and metabolism besides structural and/or functional roles in metalloenzymes protein and hormones. Trace element status influences growth and reproduction (Zn, Se), immune functions (Zn, Se, Fe), lean body mass (Cr), bone density (Cu, Zn, Cr), cognitive functions (Zn, Se), insulin sensitivity (Cr) and oxidative stress (Zn, Se, Cu, Fe). Antioxidant trace elements (Zn, Se, and Cu) are involved in cellular antioxidant defenses and protection against accelerated aging processes (Roussel, 2000).

Deficiencies of minerals in pets are uncommon as a result of the widespread feeding of complete and balanced pet foods that meet the nutrient profiles specified by expert panels. However, deficiencies may arise when the animal's intake is reduced, when the diet is poorly formulated or stored or when the animal is unable to digest, absorb or utilize the nutrient as a result of disease or genetic factors. Additionally, some of the essential minerals may lead to clinical abnormalities when consumed in excess. Dietary interactions that reduce nutrients availability can result from errors in formulation, prolonged storage or injudicious over-supplementation of an otherwise balanced diet (Watson, 1998). Thus, in companion animals, although acute deficiencies and related pathologies are scarce and pet food commercially available is supposed to be adequate to prevent deficiencies, however, sub-clinical deficits leading to decreased immune functions, impaired growth and reproduction, or sub optimal health state, cannot be ruled out.

The bioavailability of trace-elements is reduced by a high content of certain minerals (e.g. calcium), the level of other trace elements (e.g. high zinc decreases copper absorption) and sources of phytic acid (e.g. some soy products). Therefore, as the calcium level approaches the stated nutritional maximum, it may be necessary to increase the levels of certain trace elements such as zinc and copper. Because of very poor availability, iron from oxide or carbonate salts that are added to the diet should not be considered sources contributing to the minimum nutrient level (NRC, 2006).

Calcium and phosphorus : Of the minerals, calcium is required in the greatest amount and also, it is the most critical especially in terms of clinical manifestation of its deficiency. A calcium level of 0.8% has been shown to be adequate for growing dogs. However, this level has been reported to be marginal for some breeds (Alexander *et al.,* 1988; Laflemme *et al.,* 2001) particularly during the fast growing phase (particularly breeds with lower energy requirements). Therefore, a general recommendation is for a level of 1.0 g/100g DM for early growth and 0.8 g/100g DM for later growth (FEDIAF, 2007). High intake of calcium has an adverse effect on skeletal development in large breed dogs, particularly during the early growth phase. Therefore a strict nutritional maximum is recommended for foods intended for large breed puppies. It has been experimentally proved that when feeding a balanced food, calcium level as high as 1.6% DM does not cause side effects (Weber *et al.,* 2000).

Phosphorous is the other dietary mineral required in a relatively high amount in the diet. However, phosphorous deficiency occurs very infrequently in dogs and cats. In fact, excessive dietary phosphorous which accelerates the progression of renal failure is much more common. As a matter of fact, calcium deficiency results primarily when animals are fed diets high in meat and meat products, which are high in phosphorous and low in calcium and is usually expressed as skeletal abnormalities often referred to as rickets. Besides, low calcium levels during pregnancy and lactation (puerperal tetany or eclampsia) is also quite common. Inversely, calcium deficiency may also results from feeding adequate calcium without the correct amount of phosphorous that prevents adequate uptake and utilization of the calcium (Schoenmakers *et al.,* 2000). Thus it is very important that calcium and phosphorous be fed at the correct ratio of around 1.2 parts of calcium for each 1 part of phosphorous (1.2:1). Dietary Ca:P ratio is of much higher importance in puppies of less than 6 months of age (Lauten *et al.,,* 2002).

Feeding high calcium diets is often held responsible for contributing to bone problems in young, rapidly growing dogs. There does appear to be a link between the incidence of hyprertrophic osteodystrophy (HOD), osteochondritis dissecans (OCD) and hip dysplasia, and the overfeeding of calcium, especially in large breed of dogs. Growing giant-breed dogs are more susceptible to developing skeletal disorders than small-breed dogs when raised on a diet with deficient or excessive Ca content. This phenomenon may be related to differential regulation of Ca homeostasis and skeletal growth between breeds for example broken. Great Danes and Miniature Poodles (Hazewinkel and Tryfonidou, 2002; Tryfonidou *et al.*, 2003).

Magnesium : The magnesium content of pet food depends on the ingredients, but is usually not added in supplemental form. Dog and adult cat food should contain at least 0.04% magnesium. High amounts of calcium or phosphorus decrease the absorption of magnesium from the intestines, and can affect the body's magnesium balance. Magnesium deficiency is very rare - it is even difficult to demonstrate in a research setting. Symptoms of deficiency include muscle tremors and weakness, hyperirritability, and depression.

Sodium and Chloride : Sodium and chloride are found in almost all foods. Salt is added to many pet foods to increase the flavor of foods. In general, the chloride requirement is 1.5 times the sodium requirement. Adult dog foods should contain at least 0.06% sodium and 0.09% chloride. A dietary deficiency of sodium and chloride would be extremely rare in pets fed commercial pet foods. A deficiency is more likely to occur in cases of excessive losses of these two minerals from the body as in case of prolonged (or chronic) severe diarrhea and/or vomiting.

Potassium : Potassium is widely distributed in many foods so deficiencies in the diet are not likely if dogs are fed complete and balanced dog foods. Dog and cat foods should contain at least 0.6% potassium. Potassium deficiency in the body is most often due to an excessive loss rather than too little dietary intake. Like sodium and chloride, potassium deficiency can occur in animals that have chronic diarrhea and/or vomiting, burns, kidney disease, or other illnesses, which result in a loss of potassium from the body. Symptoms of potassium deficiency include cardiac arrest, nervous disorders, loss of appetite, poor growth, and weakness. Potassium toxicity generally does not occur from excessive intake as long as the kidneys are functioning normally. The potassium level in the blood, however, can reach a dangerous level in a disease called hypoadrenocorticism or Addison's disease. This is a disease in which the adrenal gland does not produce enough of the hormone that helps regulate the amount of potassium in the blood. In this context the ratio of Na:K assumes greater importance (Pak, 2000).

Iodine : Dogs can adapt over time to reasonably low intakes of iodine, and reports of deficiency in mature dogs are very few. Dogs should receive 1.5 mg of iodine daily for every kg of dog food they eat. Iodine deficiency results in sub-optimal production of thyroid hormones. Symptoms of this hypothyroidism include poor growth, hair loss, weight gain in older animals, weakness, and some behavioral changes such as irritability. Hypothyroid animals often cannot breed successfully.

Iron : Most commercial pet foods contain a highly available form of supplemental iron to help meet dietary requirements. The iron should be in a form other than iron oxide or iron carbonate, which are not good sources of bioavailable iron. Dog diets need iron at 80 mg per each kg. A deficiency in iron results in the development of anemia leading to decreased growth rate, weakness, and increased susceptibility to stress or disease. Animals with iron deficiency may also develop constipation. Puppies and kittens can be born with lower than normal stores of iron and often develop iron deficiency anemia during the nursing period if their mothers did not receive adequate iron during pregnancy.

Copper : Bioavailability of copper is affected by the presence of a number of substances which include high levels of ascorbic acid, increased levels of Ca, Zn, Fe and sulfur, and some toxic metals such as cadmium, silver, or lead. Copper deficiencies are rare in dogs and cats. Copper oxide is poorly bioavailable. In copper deficiency, an anemia can develop, and there may be abnormalities in bone development. A specific problem in copper storage can result in some dogs showing symptoms of copper toxicity. Bedlington Terriers and West Highland White Terriers have been shown to have this hereditary disorder, which causes copper to accumulate in the liver and results in hepatitis. Doberman Pinschers can also develop hepatitis with an associated accumulation of copper in the liver. The typical symptoms of toxic levels of copper in the liver include lethargy, vomiting, jaundice, and weight loss.

Zinc : Zinc is one of the essential minerals that needs supplementation in diets for dogs and cats. The zinc demands of pet animals vary by breed, genetics, life stage, nutritional status and environmental stress. Dogs and cats may also experience a higher demand for zinc under circumstances of stress, during growth periods, levels of high activity, gestation, lactation or illness. Absolute dietary deficiencies of zinc are considered rare in dogs and have not been reported in cats. However, a relative deficiency can occur in some dogs related to a decreased bioavailability of dietary zinc (soy based dry food). In un-supplemented animals, zinc ingestion correlates with protein intake (Roussel, 2000). There are several factors that influence the absorption of zinc. One of them is genetics; several breeds including Siberian Huskies, Alaskan Malamutes and Canadian Inuit have a genetic inability to adequately absorb zinc. Many of these breeds must be fed a diet that is higher in zinc to prevent zinc deficiency associated skin problems. Fibres and phytates bind zinc and reduce its absorption. Therefore, animals that are fed a diet high in plant material may have an increased risk of developing zinc deficiencies. Calcium also binds zinc, and zinc deficiencies can be produced when excess amounts of calcium are fed. Dogs or cats with inflammatory bowel disease may develop zinc deficiency because of lack of absorption.

Indeed, zinc plays a critical role in regulating many aspects of cellular metabolism, which are related with the maintenance of a healthy coat and skin. Zinc, as a cofactor for RNA and DNA polymerase is of particular importance in rapidly dividing cells, including those of the epidermis. Zinc is also essential for the biosynthesis of fatty acids and is involved in the metabolism of vitamin A. In adult pets, signs of zinc deficiency are confined mainly to the skin, but these may be accompanied by impaired growth and other abnormalities in young animals. Appetite may be depressed as a result of a diminished taste and smell. Prolonged deficiency can result in weight loss, impaired wound healing, conjunctivitis and keratitis. Zinc deficiency in the dog most commonly occurs as a skin condition that is called 'zinc responsive dermatosis'. The disease is divided into two different syndromes. One affects huskies and malamutes and the other affects puppies on zinc-deficient diets or diets that are over-supplemented with calcium. The problem may become aggravated if the animals are stressed. The usual symptoms are hair loss, and scaling and crusting of the skin around the face, head, and legs. Lesions often encircle the mouth, chin, eyes, and ears. The footpads may be scaly and the hair coat is dull and dry. Puppies fed a deficient diet may also show these symptoms but may also be lethargic, anorexic, and be prone to secondary infections.

Manganese : Manganese is essential for the proper use of protein and carbohydrate by the body, reproduction, and the action of many enzymes in the body responsible for the production of energy and making fatty acids. As with magnesium, excess calcium and phosphorus have been known to interfere with the absorption of manganese from the intestinal tract. Manganese deficiency is very rare in dogs and cats; when it does occur, newborn and young animals are more likely affected. The symptoms of manganese deficiency include poor growth, skeletal abnormalities, reproductive failure, and ataxia (loss of equilibrium).

Selenium : Selenium is an antioxidant, which functions in conjunction with vitamin E and certain enzymes to protect cells. The daily requirement for selenium is less than the requirement for any of the other trace elements. Selenium deficiencies are extremely rare in dogs and basically unknown in cats. A deficiency, however, would cause poor reproduction, puppy death, muscle weakness, and abnormalities of the heart muscle.

Vitamins

Most vitamins cannot be synthesized in the body and must, therefore, be present in the diet. A frequent intake of water-soluble vitamins is necessary since they are poorly stored in the body, with excesses being lost via the urine. The fat-soluble vitamins are stored to a much greater extent and consequently, a daily intake is less critical. However, because they are stored, the risk of toxicity arising through excessive intake is far greater with the fat-soluble vitamins. Exogenous supplementation of balanced diets and/or supplementation without considering the contribution from major food ingredients may lead to inhibition of absorption leading to adverse effects. Further, processing and storage of food leads to loss of vitamins thus it becomes difficult to ensure nutritional adequacy.

Vitamin A : Vitamin A deficiency is rare in dogs as they can convert carotene in vegetable matter to vitamin A, if needed. Besides, dogs store vitamin A in their liver, kidney and fat; so prolonged dietary deficiency must occur before symptoms appear. However, too high concentrations of fatty acids or rancid fat supplement in diet will destroy vitamin A, and may induce deficiency. Common signs of deficiency include stillbirths, spontaneous abortions, birth defects, blindness, deafness and ataxia. It may lead to anorexia, body weight loss, conjunctivitis, corneal disorders, skin lesions, respiratory ailments besides an increased susceptibility to infection. Excesses of vitamin A are equally dangerous and usually results in imbalance in bone remodeling processes, artery and vein degeneration, dehydration, central nervous system depression and joint pain.

Vitamin D : Deficiency of vitamin D occurs in association with calcium or phosphorus deficiency or imbalance. Most often the deficiency is attributed to over-supplementation (exogenous vitamin D or fish oil supplements) rather than deficient dietary formulation. Studies in Great Dane puppies showed that higher dietary vitamin D level can affect calcium absorption and may stimulate endochondral ossification disturbances (Tryfonidou *et al.*, 2002). Signs of deficiency include bone abnormalities (rickets, bone swelling and bending), lethargy, loss of muscle tone, calcification of soft tissue and muscular dystrophies. In situations of excesses, signs induce anorexia, weakness, diarrhoea, vomiting, calcification of soft tissue, excessive mineralization of long bones, dehydration, dry and brittle hair and muscle atrophy.

Vitamin E : Too high a fat diet or rancid fat destroys vitamin E, causing deficiency. Show dogs fed excessive diets of polyunsaturated fats, especially fish-oils, to improve coats will show opposite results, and induce vitamin E deficiency. The signs of deficiency are muscular dystrophies (degeneration of skeletal muscle), cardiac insufficiency, reproductive failure (stillbirths, fading-puppies), retinal degeneration and poor coat.

Vitamin C : Ascorbic acid is required for many intracellular reactions and protein synthesis, but most mammals (except man, other primates and the guinea pig) can synthesize it from glucose. Dogs also make their own vitamin C and do not require a dietary source. There is no dietary requirement for vitamin C in normal, healthy companion animals, but a dietary source may be beneficial, as it is a powerful dietary antioxidant. Hence although a deficiency may not be a problem, but supplemental vitamin C does help in overcoming stress-situations.

Vitamin B Complex : The B-complex vitamins, as co-enzymes (co-factors), are involved in normal metabolic functions, especially energy metabolism and synthetic pathways. In general, anorexia and loss of weight are common signs of deficiency of B vitamins. Raw fish contains thiaminase, which destroys thiamin and may lead to paralytic syndrome in dogs; cooking the fish destroys the enzyme. The deficiency signs include decreased appetite, constipation, weight loss, weakness, drowsiness, paralysis, seizures and anxiety. A deficiency may also lead to neurological abnormalities in puppies; damage to the nervous system and the heart in adult dogs. Riboflavin, if deficient, may induce muscular weakness, flaking dermatitis and eye lesions. Irritation and inflammation of the lips, cheeks, and throat, profuse salivation, bloody diarrhea are typical signs of niacin deficiency. Similarly, pantothenic acid deficit in diet may cause erratic food intake, sudden prostration or coma, rapid respiratory and heart rates, convulsions, gastrointestinal symptoms, and reduced antibody production. Anemia may result from deficiency of pyridoxine, cobalamin and folic acid.

Water

With approximately 70% of the lean body mass of animals being water, it is the single most important nutrient for the body. Although animals can live after losing almost all of their body fat and more than half of their protein, a loss of only 10% of body water results in death. Water is required to carry out metabolic processes and chemical reactions inside cells; it is required for regulation of body temperature besides being an essential part of normal digestion. The daily water requirement depends upon several factors like physical activity (level of exercise), body or ambient temperature, renal health, physiological state (onset of lactation) and amount of water in pet's food (commercial pet food typically may contain ~7% in dry foods to as high as ~80% in canned food). Besides, the amount of calories consumed, and the level of salt in the diets may also influence voluntary water consumption. In a thermo-neutral environment, most mammalian species need ~44-66 ml water/kg BW. Generally, for maintenance in thermo-neutral environment, the water requirement (ml) is equal to 2-3 times the DM intake of food, expressed in gram (NRC, 1985). Considering the fact that water needs appear to be highly associated with the amount of food consumed, it is further proposed that, daily maintenance water requirements in ml should be equal the animal's maintenance energy requirement in kcal of ME (Lewis *et al.*, 1967). Clean fresh water should be available at all times; when provision is made for ample amounts of water, healthy animals can effectively self-regulate their intake.

Feeding Through life Stages

Just like humans, dogs and cats pass through life stages requiring different types of food in varying amounts. It is thus important to recognize these life stages and respond to them by providing the right nutritional management.

Nursing and Young Ones

Newborn puppies and kittens receive complete nutrition from their mothers' milk for the first four weeks of life. In case the mother is ill or has an extremely large litter or doesn't produce enough milk, it may be necessary to feed a properly formulated milk replacer. Puppies generally begin eating puppy food around three or four weeks of age. By the time the pups are completely weaned at seven to eight weeks old, they should be eating their dry food consistently. During the first weeks of life, body weight may double or triple and this rapid growth will continue (although at a gradually decreasing rate) until maturity. Large amounts of energy and nutrients are required in balanced quantities to support this spectacular growth.

Puppies require up to twice the energy intake of adults and, depending on the breed, will need to be fed a properly balanced high protein food. Small breeds of dogs (~10 kg adult BW) reach mature BW by 9-12 months. As puppies, they can be fed free-choice. When food is readily available, most small-breed dogs will develop good eating habits and not become overweight. Most medium-breed puppies (adult BW between 10 and 25 kg) and all large- or giant-breed pups (>25 kg adult BW) are best fed adopting the portion-control method. If they are allowed to overeat, they can consume too many calories, grow too rapidly and develop bone growth problems evident as bowing of the front legs. Sometimes, these signs are misdiagnosed as calcium deficiency (rickets). It is thus always advisable not to overfeed in an attempt to accelerate a puppy's growth rate. Controlled feeding of a balanced diet specifically made for large- and giant-breed puppies facilitates optimal skeletal development. It is therefore, important to aim for a slower rate of growth with large and giant breed puppies.

Adults

Adult dogs require sufficient nutrients to meet energy needs and to maintain and repair body tissues. The amount of feed required by an adult dog should be based on its metabolic body size. Besides, activity levels, which vary dramatically between pets, play an important role in determining energy requirements. The major risk involved in feeding of adult dogs is overfeeding which leads to extra weight and concomitant health problems. House pets vary widely in their activity levels. An animal with a "normal" activity level should receive maintenance energy (130 kcal per $kgW^{0.75}$). This can be reduced in case of an inactive dog which may require 10 percent below maintenance, while an active pet who exercises regularly outdoors may require 20 to 40 percent above maintenance. The working canines, such as police dogs, may require 50 to 70 percent extra energy compared to maintenance depending upon work load. An animal recovering from surgery or suffering from a disease may have an increased nutritional requirement for repair, healing and fighting infection. Environment influences energy needs, and extreme hot or cold weather can increase a dog's energy needs.

Reproducing Females

Nutrition has long been recognized to influence the reproductive success in the bitch. Ideally, the correct feeding management of reproducing animals begins during growth and development of the dam and sire and continues throughout mating, gestation and lactation (Case *et al.*, 1995). The basic aim while feeding during pregnancy and lactation should be to ensure that the content as well as the balance of nutrients in the diets are carefully regulated, matching the requirements. However, so long as the diet is balanced, the increased requirement for nutrients is met when food intake is increased to meet the energy needs of the female.

Pre-breeding

It must always be remembered that the reproductive process does not begin at mating, but several weeks prior to the mating process when ovarian follicles are being recruited for the upcoming cycle (Kelley, 2001). It is therefore recommended to ensure that both the sire and dam must be in ideal health condition with optimum weight. If the dam is underweight, she may not be able to consume enough food during the ensuing gestation to meet the nutritional requirements of her own as well as the developing foetus; lack of proper nutrition in dam can result in decreased birth weight and increased neonatal mortality. Conversely, overweight conditions in dams can lead to development of very large fetuses and dystocia (Case *et al.*, 1995).

The queen or bitch should be fed a high-quality, highly digestible diet that is nutritionally adequate. Any new food, if required, should be introduced as soon as signs of proestrus are observed (Case *et al.*, 1995). In fact, pet foods of higher nutrient density is often necessary to meet the enhanced nutrient requirements of reproduction without resorting to excess food consumption, which otherwise may lead to gastrointestinal upsets or weight loss. When bitches are transitioned to a diet comprised of approximately 30% highly digestible animal-based protein and 20% fat (balanced for fatty acid content to supply an omega-6 to omega-3 fatty acid ratio in the range of between 5:1 and 10:1) approximately two weeks prior to breeding and continued throughout the reproductive cycle, such a diet resulted in fewer misconceptions, a reduced number of stillbirths and more consistent-sized litters from breeding to breeding (Kelley, 2000). During oestrus, many bitches exhibit a depression in appetite; Bebiak *et al.* (1987) in a study have observed an average depression of food intake by 17% margin occurring at and around ovulation. This short-term loss of appetite does not appear to affect fertility or litter size in normal bitches.

Pregnancy

The average duration of pregnancy in the bitch is 63 days, but her nutrients requirements do not increase appreciably until the last third of gestation when most foetal weight gain occurs. It is important, therefore, to avoid overfeeding in early pregnancy, especially the early post-breeding period, since this will lead to the deposition of unwanted fat and may predispose the bitch to problems at whelping. As a matter of fact, it is not unusual for bitches to undergo a transit period of appetite loss at approximately 3 weeks of gestation (Case *et al.*, 1995). Like the appetite depression that occurs during oestrus, this phase last only for a few days, and eventually may end up showing a dramatic increase in appetite (Kelley, 2001). This period of pregnancy parallels maternal recognition of pregnancy and embryonic implantation that may trigger these appetite changes. It is very important that the bitch be maintained on her normal routine during this period to prevent any undue stress, which could be detrimental to the pregnancy.

A gradual increase in food allowance over the second half of gestation (following 4th or 5th week of pregnancy) is however essential so that at the time of whelping the bitch's daily food intake is approximately 25 to 60% higher than her normal maintenance needs, depending on the size of the litter and the size of the bitch (Moser, 1992). It is necessary to closely monitor the BW of the bitch during the later stages of gestation to ensure that she is gaining sufficient weight. Ideally, a bitch's body weight should increase by about 15 to 25% at whelping. It is impossible to give an exact percentage of weight that a bitch should gain since the increase will vary greatly from breed to breed, even within similar adult sizes. For instance, one might expect a Golden Retriever to gain more weight than a German shepherd on an average since the former typically gives birth to larger litters. However, a good rule of thumb would be to target a 25% weight gain in the bitch by the end of week 8 (d56) post-breeding (Lepine, 1997).

A satisfactory feeding regimen would be to increase the amount of food by 15% of the bitch's maintenance ration each week from the fifth week onwards. During the week before whelping the bitch should, therefore, be eating 60% more than when she was mated. Because the additional requirements imposed by pregnancy are relatively small, they can usually be met by simply increasing the amount of the bitch's normal food, provided that it is nutritionally complete and balanced. However, in late pregnancy and particularly if the litter is large, the space occupied by the gravid uterus may be so great that the physical capacity for food intake is limited and appetite is reduced. In this case, feeding a concentrated diet, such as one designed for puppy growth, can help to ensure an adequate intake. Besides, providing several small meals per day during the last few weeks of gestation also facilitates consumption of adequate amount of food to take care of the limitation of abdominal space.

Lactation and Weaning

Lactation represents the most nutritionally demanding life stage for the female. During the first four weeks post-whelping, she must eat enough to support both herself and her rapidly growing puppies. The extra energy and nutrients needed over and above the normal intake depends on the size and age of the litter but at peak lactation (three to four weeks after whelping), she may need to eat up to four times her normal maintenance allowance. If the bitch is unable to produce enough milk or to eat the amount of food she needs, then early supplementary feeding of the puppies may be necessary if both the bitch and puppies are to thrive. To meet the high demands of lactation, a palatable, highly digestible, calorie-dense diet should be offered in several small meals or *ad libitum*. An unlimited supply of drinking water should also be provided to cater for the large volumes that may be involved in milk production. Besides, milk production is affected by protein quantity and quality in the diet and it is important that the extra food supplied contains a good quality protein. Diets should also contain some carbohydrate for optimum lactose production. The recommendation for protein assumes the diet contains some carbohydrate to decrease the risk of hypoglycaemia in the bitch and neonatal mortality. If carbohydrate is absent or at a very low level, the protein requirement is much higher, and may be double (Romsos *et al.*, 1981; Kienzle and Meyer, 1989). In other words, a proper balance and adequate supply of both protein and carbohydrate is essential for lactating bitches.

Weaning of the litter should be accomplished gradually, since an abrupt separation of bitch and puppies may lead to mastitis in the bitch and a reduction in the rate of growth of the puppies. Most puppies begin to take an interest in solid foods from about 3-4 weeks, although small amounts of soft foods may be offered from as early as two weeks of age. The age at which alternative foods may be accepted will depend largely on the size of the litter and the milk supply of the bitch but, in any event, the bitch's milk should remain the prime source of nutrients until the puppies are at least four weeks old. Once the puppies are eating well, the bitch may be separated from them for progressively longer periods to allow her milk supply to decrease. Weaning may be completed between 6-8 weeks of age and it is be advisable to cut the bitch's ration down to her maintenance level following separation from the puppies. If she has, however, lost condition during lactation, a nutrient and energy dense diet should be fed until she regains her former condition.

Geriatrics

Dogs and cats begin to show visible age-related changes at about seven to twelve years of age, depending upon breed. There are metabolic, immunologic and body composition changes. While some of these are unavoidable, others can be managed with proper dietary changes. The main objectives in the feeding an older dog or cat should be to maintain health and optimum body weight, slow or prevent the development of chronic disease, and minimize or improve clinical signs of diseases that may already be present. Cats can be initiated into a senior diet at about seven years of age. Since smaller dogs live longer and do not experience age-related changes as early as bigger dogs, size is used to determine when its time to feed a canine a senior diet in general, for small (<10 kg) and medium (10-25 kg) breeds, it is 7 years; large breeds (25-40 kg), 6 years; and giant breeds (> 40 kg); 5 years of age.

As a dog or cat ages, health issues may arise, including deterioration of skin and coat, loss of muscle mass, more frequent intestinal problems, arthritis, obesity, dental problems and decreased ability to fight off infection. Older dogs and cats have been shown to progressively put on body fat in spite of consuming fewer calories. This change in body composition is inevitable and may be aggravated by either reduced energy expenditure or a change in metabolic rate. Either way, it is important to feed a diet with a lower caloric density to avoid weight gain, but with a normal protein level to help maintain muscle mass. Senior diets that have reduced levels of protein should be avoided. Studies have shown that the protein requirement for older dogs does not decrease with age, and that protein levels do not contribute to the development or progression of renal failure. It is important to feed older dogs diets that contain optimum levels of highly digestible protein to help in maintaining good muscle mass.

Antioxidants such as vitamin E and beta-carotene help eliminate free radical particles that can damage body tissues and cause signs of aging. Senior diets for dogs and cats should contain higher levels of these antioxidant compounds. Antioxidants can also increase the effectiveness of the immune system in senior cats and dogs. Antibody response decreases as cats age. Increasing the intake of vitamin E in cats older than seven years of age can increase their antibody levels back to those seen in younger cats. Similarly, gamma-linolenic acid (GLA) is an omega-6 fatty acid that plays a role in the maintenance of healthy skin and coat. Although it is normally produced in a dog's liver, GLA levels may be diminished in older dogs.

Nutrition and Aging : Brain cells, and whole central nervous system, require huge quantities of good quality nutrients for functioning properly. Hence, diet is a key factor in the brain aging processes, and thus on the timing of the appearance of any unwanted behaviors associated with aging. An underfed pet, both in terms of diet quality and quantity, can suffer neuronal damage, in respect of neurone cell membrane metabolism and dendrite function, causing improper neural transmission, impaired neurotransmitter metabolism, storage and recycling, and worse still, synaptic loosening, neuronal death and inactivity, and associated loss of brain function and behavioural coordination.

Inappropriate feeding can also lead to degenerative pathologies as chronic liver and kidney failure, heart disease, arthritis, irritable bowel disease, disc disease, obesity, etc, with behavioural disorders occurring as a result of these diseases as well. The senses of hearing, touch, smell, taste and visual acuity and cognitive disorders can all arise due to the early onset of senility catalyzed by poor nutrition, and lead to many behavioral problems from ataxia and loss of movement co-ordination and training through to breakdowns in house-training.

Proper nutrition throughout life helps ensure that the aging process proceeds as healthily as possible. If since birth animals are fed with high quality food appropriate to their age and lifestyle they will tend to have a strong immune system, and less pre-disposition to becoming ill, and of course their overall life will be healthier and more active than those fed poor quality, inadequate or improper diets. Most of the modern day quality pet food manufacturers produce a lifestyle range of products that ensure that the needs of the animal can be met, and this is especially important in old age from a physiological and behavioral point of view.

Feeding Management

Dogs may be fed successfully in a number of ways that meet both the owner's and the animal's needs and circumstances. These methods include portion-control feeding, free-choice feeding and timed feeding.

Portion-control feeding entails measuring the pet's food and offering it as a meal, thereby controlling the amount of food that can be consumed. This method is used for weight control programs and for animals that might overeat if fed free-choice. Food can be provided in one or more meals daily.

Free-choice feeding is also known as "ad lib" feeding or "free feeding." Food is available at all times, as much as the pet wants, whenever the pet wants. Most nursing mothers are fed by the free-choice method. This method is most appropriate when feeding dry food, which will not spoil if left out.

Timed feeding method involves making a portion of food available for the pet to eat for a specified period of time. For example, the food can be placed in the dog's bowl for thirty minutes. After that time, if the pet has not consumed the food, it is removed.

However, all normal and healthy adult dogs should be fed twice daily by simply dividing the amount suggested into two meals, spaced eight to twelve hours apart. Some dogs will overeat when fed free-choice method, which can result in obesity. If a pet eats free-choice and has put on too much weight, it should be switched to portion-control feeding.

Proprietary Pet Food

Any product produced by a pet food manufacturer, whether processed, partially processed or unprocessed, intended to be ingested by pet animals after placing on the market is classified as a pet food. As per FEDIAF (2006), it can be either a complete pet food, which, by reason of its composition, is sufficient for a daily ration, or complementary pet food, which has a high content of certain substances but which, by reason of its composition, is sufficient for a daily ration only if used in combination with other pet foods. The broadest classification of proprietary pet food divides products according to processing method, method of presentation and moisture content. These categories are dry, canned and semi-moist foods.

Dry Pet Foods

Pet foods with a moisture content of less than 14% are classified as dry pet foods. Dry pet foods contain 6-10% moisture and 90% or more DM (Burger, 1988). This category includes pellets, flakes, meals, expanded chunks, biscuits, kibbles etc. Typical ingredients used include cereal grains, meat, poultry or fish products, some milk products and vitamin and mineral supplements. A certain level of starch must be included in expanded products to allow proper processing of the product. The caloric density ranges between 3000 to 4500 kcal of ME per kg on DM basis. Normally this type of pet food contains 24% (18-32) protein, 8% (8-22) fat, 46-74% carbohydrates, 1% linoleic acid and not more than 3.6% fibre. Dry dog foods are the most common type of pet food. The advantages with dry pet foods are: easy to store, less chance of spoilage and offer dental hygiene - the chewing and grinding that accompanies eating dry biscuits/pet food may aid in prevention of plaque and calculus accumulation on teeth. However, the disadvantages include lower palatability, and very low digestibility and nutrient availability in poor quality dry foods.

Semi-moist Pet Foods

Pet foods with moisture content of 14% or more and less than 60% are categorized under semi-moist pet foods.These include fresh or frozen animal tissue, cereal grains, fats and simple sugars as their principal ingredients. The soft texture of semi-moist foods contributes to their acceptability and palatability. Humectants such as simple sugars, glycerol or corn syrup bind water molecules in the food and are used to prevent contamination and spoilage. The high simple sugar content contributes to the palatability and digestibility of these products. The moisture content is 15-30% and ME content/ kg is 3000-4000 kcal on DM basis with 20-28% protein, 8-14% fat, 58-72% carbohydrates, 0.825% linoleic acid and 3% fibre on DM basis. Advantageous with semi moist foods are (i) less odour and available in convenient single serving packages, (ii) available in appealing shape and texture, (iii) do not require refrigeration before opening, (iv) relatively long shelf-life, and (v) price between dry and canned per foods. However, the inherent disadvantage is that it cannot be left for a long time in the pet's bowl because they will dry out soon.

Canned Pet Foods

Pet foods with a moisture content of 60% or more are classified as wet or canned pet foods. There are of two types canned pet foods meant for providing (a) complete and balanced nutrition, or (b) a dietary supplement in form of canned meat or meat byproduct. Complete and balanced foods may contain blends of ingredients such as muscle meats, poultry or fish by products, cereal grains, textured vegetable protein and vitamin and minerals. The second type, often referred to as canned meat products, consist of some type of meat but without supplemental vitamins and minerals. These are not nutritionally complete and are usually meant to be added to dry foods as supplement. The high fat content of canned supplement enhances the texture and palatability of the pet's diet. From a processing stand point, there are 3 types of canned foods (i) loaf, (ii) chunks or chunks in gravy and, (iii) a chunk in loaf combination. Depending on the ingredients that are used, these products can vary greatly in nutrient content, digestibility and availability. On DM basis, the caloric content ranges between 3500 to 5000 kcal ME/kg, with 20-32% fat, 28-50% protein, 18-57% carbohydrates, 0.275% linoleic acid and 1% fibre. The moisture content is usually 75%. The greatest advantage of canned pet foods is their extremely long shelf-life and palatability. But the disadvantages include their expensive nature and chances of obesity if over consumed.

Complementary Pet Food

It covers a wide range of products including: (a) products, such as a meat and biscuit combination, where each component contributes significantly to the energy content of the mixture; (b) products, which contain certain nutrients but are not designed to contribute significantly to the energy content of the mixture. The later includes treats and snacks normally given to strengthen the human animal bond and as rewards during training. Besides, tablets and conditioners are often used to balance the diet when homemade foods are given. Similarly, products such as dog chews, that are not intended to contribute to the nutritional content of the daily ration, but are given to engage the animal and can be eaten.

Human chocolate is toxic for dogs as it contains a chemical substance called theobromine, which they can't metabolize. Symptoms of consumption of human chocolate include vomiting, diarrhoea or collapse. Dogs therefore should be fed specially formulated 'chocolate' treats.

Homemade Pet Food

Home-prepared pet foods require a clear understanding of the specific nutritional needs of the pet. Although majority of dog owners in the western countries enjoy the convenience, economy and reliability of commercially produced pet foods, some owners still prefer homemade diets for their pets. In India, the situation regarding the use of pet foods is just opposite, with a vast majority of pet owners relying on homemade diets to rear their pet dogs. The major problem with this type of diets is that most of the homemade recipes have not been adequately tested for nutrient content and availability.

Nearly all of the pet population in the USA consumes some type of table food at some time in their lives, but the vast majority of pets are fed a commercially produced, complete, and balanced product accounting for 90% of their caloric intake. In some European countries, homemade foods supply an estimated 35% of the cats with 60% of their caloric intake. Some pets are fed table foods intentionally, on an occasional basis, but these foods are not of concern when they comprise less than 10% of the daily food intake of healthy pets. When the pet receives more than half its daily calories from table foods, the whole diet should then be formulated to ensure a proper nutrient intake.

In India, homemade diets constitute the mainstay of feeding and nutrition of majority pet dogs with most of the dog-owners preferring to feed their dogs according to their own convenience and perceptions (Pattanaik and Sharma, 2006). A survey of 494 pet owners visiting the selected pet clinics in three cities in northern India revealed that a total of 79.4% of the respondents were feeding homemade diets to their dogs with only 3.4% rearing their pets exclusively on commercial pet foods (Shakhar *et al.*, 2010). This is in contrast to about 90% of the pet owners in Kerala keeping their pets on homemade diets with as high as 77% pet owners relying on their own-self to decide about the feeding and nutrition of their pet dogs (Vijay Kumar *et al.*, 2004). Supplementation in terms of minerals and vitamins is restricted to only about 30% of the pet owners; however, the composition and quality of such supplements varied widely and is difficult to ascertain. In their study, Vijay Kumar *et al.* (2004) reported that a majority (93%) of the owners preferred to feed non-vegetarian foods to their pet dogs in Kerala. In contrast, about 58% pet owners in northern India on non-vegetarian (fully or partly) diets to raise their dogs (Shakhar *et al.*, 2010). A recently conducted survey, covering more than 1000 pet dogs from different parts of the country, revealed that homemade diets of varied ingredient composition are the common food offered to pet dogs (Pattanaik, 2011). These types of foods are not only deficiency but also imbalanced with respect to various nutrients to meet the requirements of healthy dog.

As India is a very vast country with varied cultures in terms of religion, socio-economic and above all food habits, the pets reared on homemade diets would automatically have access to a variety of radically different recipes offered to them. In northern India, for example, most of the recipes included milk-bread (or *roti*), or milk-dalia, or *roti*-vegetables. Similarly, in other parts of the country, rice forms the main basal diet to which varied combinations of proteins, vegetables etc are added. Supplementation of these diets with occasional fish, meat and egg can be observed in some cases, but here too, most of the times, the meat is of inferior quality (offal). The type of homemade diets used for feeding pet dogs is more often than not are imbalanced both quantitatively as well as qualitatively. There is no scientific basis on which these diets are formulated. Majority of diets are of vegetarian origin containing lot of fibre, for example. Although dog has evolved in food habits from carnivorous to omnivorous due to domestication but still its ability to digest fibre beyond 15% in diet is questionable (Yamka *et al.*, 2002) and not advised, as it leads to many gastrointestinal disorders (Rowe *et al.*, 1999). Vegetables are of no direct benefits to dogs, since they are relatively indigestible. They add bulk to diet and can provide some minerals and vitamins but a diet solely based on vegetables and *roti* becomes significantly low in proteins. The level of fiber is very high in vegetables and in households where vegetable and *roti* are offered as food on routine basis, the incidence of gastrointestinal tract problem is expected to be high.

Reasons for use of homemade diets

Public awareness of nutrition is steadily increasing, and pet owners are understandably interested in the nutrition of their pets. There is a growing segment of pet owners that are electing to prepare homemade foods for their pets. Their reasons for doing so are diverse. Many people are preparing their pet's food in their homes, out of a desire for a more natural diet, to meet some special need of the pet, to alleviate allergies, or simply out of personal preference. Some people have pets with special dietary requirements that may be hard to meet with commercial foods, such as food allergies or to support a pet with a serious medical condition that may affect the appetite. Some people feed a homemade diet because they want a source of nutrition that is free from the by-products, chemical additives, and processing found in many commercial foods.

i) *Socio-economics*: Many pet owners simply prefer to feed their pets on homemade diets because of monetary reasons. In addition to the affordability, it also lends convenience as in most of cases homemade diets constitute the table scraps or at best a portion of the owners' own food.

ii) *Preference for a natural diet:* Some pet owners simply believe that homemade diets are healthier, more natural, and can use ingredients that are natural, organic, vegetarian, or consistent with their moral or ethical beliefs. Because of their own consciousness and concern, they accept that pets must have naturally grown foods, devoid of artificial colors, flavors or preservatives, synthetic nutrient additives such as amino acids, vitamins or minerals and with ingredients (meat and grains) produced without synthetic hormones, pesticides or fertilizers for proper health.

iii) *Non-availability of commercial food*: Very often, homemade diets need to be specially formulated with a nutrient profile for the specific medical conditions. For a particular medical problem a therapeutic pet food may be available, but either the product is not palatable and thereby consumed in adequate quantities to support body weight and condition of the patient, or it is not acceptable to the owner. Alternatively, performance dogs such as sled dogs are also fed homemade diets since they require very high amounts of fat and protein that cannot be met by many commercial diets.

iv) *Desire to cook*: Some pet owners simply want to cook for their pets and are willing to spend the extra time and money required for meal preparation. Some people believe that preparing the pet's diet strengthens the human-companion bond.

v) *Allergies*: Feeding a homemade food to a pet can be a diagnostic and/or therapeutic measure in cases of dietary sensitivity and food intolerance. As per anestimate, the prevalence of adverse reactions to food (including food intolerance and food allergies) has been roughly estimated at 1% of all general dog and cat cases and is responsible for 10-20% of cases of skin disease seen by veterinary specialists.

vi) *Habit*: Some pet owners begin feeding a young or sick dog on homemade diet only to realize later that the pet will not eat any commercially prepared food and thereafter the pet continue to be raised exclusively on table foods commonly used in the household.

Classification of homemade diets

The different kinds of homemade diets being fed to pet dogs can be basically classified into three main categories.

i) *Exclusive balanced homemade diet*: This diet, which is well balanced, and nutritiously complete, contains premium protein sources, a balance of carbohydrates, proteins, fats, and fiber, and meets the animal's entire vitamin and mineral needs. People that feed this diet are truly dedicated to the health of their pet. This type of diet requires a commitment of time and money.

ii) *Supplemented homemade diet*: It usually consists of a commercial dry food, and the owner then supplements the diet with meat and some carbohydrate sources. The family leftovers usually get scraped into the pet's bowl. This diet although apparently meeting the animal's nutrient needs, may become imbalanced in situations where the table scraps account for more than 10% of the diet.

iii) *Table scrap based homemade diet*: The third type of homemade diet is the one where the owners feed their pet only table food and do not balance the diet for protein, fat, carbohydrates, minerals and vitamins.

Problems with homemade diets

Unfortunately, most homemade diets are flawed even when the compositional guidelines are followed exactly and consistently. One survey found that 90% of the homemade diets prescribed by over 100 US veterinarians were not nutritionally adequate for adult dogs or cats. Almost no homemade recipes for dogs in India have been properly tested for nutritional adequacy. The palatability, digestibility, and safety of these recipes have not been adequately and scientifically tested in animals.

i) Homemade foods are rarely balanced for micro-minerals or vitamins, and impromptu use of veterinary vitamin/mineral supplements seldom corrects the deficiencies. There is no one veterinary supplement, which can be added to homemade recipes for dogs that will meet all the micro-mineral and vitamin requirements adequately. If a homemade diet is not properly balanced it can be worse for the pet than commercial diets.

ii) Inappropriate food substitutions are another common error made by pet owners formulating their pet's diet. Many owners make their own food substitutions, without understanding the full ramifications involved, selectively omitting items due to personal preference or convenience, and make preparation errors that can result in an unbalanced formulation.

iii) Foods that owners enjoy are not necessarily the most nutritious food to offer to their pets. Owners mistakenly feed their pets according to current and popular human nutritional guidelines such as avoiding fat, cholesterol, and sodium; that too, does not constitute a complete and balanced food for the pet.

iv) Use of uncooked meat and eggs in homemade foods can be dangerous which may harbour pathogenic bacteria that would be killed during cooking.

v) Preparing a homemade diet takes more time.

vi) Careful attention to the cooking and storing of homemade diets is necessary to avoid any food borne illnesses.

vii) Homemade diets are often soft and do not provide the chewing action that is good for the teeth and gums.

viii) Once a pet gets habitual to eat home made food it may become difficult to switch it to a commercial food.

Nutritional adequacy of homemade diets

In general, veterinary nutritionists agree that healthy pets should be fed a complete and balanced, commercially prepared food. Unlike commercially available foods, homemade diets have not been adequately tested with animal feeding trials or laboratory analysis to confirm nutrient content and nutrient availability. Homemade diets are often crudely balanced and may not achieve satisfactory palatability, digestibility or safety. A study by Roudebush *et al.*, (1994) reported that 90% of homemade diets used for managing adverse food reactions were not nutritionally adequate.

Nutritionally responsive diseases are rarely seen in dogs and cats fed good-quality commercial rations or nutritionally balanced homemade diets. In contrast, dog or cat foods on homemade diets derived from a single food item are not nutritionally satisfactory and may predispose the pets to a number of diseases. For example, feeding raw freshwater fish to cats can induce a thiamine deficiency. Feeding liver can induce vitamin A toxicity in both dogs and cats.

The most common errors with homemade diets include deficiency of protein, and the formulation of diets that are deficient calories, calcium, vitamins and microminerals. Deficiency of protein, either due to unpalatable diet of low-protein concentration or poor quality dietary (vegetarian) protein resulting in decreased digestibility or due to dietary imbalance (too much fat or carbohydrates in diet), induces poor growth and body condition, pot-belly, poor muscle tone or development, anemia, reduced immunity and poor wound healing. Diets with low caloric density in case of puppies, lactating bitches and working dogs may result in energy deficiency, which is manifested as pot bellied condition with poor muscle tone. Dogs do not need a large amount carbohydrate to be healthy (as a rule, dogs should receive <12g digestible carbohydrate per kg live weight); a diet low in carbohydrates and high in protein is an ideal diet. Diets high in carbohydrates take a long time to digest, produce voluminous smelly stools and gas. They also build up tartar on dog's teeth, making the gums sore and breath smelly. On the other hand, feeding the pet dogs with human surplus food (table scraps), frequently starch-derived and fatty meat (or leftover curry), may predispose the dogs to obesity.

Another common mistake is the incorporation of too much or too little calcium, both of which affects bone development. Too much calcium has been shown experimentally to increase the incidence of bone lesions. Pups fed homemade diets need careful calcium supplementation to avoid excesses. Feeding predominately meat or even a meat and rice diet to dogs can induce calcium deficiency and nutritional secondary hypoparathyroidism. High quantities of meat, coupled with calcium deficiency result in abnormal calcium to phosphate ratios. Commonly used meat and carbohydrate ingredients contain more phosphorus than calcium, and these diets can have an inverse Ca:P ratio as high as 1:10.

Research on homemade diets

The quantum of research available on the nutritional adequacy of homemade diets is scarce. This is mainly due to the fact that it is more often than not a characteristic of Indian pets but the pet nutrition research in India is still at infancy. However, whatever little literature available only confirms the generally accepted perception that homemade diets are highly imbalanced to take care of the nutritional needs of pet dogs. Most of the ingredients in typical western homemade diets are meat scraps, cooked meat, raw meat, vegetable, bread, biscuits, cakes, rice, potato, milk etc. One Austrian study comparing between homemade food and commercially manufactured pet food (CMP) reported that homemade diets were significantly low in Ca and P and in Ca:P ratio than both CMP and AAFCO recommendations. The homemade diets were also lower in potassium, zinc and copper, and fat-soluble vitamins A, D and E. They were higher in total saturated fat and lower in total polyunsaturated fat than CMP (dry extruded food). They were energy dense, but without an increased nutrient density (Streiff *et al.*, 2001). Rice and wheat are the most favoured cereal sources commonly used in dog diets. In a study with Spitz dogs it was shown that maize, sorghum and pearl millet are not as effectively utilized as rice in home cooked diet (Kore *et al.*, 2009).

Rearing of dogs on homemade diet comprising of chicken and basmati rice reported to induce Ca malnourishment, providing 0.22 g Ca vs. the daily requirements of 0.6 g (Diquelao *et al.*, 2000). Dogs fed on high Ca diet without proportionally higher P are reported to become hypercalcaemic and hypophosphataemic, and had severe disturbances in skeletal development as well as growth (Schoenmakers *et al.*, 2000). In a study comparing the metabolic profile of dogs fed on commercial, homemade or mixed ration, Gonzalez *et al.* (2003) have reported lower availability of protein based on the low contents of plasma albumin and/or urea. Further, dogs fed with mixed diets showed higher glucose and cholesterol levels suggestive of a high caloric intake and a risk of obesity. A group of Walker Hounds and Beagles fed on a diet of table scraps developed slow, progressive loss of vision, which upon investigation pointed towards dietary vitamin E deficiency (Davidson *et al.*,, 1998). On the other hand, optimization of nutrient profile of homemade diet to match the requirement could be an effective strategy to provide complete nutrition; studies by Pawar *et al.* (2008; 2011) demonstrated that optimization of nutrient profile of rice-milk based homemade diet induces positive effects on growth, gut health indices and humoral immune response of Spitz pups.

While attempting to assess the nutritional adequacy of the homemade diets as a pert of an ongoing research project at Indian Veterinary Research Institute, the major obstacle encountered was the great variation of the combinations as well as the typicality of the food ingredients found to be used for feeding of the pet dogs. But attempts were made to club together these diverse food combinations into fewer major categories. The specified categories only constituted the basal components used for feeding the pets for most of the time. It was quite understandable that the pet owners quite often change the combination or even add novel ingredients to the set combination, depending upon a multitude of factors involving personal, social, economic as well as logistical reasons. The problems spelled out above notwithstanding, the nutritional attributes of the selected dietary combinations can be ascertained, with some degree of approximation though, with the help of food composition tables. As no data is available on the nutritional quality of various food ingredients for dogs as such, the data available for human foods may be taken onto consideration.

In such a study done in parts of northern India, we have classified all the observed homemade recipes into five broad classes viz. (i) milk-bread, (ii) milk-bread with vegetables, (iii) milk-bread with non-vegetarian (egg and/ or meat) components and sometimes with additional vegetables, (iv) milk-bread-egg/meat-with or without vegetables but with pet foods, and (v) exclusive milk-pet food. A striking feature that emanates from these findings is that all the pet owners are using milk as an indispensable component of the food for their pet dogs. However, the quantity of milk offered in many instances may not suffice the entire nutritional needs of the animal. Further, as age increases, the capacity to digest milk products decreases in dogs; this eventually may lead to high incidence of gastrointestinal disorders with recipes containing milk.

Bread-milk constituted one of the most used food combination for about a quarter of the pet population surveyed. Although milk is a good source of protein and fat as well, but it lacks iron, copper and vitamin C. Bread is a good source of energy but lacks lysine. It compensates for the lack of iron in milk, but vitamin C is absent in both. Nutritional evaluation of a bread-milk diet with or without additional egg in Mongrel pups revealed that in either case it is inadequate to meet the requirements for energy, protein, calcium, phosphorus and zinc (Shakhar, 2005). The other common combination of food for pet dogs was bread-milk with vegetables. The amount of vitamins and minerals is expected to vary with the composition of vegetables being used to supplement the basal diet. But in general, they are good source of vitamin C along with iron, and thereby can compensate for the lack of both vitamin C and iron on the bread-milk diet. But in terms of energy, they often fail to reach the recommendation. Vegetables are a fairly good source of B vitamins but these may be destroyed during cooking. Further, dogs may obtain some of the dietary precursor of vitamin A from vegetable sources in the form of beta-carotene. Fibre is another aspect associated with vegetables, which needs careful consideration depending upon the individual vegetable being used for supplementation. Increased dietary fibre dilutes the caloric content of food, induce satiety and thereby reduce voluntary intake of (food) energy (Jewell *et al.,* 2000; Shakhar *et al.,* 2007). Shakhar (2005) while experimentally validating the nutritional adequacy of a bread-milk-vegetables diet with or without pulses, observed that neither of the diets was able to suffice the energy, protein, Ca, P and Zn requirements of Spitz pups.

Supplementation of the bread-milk basal diet with occasional feeding of egg or meat is quite common. Eggs provide very good quality protein. The number of eggs given to the pets varies with different situations, and so is the nutritional adequacy of this combination. The supplementation of meat to the above combinations has its own merits and demerits. It has been a tendency in part of most of the pet owners to provide low quality of meat containing mostly offals not fit for human consumption because of monetary considerations. This entails for a situation where there is no control over the maintenance of a fixed quality. As a result, the proportion of fat, muscles and quite often bones vary widely, thereby influencing the overall nutritional quality of meat vis-à-vis the requirement of the pet dogs. A similar situation was encountered while establishing the nutritional adequacy of rice-meat based diet with added vegetables (Shakhar *et al.,* 2007). A sizeable population among the pet owners uses diets containing pulses. Pulses, in general, are good sources of protein; however the quality of the same cannot be compared with that of animal proteins. But they can be used to complement the cereals with respect to the lower level of lysine characteristics of most cereals including wheat and rice. Pulses serve as the sole source of protein under most situations in homemade dog diets; utilization of protein from such sources depends upon the presence of other compounds such as structural and non-structural carbohydrates (Nerinich *et al.,* 2001), trypsin inhibitors, phytates and oligosachharides (Fan *et al.,* 1995). Studies conducted using red gram or lentil as replacement for soybean meal has shown that they may effectively used to partially, if not fully, replace soybean meal protein in the diets of adult dogs without any adverse impact on the lower gut fermentative indices or even the total tract digestion (Pattanaik and Kore, 2009). However, soybean meal could replace soy nuggets in the homemade diet of adult Spitz dogs without any significant effects in nutrient utilization and blood metabolic profile (Pawar and Pattanaik, 2008).

Nutrition for Health

Clinical nutrition is a rapidly developing discipline, relating nutrition to health, and clinical nutrition of pets is no exception. As a result, instead of simply aiming to cover a pet's nutritional requirements, the aim of nutrition now is to improve an animal's overall health by anticipating potential threats which may affect its well-being and longevity. Nutrition plays a fundamental role in determining the health of any animal, and this applies to pets as well; thus a correctly balanced diet is highly essential to avoid diseases. Equally important is the nutritional needs of animals in disease conditions. Each disease process has its own impact on the metabolism of specific nutrients, and this has to be taken into care while formulating diets for specific disease conditions. In the last three decades the development of diets for dogs of different types and at different physiological stages, and the use of prescription diets to support medical therapy have improved the health and wellbeing of dogs significantly. In this connection nutrition research has shifted its focus to bioactive food components that not only help ensure adequate nutrition, but may provide specific health benefits as well. Bioactive components of food origin can be defined as substances, both nutrient and non-nutrient, which may exert regulative activities beyond basic nutrition. In particular, food-derived bioactive proteins and peptides are claimed to be health-enhancing components used to reduce the risk of disease or to enhance a certain physiological function (Meisel, 2007). Consequently, nutrition research world over is focused to exploit the beneficial effects of host of food and non-food origin compounds, broadly categorized as nutraceuticals, for maximizing health and wellbeing of human and animals. Although a detailed discussion on these aspects is out of the purview of this topic, but research in pet nutrition is being carried out targeting various groups of nutraceuticals including prebiotics, probiotics (or their combination as synbiotics), antioxidants and phytochemicals and botanicals.

Pet Food Evaluation

Nutritional studies to evaluate pet foods can be done by two methods viz. indicator method and quantitative collection method (AAFCO, 2007). The indicator shall be uniformly mixed in a quantity of food sufficient to feed all animals for the duration of the pre-collection and collection periods. Chromic oxide is most commonly used as an indicator; approximately 0.25% of a high quality chromic oxide (Cr_20_3) free of soluble chromium shall be mixed with the food. A minimum of six fully grown animals at least one year of age shall complete the test. The animals shall be in good health and of known weight, sex and breed. Animals shall be individually housed during the trial (collection period). The feeding shall consist of two phases. The first phase shall be the pre-collection period of at least three days for dogs and five days for cats (Nott *et al.*, 1994) with the objective of acclimatizing the test animals to the diet and adjusting food intake, as necessary, to maintain body weight. The second phase shall be the total collection period; faeces and possibly urine will be collected during at least four days (96 hours) for dogs and five days (120 hours) for cats.

The determination digestible energy (DE) and protein (DP) is based on assays of the gross energy or crude protein consumed minus the energy or crude protein in the faeces. Digestible fat, ash and dry matter are calculated in the same way as digestible protein. Metabolizable energy is determined based on assays of the gross energy consumed minus the energy lost in faeces and in the urine. In case urine is not collected, ME value of diet is calculated from DE by using correction factor for energy lost in urine viz. 1.25 kcal or 5.23 kJ/g DP for dogs and 0.86 kcal or 3.60 kJ/g DP for cats (Kienzle *et al.*, 1998). ME (kcal/g) = DE - (DP x correction factor for energy lost in urine).

The ME content of any particular diet or ingredient can be determined by feeding trial or by mathematical calculation. Through feeding trial, it can be done by routine procedure that involves use of test animals, and faeces and urine collection over a pre-designated time period. Subsequently, determination of gross energy content of the feed, faeces, and urine allows direct calculation of ME [ME (kcal/g) = $(GE_{food} - GE_{faeces} - GE_{urine})$ / gram of food consumed]. Mathematical model entails calculation of a food's ME from its analyzed contents of carbohydrate, protein and fat. In human foods, the Atwater factors of 4, 9 and 4 kcal/g are commonly used to estimate ME values of carbohydrate, fat and protein, respectively. These factors are arrived at by multiplying the GE (kcal/g) values of carbohydrate (4.15), fat (9.40) and protein (5.65) with their respective estimated digestibility coefficients (96% for carbohydrate and fat, and 91% for protein), which in effect accounts for the digestive and urinary losses. But considering the fact that digestibility of many pet food ingredients is lower than the digestibility in case of humans, (NRC, 1985) suggested that digestibility coefficients of 85, 90 and 80 percent be used for fat and protein carbohydrates, for dog foods. The resulting factors (3.5, 8.5 and 3.5 for carbohydrate, fat and protein, respectively, referred to as *modified Atwater factors,* are thus used for calculating ME value of pet foods or their ingredients. Because this Atwater calculation method uses averages, it may underestimate the ME content of foods that contain highly digestible protein sources and low levels of indigestible fibre, and overestimate those that have less than average digestibility. For all these calculation NFE is taken as carbohydrate.

Conclusion

A well-coordinated nutrition, health care, and management program is required to optimize health of pet animals. A proper nutrition program is paramount for these animals to have adequate health. When proper nutritional programs involving adjustment of nutrient levels for metabolic needs for maintenance, growth, reproduction, and lactation are implemented, optimal health can be ensured. However, feeding of pet dogs under homemade diets needs special consideration so as to make them complete and to take care of the nutritional requirements. Besides areas involving therapeutic diets and nutraceuticals also constitute prime researchable issues for ensuring their integration into feeding for health of pets.

References

AAFCO (2007). *In: Official Publication - Association of American Feed Control Officials Inc., pp.* 160-165.

Alexander JE, Moore MP, Wood LLH (1988). *Modern Veterinary practice,* 31: 144-148.

Bauer *et al.,* (2006). *J. Nutr.,* 136: 1991S-1994S.

Bauer J.E., Heinemann K.M., Bigley K.E., *et al.* (2004). *J. Nutr.,* 134 (8S): 2035S-2038S.

Blum JW, Zentek J, Meyer H. (1992). *J Vet Med A Physiol Pathol Clin Med.,* 39: 568-574.

Hall JA, Wander RC, Gradin, Jewell DE (*1999*). *Am. J. Vet. Res.,* 60 (3): 319-327.

Heinemann KM, Bauer JE. (2006). *J. Am Vet Med Assoc.,*228 (5): 700-705.

Hemsworth, S. and Pizer, B. (2006). *Eur J Oncol Nurs.,* 10(2):117-127.

Hernot, D.C., Dumon, H.J., Biourge, V.C. *et al.,* (2006). *Am J Vet Res.,* 67(2): 342-347.

Kelley, R., Lepine, A. and Morgan, D. (2005). Improving puppy trainability through nutrition. In: 50th Congresso Nazionale Multisala SCIVAC, 2005 – Rimini, Italia (Source: www.ivis.org)

Kienzle, E., Meyer, H. (1989). In : Burger, I.H., Rivers IPW, eds. Nutrition of the dog and Cat. Cambridge, U.K. Cambridge University Press, 243-257.

Kienzle, E. and Rainbird, A. (1991). *J. Nutr.,* 121(11S): S39-S40.

Laflamme DP. *Supplement to Compendium on Continuing Education for the Practicing Veterinarian 2001;* 23 (9A): 66-69.

Lindsay, S., Entenman, C., Chaikoff, I.L. (1948). *Arch. Path.,* 45: 635-638.

NRC, (2006). The National Academic Press, Washington, DC.

Parslow, R.A., Jorm, A.F., Christensen, H., Rodgers, B. and Jacomb, P. (2005). *Gerontology* 51:40-47.

Pibot, P. (2007). *Veterinary Focus,* 17(2): 40-44.

Romsos, D.R., Palmer, H.J., Muiruri, K.L., *et al.,* (1981). *J. Nutr.,* 111: 678-689.

Roussel, A.M. (2000). *Revue Méd. Vét.,* 151(7): 637-642.

Scott, D., Miller, W., Griffin, C. (2001). *In: Small Animal Dermatology, Saunders, Philadephia,* 6: 1-70.

Tryfonidou MA, Stevenhagen JJ, Van den Bemd GJCM, *et al.,* (2002). *J. Nutr.* 132: 2644-2650.

Wander R.C., Hall, J.A., Gradin, J.L., *et al.,* (1997). *J. Nutr.,* 127: 1198-1997.

Watson, T.D.G. (1998). *J. Nutr.,* 2783S-2790S.

Weber, M., Martin, L., Dumon, H., *et al.,* (2000). *J. Vet Int. Med;* 14 (May/June): 388 Abstr. 243.

Wood, L., Giles-Corti, B. and Bulsara, M. (2005). *Soc Sci Med.,* 61(6):1159-1173.

□□□

Animal Nutrition, 2012
eds. Dr. (Mrs.) Usha R. Mehra et al., pp. 259-277
Satish Serial Publishing House e-mail : info@satishserial.com; website : www.satishserial.com

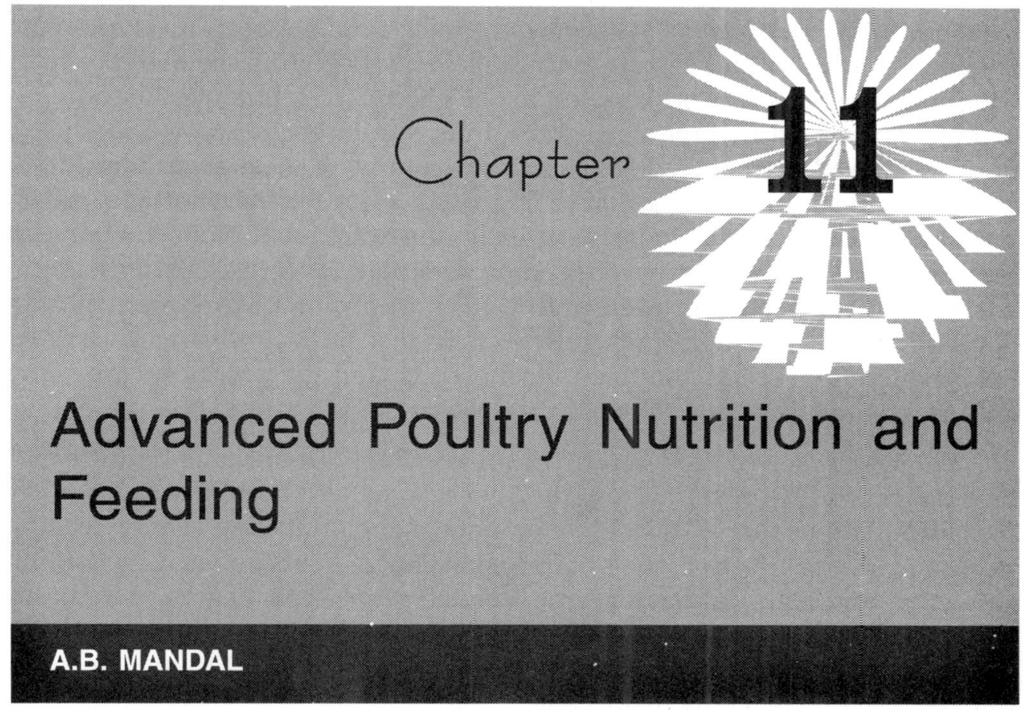

Chapter 11

Advanced Poultry Nutrition and Feeding

A.B. MANDAL

Poultry production has gained momentum during the last five decades. Consequently, it has taken the shape of full-fledged industry. At present, this industry has emerged as the most dynamic and fastest expanding segment in animal husbandry sector. The performance of birds in terms of meat and egg production has also improved significantly. The cost of feed accounts for 65-70% of broiler and 75-80% of layer production cost and a major means of manipulating the production cost. The feeding cost alone being the major constraint in poultry enterprise, every effort is directed to maintain feed quality, contain feed cost and utilize every bit of the feed to convert into food for the mankind. The cost, easy availability and nutritional quality of feed coupled with genetically potent feed efficient stocks to produce safe food from poultry are the need of time.

Feed Resources

The availability and cost of maize and soybean meal generally determines feed cost. The countries producing maize and soybean meal produce broilers with low feeds cost. However, there has been shortage of these two major feedstuffs. To overcome such shortage of maize and soybean meal alternate feedstuffs like nutritious cereals (pearl millet and sorghum), cereal byproducts (rice polish or rice bran, broken rice, maize gluten, rice gluten), other oilcakes or meals (mustard or rapeseed, groundnut, sunflower, sesame and cluster bean meal) and animal feed sources (meat-cum bone meal, meat meal, liver meal, fish meal, blood meal) are being used to buffer the shortage. Again production of foodstuffs fluctuates greatly due to frequent monsoon failures, low productivity, insects, weeds, environmental concerns, cost efficiency, sustainability, declining area under cultivation, etc. Moreover, human population is increasing significantly; certain feedstuffs are being diversified for production of foods, bio-fuels, alcohols, etc. and the producers are being encouraged for diversion towards production of cash crops.

Large number of feed resources are available in variable quantity for feeding, however, only a narrow range of raw materials are used in poultry feed formulations due to lack of reliable data on their nutritive quality, feeding value and safe or effective levels of inclusion. Maize, soybean meal, groundnut extraction and fishmeal have been evaluated with a fair degree of accuracy and reliability but database is limited for other ingredients. There should be database of nutrient contents, digestibility/availability of different nutrient, safe/effective level of inclusion and presentation form of feed for feeding. The proximate composition, toxicants, amino acid composition and metabolizable energy values of different cereals and oilseed residues have also been analyzed and their effective levels maize-soybean meal or in maize-pearl millet-soybean meal or maize-sorghum-soybean meal based diets (Tyagi *et al.*, 2004ab). Moreover, most of the feedstuffs in their native state harbour one or more of the anti-nutritive substance(s). Cereal by-products and oilseed residues, usually constituting about 50% of poultry diet, are also not an exception in terms of non-starch polysaccharides and anti-nutritional factors. Low and variable content of metabolizable energy and fibre in diet many times have led to poor feed conversion efficiency, more excreta output, nutrient loss through excreta and excessive foul odor in poultry house. There is, therefore, both a need and scope for improvement in the nutrition of poultry through enhancing nutrient availability. There is scope of utilization of the other cereals and oilseed residues in combinations within their safe levels to replace maize partially or completely and soybean meal partially. However, the effective combinations (cereal mixture, protein mixture and protein-cereal mixture) are required to be identified through biological trials. The recent findings on utilization of different cereals and oilseed residues have been encouraging (Tyagi *et al.*, 2004ab, Kumar *et al.*, 2005). The combinations of maize, pearl millet and sorghum @ 33% each or maize, pearl millet, sorghum and finger millet @ 25% each could support the broiler growth and feed efficiency. Similarly, combination of maize (50%), sorghum (25%) and pearl millet (25%) or combinations of maize sorghum and pearl millet 33% each provided economical gains in commercial broilers. Moreover, these nutritious cereals can safely be used as part or solely as dilutor of protein-mineral concentrates used in broiler feeding after 3 or 4 weeks of age. The combinations of maize sorghum and pearl millet at 33.3% each provided gain and feed conversion efficiencies similar to maize based diet. Inclusion of rapeseed meal and sunflower seed meal each at 10% level replacing soybean meal supported optimum growth and feed conversion efficiency and reduced cost of production of edible meat. Similarly, combination of rapeseed meal and sunflower seed meal at 10% each replacing 67% of soybean meal resulted in similar growth and feed conversion efficiency as obtained in diet with soybean meal as sole source of vegetable protein. Combination of groundnut meal and niger meal in 75:25 ratio was found to be suitable for economic egg production. Solvent extracted rapeseed meal (RSM) and un-decorticated sunflower seed meal (SSM) could safely be included up to 10 and 5% level, respectively, replacing part of soybean meal in maize or maize-pearl millet based diet. However, combination of maize and pearl millet in a ratio of 1:1 and soybean meal alone or with RSM or SSM yielded apparently better performance than maize with soybean meal. Use of RSM or SSM in broiler starting diets based on sorghum or finger millet may be restricted. However, these meals can be used at 5 or 10% levels in sorghum or finger millet based finisher diets (4-6/7wk of age). Replacement of 50% of dietary maize with pearl millet, and soybean meal with combination of rapeseed meal (solvent extracted) and sunflower seed meal un-decorticated, (solvent extracted), each at 5 or 10% level of diet supported optimum growth, feed utilization efficiency and meat production in broiler chickens. Inclusion of 30% (w/w) pearl millet, 5% (w/w) rapeseed meal and 10% (w/w) sunflower seed meal or 30% pearl millet, 10% rapeseed meal (RSM) and 10% sunflower seed meal (SSM) replacing maize and soybean meal (SBM) partially rendered economic broiler production. The alternate vegetable feed resources are generally deficient in one or more amino acids. However, the critical amino acids (lysine, methionine and threonine) are available commercially for supplementation to ensure improved utilization of protein and feed. Again, the cost of lysine generally fluctuates based on soybean meal prices, being soybean meal rich in lysine. Some of the ingredients (sesame meal, maize gluten meal and rapeseed meal) are relatively rich in methionine (Mandal *et al.*, 2004b), thus judicious use of these ingredients along with (SBM) may reduce some amount of methionine supplementation in diet saving national money as large amount of methionine is imported in India.

Table 1 : Nutrient composition (%) and apparent metabolizable energy (kcal/kg) value of major feed ingredients

Ingredient	CP	EE	CF	AIA	Ca	Total P	AMEn
Red sorghum	9.60	3.46	4.35	1.72	0.02	0.16	2738
Brown sorghum	10.90	2.65	1.66	0.39	0.05	0.17	2999
White sorghum	10.91	2.57	1.11	0.16	0.15	0.30	2970
Finger millet	7.075	1.11	4.56	2.86	0.31	0.20	——
Pearl millet	12.40	4.23	4.31	0.52	0.12	0.12	2715
Maize	9.74	3.30	2.35	0.35	0.18	0.22	3352
Soybean meal	46.90	1.44	7.58	2.31	0.56	0.95	2440
Rice bran, (solv. ext.)	15.09	1.22	12.46	4.51	0.37	1.35	2034
Fish meal	45.88	4.79	3.42	9.84	5.85	2.58	——
Rapeseed meal (solv. ext.)	38.38	1.17	7.81	1.57	0.65	1.23	2051
Sunflower seed meal-(solv.ext.)	30.14	0.89	25.32	0.70	0.39	0.34	1510
Ground-nut cake (solv. ext.)	43.85	0.61	6.47	2.40	0.60	0.48	2230
Wheat	10.62	2.46	2.83	1.23	0.12	0.32	3107

CP = crude protein, EE = Ether extract, CF = crude fibre, AIA = acid insoluble ash, Ca = calcium,P=phosphorus,AMEn=apparent metabolizable energy

Table 2 : Essential amino acid contents (% of crude protein) of some common feedstuffs

Amino acid	Pearl millet	Sorg-hum	Maize	DO RB	RS M	SS M	SB M	GN C	MB M	FM
Methionine	2.31	1.89	2.15	2.30	1.87	2.29	1.42	1.10	1.32	2.86
Cystein	1.84	1.79	1.99	2.43	2.42	1.64	1.52	1.09	1.32	0.86
Lysine	3.27	2.59	2.71	4.73	4.83	3.68	6.20	3.10	5.05	6.50
Threonine	3.87	3.40	3.65	4.32	4.02	3.68	4.03	2.91	3.30	4.40
Arginine	4.82	4.06	4.40	8.31	6.36	8.04	7.51	10.14	6.31	6.98
Isoleucine	3.96	3.89	3.44	3.92	3.79	3.98	4.45	4.40	2.91	3.84
Leucine	9.53	12.54	13.09	7.98	6.65	6.25	7.50	6.68	6.31	7.44
Valine	5.21	4.77	4.54	6.08	4.80	4.80	4.56	5.00	4.43	5.14

DORB=deoiled rice bran meal, RSM= rapeseed meal, SSM= sunflower seed meal, SBM= soybean meal, GNC= ground nut cake, MBM =Meat cum bone meal, FM = Fish meal

Table 3 : True amino acid digestibility values of some of the feed ingredients

Amino acid	Maize	Wheat	Sorghum	DO RB	SB M	Soya full fat	GNC	Sesame meal	Sunflower meal	FM	Meat meal
Lys	77.8	81.0	78.0	78.5	89.5	80.9	83.0	88	84.0	88.3	79.0
Met	89.5	87.0	89.0	76.8	90.8	86.5	88.0	94	93.0	90.4	85.0
Cys	84.0	87.0	83.0	65.7	81.7	76.4	78.0	82	78.0	73.7	58.0
Met+ Cys	86.0	-	-	69.2	86.5	81.5	-	-		-	-
Arg	85.6	88.0	74.0	85.7	90.6	70.4	84.0	92	93.0	89.7	85.0
Thr	75.5	83.0	82.0	71.3	84.7	88.7	82.0	87	85.0	86.0	79.0
Ile	80.4	88.0	88.0	81.7	88.5	83.6	91.0	92	90.0	89.1	83.0
leu	91.4	91.0	94.0	77.5	88.4	90.5	92.0	91	91.0	89.8	84.0
Val	80.0	86.0	87.0	80.4	86.7	83.9	88.0	91	86.0	86.7	82.0
Phe	88.3	92.0	91.0	77.0	88.7	83.8	94.0	93	93.0	88.2	84.0
His	94.0	91.0	87.0	82.0	87.0	91.1	83.0	89	87.0	85.9	80.0
Trp	-	-		-	87.5	83.5	-	-	-	89.7	-

Table 4 : Total phosphorus (%), phytic acid (%), tannin (%) and glucosinolates contents in test ingredients

Ingredients	Total P	Non phytate P	Phytate P	Phytate P %, P	Phytic acid	Tannin	Glucosin -olates (µmole/g)
Sorghum (red)	0.29	0.1	0.19	65	0.67	1.86	-
Sorghum (yellow)	0.23	0.08	0.15	65	0.53	0.57	-
Sorghum (white)	0.30	0.09	0.21	70	0.74	0.32	-
Pearl millet	0.31	0.08	0.23	74	0.82	-	-
Groundnut meal	0.62	0.15	0.47	76	1.66	-	-
Soybean meal	0.90	0.34	0.56	62	1.98	-	-
Sunflower seed meal	0.89	0.45	0.44	49	1.56	-	-
Rapeseed meal (solv.ext.)	1.29	0.56	0.73	57	2.58	-	105±4.3
Maize	0.39	0.14	0.25	64	0.89	-	-
Rice bran (solv.ext.)	0.58	0.10	0.48	83	1.70	-	-

Phytic acid content was calculated by assuming that it contains 28.2% P.

Feed Processing

Feed manufacturing technology has gone revolutionary changes from hand mixing to a vertical mixer system and ultimately to the fully automatic computer compatible modern feed-manufacturing units. However, all the compounding processes are in operation depending upon the flock size and economic status of the producers. The loss of the nutrients through excreta, microbial load in feed and the cost of the production could be minimized through suitable processing of feed. Many incriminating factors of feed are also destroyed due to processing. The production of crumbles and pellet feeds, especially for broilers, are in increasing trend. Steam pelleting and or extrusion are much more effective to reduce microbial contamination in feedstuffs and in *Salmonella* control. Pelleting also provides scope for utilization of high fibre feed resources. Pelletisation of feed improves their efficiency for growth and egg production and the improvement was progressively greater as the fibre level in the diet increased (Bearse *et al.*, 1952), attributed to increased density of diet (in pellet or crumble in comparison to mash form) and energy utilization.

Optimizing and Updating Nutrient Requirements

Supply of essential nutrients in adequate quantities to poultry is primarily considered to obtain an optimum growth, production and/or reproduction. Energy and protein are two major items of poultry mash that need special consideration as both can bring a continued and increased production of eggs and meat with an entry of improved genetic stock. Application of ideal protein concept and meeting amino acids requirements in terms of digestible in practical feed formulation (Bhanja and Mandal, 2005) may help in utilizing costlier proteinic ingredients and thus in reducing feed cost as feed, if formulated with minimum requirements based on digestible amino acids rather than total, the total amino acids could be adjusted downward by 10% (Waldroup, 2001). Moreover, ideal protein system reduces nitrogen excretion, soil and water pollution and stress to the birds. Remarkable results are being obtained in performance of broilers through manipulations of dietary energy and amino acids especially lysine and methionine. The white meat contained 74.41% moisture, 23.40% protein, 0.80% fat, 1.14% ash, 0.005% calcium and 0.273% phosphorus, while red meat contained 75.26% moisture, 19.11% protein, 4.12% fat, 1.04% ash, 0.005% calcium and 0.186% phosphorus. Breast meat was 21.94% of live body weight and breast meat gain to mass of cut carcass was 29.70%, while leg and thigh meat to live weight was lower at 15.57%, while the leg and thigh meat to cut carcass weight was 21.09% (Alibegovic, *et al.*, 2003). Therefore, the nutritional factors that are influencing breast meat development will also improve quantitative meat yield and nutritive value of meat. Nutritional manipulation may result 2 to 5% more breast yield. Narrower dietary energy to protein ratio, slightly higher methionine, lysine, or formulation of diet based on available amino acids influence the breast yield. Similarly, methionine, linoleic acid and choline, total protein in diet may alter egg size.

In addition "requirements' have generally been established as that level of nutrient that gives maximal response in terms of growth and egg production. It is required to characterize the response to nutrients using criteria other than body weight or feed conversion to allow estimation of economic performance. The nutritional requirements differ due to several factors such as management practices, genetic make up, environmental temperature, metabolic and behavioural characteristics (NRC, 1981). Substantial differences also exist in the estimates of nutritional requirements for chicken and other poultry species of tropical countries from that of temperate climate. Moreover, no set of nutrient recommendations should be accepted as universal. The persons responsible for feed formulation must carefully evaluate local conditions in relation to ingredient variability, quality of ingredients, consistency of feed mixing and delivery system that affect the amount of nutrient that should be present in the diet. Except calcium and phosphorus, less emphasis has been given on requirements and bioavailability of other essential minerals, and also for vitamins of feed origin. The performance of birds employed in nutritional experiments does not always corroborate with the performance of exotic birds under commercial production systems. Therefore the validity of such results under commercial poultry production system some times becomes questionable.

The norms of feeding of diversified poultry species other than chicken like ducks, turkey, guinea fowl, quails etc. need to be explored. Scanty information (Elangovan *et al.*, 2004c, Mandal *et al.*, 2005a) is available on nutritional requirements of native chickens or strains developed for backyard poultry for sustainable low input rural poultry production. Efforts are being made to expand village poultry and organic poultry production. Though, extra care is not required in feeding and nutrition when the birds are being reared under conventional backyard rearing system with very few birds, but for intensified farming even under scavenging/backyard rearing system with sizable number of birds definitely require supplementary feeding to augment their production level. Generally they suffer from availability of less feed rather than the deficiency of micronutrients and have the potentiality to produce more, provided supplementary packages are developed.

The high correlation between broiler body weights in the first 6 days and at 6 to 7 weeks of age gives strong evidence of the importance of a good start to good overall performance in commercial broilers. Early nutrition of chicks appears to play a significant role in poultry production and profitability. *In ovo* supplementation of amino acids (Bhanja and Mandal 2005) and other micronutrients also provides scope for early post-hatch anatomical and functional growth of digestive system, post-hatch body weight and immunity.

Table 5 : Nutrient's requirement of broilers as per cent or unit per kg diet (90% DM) as suggested by NRC (1994) and modified at different energy levels (2900 & 3000 kcal/kg)

		0-3 wk			3-6 wk			6-8 wk	
Energy	**kcal**	**3200**	**3000**	**2900**	**3200**	**3000**	**2900**	**3200**	**3000**
CP	%	23.0	21.56	20.84	20.0	18.75	18.10	18.0	16.9
Lysine	%	1.10	1.03	1.00	1.00	0.94	0.91	0.85	0.80
Methionine	%	0.50	0.47	0.45	0.38	0.36	0.35	0.32	0.30
Threonine	%	0.80	0.75	0.725	0.74	0.70	0.68	0.68	0.64
Calcium	%	1.00	0.94	0.91	0.90	0.84	0.81	0.80	0.75
NPP	%	0.45	0.42	0.41	0.35	0.33	0.32	0.30	0.28
Sodium	%	0.20	0.19	0.18	0.15	0.14	0.14	0.12	0.11
Chloride	%	0.20	0.19	0.18	0.15	0.14	0.14	0.12	0.11
Copper	mg	8.0	7.5	7.25	8.0	7.5	7.3	8.0	7.5
Manganese	mg	60	56	54	60	56	54	60	56
Zinc	mg	40	37.5	36.25	40	38	37	40	37.5
Vitamin A	IU	1500	1400	1360	1500	1400	1350	1500	1410
D_3	ICU	200	190	180	200	190	185	200	188
E	IU	10	9.5	9.0	10	9.5	9.2	10	9.4
Thiamin	mg	1.80	1.70	1.60	1.80	1.70	1.64	1.80	1.69
Riboflavin	mg	3.6	3.37	3.26	3.6	3.38	3.27	3.0	2.8
Pyridoxine	mg	3.5	3.28	3.17	3.5	3.3	3.19	3.0	2.8
Vitamin B_{12}	mg	0.01	0.009	0.009	0.01	0.01	0.01	0.007	0.007
Niacin	mg	35	33	32	30	28	27	25	23.5
Choline	mg	1300	1200	1180	1000	940	910	750	700

* Values of requirements under 3200

Table 6 : The requirements of total and digestible amino acids for broilers (DegussaAG)

		Total amino acid basis			Digestible amino acid basis		
Nutrients	**Unit**	**0-3 wk**	**3-6 wk**	**6-9 wk**	**0-3 wk**	**3-6 wk**	**6-9 wk**
AMEn	Kcal/kg	3150	3200	3250	3150	3200	3250
Protien	%	21.0	20.0	18.0	21.0	20.0	18.0
Lysine	%	1.28	1.22	1.05	1.15	1.08	0.92
Methionine	%	0.56	0.52	0.44	0.52	0.48	0.40
Met +Cys	%	0.96	0.92	0.81	0.84	0.81	0.72
Threonine	%	0.84	0.80	0.72	0.71	0.68	0.60
Tryptophan	%	0.21	0.20	0.18	0.18	0.17	0.16
Arginine	%	1.34	1.28	1.10	1.20	1.14	0.99

Table 7 : Nutrients requirements (% or per kg diet, 90%DM) of starting and growing pullets of white-egg-laying strains as per NRC (1994) or modified on energy basis

Nutrients	Unit	NRC (1994)				NRC (1994), modified			
		0-6 wk	6-12 wk	12-18 wk	18wk - 1st egg	0-6 wk	6-12 wk	12-18 wk	18 wk -1st egg
Energy	kcal	2850	2850	2900	2900	2700	2600	2650	2700
CP	%	18.0	16.0	15.0	17.0	17.0	15.0	14.0	16.0
Lysine	%	0.85	0.60	0.45	0.52	0.81	0.55	0.41	0.48
Methionine	%	0.30	0.25	0.20	0.22	0.28	0.23	0.18	0.2
Threonine	%	0.68	0.57	0.37	0.47	0.65	0.52	0.34	0.44
Linoleic acid	%	1.0	1.0	1.0	1.0	0.95	0.9	0.9	0.93
Calcium	%	0.90	0.80	0.8	2.0	0.85	0.73	0.73	1.86
NPP	%	0.4	0.35	0.30	0.32	0.38	0.32	0.27	0.3
Sodium	%	0.15	0.15	0.15	0.15	0.14	0.14	0.14	0.14
Chloride	%	0.15	0.12	0.12	0.15	0.14	0.11	0.11	0.14
Copper	mg	5.0	4.0	4.0	4.0	4.75	3.65	3.7	3.72
Manganese	mg	60	30	30	30	57	27	27.5	28
Zinc	mg	40	35	35	35	39	32	32	33
Vitamin A	IU	1500	1500	1500	1500	1420	1370	1370	1400
D_3	ICU	200	200	200	200	190	182	185	186
E	IU	10	10	5	10	9.5	9.12	4.6	9.3
Thiamin	mg	1.0	1.0	0.8	0.8	0.95	0.91	0.73	0.75
Riboflavin	mg	3.6	1.8	1.8	2.2	3.4	1.64	1.65	2.05
Pyridoxine	mg	3.0	3.0	3.0	3.0	2.8	2.74	2.75	2.8
Vitamin B_{12}	mg	0.009	0.003	0.003	0.004	0.009	0.003	0.003	0.004
Folic acid	mg	0.55	0.25	0.25	0.25	0.52	0.23	0.23	0.23
Niacin	mg	27.0	11.0	11.0	11.0	26	10	10.05	10.2
Choline	mg	1300	900	500	500	1230	820	460	465

Table 8 : Nutrients requirements (% or unit/kg, 90% DM basis) of starting and growing pullets of brown-egg-laying strains NRC (1994) or modified from NRC (1994)

Nutrients	Unit	Brown-egg-laying strains				Modified levels			
		0-6 wk	6-12 wk	12-18 wk	18wk -1st egg	0-6 wk	6-12 wk	12-18 wk	18wk - 1st egg
Energy	Kcal	2800	2800	2850	2850	2600	2600	2600	2650
CP	%	17.0	15.0	14.0	16.0	15.8	13.9	12.8	14.9
Lysine	%	0.8	0.56	0.42	0.49	0.7	0.5	0.4	0.5
Methionine	%	0.28	0.23	0.19	0.21	0.3	0.2	0.2	0.2

Contd...

Threonine	%	0.64	0.53	0.35	0.44	0.6	0.5	0.3	0.4
Calcium	%	0.90	0.80	0.80	1.80	0.8	0.7	0.7	1.7
NPP	%	0.40	0.35	0.30	0.35	0.4	0.3	0.3	0.3
Sodium	%	0.15	0.15	0.15	0.15	0.1	0.1	0.1	0.1
Chloride	%	0.12	0.11	0.11	0.11	0.1	0.1	0.1	0.1
Copper	mg	5.0	4.0	4.0	4.0	4.6	3.7	3.6	3.7
Iodine	mg	0.33	0.33	0.33	0.33	0.3	0.3	0.3	0.3
Iron	mg	75	56	56	56	69.6	52.0	51.1	52.1
Manganese	mg	56	28	28	28	52.0	26.0	25.5	26.0
Zinc	mg	38	33	33	33	35.3	30.6	30.1	30.7
Vitamin A	IU	1420	1420	1420	1420	1320	1320	1295	1320
D_3	ICU	190	190	190	280	176	176	173	260
E	IU	9.5	4.7	4.7	4.7	8.8	4.4	4.3	4.4
Thiamin	mg	1.0	1.0	0.8	0.8	0.9	0.9	0.7	0.7
Riboflavin	mg	3.4	1.7	1.7	1.7	3.2	1.6	1.6	1.6
Pyridoxine	mg	2.8	2.8	2.8	2.8	2.6	2.6	2.6	2.6
Vitamin B_{12}	mg	0.009	0.003	0.003	0.003	0.003	0.003	0.003	0.003
Niacin	mg	26.0	10.3	10.3	10.3	24.1	9.6	9.4	9.6
Pantothenic acid	mg	9.4	9.4	9.4	9.4	8.7	8.7	8.6	8.7
Choline	mg	1225	850	470	470	1138	789	429	437

Feed Additives and Nutraceuticals

Presently, feed additives have assumed a position of prime importance. Poultry strains employed in well-organized production system are more prone to stressors, infections and diseases, and thus they require better managemental practices and welfare. Besides, attempts are also being made to improve the physical appearance, consistency, nutritive quality, shelf life and texture of diet. Keeping this in view, the use of appropriate feed additive(s) in poultry feeding has become obligatory. Not only profitable production, but also the feed additives have made it possible to provide more eggs and meat that would not be possible without them. The feed additives, administered orally in relatively small amount for improving intrinsic value of the nutrient mix, have been renamed (Rosen, 1996), as micro-feeding stuffs. For convenience sake, those have been classified as nutrients, pro-nutrients, conditioners and prophylactics in order to specify their nature, scientific functions in nutrition science, to improve their public image and to facilitate standardization of terminology and use in international regulations. Another term "nutraceutical products" has also been introduced to define substances produced in a purified or extracted form, and which on administration provide or stimulate production of raw materials required for normal bodily functions. The additives hold great promise in the feeding of poultry includes antibiotics, antioxidants, synthetic micronutrients, enzymes, prebiotics, probiotics, anticoccidials, mould inhibitors, herbal products, etc.

Antibiotic compounds have been employed as feed additive in low concentrations throughout the world for nearly 50 years to promote growth and feed conversion efficiency in broilers and increasing egg production in layers. There are evidences that some antibiotics when used as feed additive help the birds to overcome from low level of infection normally present continuously even at some of the well organized poultry units. The effect of antibiotics is more pronounced when the animals are kept under unhygienic condition and are fed relatively vitamins and/or amino acid imbalance/ deficient diet. However, there has been general awareness that low concentration of antibiotics may favour proliferation of antibiotic resistant microorganisms, which have serious consequences for disease control in humans and animals. The use of antibiotics as feed additives has been banned or efforts are being made to ban in many countries, but the experience has not been always satisfactory, as the disease incidence has been increased resulting much more use of therapeutic antibiotics. The antibiotics are classified as feed antibiotics and therapeutic antibiotics to curb the use of therapeutic antibiotics at sub-therapeutic levels for animal production. Efforts are being made to replace antibiotics through proper nutrition of management that will lead to microbiological control and augmenting gut health allowing for more consistent production responses in the absence of antibiotics. Supplementations of high quality ingredients, whole grain cereals, live microbial additives and fermentable sugars (prebiotics), processing/ sterilization of feeds, acidifiers are some of the alternatives to minimize the use of antibiotics.

The purpose of using probiotics has been primarily to establish normal intestinal flora to prevent or minimize the disturbances caused by enteric pathogens and secondarily to serve the function of antibiotic feed additives because there has been so called public mood against the use of antibiotic feed additives in diet of animals. Probiotics especially the lactobacilli and *Bacillus cereus* are important in the development of immuno-competence against enteric infections. However, the probiotics are not substitute of antibiotics in birds with serious infections but are useful in restoring the normal bacterial population that was otherwise altered due to administration of antibiotics. They are active against a wider range of conditions when multiple - strain preparations are used. The possible mode of action of probiotics has been reviewed (Mandal and Verma, 2000a).

Certain non-digestive feed components (prebiotics) like galacto-oligo-saccharides, fructo-oligo-saccharides, mannan-oligo-saccharides and lactose derivatives have all been tried in chickens, rabbits and other monogastric animals to combat colonization of pathogens (*Salmonella* spp., *Escherichia coli, Vibrio cholera, S. typhimurium, S. enteridis* etc.). Legumes like soybean and oil palm kernel are the most common sources of oligo-saccharides. The effect of prebiotics on performance of broilers and layers are inconsistent (Gujral *et al.*, 2005ab). Addition of mannan-oligosaccharide in conventional maize-soy diet did not influence the growth performance of broilers reared in battery cages, but was helpful in reducing the total viable counts and enteropathogens of intestine and total viable counts of meat samples.

Available reports from the European countries (Bedford 1995) indicated improvement in nutritive value, feed utilization, body weight gain and reduction in excreta volume following the supplementation of poultry diets with microbial non-starch polysaccharidases such as cellulases, pectinases, hemicellulases, arabinoxylanases,and beta glucanases. Autolysis of native phytate phosphorus present in some of the feedstuffs like wheat and wheat bran rich in endogenous phytase activity by water soaking not only hydrolyzed phytate P into inorganic P in a considerable amount but it improved the performance and utilization of phosphorus by the birds (Tyagi *et al.*, 1997). Tyagi *et al.* (1999) found that the supplemental vit. D_3 at 600 ICU/Kg in diets rich in endogenous phytase was optimum for normal blood Ca and P content and also for a proper bone development and mineralization in fast growing broiler chicks. Supplementation of diet with microbial phytase (Sebestian *et al.*, 1998) also tended to increase availability of phytate-bound phosphorus, calcium, zinc, copper, crude protein and amino acids. Such enzymes act by removing or decreasing deleterious incriminating factors, increasing saccharification of non-starch polysaccharides, exposing nutrients to the digestive processes through breaking down cell walls, augmenting host enzymes though exogenous supply. They also decrease manure output and improve health of birds through manipulation of gut ecology. Extensive studies have been conducted in India using commercial feed grade enzymes but responses have rather been inconsistent (Reddy *et al.*, 1999). Improvements in body weight gain and FCE and digestibility of fibre components have been observed in certain experiments but discouraging results have also been reported. Similarly a series of experiments have been conducted in our experimental station (Mandal *et al.*, 2004d, Elangovan *et al.*, 2004ab) employing NSP enzymes in various maize-soya, pearl millet, sorghum, finger millet, mustard cake and un-decorticated sunflower seed meal based diets in broiler chickens and Japanese quails. The preparation was analyzed and found to contain sufficient enzyme activities. The AMEn values of rapeseed meal did not improve on enzyme supplementation. However, AMEn values of sunflower seed meal significantly increased on enzyme supplementation from

6.1 MJ to 6.5 MJ/kg dry matter (Mandal *et al.,* 2004b). There was marginal (about 3 to 3.5%) improvement in growth in pearl millet based diets during starting phase, in finger millet, and in sunflower seed meal based diets during both the phases. However, on repeated trials on maize-soya-deoiled rice bran diets for three times in broiler chickens, twice in Japanese quails and twice in native chickens, enzyme supplementation did not prove beneficial in terms of growth or feed conversion efficiency. The differences in effectiveness of the products could be explained in terms of variations in application rate of the enzyme preparation, its composition in terms of enzyme activities, nature of feed non-starch polysaccharide and their chemical linkages, etc. The enzyme preparations imported from European countries have mainly been formulated for specific non starch polysaccharide (s) present in barley, wheat, rye and some vegetable proteins, as has been claimed accordingly. Moreover, the preparations are not always tested for the activity of different enzymes present in it before use. There are no measures of quality control or regulation regarding their use. Certain feed ingredients also require specific enzyme(s) depending upon proportion of non-starch polysaccharides present in it. However, the ultimate commercial values of enzymes as feed additive will depend upon economical consideration.

Nutrition in Diseases and Immunity

The present strategies towards control of diseases have been a joint approach including vaccination programmes, selective breeding for augmenting disease resistance capacity of birds, improved management to curtail environmental stresses to a minimum level, and nutritional management as the control measure of various infectious diseases through vaccination alone has proved many times ineffective. With the emergence of newer information on nutrition-disease interrelationships, there is scope for devising therapeutic diets suitable for interacting synergistically with infection and diseases and stimulating immuno-responsiveness towards pathogens. As the feeding of poultry is under control, there is ample scope for utilizing the suitable recommendations through dietary manipulation. With the advent of more knowledge (Mandal *et al.,* 2001) on interaction of nutrition with infection, immuno-competence, management of mycotoxins, it is obvious that nutrition may play important role in disease management favouring organic chicken production. There is an interaction between one or more nutrients towards the artificially induced or naturally occurring disease/infection. Nutrients interact with bacterial, viral and protozoal pathogens either synergistically or antagonistically include protein/amino acids and energy/fish oil (Korver *et al.,* 1997); vitamin A (Sijtsma *et al.,* 1989); vitamin D3 (Huff *et al.,* 2000); Vitamin E and selenium (Colnago *et al.,* 1984); vitamin K (Ryley and Hardman

1978); vitamin C (Mckee and Harrison, 1995); iron (Hill and Smith, 1974); zinc and calcium (Khanagwal *et al.*, 2000ab). Dietary composition impacts immune function of the chicken. As research in the area of nutritional immunology has increased, it is becoming apparent that nutrient needs for immunity do not coincide with those for growth or skeletal tissue accretion. Click (1977), in a review reported the development and functions of the chicken's humoral immune system and indicated a limitation in understanding of avian immune system and environmental factors. This led to research in chickens to evaluate the humoral immune system (Click *et al.*, 1981) and cellular immune system (Click *et al.*, 1983) in the presence of a calorie-protein deficiency. Proper functioning of the immune system depends upon the availability of nutrients, the precursors for cell growth and activity. Impaired nutrition is associated with reduced capacity of host to form specific antibodies; decrease in the phagocytic activity; interference with production of non-specific protective substances; reduced non-specific resistance to bacterial toxins; altered tissue integrity; diminished inflammatory response, collagen formation and wound healing, decreased antibody affinity and complement system; and variable endocrine activity. The nutrients which have immuno-modulating effect include protein and energy (Praharaj *et al.*, 1999); methoinine (Swain and Johri, 2000); Vitamin A (Friedman and Sklan, 1997); Vitamin E and Se (Hooda *et al.*, 2005); Vitamin C (Amakya-Anim *et al.*, 2000); sodium (Pimental and Cook, 1987); and trace elements like zinc, iron, copper and manganese (Dardenne, 2002).

About 25% of world's cereals are contaminated with known mycotoxins. Mycotoxins present in poultry feeds cause serious adverse effects on production and health. Feeding of high protein, methionine or cysteine through diet decreased the growth depression effect of aflatoxins. Synthetic antioxidants (butylated hydroxytoluene, ethoxyquine,and ß-naphthoflavone) stimulated detoxification enzyme system in liver. Selenium, a component of glutathione peroxidase, promoted the clearance of toxin by enhancing the formation of water-soluble conjugated form of aflatoxin. Supplementary vitamin C was beneficial in counteracting toxic effects of T_2 toxin in hen but had no beneficial effect on aflatoxins. High fat or fibre containing diets also reduced the toxicity of aflatoxins (Devegowda, 1998). Though the incidence of mycotoxins in conventional materials like maize, ground nut cake etc. is high, alternate feed ingredients are not an exception as considerable proportion of millets and milling by-products were found to contain aflatoxin (Raju *et al.*, 2004b). Feeds contaminated with mycotoxins, if fed to birds, reduce feed intake, weight gain (Raju and Devegowda 2002) and egg production (Rogers *et al.*, 1991).

Quality Poultry Products

Hofman (1994) briefed the meat quality as 'the totality of all properties and characteristics of meat that are important to its nutrient value, acceptability and human health and processing. Nutrition or feeding of birds influences meat qualities in terms of nutritive value, acceptability, human health and processing safe guarding interest of producers, processors and consumers. The role of nutrition in meat quality has recently been reviewed by Mandal (2005). There are growing public concern over consumption of eggs being high in cholesterol (200-300mg) and poultry meat with more of saturated fatty acids and cholesterol. It may be of economical advantage for the producer to market eggs with low cholesterol and meat with low fat. Numerous nutritional factors have been demonstrated to alter cholesterol deposition in egg (Griffin, 1992). Cholesterol content of egg yolk may be altered by about 25% through manipulation of dietary fat/energy and cholesterol (Sutton *et al.*, 1984). Dietary fiber and administration of certain drugs and herbal preparations (Sharma *et al.*, 2005) also reduce yolk cholesterol concentrations but only marginally (5-15%). However, it will be commercially viable only when egg cholesterol is reduced (50%) to a level of 125 to 150 mg/egg. Another approach has been to let the hens lay egg enriched with omega-3 fatty acids (n-3 polyunsaturated fatty acids, docosohexaenoic acid and icosapentaenoic acid). The flaxseed and fish oil are the rich sources of omega-3 fatty acids and are being used to enrich eggs with these acids. The eggs are the good sources of conjugated linoleic acid (CLA), which may further be enriched with this acid. Hens fed with approx.125 mg CLA produced eggs with 18 mg CLA (Jones *et al.*, 2000).

The other major concern of people producing broilers is the excessive accumulation of carcass fat, particularly in the abdominal area. This fat is generally disliked by consumer and represents a waste product to the processor. High-energy excessive diets are frequently blamed for the deposition of fat though increasing the ratio of amino acids to energy in diet reduces fat deposition but increases cost of production (Waldroup, 2001). Supplementation of lysine, glycine, methionine, tryptophan and amino acid mixtures in poultry diets reduced body fat deposition (Takshashi *et al.*, 1994). Increasing total sulphur amino acid content (TSAA) from 0.70% to 0.95% of the diet reduced the abdominal fat content of the carcass from 4.00% to 3.30%. Poultry meat is highly susceptible to oxidation in frozen storage. The stability of the meat has been correlated with the tissue concentration of alpha-tocopherol, the supplemented tissues being more stable in cold store (Lin *et al.*, 1989). For poultry, levels of 7 g alpha tocopherol per kg in muscle are recommended to prolong the keeping quality of meat. The supplementation of broilers diet with higher concentrations of Vitamin E (225 IU) and inorganic selenium

(0.5 mg/kg) during 4 to 7 weeks of age resulted in maximum meat stability up to 3 months of storage at -18°C (Tyagi *et al.*, 2005).

References

Alibegovic-Zeic F., Gagic, A., Piplica, S., Aklovica, F., Residbegovic, E., Kavazovic, A. and Crnkic, C. (2003). *Veterinaria Sarajevo* 52: 137-146.

Amakye-Anim, J., Lin, T.L., Hester, P.Y., Thiagarajan, D., Watkins, B.A. and Wu, C.C. (2000.) *Poul. Sci.,* 79:680–688.

Bearse, G.E., Berg, L.R., Mc Clary, C.F. and Miller, V.L. (1952). *Poul. Sci.,* 31: 907-911.

Bedford M R. (1995). *Anim. Feed Sci. Technol.,* 53: 145-155.

Bhanja, S.K. and Mandal, A.B. (2005). *Asian-Aust. J. Anim. Sci.,* 18: 524-531.

Bhanja S.K., Mandal, A.B. and Goswami, T.K. (2004a). *Indan. J. Poul. Sci.,* 39: 212-218.

Bhanja S.K., Mandal, A.B. and Johri, T. S. (2004b). *Ind. J Poul. Sci.,* 39: 105-111.

Boa-Amponsem K., O'Sullivan N.P., Gross, W.B, Dunnigton, E.A. and Siegel, P. B. (1991). *Poul. Sci.,* 70: 697-701.

Chesson A. (1993). Feed enzyme. *Anim. Feed Sci Technol.,* 45: 65-79.

Chesson A.(1987). Supplementary enzymes to improve the utilization of pig and poultry diets. In: *Recent Advances in Animal Nutrition.* pp. 71-89. (Ed.) W Haresign and D A Cole., Butterworth, London.

Click, B., Day, E.J. and Thompson, D. (1981). *Poul. Sci.,* 60:2494-2500.

Click, B., Taylor, R.L. Jr., Martin, D.E., Watabe, M., Day, E.J. and Thompson, D. (1983). *Poul. Sci.,* 62:1889-1893.

Click B. (1977). *Internat. Rev. Cytol.* 48:345-402.

Colnago, G.L., Jensen, L.S. and Long, P.L. (1984). *Poul. Sci.,* 63: 1136-1140.

Dardenne M. (2002). *European J. Clinical Nutr.,* 3: 20-23.

Deo, C., Elangovan, A.V., Mandal, A.B., Singh, D.P. and Shrivastava, H.P. (2004a). *Indan. J. Anim. Nut.,* 21: 73-76.

Deo, C., Elangovan, A.V., Mandal, A.B., Singh, D.P. and Shrivastava, H.P. (2004b). *Indan. J. Poul. Sci.,* 39: 25-32.

Devegowda, G., Raju, M.V.L.N., Afzali, N. and Swamy, H.V.L N. (1998). *Proceedings of 14th Alltech's Annual Symposium on Biotechnology in the Feed Industry* pp. 241-255.

Elangovan, A.V., Mandal, A.B., Tyagi, K. Pramod, Tyagi, K. Praveen, Toppo, S. and Johri, T.S. (2004a). *J. Appl. Anim. Res.,* 26: 33-38.

Elangovan, A.V., Mandal, A.B., Tyagi, Praveen, K., Tyagi, Pramod K., Toppo, S. and Johri, T.S. (2004b). *J. Sci. Food and Agri.,* 84: 2028-2034.

Elangovan, A.V., Deo, C., Mandal, A.B, Singh, D.P. and Shrivastava, H.P. (2004c). *Indan. J. Poul. Sci.*, 39: 61-65.

Friedman, A. and Sklan, D. (1997). *World's Poul. Sci. J.*, 53: 185-196.

Griffin H D. (1992). *World's P. Sci. J.*, 48: 101-111.

Gujral, D., Shrivastav, A.K., Elangovan, A.V., Mandal, A.B. and Tyagi, Pramod K. (2005a). *Proc. Indan. Poul. Sci. Assoc., p.* 213.

Gujral, D., Shrivastav, A.K., Elangovan, A.V., Mandal, A.B. and Tyagi, Pramod K. (2005b). *Proc. Indan. Poul. Sci. Assoc.*, p. 214.

Hill, R. and Smith, I.M. (1974). In: *Trace element metabolism in Animals.* pp. 641-643. (Ed.) Hoekstra W G, Suttle J W, Ganther H E and Mertz W. Univ. Park Press, Baltimore, Maryland.

Hofman, K. (1994). *Fleischwirtsch International* 2:3-12.

Hooda, S., Tyagi, Praveen, K., Tyagi, Pramod, K. and Sharma, D. (2005). *Indan. J Poul. Sci.*, 40: 33-36.

Huff, G.R., Huff, W.E., Balog, J.M. and Rath, N.C. (2000). *Poul. Sci.*, 79: 672-679.

Jones, S., Ma, D.W.L., Robinson, F.E., Field, C.J. and Clandinin, Thomas M. (2000). *J. Nutr.*, 130: 2002-2005.

Khanagwal, P., Ghosh, J.D. and Mandal, A.B. (2000a). *Indan. J. Anim. Sci., 70:* 519-522.

Khanagwal, P., Mandal, A.B. and Ghosh, J.D. (2000b). *Indan. J. Anim. Sci.,* 70: 89-91.

Korver, D.R., Wakenell, P. and Klasing, K.C. (1997). *Poul. Sci.*, 76: 1355-1363.

Kumar Vinod, Elangovan, A.V. and Mandal, A.B. (2005). *Asia-Austral. J. Anim. Sci.*, 18: 538-544.

Lin, C.F., Gray, J.I., Asghar, A., Buckley, D.J., Booren, A.M. and Flegal, C.J. (1989). *J. Food Sci.*, 54: 1457-1469.

Mandal, A.B. and Verma, S.V.S. (2000a). Use of Microbial feed additives in poultry feeding. In: *Feed Microbiology.* pp. 91-98 (Ed.), Chaudhary LC, Agarwal N, Kamra D N, Agarwal D K. CAS in Animal Nutrition, IVRI, Izatnagar.

Mandal, A.B., Deo, C., Elangovan, A.V., Singh, D.P. and Shrivastava, H.P. (2005a). *Anim. Nutr. Feed Tech.*, 5: 117-124.

Mandal, A.B., Elangovan, A.V. and Verma, S.V.S. (2001). *Anim. Nutr. Feed Technol.*, 1: 19-38.

Mandal, A.B., Pathak, N.N. and Singh, H. (1999). Energy and protein requirements of guinea keets (*Numida meleagris*) as meat bird in a hot-humid climate. *J. Sci. of Food Agri.*, 79: 523-531.

Mandal, A.B., Tyagi, Pramod, K., Tyagi, Praveen, K. and Elangovan, A.V. (2004d). Utilization of nutritious cereals and byproducts of oilseed based cropping systems for poultry production. *NATP Technical Bulletin*, Central Avian Research Institute, Izatnagar.

Mandal, A.B. (2005). Nutritional manipulation for improving poultry meat quality. In: Training manual on Recent advances in poultry and egg processing and quality assessment of poultry products. CARI, Izatnagar pp. 11-14.

Mandal, A.B., Yadav, A.S., Johri, T.S. and Pathak, N.N. (2004b). *Nutrition and disease management of poultry*. International Book Distributing Agency, Charbagh, Lucknow.

Mckee, J.S. and Harrison, P.C. (1995 *Poul. Sci.*, 72: 1772-1785.

NRC (1981). *Effect of environment on nutrient requirements of domestic animals*. pp. 109. National Academy Press, Washington D C.

NRC (1994). *Nutrient requirements of Poultry*. National Academy Press, Washington D C.

Pimental, J.L. and Cook, M.E. (1987). *Poul. Sci.*, 66: 2005-2010.

Praharaj, N.K., Reddy, M.R., Rama, Rao, S.V., Shyam, Sunder. G. and Reddy, B.L.N. (1999). *Archiv fur Geflugelkunde* 63: 1-8.

Raju, M.V.L.N. and Devegowda, G. (2002). *Asian-Austral. J. Anim. Sci.*, 15: 1051-1056.

Raju, M.V.L.N Gowda, N.K.S., Sapcota, D. and Saxena, N. (2004b). Report submitted to AED (RF).

Reddy, V.R., Rao, S.V., Rao, P.V.N., Rao ,M. H. and Reddy, V.R. (1999). Enzymes in Poultry Nutrition – Current Approach. Proceedings *of the IX Animal Nutrition Conferenc*. pp 32-36.

Rogers, S.R., Pesti, G.M. and Wyatt, R.D. (1991). *Poul. Sci.*, 70: 307-312.

Rosen, G.D. (1996). *World's Poul. Sci. J.*, 52: 53-57.

Ryley, J. F. and Hardman, L. (1978). *Parasitol.*, 76: 11-20.

Sebestian, S., Touchburn S.P. and Chavez, E.R. (1998). *Poul. Sc. J.*, 54: 27- 45

Sharma, R.K., Elangovan, A.V., Mandal, A.B. and Shrivastav, A.K. (2005). *Proceed.s of the Indan. Poul. Sci. Association* p. 75.

Sijtsma, S.R., West, C.E., Rombout, J.H.W.M. and Van der Zijpp, A.J. (1989). *J. of Nutri.*, 119: 932-937.

Sutton, C. C., Muir, W.M. and Mitchell, G E. (1984). *Poul. Sci.*, 63: 972-980.

Swain, B.K. and Johri, T.S. (2000). *Brit. Poul. Sci.*, 41:83-88.

Takahashi, K., Konashi, S., Akiba, Y. and Horiguchi, M. (1994). *Anim. Feed Sci. and Tech.*, 65: 244-250.

Tyagi, K. Pramod, Mandal, A.B., Elangovan, A.V., Tyagi, K. Praveen, Johri, A. and Kaur, S. (2004b). *Anim. Nutri. and Feed Technol.*, 4: 153-160.

Tyagi, K. Pramod, Mandal, A.B., Elangovan, A.V., Tyagi, K., Praveen, Johri, A. and Kaur, S. (2004a). *Indan. J. Poul. Sci.*, 39: 131-135.

Tyagi, K. Praveen, Tyagi, K. Pramod, Singh, R.P, Elangovan, A.V. and Mandal, A. B. (2005). *Anim. Nutr. Feed Technol.*, 5: 53-60.

Tyagi, Pramod, K., Verma, S.V.S., Tyagi, Praveen, K. and Singh, K.B. (1999). Efficacy of dietary endogenous and microbial phytase supplemented with or without 1-25 dihydroxycholecalciferol on the performance of broiler chicks. *Proceedings of XIX Conference and Symposium of Indian Poultry Science Association* p. 99.

Waldroup, P.W. (2001). *Feedstuffs,* 73: 56-65.

□□□

Animal Nutrition, 2012
eds. Dr. (Mrs.) Usha R. Mehra et al., pp. 279-287
Satish Serial Publishing House e-mail : info@satishserial.com; website : www.satishserial.com

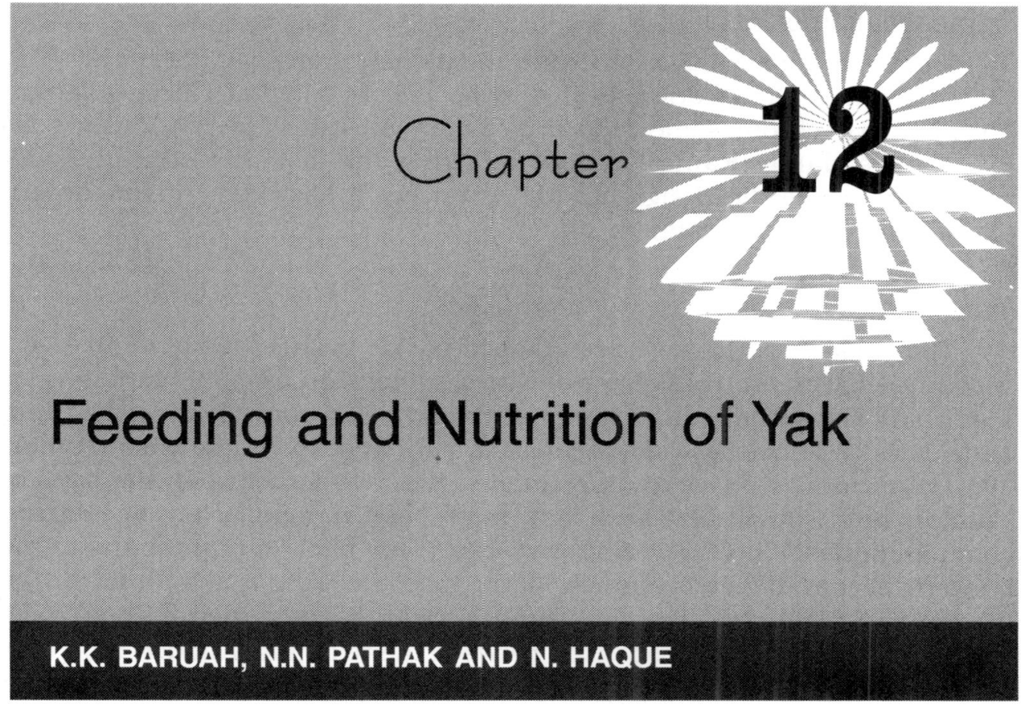

Chapter 12

Feeding and Nutrition of Yak

K.K. BARUAH, N.N. PATHAK AND N. HAQUE

The yak is one of the important gift of God for the service of mankind. The yak (*Poephagus grunniens* or *Bos grunniens*) belong to the order Artiodactyla, family Bovidae, sub family *Bovine* genus *Bos* and species *grunniens* and *mutus*. Yaks are multipurpose ruminant animals adapted for living at high altitudes above 3000 metre mean sea level (MSL). Yak (*Bos grunniens*) was domesticated from the wild yak (*Bos mutus*) which is still found in remote mountain of Quinghai–Tibet plateau as well as neighbouring regions. The yak is found at very high altitude of Himalayas viz. Tibetan plateau and entire Indian territory extending from north-west frontier area (NWFA) to north-east frontier area (NEFA), western China, Pakistan, Northern Afghanistan, Bhutan, Mangolia, Nepal and Soviet Union. Yaks are highly valued by Himalayan peoples because of its contribution to human economics as meat, milk, wool, leather, dung, and as pack animal. Of the 14.2 millions domesticated yaks in the world about 13.3 millions are found in China whereas of the sixty five thousand population of yak in India 9, 2, 47, and 7 thousand are found in Arunachal Pradesh, Himachal Pradesh, Jammu and Kashmir (Ladakh region) and Sikkim, respectively (Annon, 2003). Moreover, a small population of domesticated yaks are also found in Uttarakhand beyond Badrinath and Kedarnath along the Tibet border (Pathak, 2009).

Domestication of Yak

The yaks were domesticated during late new stone age (2008-2300 BC). They are believed to be domesticated by people of Quinghai-Tibetan-Plateau. The number of chromosomes in yaks is similar with cattle (2n=60). This species is inter-breedable (Ramesha, 2008). During the last three decades yak population has declined significantly and hence it has been a great concern to the rearers and its planners.

Types of yak in India

The yaks of world have been named on the basis of their country viz., Indian yaks, Chinese yaks, Nepalese yaks, Mongolian yaks, Bhutanese yaks, Pamir and Caucasian yaks. However, Indian yaks were distinguished into Ladakh yaks, Himachal yaks, Arunachal yaks and Sikkimese yaks (Pathak, 1994). Sikkimese yaks were differentiated into two varieties on the basis of their location in Sikkim and they have been named after the rearing communities as "Bho" and 'Aho' varieties. The 'Bho' yaks are found in the western part and they are much larger than the 'Aho' yaks found in the eastern part of Sikkim. The two varieties could maintain their original traits due to natural barrier of a hot zone between the two hills (Khera *et al.*, 1978). Indian yaks have been categorized into five types on the basis of their morphological traits viz., common type, Bisonian type, Bareback, white and Hairy forehead (Pal, 2004). Probably bareback condition might be due to deficiency of trace minerals in that region.

Purpose of Yak Rearing

The following purposes have been considered for the domestication of yaks by the nomadic communities inhabiting high altitudes of Pamirs, Tibetan plateau and Himalaya. (Baruah and Pathak, 2009).

- Production of high energy-high protein milk for human consumption.
- Production of edible flesh of high quality protein and fat.
- Capability of utilizing scanty herbages for food production at high altitudes.
- Regular supply of dung for fuel at places where it was very difficult to obtain fire wood.
- Supply of long and coarse hairs for preparing ropes and carpets and utilization of soft under coat for the manufacture of fabrics for warm cloths.
- Availability of hides for the preparation of tents, shoes and other goods for domestic uses.

- Heavy horns are used for the manufacture of milking pails and other articles. Now a days variety of decoration articles are made from the horn.
- There was a great demand of bushy tail in olden days. Stalked on wooden handle mounted with carved silver cover the chawar of yak tail is used in temples and royal families and also at important ceremonies in many countries like India, Bhutan, Nepal, Tibet, Turkey, China and Mongolia.
- One of the most important purpose of yak domestication is the production of useful hybrids of yak with cattle and mithun. Hybrids produce more milk, fat and flesh and the males are also better draught animals (Ivanova and ljubimov, 1951; Sharma, 1954; Schulthess, 1967).

Feeding Behaviour

Very little is known about the feeding of yaks. In early summer when the pasture is covered with lush growing long grasses, tongue is more actively utilized for ingestion whereas on pasture of short grasses, lips and incisor teeth are active. However, during the winter season when the pasture is covered with thick layer of snow, yaks mostly use hoof, horn, head and muzzle for digging the snow layers, to access the wilted vegetation. Probably this is helped by sensitively developed olfactory organs. In one of the observations it has been reported that the grass with height of 15 cm is reduced to 2.6 - 5.2 cm by grazing (Wiener *et al.*, 2003). During scarcity period the yaks continue to consume even stems and leaves from the residual wilted grasses available in spring season. Yak can graze very close to the surface of alpine meadow. This grazing is possible due to anatomical peculiarities in muzzle and lips, which help them in prehension. Strong and sharp edge incisor teeth help in intake of coarse roughage during cold season.

Factors Affecting the Grazing Behaviour

There are several factors which affect the grazing behaviour. (Baruah and Pathak, 2009).

Herbage Cover and Season

During hot and humid season when lush growing pasture is available they spend relatively less time to satisfy their appetite whereas in winter they are required to spend much more time in search of feed. Therefore, the energy spent is higher in comparison to hot season.

Grazing Time

The grazing time normally varies from 34 to 80 per cent of the total time available for grazing. The remaining time is spent in walking, resting, drinking and mastication.

Growing and Lactating Yaks

Lactating and growing yaks spend more time in grazing due to their higher nutritional demands for supporting their active productive function. However lactating animals with calves on foot are frequently disturbed due to suckling by young calves.

Climate Change

During snowfall and hail storms yaks run over the pasture at a very high speed (about 3400 m/hour).

Herd Density

The number of yaks per unit of land influences the grazing time due to competition for biomass. As the number of yak increases grazing time increases.

Aggressiveness of Animals

Aggressive animals do not allow other to graze in their surroundings.

Feed Resources

During winter in Ladakh region it is a common practice of feeding 'oal' a variety of Lucerne hay as a supplementary feed for vulnerable group of young calves, pregnant animal and lactating cows.

Nutrition of Yak

The yaks receive their nutritional supply through grazing on alpine pastures and other harbages of high altitudes. In yak breeding zones of Arunachal Pradesh and Sikkim, yaks feed on different natural harbeges of the region for the nutritional supply. Proximate composition of some of the harbages (Table 1) indicates satisfactory nutrient density. In Arunachal Pradesh the yaks are grazed in defined restricted area due to restriction imposed on the movement of yaks by different tribal clans. Besides, small patches of herbages scattered on the stiff hilly region are used for the grazing of yaks. In winter months, yak herders stay in the village and graze the yaks on adjoining pasture lands. Overgrazing has resulted in the deterioration of pasture land to a great extent. Yak also consumes tender branches of shrubs. They generally avoid poisonous or thorny plants. But during lean period due to acute shortage of green they graze on poisonous weeds and suffer from poisoning. New born calves follow their dams during pasture grazing, but separated from their dams during night and stormy weather, and provided protection in tents (Singh, 1987). Supplemental feeding is given only to the yak cow. In India, yaks loose 25-30% of their body weight during winter due to inadequate fodder (Pal, 2004). Similar winter loss in the body weight of Chinese yaks has been reported and it was 15.8 to 26 per cent of the body weight in steers of 1-4 years of age, when the grazing was not supplemented by stall feeding (Rong-Chang, 1985).

Performance of Yak

Inspite of inadequate fodder resources a high growth rate is obtained through grazing on pasture during the summer season in different regions of yak breeding tract. The calves of Pamir yaks born at the high altitudes at 2500-3700 m above the sea level averaged 135 kg at 6 months of age, which was equivalent to about 667 g daily gain in body weight (Mochalovskii and Adbusalamov, 1973). In the yak calves of Kirgiz regions, daily gain in body weight ranged from 370-427 g (Abdykerimov and Denisov, 1970). In Arunachal yaks a growth rate of 450 g per day with feed conversion ratio of 8.58 has been reported (Saikia, *et al.*, 2009).

The total lactation yield at organized farm (NRCY) ranged from 254.73 to 888.43 kg (461.27 ± 42.53) in a lactation length ranging from 280 to 480 days. However, in migratory system the lactation length is shorter (150 to 240 days) and milk yield ranged from 180 to 315 kg per lactation. The average daily milk yield in yak cows in Nepal, China and India ranged from 1.0 to 1.64 L (Jest, 1976; Zhenkang and Tianshui, 1980; Jain and Yadav, 1985). But average milk yield in yak cows in Pamir was 2.5 L (Dor, 1976). Yak milk contains water (81.85%), protein (5.94%), fat (7.5%), total solids (17.93%) and solid not fat (11.50%). The milk is slightly acidic. The meat samples from shoulder region was analysed and found to contain water 68%, protein 20%, fat 7%, ash 5.1%, calcium 1.28% and phosphorus 1.08%. The nutrient composition of yak meat is comparable well with meat of other species, but high in fat content. The yak meat is tender and had greater proportion of interstitial fat. The flesh fibres are finer than those of beef and resembles mutton fibres.

Rate of Passage

The rate of passage of ingesta through the gastro-intestinal tract of yaks is much slower in comparison to cattle. Average retention time of feeds in the gastro-intestinal tract of yaks is about 78 hours. It is similar to 79 hours in the bison but 9-13 hours more than in cattle on the some feeding regimen. Longer retention time of feeds in the gastrointestinal tract of the yaks is a very important factor in the utilization of nutrients of the feeds. This provides more opportunity for the action of the digestive microbial enzymes of the gut and longer time for the absorption of the digested nutrients. This is also advantageous for the more efficient utilization of dietary nitrogen available as non-protein nitrogen through recycling (Schaffer *et al.*, 1978). Under natural feeding on pastures it may be possible that the feed retention time is further increased due to less availability and fibrous nature of the herbages.

Water Requirement

Perhaps quantitative estimate is not available for the water requirement of yaks for drinking. However, yaks like to drink running water and satisfy their thirst by eating snow in the winter. In bright summer days they like to take bath in streams for several hours.

Protein Requirement

Scanty informations are available about the protein requirement of yaks. Saikia *et al.* (2007) reported that protein requirement of yaks was 75 per cent of Kearl (1982) requirement of growing cattle for 500 g daily body weight gain. The average daily gain of 401 ± 0.02 g and FCE of 9.70 ± 1.56 have been recorded. In another study rumen degradable crude protein requirement for maintenance in growing yak was found to be around 6.09 g per kg metabolic body weight (Wiener *et al.*, 2003).

Energy Requirement

Very little information is available about the energy requirement. The metabolizable energy requirement for maintenance (MEm) in growing yak was found to be 460 kJ per kg metabolic body weight per day (Wiener *et al.*, 2003).

Mineral Requirement

No information is available about the mineral requirement of yak but there is a possibility of mineral deficiency due to non-availability of feed during winter months and also leaching during summer in draining water of melted snow.

Carotene Utilization

The conversion of carotenes into vitamin A activity is less efficient in yaks as in cattle. It is evident from the high yellow pigmentation of butter fat in the yak milk.

Table 1 : Proximate composition of some top feed of high altitude for yak.

Name of forage	Crude protein	Ether extract	Crude fibre	Total ash
Barhar (*Artocarpus lakoocha*) (T)	13.74	1.70	27.58	12.72
Dudhilo (*Ficus nemoralis*) (T)	9.98	1.06	16.68	11.20
Gineri (*Premna mucronata*) (T)	16.01	1.64	32.40	8.98
Kabra (*Ficus infectoria*) (T)	14.89	2.68	49.84	8.76
Kamli (*Bohmeria macrophylla*) (T)	16.54	1.36	36.82	14.96
Bat (*Ficus bengalensis*) (T)	11.90	2.16	40.66	11.12
Chiple (*Reevesia pubescens*) (T)	19.43	2.64	44.50	14.71
Khasre (*Ficus hirta*) (T)	16.80	1.22	21.86	16.60
Katush (*Castonopsis tribuloides*) (T)	11.83	3.14	43.90	6.22
Gayo (*Bridelia retusa*) (T)	11.99	1.02	24.00	10.47
Jhingani (*Eurya japonica*) (T)	9.66	4.92	17.36	6.06
Lali (*Ampora wallichi*) (T)	11.57	1.66	18.98	7.23
Pipli (*Exbucklandia populnea*) (T)	6.81	1.74	20.20	7.83
Melato (*Macranga nepalensis*) (T)	16.75	2.88	14.74	5.00
Lutekhanyum (*Ficus elevata*) (T)	17.69	1.04	28.24	14.34
Sirish (*Aldizia lebbek*) (T)	14.74	0.74	40.74	6.58
Rubber (*Ficus elastica*)	7.44	2.46	30.02	10.10
Tanki (*Bauhinia purpurea*) (T)	16.15	3.28	36.76	9.70
Nik-Narre (*Orechnide integrifolia*) (T)	16.40	3.46	21.30	5.60
Yaal (*Trema orientalis*) (T)	10.60	1.39	25.60	6.20
Haara (*Macrenga denticulata*) (T)	13.90	3.69	21.30	5.60
Sechoninch (*Sauruia roxberghii*) (T)	11.20	2.30	23.50	4.00
Tokku (*Ficus elmerii*) (T)	9.60	2.05	26.90	9.70
Taao (*Ficus roxberghii*) (T)	15.50	1.10	25.7	9.10
Poprarr (*Rhyngopticum ellipticum*) (T)	14.75	1.30	21.60	12.50
Khussu (*Ficus glomerata*) (T)	16.30	2.80	17.30	17.50
Kuchin (*Ficus variolosa*) (T)	17.40	1.80	17.25	16.20
Dayy-Dassa (*Osbekia neplansis*) (S)	13.90	2.03	18.12	13.05
Rubdi/Rubdikk (*Phegopteris auritica*) (S)	9.90	1.30	17.20	10.30
Kullu/Kullung (Kol/Jungle banana) (*Musa paradiasica*) (H)	6.60	0.70	22.30	10.60

Contd...

Thazza (*Thysoleuna maxima*) (H)	6.40	2.30	22.50	12.40
Aay/Aaing (*Dendrocalamus hamiltonii*) (H)	12.40	1.30	26.30	14.30
Missir (*Carex crusiata*) (H)	8.30	1.49	21.30	19.60
Riem Terr (*Peuraruia* sps.) (C)	11.80	3.02	27.02	16.20
Reich (*Terr enthada porseatha*) (C)	16.40	3.50	21.50	20.40
Blemkar (*Buddlija asitica*) (T)	14.00	0.66		
Domkar (*Symplocus racemosa*) (T)	11.03	1.86		
Salyx (*Salyx humboldtiana*) (T)	14.45	2.34		
Sylulii (*Acer campbellii*) (T)	15.05	1.54		
Maar (*Costanpsis* spp.) (T)	11.90	1.04		

T= Tree fodder , S= Shrub, H= Herb, C= Creeper
Source: Annual Report NRC on Yak (01-02, 04-05)
Heli, *et al.*, (2009). Indian J. Anim Sci.79 (1): 87-88

Salt Feeding

Yaks have great craving for salt. This habit has been used to attract the animal and they return from the pasture to obtain their salt on the fixed day and time. Salt is fed at weekly or fortnightly intervals.

Strategic Supplementation

Since adequate informations are not yet available on different aspects of nutrition, it may be advantageous to provide some supplements of proteinous feeds and complex mineral mixture to take care of deficiency, if any.

References

Abdykerimov, A.A. and Denisov, V.F. (1970). *Trudy kirgiz sel, khoz. Inst. Ser. Zoovet.*, 15(3): 115-118.

Anon (2003). 17th livestock census Report, Ministry of Agriculture, Govt. of India, New Delhi.

Annual Report, 01-02. NRC on Yak, ICAR, Dirang, Arunachal Pradesh.

Annual Report, 04-05 NRC on Yak, ICAR, Dirang, Arunachal Pradesh.

Baruah, K.K. and Pathak, N.N. (2009). Proc. International Conference on Yak Husbandry challenges and strategies, 20-22 April, 2009 at NRC on Yak, Dirang, A.P.

Dor, R. (1976). The yak in the Pamir.In Ethnozootechnie, 5:126-132.

Heli, T. Thakuria, Sarma, D.N., Mili, D.C. and Baruah, K.K. (2009). *Ind. J. Anim. Sci.* 79 :87-88.

Ivanova, V.V. and Ljubimov, I.M. (1951). *Sovetsk. Zootek*, 3: 26-37.

Jain, Y.C. and Yadav, R.S. (1985). *Ind J. Anim. Sci.*, 55: 223-224.

Jest, C. (1976). Yak breeding in the Nepalese Himalayas. Ethnozootechnie, 15:78-90.

Khera, R.C., Paljor, S., Goley, M.M., Katiyar, R.D., Sharma, P.P. and Jawa, A.K. (1978). Animal production in Sikkim. Dept. of Animal Husbandry, Govt. of Sikkim. Gangtok.

Kearl, L.C. (1982).Nutrient Requirement of ruminants in taluniv.Logan.developing countries.Int.Feedstuff Utah Agr.Exp.Sta.Utah.Staluniv, Logan.

Mc.Dowell, R.E. (1986). Feed source/Animal interactions as production determinants. Farm Animals, 1:1.

Mochalovskii, A. and Abdusalamov, Sh. (1973). Molochnos i Myasnoe skot. No. 8:21.

Pal, R.N. (2004). Yak husbandry in India: A perspective. Pashudhan.Vol. 19 (10): 1

Pathak, N.N. (1994). An Introduction to yak husbandry, Pub. No. 26, IVRI, Izatnagar.

Pathak, N.N. (2009). Personal communication.

Ramesha, K.P. (2008). NRC on yak, Dirang Arunachal Pradesh

Rong-Chang. Z. (1985). *World Anim. Rev.*, 54: 24-29.

Saikia, A. and Baruah, K.K. (1987). Indo-vision Pvt. Ltd., Gaziabad.

Saikia, P.K., Saikia, B.N., Ghosh, M.K., Baruah, K.K., Chakravarty, P. and Bhattacharya, M. (2007). Proc. VI Biennial Conf. of Animal Nutrition Assoc. Jammu, 15-17 Sept., 2006.

Schaffer, A.L., Young, B.A. and Chimwano, A.M. (1978). *Canad. J. Zool.*, 56: 2355-2358.

Sharma, G.P. (1954). *Indian farming*, 3 (II): 24-26.

Shculthess, W. (1967). *World Rev. Anim. Prod.*, 3 (13): 88-97.

Singh, U.B. (1987). *Ind. Vet. Med. J.*, 11:125-127.

Wiener, G., Jianlin, H. and Ruijun, L. (2003). The yak. 2nd ed. Pub., FAO, Bangkok, Thailand.

Zhenkang, Han and Tianshui, Lu, (1980). *J. Nanjink Agril. Coll.* No. 1: 137-146.

□□□

Animal Nutrition, 2012
eds. Dr. (Mrs.) Usha R. Mehra et al., pp. 289-304
Satish Serial Publishing House e-mail : info@satishserial.com; website : www.satishserial.com

Feeding and Nutrition of Mithun

N. HAQUE, SAROJ TOPPO, H. RAHMAN AND K.K. BARUAH

Mithun (*Bos bobis frontalis*) is domesticated from wild gaur and found mainly in the Northeastern Hill Region of India. It is also found in Bhutan, China, Myanmar and Bangladesh (Simoons, 1984). Mithun belongs to the order Artiodactyla, Sub-order Rumentia, family Bovidae and tribe Bovinae. Bohlken (1958) classified Bovinae in three groups *viz.*, Bovina (cattle), Bubalina (Asian buffaloes) and Syncerina (African buffaloes). Bovinae is further classified into four genera viz., *Bison*, *Bos*, *Bibos* and *Poephagus*. However, many authors consider *Bos* as a genus and *Bibos* and *Poephagus* as subgenus of *Bos*. Mithun comes under subgenus Bibos. The other members of this sub - genus is Indian gaur (*Bos bibos gaurus*), Malayan gaur (*Bibos gaurus sondaicus*), banteng (*Bibos banteng*) and kouprey (*Bibos sauveli*).

Mithun is reared in semi-wild state under free-range condition at various altitudes between 300 to 3000 m asl without resorting any scientific feeding programmes. The animal is used as a sacrificial animal by the tribal communities in the NEH Region and other adjoining countries. It yields leanest meat among all the bovine species. Mithun is an underutilized resource and its production potential has not yet been ascertained through scientific feeding, breeding and management practices. Basic information is largely lacking and only a little information is available on its feeding habit, feed intake, growth rate and nutrient utilization.

Types of Mithun

In India, two types of mithuns are found namely Nagami and Arunachali (Verma, 1996). They are distinguished based on their body conformation, shape of the forehead, body weight, coat colour, hair pattern, *etc.*

Nagami

Nagami mithun found in Nagaland and Manipur, are large in size and body weight of adult animal varies from 400 to 500 kg. Animals are mostly used for meat purpose, sacrificed during religious ceremonies. However, in Manipur it is also used as milch animal.

Arunachali

Arunachali mithun has been classified into 3 groups, namely Aka, Nishi and Adi depending on their coat colour, body size and conformation. Nomenclature has been made based on the tribes owning them (Gupta *et al.*, 1999). There are several micro-agro-climatic zones in the state of Arunachal Pradesh where environmental conditions are highly variable. Moreover, exceptionally rough and rugged terrains make this hill-state a most difficult one for communication and transport. Due to these reasons mithun populations have been bred in isolated geographical boundaries and in different environmental conditions for centuries, with no record of mixing together. This resulted with wide variation in horn pattern, body conformation and size, colour pattern and production traits from one population to other (Verma, 1996; Arora, 1998).

Aka Mithun

These mithuns are reared in the East Kameng district by the Aka tribe. Similar type of mithun is also reared by Monpa and Shredukpen tribes of West Kameng and lower ranges of Twang district. Piebaldness and different colour types are observed in this class of Mithun.

Nishi Mithun

Mithuns available in the Upper Subansiri, Lower Subansiri and Papum Pare districts mainly owned by Nishi (Dafla) tribe are called Nishi mithun. These are also reared by Apa Tani and Hill Miri over this region, however, smaller in number. Nishi mithuns are white in colour with black or brown patches or vice versa. The size of Nishi mithun is larger than Aka type but with loose body conformation.

Adi Mithun

These mithun are of uniform colour, either black or brown with white stockings on legs. This might have been resulted due to intensive selection of the animals for sacrificial purpose by the Adi tribes of Upper, East and West Siang districts. These animals are smaller in size than Aka and Nishi type of mithuns.

On a very broad term, mithuns are also classified as Nagamese, Arunachal, Manipur and Mizoram type. The average birth weight of mithun calf is 18.88 ± 2.67 kg and at maturity (at 20 months of age) is 310.45 ± 54.60 kg as reported in the farms of National Research Centre on Mithun, Medziphema, Nagaland. The Arunachal strain is having highest body weight at maturity (20 months of age) followed by Nagaland, Mizoram and Manipur strains. The heritability estimate of maturity weight is 0.11 ± 0.23, indicates that it is dependent much on feeding and management rather than genetic factors (Annual Report, 2007-08). Average birth weight of male calves in the Regional Hill Cattle Breeding Farm at Sagali, Arunachal Pradesh varies from 17.5 to 19.5 kg and in female 16.5 to 18.5 kg (Heli, 1997). However, it is also reported to be varied between 20 to 25 kg which is nearly 5.5 to 6 per cent of dam's weight (Gupta *et al.*, 1999).

Milking of mithun is not very common, but in recent years nutritional importance of milk has been recognized and milking started. Mithun milk contains 5 to 8 per cent fat, 0.8 per cent ash, 4 to 5 per cent lactose and 3.5 to 4 per cent protein. Milk yield ranges from 2 to 6 kg daily and lactation period lasts for 6 to 8 months and nursing of calves may continue after 6 months also (Baruah *et al.*, 1980, Pathak and Baruah, 1980). Arunachal strain shows better status for different milk production traits than the other genetic groups of mithun. It has the lactation length of 286.33 ± 13.38 days with average milk yield 1432.00 ± 128.88 g. Nagamese mithun has the lactation length of 175.33±38.88 days with average milk production 921.50 ± 105.23 g per animal per day (Bhusan *et al.*, 2005). Though average milk production in mithun is low, it is of superior quality with high fat content (8 to 13%). In Bhutan, mithun has been used for crossing with Siri cattle. The hybrid males (Bjatsha) produced are ideal for ploughing and hybrid females (Bjatsham) yield better milk with high fat content than native Siri cow.

The wide variation in the characteristics of Mithun might be due to their distribution over a large geographical area and bred in isolated condition for many centuries. It provides an opportunity for selection of mithun correlating their genotypic, phenotypic and economic traits. Few attempts have already been made to differentiate mithun populations available in different pockets throughout the NEH Region (Annual Report, 1992-93; Gupta *et al.*, 1999).

Natural Habitats

Mithuns prefer areas with mild environmental temperature, high rainfall and medium humidity. The highest density of mithun is observed in East Siang, East Kameng and parts of lower Subansiri districts where average rainfall is between 3310 and 4724 mm along with high humidity (Verma, 1990). However, there are some areas in Arunachal Pradesh where rainfall is even on higher side but mithun population is much less. It might be due to higher level of humidity and also high temperature in the zones (Gupta *et al.*, 1999). On the other hand, areas with low environmental temperature coupled with low rainfall is also not suitable for mithun as has been evidenced in Twang and Dirang Dzong areas of the West Kameng district where mithun population density is only $0.7/km^2$.

Mild temperature with high rainfall and medium humidity in evergreen forest areas are suitable for growth of trees with broad leaf which constituted one of the major components of fodder sources for mithun. However, in the areas where environmental temperature as well as rainfall are comparatively lower along with the increase in elevation evergreen forests are replaced by alpine and sub-alpine meadows which are suitable for sheep, yak and goats. High rainfall along with high environmental temperature and humidity favours for development of evergreen tropical vegetation. However, such areas are also not preferred by mithun though suitable fodder for them are abundant. Probably high environmental temperature and humidity during monsoon are not preferred by mithuns.

Mithuns are available as lower elevation as 300 m in Bandarban district (Bawon Zo) in the Chittagang hills in Bangladesh and at higher elevation of 3000 m in Arunachal Pradesh. They are basically shed loving animals. Shed seeking during summer might be attributed to heat stress. It indicated by Larkin (1954) that heat stress in animals might be the effect of both temperature and humidity and their interaction with genotype. So determination of thermo neutral zone and fasting heat production (basal metabolic rate) in different types of mithun might give some insight about their tolerance to heat stress in relation to their colour patterns and distribution.

Feeding behaviour

Though mild temperate zone is preferred by mithun, a small population is also observed in tropical and temperate zones. Mithun habitat areas, especially in the subtropical to mild temperate zones are covered with moist/ rain forests. These forests are rich in wide variety of flora in terms of tall trees in the first tier and tall shrubs, evergreen herbs and vines in the second tier. A variety of grasses are observed on the ground while creepers with broad leaves are wrapped around big trees. Mithuns prefer to browse on leaves and twigs of trees and shrubs and graze on long grasses. Broad-leaf trees like *Ficus hookerii* are in their preference list. Mithun may travel long distance in search of preferred species of forages. When mithuns are offered cut oat fodder and leaves and twigs of *F. hookerii* at a time, they are attracted by *Ficus* leaves and twigs rather than oat fodder. They consume *Ficus* leaves with greater relish. Mithuns follow a routine system of browsing and grazing. They browse along the edges of forests in the morning, go to deeper part as the day progresses and prefer to stay under shade in a sunny day. However, in the afternoon when environment is cool can be seen grazing in the often forest cleanings or in the abandoned jhum (Gupta *et al.*, 1999).

As grazer they are very much selective and prefer certain species of herbage, stages of growth and particular parts of the forage and found to be concentrated in a particular area of forest abundant in particular species of plant.

Studies on the vegetations in the forest of Phek district of Nagaland conducted by National Research Centre on Mithun indicated that 91.58% of grasses, 83.30% of herbs, 70.77% of shrubs and 80.47% of tree leaves out of 107, 18, 79 and 129 numbers of species, respectively were consumed by mithun. Major grass species include *Arundinella sp., Borrena hirticulata, Curculigo secusvata, Cynodon dactylon, Dimeria sp., Imperta cylindrica, Phragmites sp., Setaria palmifolia* and *Thysanolaena agrostis*. The herbs available are *Persiceria nepalensis, Galinsoga perviflora, Artemisia vulgaris, Ageratum conzoides, Crystella parasitica, Eupatorium sp., Polygonium chinensis, Jasminum sp., etc*. These grasses and herbs are rarely available in pure stand in sizable area. In composite form, percentage of species available as well as their chemical composition varies with seasonal changes. The predominant species available during monsoon are *Setaria palmifolia, Cynodon dactylon, Thysanolaena agrostis, Artemisia vulgaris, Persicaria nepalensis, Galinsogo perviflora, Ageratum conzoides, Crytella parasitica* and *Heydyatis scandens*. The predominant species available during winter are *Thysanolaena agrostis, Setaria palmifolia, Eupatorium sp., Ageratum conzoides* and *Crystella parasitica*. Majority of the mentioned species are available through out the NEH region (Balaraman and Goley, 1991 and Heli, 1996).

Common fodder trees available through out the NEH Region and majority of which consumed by mithun are: *Acer laevigatum, Adenosacme longifolia, Albizzia sp., Alnus nepalensis, Amoera wallichii, Arotocarpus lakoocha, Bauhinia purpurea, Bauhinia variegata, Brassiopsis mitis, Bridelia retusa, Dacynia indica, Debrogesia longifolia, Desmos longiflorus, Emblica officinealis, Exbucklandia populnea, Celtis tetrandra, Erytharia stricta, Eurya accumenata, Ficus bengalensis, Ficus benjaminia, Ficus cunia, Ficus dalhousiae, Ficus elevate, Ficus elmeri, Ficus hookerii, Ficus hirata, Ficus hispada, Ficus infectoria, Ficus nemoralis, Ficus religiosa,*

Goruga pinnata, Grevia elastica, Gmelina arborea, Lagerstroemia speciosa, Leea indica, Litsea citrada, Litsea polyantha, Macranga denticulata, Meliosma pinnata, Morinda angustifolia, Morus alba, Morus levigata, Mussanda roxburghii, Orecocnide integrifolia, Oroxylum indicum, Prunus ceresoides, Prunus persica, Polyanthus sp., Rhaphidosphora sp, Sabia sp, Saraina panduana, Saurauia nepalensis, Scheffelera sp., Spondius pinnata, Stereosper tetragonium, Syzyjium sp., Terminalia bellerica, *Trevesia sp.* and *Turpinia nepalensis*. Important shrubs which are of choice of mithun are *Amomum sp., Borrena hirticulata, Callicarpa vestita, Chlerondendron sp., Dendrocalamus sp., Hibiscus chinensis, Hibiscus subdereffa, Osbekia nepalensis, Polygonum chinensis, Pouzolzia sp., Quix sp., Sarcochlamys pulcherrima, Solanum nigrum, Stereospermum chelonoedes, Urtica sp., etc.* Generally preferred grasses are *Alloteropsis semialata, Arundinella sp., Axonopus compressus, Avena sativa, Borrena hirticulata, Carex cryciata, Commelina bengalensis, Curculigo secusvata, Cynodon dactylon, Dimeria sp., Imperta cylindrica, Oplismenus compositus, Phragmites sp., Pogonetherum crinitum, Schizostachyum sp., Setaria palmifolia* and *Thysanolaena agrostis* and creepers are *Alternanthera sesiles, Cissus assamina, Jasminum sp., Melothria sp., Phaseoulus sublabatus* and *Vites sp.* in the state of Arunachal Pradesh, Manipur, Mizoram and Nagaland. The preferred herbs are *Borrena hirticulata, Impatiens sp.* and *Plantago major* and tuber was *Ipomea batatus* (Heli, 1996; Haque *et al.*, 2008; Prakash *et al.*, 2008). The chemical composition of grasses, creepers, shrubs and tree fodders consumed by mithun in the state of Arunachal Pradesh, Manipur, Mizoram and Nagaland is presented in Tables 1, 2, 3 and 4, respectively.

Agricultural and forest by-products that are relished by mithun are banana leaves and stalks, pineapple leaves, potato haulms, rotten tubers, sweet potato vines, tapioca waste, brewery waste (processed millet grains), tubers, *etc.*, (Gupta *et al.*,1999). Paddy is the major cultivated crop in NEH Region of India. Nevertheless, due to lack of awareness and practice of feeding paddy straw to ruminants especially to mithun, farmers allow paddy straw to be decomposed in fields (Prakash *et al.*, 2007).

The primitive agricultural practice in NEH region is one of the most important factor for dwindling natural vegetation. This is also responsible for decreasing the carrying capacity in the locations of jhumland (Pal and Bujarbaruah, 2002). Due to hilly terrain and high rainfall, the mithun habitat is prone to soil erosion that in turn affects the overall nutrient dynamics in the soil-plant-animal *continuum*. In deciduous trees. The nutrient composition of leaves significantly varies with maturity and in different seasons due to leaching and transport of nutrients (Guha and Mitchell, 1966; Kenworthy, 1973).

Table 1 : Chemical composition (%DM basis) of different foliages collected from Arunachal Pradesh

Botanical name	CP	EE	CF	NFE	Ash
Tree fodder					
Celtis sp	10.6	1.39	25.6	56.2	6.2
Ficus fistulosa	13.3	1.46	21.4	58.7	5.1
Ficus hirta	15.1	1.99	12.5	62.4	8.0
Leea indica	16.2	2.68	25.6	48.4	7.1
Macranga denticulata	13.9	3.69	21.3	55.5	5.6
Magnolia pteroocarpa	11.5	1.75	23.2	57.5	6.0
Mussanda roxyburghu	9.97	2.29	24.6	52.8	10.3
Oreocnite integrifolia	16.4	3.43	21.3	53.2	5.6
Saurauia roxyburglis	11.2	2.30	23.5	59.0	4.0
Sterculia villosa	14.4	1.05	21.4	56.8	6.3
Shrub					
Angiopetris evecta	15.7	2.11	15.6	61.5	5.0
Brassaiopsis hainla	8.95	1.80	12.4	68.9	7.9
Costus specious	11.9	3.73	13.5	64.3	6.5
Crassocephalum crepsoids	14.2	1.65	20.3	56.7	7.1
Litsea cubeba	20.1	5.43	14.8	52.6	7.0
Melastomia sp	13.7	1.99	25.6	53.9	4.8
Phegopeteris auritica	19.0	1.66	15.6	54.7	9.0
Piper peticellosum	19.3	1.86	14.9	56.6	7.3
Polygonum runcinatum	10.2	1.78	12.3	71.1	4.6
Solanum kurzu	25.7	3.09	16.5	45.8	8.9
Pilea glaberrima	18.1	2.39	14.5	57.7	7.3
Creeper					
Thunbergia sp	13.9	2.96	11.7	64.7	6.7
Grass					
Hedychium flavum	13.0	2.18	16.5	60.3	8.0
Hedychium spicatum	11.5	2.79	17.8	61.1	6.8
Larex polycephala	6.81	2.10	15.6	67.4	8.0
Pinnaga gracilis	11.8	2.46	15.4	65.4	4.9
Thysanolaena sp	5.13	1.66	14.6	71.6	7.0
Wallichia densiflora	6.97	3.10	16.3	66.4	7.2

Table 2 : Chemical composition (%DM basis) of different foliages collected from Manipur

Botanical name	CP	EE	CF	NFE	Ash	CT
Tree fodder						
Bauhinia hookeri	16.5	1.19	24.8	48.3	9.25	11.1
Callicarpa arborea	16.9	3.29	21.7	52.4	5.69	2.47
Callicarpa macrophylla	9.51	2.80	25.7	57.1	4.86	5.97
Ficus hirta	18.4	2.97	16.7	48.2	13.7	7.79
Ficus incurva	13.3	1.42	19.8	56.0	9.42	2.43
Ficus silhetensis	11.1	2.06	21.3	55.4	10.2	2.18
Gentiana spp	15.5	2.58	15.2	50.3	16.4	4.9
Leucosceptrum canum	18.6	3.05	18.5	52.3	7.44	4.90
Sarcochlamys pulcherrima	14.5	2.64	23.7	41.5	17.6	8.11
Sauriara panduana	10.8	1.69	17.2	64.3	6.00	1.94
Verbena spp	17.7	4.00	15.1	51.2	11.9	4.92
Shrub						
Elastostema spp	11.2	1.47	14.2	51.2	21.8	1.65
Musa spp	9.91	1.49	18.6	56.5	13.5	4.28
Passiflora foetida	12.9	2.95	28.7	47.0	8.38	2.59
Rubus spp	16.9	1.79	23.1	51.4	6.85	6.96
Solanum spp	23.8	1.77	15.1	50.5	8.80	5.56
Tithonia rotundifolia	15.2	1.52	12.0	51.3	19.9	1.80
Urena lobata	14.2	1.31	17.4	54.2	12.8	2.18
Urtica dioica	26.3	2.32	28.4	27.5	15.5	7.57
Vitex spp	12.9	2.30	29.4	45.1	10.3	5.78
Creeper						
Herpetospermum spp	22.9	2.29	24.5	34.5	15.7	4.90
Grass						
Cynodon dactylon	8.86	2.80	33.3	46.4	8.67	4.53
Imperata cylindrica	7.04	1.00	37.9	48.1	5.85	1.85
Neyraudia reynaudiana	9.23	1.55	33.8	56.1	5.85	2.18
Thysanolaena agrostis	14.8	2.19	37.6	36.6	8.84	7.54

CT = Condensed tannin, Annual Report (2007-08)

Table 3 : Chemical composition (%DM basis) of different foliages collected from Mizoram

Botanical name	CP	EE	CF	NFE	Ash	CT
Tree fodder						
Bides didernata	18.2	1.63	13.5	55.9	10.7	2.8
Boehmeria platyphylla	11.7	0.90	18.0	51.2	18.1	4.2
Callicarpa arborea	13.9	2.66	40.3	39.0	4.14	7.3
Canthium glabrum	12.4	1.53	20.7	59.1	6.26	8.5
Ficus articulata	15.5	2.39	34.8	34.1	13.1	2.3
Ficus prostrata	13.2	1.42	11.1	64.9	9.39	4.6
Gmelina arborea	20.6	1.82	55.4	15.2	6.95	4.0
Trema orientalis	9.47	1.60	18.4	59.3	11.2	6.8
Sarcochlamys sp	13.9	1.59	20.0	51.9	12.5	3.6
Shrub						
Chromolena odorata	17.2	2.29	15.0	56.4	9.16	6.0
Debregeasia longifolia	10.6	1.93	15.6	58.8	13.1	7.2
Erianthus longisetosus	10.1	1.55	30.3	50.0	7.91	9.6
Manihot esculenta	17.9	4.97	19.2	50.2	7.60	7.7
Mussaenda sp	14.7	2.78	18.2	54.9	9.32	2.7
Grass						
Cynodon dactylon	8.85	0.98	36.1	47.0	7.04	4.3
Dendrocalamus hamiltonii	26.8	2.14	29.6	29.8	11.7	3.8
Hedyotis scanden	16.4	1.78	23.1	47.9	10.8	2.4
Polygonum chinensis	12.6	0.53	29.8	48.6	8.48	1.5
Thysanolaena maxima	10.1	2.69	35.0	42.4	9.76	6.0

CT = Condensed tannin Annual Report (2007 – 08)

Table 4 : Chemical composition (%DM basis) of different foliages collected from Nagaland

Botanical name	CP	EE	CF	NFE	Ash
Tree fodder					
Adenosacme longifolia	28.3	2.5	12.1	49.6	7.5
Alnus nepalensis	14.7	1.50	32.6	44.2	6.92
Bauhinia variegata	15.1	2.15	34.2	42.6	5.86
Bisehafia sp	7.37	1.92	18.2	65.0	7.5
Bridelia tomentosa	11.7	2.50	26.8	52.7	6.3
Desmos longiflorus	13.5	1.51	14.6	61.2	9.1
Emblica officinalis	7.75	2.6	36.2	48.6	4.8

Contd...

Eurya accumenata	7.9	1.2	17.6	69.5	4.8
Ficus bengalensis	15.2	1.6	26.7	49.8	6.7
Ficus dalhousiae	11.9	2.47	22.5	58.7	4.36
Ficus elmeri	22.5	2.79	18.5	49.2	6.96
Ficus hirta	18.0	2.9	21.2	50.1	7.8
Ficus religiosa	13.6	2.6	16.2	61.2	6.4
Lagerstroemia sp	23.1	2.1	18.1	49.4	7.3
Leea indica	14.5	2.6	19.7	53.8	9.4
Litsea citrada	12.2	1.8	26.3	52.5	7.2
Macaranga denticulata	19.7	2.6	22.3	46.5	8.9
Morinda anguistifolia	10.3	1.4	23.3	58.2	6.8
Oroxylum indicum	19.8	1.9	27.2	44.8	6.3
Phylanthus sp	13.7	5.5	25.6	47.7	7.5
Rubia foetida	11.8	3.6	25.6	50.2	8.8
Saraina panduana	10.0	3.8	23.2	55.4	7.6
Sarcochlamys pulcherrima	10.4	4.4	16.5	60.8	7.9
Scheffelera sp	11.3	3.48	18.9	59.2	7.10
Spondias pinnata	19.4	2.0	17.8	52.3	8.5
Terminalia bellerica	17.0	4.6	31.2	40.8	6.4
Trevesia sp	16.2	1.17	21.3	51.0	10.3
Mallotus sp	11.8	2.22	26.5	51.6	7.8
Murus sp	22.2	2.8	25.6	44.5	4.9
Mussanda roxburghii	11.6	1.4	33.2	48.2	5.6
Shrub					
Ammomum sp	13.0	2.5	32.4	44.5	7.6
Callicarpa vestita	21.6	2.10	18.7	49.3	8.21
Chlerondendron sp	15.8	4.52	31.2	40.6	7.80
Hibiscus chinensis	21.4	3.3	21.6	47.8	5.9
Hibiscus subdereffa	24.1	4.8	18.6	43.7	8.8
Osbekia sp	14.9	2.3	12.6	63.3	6.9
Polygonum chinensis	15.4	4.8	16.5	56.9	6.4
Pouzolzia sp	14.6	2.62	25.9	51.5	5.38
Quix sp	12.2	1.25	25.6	53.8	7.1
Rubus sp	14.2	3.6	14.7	59.4	8.1
Solanum nigrum	12.1	3.4	31.9	44.7	7.9
Urtica sp	20.6	2.48	12.0	56.7	8.19
Grass					
Alloteropsis semialata	6.72	1.61	25.6	55.7	-
Avena sativa	8.7	3.5	18.5	60.4	8.9
Axonopus compressus	7.87	2.14	25.6	54.8	9.5

Contd...

Carex cryciata	7.75	2.30	21.0	58.7	10.2
Commelina bengalensis	14.7	3.4	22.5	49.2	10.2
Oplismenus compositus	12.9	4.10	22.3	53.6	7.1
Pogonetherum crinitum	11.2	1.8	22.1	59.3	5.6
Schitostachyum sp	8.9	2.1	31.8	51.3	5.9
Creeper					
Alternanthera sesiles	19.1	2.1	14.6	55.7	8.5
Cissus assamina	12.8	2.12	16.2	58.5	10.3
Jasminum sp	11.5	2.33	14.5	65.2	6.40
Melothria sp	12.6	2.60	16.3	58.4	10.1
Phaseoulus sublabatus	14.4	3.10	20.1	54.5	7.9
Vites sp	12.7	3.2	16.5	55.3	12.3
Herb					
Borrena hirticulata	16.0	1.9	22.3	50.7	9.1
Impatien sp	11.4	2.56	19.4	58.6	7.98
Plantago major	6.80	1.12	15.6	66.2	10.2
Tuber					
Ipomea batatus	16.8	1.47	18.9	59.4	3.4
Manihot esculenta	29.5	2.93	16.3	43.8	7.4

Annual Report (2005-06), Prakash *et al.*, (2006).

Table 5 : Micronutrients in the forages of NEH region (mg/kg)

Botanical name	Fe	Mn	Zn	Cu	
Trema orientalis	233 ± 5	74 ± 10	433 ± 13	14 ± 1.0	Nagaland
Lagerstromea speciosa	120 ± 4	157 ± 4	46 ± 5	10 ± 0.6	Nagaland
Ficus hookerii	528 ± 18	115 ± 5	70 ± 2	10 ± 0.7	Nagaland
Thysanolaena agrostis	137 ± 18.3	210 ± 41.7	35 ± 3.2	9 ± 0.5	Sikkim
Eupatorium sp	462 ± 34.4	24 ± 3.2	42 ± 2.8	11 ± 0.8	Sikkim
Artocarpus lakoocha	78 ± 6.8	184 ± 11.6	35 ± 2.5	8 ± 0.6	Sikkim
Reevesia pubescens	139 ± 11.3	119 ± 8.4	50 ± 5.6	20 ± 1.5	Sikkim
Brassiopsis mitis	56 ± 3.2	37 ± 2.1	28 ± 1.4	11 ± 0.6	Sikkim
Setaria palmifolia	234 ± 45.7	57 ± 2.7	45 ± 3.1	12 ± 1.5	Sikkim
Ageratum conzoides	295 ± 15.5	115 ± 9.5	110 ± 8.9	19 ± 1.2	Sikkim
Ficus infetoria	54 ± 4.2	32 ± 3.1	14 ± 1.1	11 ± 0.7	Sikkim
Ficus hoookerii	118 ± 20.0	139 ± 23.6	26 ± 1.2	10 ± 1.2	Sikkim
Polygonum nepalensis	290 ± 25.9	88 ± 6.7	62 ± 3.5	10 ± 0.5	Sikkim

Feed Intake

Incorporation of green fodder (napier and *Lagerstroemia speciola*) in paddy straw and concentrate based total mixed ration up to 30%, the dry matter intake is 2.70% of its body weight and 98.7 g per kg metabolic body weight per day (Prakash *et al.*, 2007). However, in intensive system the intake of dry matter on jungle grass based ration with supplementation of 2.0 kg rice bran fortified with 1% mineral mixture and 1% common salt, is 6.86 and 6.09 kg in male and female mithun calves, respectively which correspond to 2.98 and 2.53% of the body weight (Pal *et al.*, 2004). On feeding a ration comprised of 50% concentrate and 50% roughage (tree leaves of *Ficus hirta, Debrogesia longifolia, Lagerstroemia speciosa* and *Litsea sp.*, 2 parts and paddy straw, 1 part) average dry matter intake was 4.93 ± 0.21 and 4.74 ± 0.21 kg in male and female mithun weighing 230 and 221 kg, respectively. It corresponds to 101.1 ± 4.93 and 98.3 ± 3.33 g per kg metabolic body size per day (Annual Report, 2007-08).

Energy Requirement

No data is available regarding energy requirements (digestible energy / metabolizable energy/net energy) for maintenance, growth, lactation, etc. It is mentioned earlier that there is lot of variation among different strains of mithun in terms of milk yield, adult body weight, growth rate, etc. It provides an opportunity for selection of these animals in terms of efficient meat producer.

Lower energy requirement per kg metabolic body size for maintenance might be used as one of the basic tools for selection of mithun for better growth rate. Higher milk yield in beef cattle is positively correlated with higher energy requirement for maintenance. It indicates that the higher the milk yield in mithun, the lower is the efficiency of utilization of energy in terms of growth. Beef cattle with higher milk yielding capacity has 11% higher metabolizable energy requirement for maintenance compared to low yielder (Montano-Bermudez *et al.*, 1990). Cattle having a greater propensity to deposit fat subcutaneously, are better able to increase thermal insulative efficiency and are more tolerant and adaptable to cold environment (Webster and Young, 1970). It explains about lower maintenance requirements for low milk yielder. Comparative study regarding efficiency of utilization of energy in different strains using roughage as well as concentrate based diets is imperative to make mithun rearing a viable proposition in commercial line.

Protein Requirement

No data is available regarding requirements of protein for different purposes in mithun. However, mithun might have developed some capacity to detoxify or nullify the effects of some antinutritional factors like tannins as it is mainly dependent on fodder rich in these factors, in natural condition. tannins affect digestion and utilization of protein. So during determination of requirements of protein in mithun for different purposes these factors must be taken into account.

Mineral Requirements

Meager information is available on seasonal micronutrient dynamics of the evergreen tree fodder in the NEH region. The topography of this region is undulating. In such area leaching is very common phenomenon due to heavy rainfall (Kleinman *et al.*, 1996) and soils are prone to mineral deficiency which could also affect the vegetation (Prasad *et al.*, 1986). Craving for salt is more pronounced in *Bibos* species viz. mithun, gaur, bentang and koupray than other large size hoofed wild animals (Wharton, 1957). Information regarding requirements of various macro and micro-minerals and their availability during free-grazing condition in mithun is inadequate. Various hypotheses have been presented regarding this including a) hunger for particular mineral and sodium chloride, b) want of some trace minerals, *etc*. However, it is reported that nutrient content is adequate in most of the foliages (out of 16) consumed by mithun under free-grazing system, except sodium (Prakash *et al.*, 2009). This could be the reason, why the mithuns reared under free-grazing condition often exhibit the salt licking behaviour in contrast to those kept under confined condition. The content of Fe, Cu, Mn and Zn in some fodder available in NEH region is presented in Table 5. The level of Fe, Mn and Zn is found to be higher in all the fodder but level of Cu is within the normal range when prescribed normal range is considered to be 30-50, 20-40 and 07-11 mg per kg for Fe, Mn, Zn and Cu, respectively (McDowell, 1997). The importance of mineral elements to the health and well-being of animals has been recognized for centuries (Underwood, 1956).

Water Requirement

Data on water requirement is very meager. Growing mithun calves consume about 15.18 litres of water per 100 kg body weight (Pal *et al.*, 2008). However, environmental temperature has a significant effect on it. Drinking water consumption per unit of body weight is higher in summer than in winter. Supplementation of concentrate feed on free grazing animals increases water consumption. It is estimated that mithun calves consume 4.30 litres of water per kg dry matter intake.

Growth Rate

In paddy straw and concentrate based total mixed ration, supplementation of green fodder (napier and *Lagerstroemia speciola*) up to 30%, the growth rate and feed conversion efficiency were 561 g and 9.36 kg DM per kg gain, respectively. It is also reported that mithun can be reared successfully in the intensive system (Prakash *et al.*, 2008a). However, in intensive system the average daily gain on jungle grass based ration with supplementation of 2.0 kg rice bran fortified with 1% mineral mixture and 1% common salt, is 371 and 306 g, in male and female mithun calves, respectively (Pal *et al.*, 2004). Male mithun calves showed 548 g average daily gain on feeding a ration containing *Borrena hirticulata* 300 g, rice straw 300 g and concentrate 400 g per kg in intensive system (Prakash *et al.*, 2008). Average daily gain is observed to be 602 ± 44 and 554 ± 9.03 g in male and female mithun calves respectively, fed on a ration comprised of 50% concentrate and 50% roughage (tree leaves of *Ficus hirta, Debrogesia longifolia, Lagerstroemia speciosa* and *Litsea sp.*, 2 parts and paddy straw, 1 part) (Annual Report, 2007-08).

In case of beef cattle, economic pressure to improve production efficiency has prompted the researchers, to evaluate the performance of different types of cattle and methods used, to produce high quality meat with higher yield. Feeding grain diets to cattle is generally considered to yield meat that is more tender, flavourful and juicy than that of forage-fed cattle. However, feeding of grain based diet results with excess fat deposition (Dikeman *et al.*, 1985). In this way feeding grain based diet is inefficient as fat deposition is energetically more expensive than protein synthesis on a tissue weight basis (Thorbeck, 1977). Feeding cattle for maximum rate of gain, results in improved feed efficiency because of dilution of maintenance requirements (Dikeman, 1973). Therefore, feeding for maximum rate of gain and terminating the feeding period when cattle have deposited a minimum amount of trimmable fat, result in optimal feed efficiency.

Tenderness of meat is an important parameter for evaluation of meat quality. After slaughter of animals, reduced proteolysis of myofibrilar proteins due to reduced activity of μ-calpain and m-calpain, or in the other way over-activity of their inhibitor, calpastatin, produce less tender meat. So suitable feeding strategy and selection of mithun strain having less capastatin content in their meat should be taken into account besides consideration of growth rate, milk production and other economic traits for viable mithun production system.

References

Annual Report (1992-93). Annual Report, National Research Centre on Mithun, Jharnapani, Medziphema, Nagaland.

Annual Report (2005-06). Annual Report, National Research Centre on Mithun, Jharnapani, Medziphema, Nagaland.

Annual Report (2007-08). Annual Report, National Research Centre on Mithun, Jharnapani, Medziphema, Nagaland.

Arora, C. L. (1998). Less used animals: yak and mithun – an overview. Indian Journal of Animal Sciences, 68 (Special Issue): 735-742.

Balaraman, N. and Goley, M. M. (1991). Livestock Production in Sikkim. Sikkim Science Society, Gangtok, pp. 1-259.

Baruah, K. K., Ahmed, S. U., Pathak, N. N. and Sharma, P. K. (1980). *Dairy Guide*, 2: 25.

Bhusan, S., Rajkhowa, C., Bujarbaruah, K. M. (2005). Productive traits of mithun (*Bos frontalis*) and their correlations. *Ind. J.of Anim. Sci.*, 75: 971-973.

Bohlken, H. (1958). Vergleichende untersuchungen an wildrindern. Zoologische Jahrbücher, 68: 113-202.

Dikeman, M. B. (1973). Relationship of efficiency of live weight gain and body composition during growth of domestic animals. 26th Proceedings of Reciprocal Meat Conference, 26: 167.

Dikeman, M. E., Dayton, A. D., Hunt, M. C., Kastner, C. L., Axe, J. B. and Ilg, H. J. (1985). Conventional versus accelerated beef production with carcass electrical stimulation. *J. Anim. Sci.*, 61: 573-583.

Guha, M. M. and Mitchell, R. L. (1966). The trace and major element composition of deciduous trees. II. Seasonal changes. *Plant and Soils*, 24: 90-112.

Gupta, S. C., Gupta, Neelam and Nivsarkar, A. E. (1999). Mithun – A Bovine of Indian Origin, Indian Council of Agricultural Research, Krishi Anusandhan Bhavan, Pusa, New Delhi, pp 1-328.

Haque, N., Toppo Saroj, Rahman, H. and Bujarbaruah, K. M. (2008). Feed and fodder resources of Northeastern India. All India Dairy Business Directory (Dairy Year Book 2008). Sadana Publishers and Distributors, G. T. Road, Ghaziabad, New Delhi, pp. 132-142.

Heli, T. (1996). A study on the browsing and natural fodders of mithun: An important browsing animal of Arunachal Pradesh. *Arunachal Forest News*, 13: 14-16.

Heli, T. (1997). Mithun breeding farm at Sagalee: An overview. *Arunachal Rev.*, 1: 6-8.

Kenworthy, A. L., (1973). Plant analysis as an aid in fertilizing orchards. In: Welsh, L. M. and Beaton, J. D. (eds). Soil Testing and Plant Analysis, Soil Sci. Society of America, Madison, pp. 381-392.

Kleinman, P. J. A., Bryant, R. B. and Pimentel, D. (1996). Assessing ecological sustainability of slash-and-burn agriculture through soil fertility indicators. *Agro-Journal*, 88: 122-127.

Larkin, F. M. (1954). Observation on the grazing behaviour on beef cattle in tropical Queensland. *Queensland J. Agric. Sci.*, 11: 115-141.

Montano-Bermudez, M., Nielsen, M. K. and Dietscher, G. H. (1990). *J. of Anim. Sci.*, 68: 2279-2288.

Pal, D. T. and Bujarbaruah, K. M. (2002). *Ind. J. of Anim. Sci.*, 72: 1001-1003.

Pal, D. T., Dhali, A., Mondal, S. K., Rajkhowa, C. and Bujarbaruah, K. M. (2008). *J. of Mountain Res.*, 5: 178-188.

Pal, D. T., Singh, A.S., Kezhavituo Vapru and Bujarbaruah, K. M. (2004). Growth performance and nutrient utilization in male and female mithun calves on green forage based diet. *Trop. Anim. Health and Prod.*, 36: 655-661.

Pathak, N. N. and Baruah, K. K. (1980). *Sci. Rep.*, 17: 483.

Prakash, B., Dhali, A., Mech, A., Khate, K., Moaakum, H. and Rajkhowa, C. (2008). *Livestock Sci.*, 117: 263-269.

Prakash, B., Dhali, A., Mondal, M., Sangtam, M., Khati, K., Rathor, S. S. and Rajkhowa, C. (2008a). *J. Anim. Physiol. and Anim. Nutri.*, 92: 591-596.

Prakash, B., Dhali, A., Rathore, S. S., Das, K. C., Walling, I., Vupru, K., Mech, A., Baruah, K. K. and Rajkhowa, C. (2009). *Anim. Feed Sci. Technol.*, 150: 223-229.

Prakash, B., Mondal, M., Rongsensusang, A., Hannah, K. and Rajkhowa, C. (2006). *Livestock Res. Rural Devel.*, 18: 119.

Prasad, R. N., Singh, A. and Verma, A. (1986). *Ind. J. Soil Conser.*, 14: 66-72.

Simoons, F. J. (1984). Evolution of Domesticated Animals. Longman, London, UK, p. 34.

Thorbeck, G. (1977). *Nutrition and Metabolism*, 2:105

Underwood, E. J. (1956). Trace Elements in Human and Animal Nutrition. Academic Press, New York.

Verma, N. D. (1990). Mithun and its habitat. In Proceedings of the National Watershed Development Project for Rainfed Area, Guwahati.

Verma, N. D. (1996). Mithun - a magnificent *Bos* species. In: Gupta, P. R. (Ed). Dairy India, A - 25, Priyadarshni Vihar, Delhi, pp. 180-181.

Webstar, A. J. F and Young, B. A. (1970). Breed and strain differences in the cold tolerance of young cattle raised in different environments. Univ. Alberta, Edmonton, Can. University of Alberta. Annual Feeders' Day Report, 49: 37.

Wharton, C. H. (1957). An Ecological Study of the Kouprey - *Novibos sauveli* (*Urbain*). Philippines (Republic) Institute of Science and Technology, Monograph No 5, Bureau of Printing, Manila, pp. 1-107.

□□□

Animal Nutrition, 2012
eds. Dr. (Mrs.) Usha R. Mehra et al., pp. 305-328
Satish Serial Publishing House e-mail : info@satishserial.com; website : www.satishserial.com

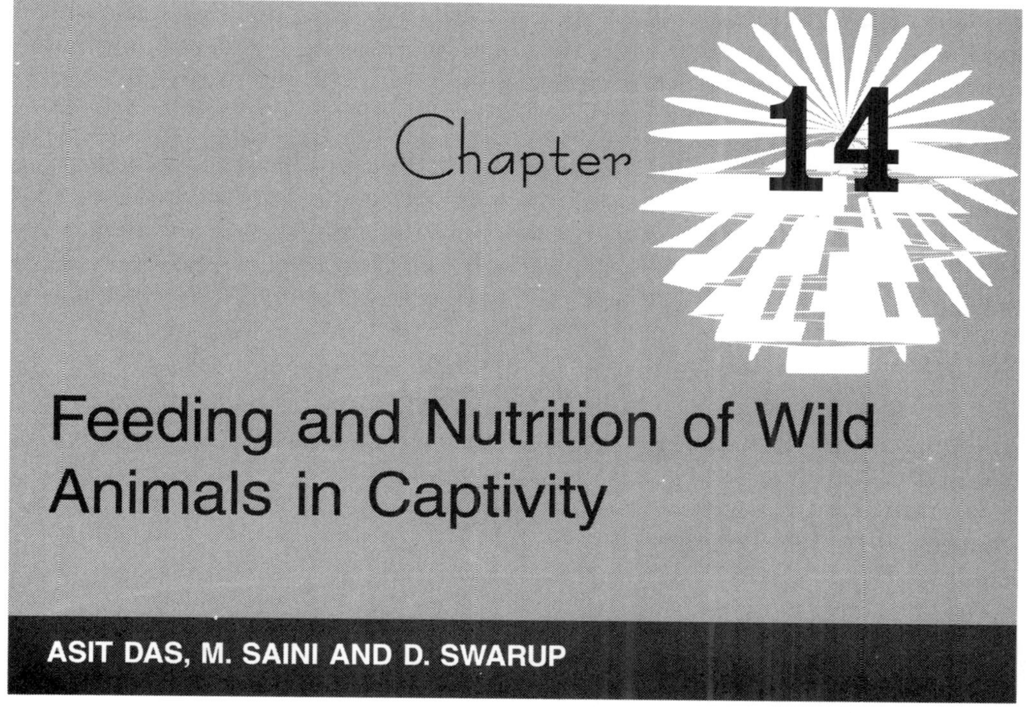

Chapter 14

Feeding and Nutrition of Wild Animals in Captivity

ASIT DAS, M. SAINI AND D. SWARUP

The science of nutrition is an integral component to the management of zoo animals and must be addressed in a scientific and professional manner. The challenge of a zoo nutrition programme is to provide a nutritionally balanced diet, which reasonably stimulates natural feeding behaviour and which is consistently palatable to the animals. The goal of a zoo nutrition programme differs vastly from those of livestock or pet nutrition. Zoo nutrition must facilitate the captive animal management goals of reproduction, longevity, good health and behavioral normality. Any nutritional programme also must consider the psychological and physiological needs of species that have evolved under diverse environmental conditions. Zoo nutritionist must ensure that the animals may get sufficient opportunity to choose their diet according to seasonal, physiological, environmental or individual needs.

The most obvious challenge in providing optimum nutrition to captive exotic or native wildlife is the lack of known requirements. In most of the zoos, animals are fed empirically based upon whether they are herbivore, omnivore or carnivore. However, such a practice is not scientific considering the fact that many herbivores will gnaw and carnivores like panda will thrive on completely vegetarian diet. Such empirical feeding practices followed in most of the zoos may either lead to under or overfeeding which may ultimately result in various health hazards, reproductive disorders and reduced life-span.

The pioneer work of Sanyal (1892) forms the very basis of feeding of zoo animals in India. Diets of zoo animals are developed on the basis of food preferences of the free ranging animals, domestic animal data and experience of the keeper. As a result, such diets are empirical and cause lots of nutritional problems which will be discussed in this chapter. Of late, with the effort of (CZA), Arora (2001) compiled the feeding schedule of zoo mammals practiced in different zoos in the country. It is evident from that compilation that inter-zoo variation in feeding schedule is very high. Hence, it is necessary to prepare a standard diet schedule for zoo animals, which could be uniformly used across the country. Such a diet schedule should provide all the nutrients in optimum quantity so as to improve general health, immunity, life span and chances of captive breeding.

Principles of Zoo Animal Nutrition

Like domestic and pet animal diet, zoo animal feed is composed of major nutrients like carbohydrates, protein and fat and specific nutrients like amino acids, fatty acids, minerals and vitamins. The major components of zoo animals feed are measured as proximate principles, which provide reasonably good estimates for the nutrient composition of the diet. However, for highly fibrous diet, this method of analysis poses some problem and a different method for estimation of fibre, as suggested by Van Soest *et al.* (1991) is followed. In this chapter, the nutritional significance of major constituents of feed will be discussed first, followed by minerals and vitamins.

Water

Wild animal meet their water requirement from drinking it as liquid water, preformed water in the feeds and fodder, and also from the metabolic water. Oxidation of 100g of protein, carbohydrate and fat yields 42, 60 or 108 g of metabolic water, respectively. The moisture in food is important source of water for many animals. Free ranging kangaroo rats, ground squirrels, peccaries, antelope, wallabies, a small fox like carnivore of Sahara desert, numerous carnivorous and insectivorous birds and mammals have been able to meet their water requirement from preformed and metabolic water (Robbins, 1992). Water is lost from the body in urine, faeces, and milk, and by vaporization through lungs and skin. In species that drink water, it is usually 2-5 times of dry matter intake (Fowler, 1986). Water consumption in Indian rhinoceros was 3.5-5.2L/kg DM (Clauss *et al.*, 2005), whereas an elephant can drink upto 200L of water daily (Holdo *et al.*, 2002). Several major physiological differences exist between birds and mammals that affect water requirement. Because of their intense metabolism and corresponding high rate of pulmocutaneous water loss, small passerines generally dehydrate during flight at air temperature above 7°C. Water loss during prolonged non-stop migration by birds may actually limit their flight. High evaporative water loss in birds is partially balanced by their reduced urinary excretion relative to mammals. Urea excretion in mammals require 20-40 times more water than is required to excrete similar amount of uric acid in birds.

Carbohydrates

The carbohydrate in foods includes simple sugars, complex sugars and polymeric compounds, such as starch, hemi-cellulose and cellulose. As hemi cellulose and cellulose are resistant to enzymatic digestion, they are considered as part of fibre (Van Soest, 1994).

Even though carbohydrates are the largest source of energy for most of the captive animal diet, they are not dietary essentials, if the supply of glucogenic precursor like propionate and glucogenic amino acids is ensured. Liver can synthesize glucose from these substances in most of the mammalian species. Glucose is required in erythrocyte, medulla of kidney and central nervous system, although central nervous system can also use ketone bodies to some extent. Under anaerobic conditions, glucose is the only potential source of energy.

Fibre in human being is commonly referred as dietary fibre, whereas fibre in wild herbivores is commonly measured as neutral detergent fibre (NDF) and acid detergent fibre (ADF) or both. Dietary fibre is a mixture of cellulose, hemicellulose, gum, pectin, enzyme resistant starch and lignin, whereas detergent method of analysis describes the structural carbohydrates. By far, cellulose is the most abundant organic substance in the earth. Neutral and acid detergent fibres (as estimated by the method of Van Soest *et al.*, 1994) are important source of nutrients for herbivores. Even omnivorous species like man and pig can utilize sizeable amount of this fibre. NDF concentration of free ranging Gorilla diet was 46% (Roger *et al.*, 1990), for orangutan it was 56% (Knott, 1999) and in lemur diet it was 40% (Dempsey *et al.*, 2002). Most of the fruits and vegetables used in captive animal diet are cultivated for human taste and contain more soluble sugars and less fibre, in comparison to those fruits and foliages found in their natural habitat (Schmidt *et al.*, 2005).

Mammals lack the enzyme cellulase. However, pregastric and postgastric fermenters harbour microbiota which ferment cellulose and volatile fatty acids (VFA) are produced. Monkeys generally obtain 30% of their energy from VFA, in comparison to about 6-10% in human being (Schmidt *et al*, 2005), In case of elephant, VFA produced in the hindgut can account for 100% of the basal metabolism. Concentration of total VFA was 120 and 75 mmol/l in elephant and rhino, respectively (Jenson, 1986). Methane production in both the species was much lower than the ruminant livestock.

VFAs absorbed by the forestomach of wild ruminants accounted for 21-75% of digestible energy intake. The average pH of rumen liquor of Sika deer was 6.1 and total VFA content was 114.6 mmol/l (Li and Qin, 1991). Mean retention time in the digestive tract was shorter in deer than in cattle. In addition, the rate of post-ruminal passage in deer was lower. The digestibility of dry matter, organic matter, crude protein and fibre in deer were significantly lower than in cattle (Asano *et al.*, 2005). However, digestibility of nutrients was much higher in Indian spotted deer and black buck (Garg, 1996; Arora, 2001; Suresh, 2008). Rumen fluid of mule deer and elk contained $11x10^9$ and $67x\ 0^9$ bacteria/ml of rumen fluid (McBee *et al.*, 1969). The concentration of total volatile fatty acids in the rumen was significantly higher in deer than in cattle. The molar percentage of acetic acid was lower and that of valeric acid was higher in deer. The number of protozoa was somewhat higher in deer (Asano *et al.*, 2005). Rumen fermentation (and apparent digestibility) was much higher in deer fed chicory than in deer fed perennial ryegrass (Kusmartono *et al.*, 1997).

Protein

Proteins are indispensable to maintain life as they perform many specialized functions in the body. They serve as enzymes, antibodies, transporting agents, buffers, osmotic regulators and hormones, besides being the structural components of body. Hair and horns may contain up to 99% protein on DM basis. Antler of spotted, hog and swamp deer contained 35.16, 36.50 and 31.99 % protein, respectively (Pathak *et al.*, 2001). Approximately, 22 amino acids constitute the building blocks of proteins. These amino acids must be present in appropriate amount and proportion for synthesis of protein. Otherwise, protein synthesis will be impaired, followed by impaired health and production. Much of a mammal's protein requirement is actually requirement for essential amino acids, although dietary proteins also supply other non essential amino acids that are used as a source of organic nitrogen for synthesis of tissue proteins. Of the ten essential amino acids, the part of methionine requirement can be met through cystine and phenylalanine through tyrosine. Domestic cat and other felids require free amino acid taurine in the diet (Howard *et al.*, 1987). Lysine, tryptophan and S-containing amino acids are quite low in vegetable protein, a fact that must be considered in formulating pelleted feeds. Ruminants and other herbivores with pregastric fermentation obtain essential amino acids from microbial protein and hence, may not require dietary source *per se*.

Fat

Mammals do not have a dietary requirement for fat *per se*, although they do require certain essential fatty acids. Linoleic acid meets the essential fatty acid requirement of most animals that have been studied, although domestic cat and other specialized carnivores require arachidonic acid, as well. Fat sources are used in manufactured feed to improve palatability (especially for carnivores), to increase energy content and to facilitate the manufacturing process as lubricants.

Minerals

Calcium and Phosphorus

Over 98% of the body's calcium (Ca) and about 80% of the body's phosphorus (P) are stored in bone, teeth and skeleton. Ca and P are required in large amounts, relative to other macrominerals. In addition to their critical structural role, Ca is essential for blood clotting, muscle contraction, transmission of nerve impulses, regulation of the heart, secretion of hormones, enzyme activation and stabilization. Leguminous green fodders are very good source of calcium. Hardened deer antlers contain about 22 per cent calcium and 11 per cent phosphorus.

The apparent absorption coefficient for Ca ranges from 60-83% in case of rhino (Clauss *et al.*, 2005) and 40-60% in elephants (Clauss *et al.*, 2003). Endogenous faecal Ca loss was calculated as 5.1 mg Ca/kg BW/day in rhino and 6.6 mg in elephant (Clauss, *et al.*, 2003). In such situation, absorption of a large proportion of Ca through GI tract, and excretion of the surplus via the kidney and urinary tract could overload with excess of Ca causing urolith.

The P is widely distributed in soft tissue and is required to drive multiple metabolic and energy reactions within and between cells. As phosphate, it helps to maintain osmotic and acid-base balance. As a component of deoxyribonucleic and ribonucleic acid, P is involved in cell growth and differentiation. As a phospholipid, it contributes to cell-membrane fluidity and integrity. Through involvement in creatine phosphate, adenosine triphosphate (ATP), and other phosphorylated compounds, P plays a vital role in energy transfer and used during gluconeogenesis, fatty acid transport, amino acid and protein synthesis, and activity of the sodium-potassium pump. Early responses to low dietary P include a decline in plasma inorganic P concentration and an increase in plasma alkaline phosphatase activity. If the deficiency is sufficiently severe or prolonged, abnormalities of the bones and teeth can be expected, growth will be slow in the young, and appetite will be depressed; and pica (deprived appetite) will be seen in some domestic and wild animals.

The apparent absorption coefficient for P was between - 12 and 29% in rhino and 10-30% in Asiatic elephant (Clauss *et al.*, 2003). Concentrates usually contain more P. Endogenous P losses were 10 mg/kg BW for rhino and 6.0mg/Kg BW for Asiatic elephant.

The metabolism of Ca and P is interrelated. These two minerals are considered simultaneously when designing or evaluating a ration. The actual amount of calcium and phosphorus required by elk increased greatly during growth, lactation and antler growth. A minimum of 0.7% Ca and 0.4% P is suggested for elk rations. Ca to P ratio of at least 1.5 to 1 is needed. However, maximum tolerable range of Ca:P in deer is yet to be established (Deerfarmer, 2003). A diet of 0.64% Ca and 0.56% P is necessary for antler growth. Stags can store minerals in their skeletons, and transfer them to the antlers when needed. In fact, during antler mineralization, male deer undergo osteoporosis. The minerals lost from the bones are replaced from the diet after the antlers are hardened. Yearling hinds and stags have high nutritional demands for skeletal growth. Yearling stags have the added nutritional demand to grow their first set of antlers. Stags require high levels of Ca, P, trace minerals and protein for antler growth (Bass Pro., 2006-07).

Ca levels are relatively high in hay, especially legumes, but P content is quite low. Grains are being relatively rich in P and poor in Ca. However, rations comprised of hay/haylage and natural grains and oilseeds or meals will not provide enough minerals and vitamins. Access to browse (twigs and leaves) improves natural mineral intake on pastures. Elk, unlike sheep, require supplemental copper (Deerfarmer, 2003).

Magnesium

Magnesium (Mg) is closely related to Ca and P in function and distribution in the body. This mineral is known to activate at least 300 different enzymes. Mg is essential for energy metabolism, transmission of the genetic code, membrane transport and nerve impulse transmissions.

Sodium, Potassium, Chlorine and Sulphur

Sodium is the most important extracellular cation. About 30-40% of body sodium reserve is found in bone. Sodium is required for active transportation of amino acids and glucose into the cell. Sodium requirement varies from 0.08 - 0.3% of the diet. Most of the feeds and fodder available in the natural habitat of elephant is reported to be deficient in sodium (Rode *et al.*, 2006) which compels them to raid crop. Potassium is the major intracellular cation which is involved in acid base balance, osmotic balance and cell membrane potential. Potassium requirement is 0.2-0.8% in the diet. Chlorine is concentrated in the extra cellular fluid. Its requirement is 0.1-0.3%. Chlorine is also secreted in gastric juice and regulates osmotic pressure. Sulphur is a constituent of amino acid and protein, connective tissue. It is involved in transmethylation and maintaining of redox potential.

Iron

Iron (Fe) is an essential component of such proteins as hemoglobin, myoglobin, and ferritin; and some enzymes require Fe as a cofactor. Fe in heme allows the transport of oxygen to tissues (haemoglobin), transitional storage of oxygen in tissues (myoglobin), and the transport of electrons through the respiratory chain (cytochromes). Biological functions that depend on Fe include energy metabolism, neurotransmitter synthesis, connective tissue metabolism, immune function, thyroid hormone metabolism, and thermogenesis. Approximately, 60% of body Fe is present as haemoglobin. Apart from this vital function, Fe is involved in the oxidative mechanism of the cells. Being a part of cytochrome enzymes Fe participates in the electron transfer chain. Fe is involved in some basic biochemical processes in the tissues as a part of flavoprotein enzyme.

Copper

Copper (Cu) is associated with a number of proteins, including many important enzymes. The Cu-containing enzymes are commonly divided into amine oxidases, ferroxidases, cytochrome c oxidases, dopamine β-hydroxylase, superoxide dismutases, and tyrosinase. The known Cu-binding proteins are metallothionein, albumin, transcuprein and blood-clotting factor.

Zinc

Zinc (Zn) is the most abundant of intracellular trace elements and is involved in structural, catalytic, and regulatory roles. Over 200 enzymes with diverse functions have been found which have zinc as prosthetic group. Zn is involved in the metabolism of carbohydrate, protein, lipids, and nucleic acids (DNA and RNA polymerase and thymidine kinase).

Iodine

Iodine is an essential component of thyroid hormones thyroxine (T_4) and triiodothyronine (T_3), which regulate the rate of energy metabolism in the body. Iodine requirements may be elevated in animals consuming goitrogenic substances, which interfere with iodine metabolism. The cyanogenic goitrogens include the thiocyanates derived from cyanide in white clover and the glucosinolates found in some forages, such as kale, turnip and rape. These goitrogens impair iodine uptake by the thyroid, and their effect can be overcome by increasing dietary iodine. Clinical signs of iodine deficiency may not be apparent for up to one year after the iodine deficient diet is initiated.

Selenium

A number of proteins contain Se and are called simply Se-containing proteins. This Se is often found in selenomethionine and the proportion of Se in Se-containing proteins is usually related to the relative proportions of methionine and selenomethionine. Unlike many other trace minerals, the range between dietary toxicity and deficiency is quite narrow. Se is required in the body for the synthesis of an enzyme that breaks down harmful oxidizing agents. Se and vitamin E are somewhat related because vitamin E protects cells from the harmful effects of the oxidizing agents. Therefore, a deficiency of either Se or vitamin E will increase the requirement for the other.

Vitamins in Wildlife Nutrition

General functions and metabolic functions of the fat and water soluble vitamins have been discussed elaborately by Robbins (1992). All the fat (Vitamin A, D, E and K) and water soluble vitamins (thiamin, riboflavin, pentothonic acid, niacin, folic acid, biotin and cyanocobalamine) are reported to perform vital metabolic functions and are dietary essential for most of the mammals. However, anaerobic bacteria can synthesize vitamin K and all the water soluble vitamins except choline and vitamin C.

Vitamin A

Vitamin A is found in animal tissues and not in plant tissues. However, its precursor (carotene and carotenoids) are widely distributed in the plant tissue. Provitamins-A are converted into vitamins by the enzymatic action in liver and intestinal mucosa. However, felids can not convert β-carotene to vitamin A. Thus, preformed vitamin A is a dietary essential in feline diet. Dietary vitamin A requirement ranges from 2000 to 10,000 IU/kg diet.

Vitamin D

The antirachitic vitamin occurs in two major forms (Vitamin D_2, ergocalciferol and vitamin D_3, cholecalciferol). Human, cattle, old world primates and rats can utilize both forms of the vitamin effectively, whereas, new world primate uses vitamin D_2 less efficiently than vitamin D_3. Birds, reptiles, amphibians and fish require vitamin D_3 and can not utilize vitamin D_2. The divergence of mammals from the other vertebrate taxa in the utilization of vitamin D_2 has been suggested as an evolutionary response in primitive insectivorous to being nocturnally active. Diurnal concealment would reduce the opportunity for the production of adequate vitamin D_3 by irradiation, consequently, requiring the utilization of dietary sources, since vitamin D is not normally stored in the body of terrestrial vertebrates.

Vitamin E

There are 8 natural compounds with vitamin E activity, tocopherol being the most potent one. All plant materials are rich source of vitamin E. In animal tissues they serve as the defense mechanism against peroxidation of unsaturated fatty acids in membrane lipid. Requirement range varies from 15 to 100 IU/kg for most of the wild mammals.

Vitamin K

The metabolic function of this vitamin is clotting of blood. As mentioned earlier, microbes can synthesize vitamin K. The green leaves are also very good sources of vitamin K.

Water Soluble Vitamins

Thiamin

Thiamin pyrophosphate is the co-factor for reaction involving oxidative and non-oxidative decarboxylation. Leafy forages and green plants are good sources of thiamin.

Riboflavin

Riboflavin as flavine mononucleotide adenine dinucleotide is involved in oxidation-reduction reaction in electron transport chain in mitochondria. Leafy vegetable is very good source of riboflavin. When animals (particularly, non ruminants) are fed higher amount of concentrate, there may be deficiency of riboflavin. Requirement varies from 2-4 mg/kg diet.

Pantothenic Acid

As co-enzyme A pantothenic acid is involved in transfer of acyl group for synthesis of steroid, heme and fatty acid. Leafy forages and animal tissues are good sources; conversely, maize and rice are poor source. Deficiency may be seen when diet contains large proportion of cereals, particularly in those animals in which microbial synthesis is minimum.

Niacin

Both nicotinamide and nicotinic acid have equal niacin activity. Greens are good source of this vitamin. Green leaves also have good amount, but most are bound and not available to the animals. As NAD and NADP, niacin is involved in a lot of vital oxidation-reduction reactions. Niacin requirement ranges form 10-30 mg/kg diet.

Vitamin B_6

Pyridoxine, pyridoxal and pyridoxamine are inter-convertible and have equal vitamin B_6 activity. Pyridoxal phosphate is involved in deamination and transamination. Most of the feedstuffs are good source of this vitamin. Requirement is 1-2 mg/kg diet.

Biotin

Even though cereal grains are good source of this vitamin, bioavailability is doubtful. Animal products are moderately good source, whereas yeast is a very good source of the vitamin. As a co-enzyme, the vitamin is involved in regulation of transketolase and fat metabolism. Biotin requirement ranges from 100-300 μg/kg diet.

Vitamin B_{12}

Cyanocobalamine, hydroxyl cobalamine, acquocobalamine and nitrocobalamine are large molecules containing Co and P in 1:1 ratio. All these compounds have vitamin B12 activity and can be synthesized by gut microflora. Requirement varies from 5 -25 μg/kg diet for most of the wild mammals.

Ascorbic Acid

The development of synthetic capability of ascorbic acid and its transition within different organs of the body follows an interesting phylogenic scale. Invertebrates and fish lack the synthetic capability and are thus, dependent on dietary sources. Amphibians, reptiles, most birds and monotremes synthesize ascorbic acid in kidney. Approximately, one half of the passeriforms (bulbul, asian paradise fly-catcher, black hooded oriole, flower-pecker, crimson sunbird, some shrikes and barn swallow) are unable to synthesize the vitamin and therefore, totally depend on the dietary source. The remaining passeriform (sparrow, jungle myna, Asian pied starling and magpie robin) synthesize ascorbic acid in the liver, whereas Indian house crow and common myna synthesize ascorbic acid in both liver and kidney. Most mammals synthesize ascorbic acid in liver, but a few including primates, bats, guinea pigs and possibly cetacean lack a synthetic ability. Thus, the ability to synthesize ascorbic acid appeared initially in the kidney with the evolution of terrestrial vertebrate life forms and was later either transferred to the liver or lost.

Comparative Digestive Anatomy of Wild Herbivores

In the evolution of herbivores, there was failure to develop enzymes capable of degrading cellulose and other complex plant polysaccharides. To overcome this handicap, herbivores have developed a synchronized relationship with microorganisms. Two major types of herbivores have evolved. Ruminants and ruminant like animals, which are pregastric fermenter and another group of animals in which fermentation takes place in the hindgut.

Ruminants

Ruminant stomach has four parts: rumen, reticulum, omasum and abomasum. Different ruminant species include all deer, antelopes, wild buffalo, wild bison, Himalayan and Nilgiri Tahr, mountain sheep (Bhoral, Nayan, Blue sheep), mountain goats (Goral, Serow), okapi, giraffe, gazelle, eland, nilgai, wild beast, etc. Again ruminants have been divided into 3 groups as follows:

Concentrate Eaters: They prefer fruits and foliages. The fore-stomach compartment comprises 6-8% of body weight when full. Most of the deer and antelopes fall in this category.

Bulk Feeders: They prefer high fiber diet. The fore-stomach comprises of 12-14% body weight in bison, gaur and wild buffalo.

Intermediate Feeders: Nilgai, elk and wilde beast belong to this category. The fore-stomach comprises of 8-10% body weight.

Non-Ruminant Pre-Gastric Fermenters

Kangaroos, wallabies, peccaries, hippopotamus and certain colobines (Asiatic langurs) have a voluminous compartmentalized or sacculated fore-stomach. The fore-stomach fermentation chamber is approximately, 86, 92 and 95% total weight of gastro-intestinal tract in peccaries, kangaroos and hippopotamus, respectively.

Diet of the colobines primarily consists of leaves, fruits and seeds, leaves contributing more than 50% of the total diet (Yeager *et al.*, 1997). The compartmentalized fore-stomach harbours microbes which ferment complex polysaccharides and produces VFA and microbial mass similar to ruminants. However, it seems that the fibrolytic activity of the microbes is much stronger than the ruminant livestock, as DM digestibility as high as 82% (Edwards, 1999) and NDF digestibility as high as 81% has been recorded in langurs (Edwards, 1999).

Post Gastric Fermenters

Relative capacity of large intestine is 11-12.5% in ruminant herbivores, 60-65% in non ruminant herbivores, 35-38% in omnivores and 14-16% in carnivores. Zebra, wild ass, tapirs, rhinoceros, elephant, wild hare and pica have capacious, sacculated large intestine and compartmentalized caecum. We can call these animals as caecal fermenters.

Wild pigs have moderately large caecum, but a very large sacculated colon (colon fermenters). Significant amount of microbial fermentation takes place in the hind gut. Post gastric fermenters depend on large intestine for digestion of fibre. The hindgut content in caecum and colon of an elephant is 11% (Van Hoven *et al.*, 1981). Energy derived from the large intestine can meet 100, 26-30 and 30% of dietary energy requirement in elephant, monkey and wild hare (Van Hoven *et al.*, 1981, Milton, 1981), respectively.

Nutrient Requirements

The daily nutrient requirement of an animal is influenced by its body size, physiological state, activity level, age, health status and other factors. Animal nutritionists usually express nutrient requirement as a percentage or as a concentration, however, it is more precise to express it on the basis of energy density, since, under normal circumstances animals will adjust their food intake to meet their calorie requirements. We can rarely achieve precision when feeding zoo animals because of the uncertainty of level of intake. Under normal circumstances, animals will not consume energy in excess of their requirement. However, obesity in pets and zoo animals is not uncommon. Zoo animals in a group situation tend to be fed in excess of their requirements in order to ensure that the youngest or most subordinate animals obtains sufficient food, but some dominant animals may consume energy in excess of their requirement and become obese. In contrast, low level of food intake may occur in animals that experience severe seasonality in food intake in the wild. Even in captivity, the effect of photoperiod, temperature and other factors may induce period of chronic energy deficit and weight loss attributable to depressed intake (Ofteadal and Allen, 1997).

Energy Requirement

Animals consume food primarily to satisfy their energy demand. The maintenance energy requirement of an animal is calculated as basal metabolic rate (BMR) measured as energy expenditure of resting body function at post absorptive stage in a thermo-neutral zone. The following equation developed by Kleiber is used to measure BMR in eutharian mammals.

$BMR = 70BW^{0.75}$; whereas, BMR is measured as Kcal/d and BW is expressed in kg.

A number of desert rodents, fossorial rodents, arboreal leaf eaters and desert carnivores have a BMR, lesser than the expected based on Kleiber's equation, whereas marine mammals, mustelids, lagomorphs, shrews and voles have higher than the expected BMR (Robbins, 1992). The marsupials have a mass co-efficient of 48.6. Heusner (1982) advocated the use of mass exponent of 0.67 instead of 0.75. Recently, Nagy (2001) has measured the feeding rate (intake of both dry matter and fresh matter) by 79 species of mammals, 95 species of birds and 55 species of reptiles. The resulting exponential equations can be used to predict food requirement with varied (60-95%) degree of success.

As BMR is difficult to measure in wild animals, Nagy (2005) suggested use of field metabolic rate (FMR) for deriving energy requirement for wild animals. The FMR of 229 terrestrial vertebrates were measured using the doubly labeled water method. Daily rate of energy expenditure was as low as 0.23 KJ per day in Gecko, to as higher 52500 KJ per day in seal. Endothermic mammals and birds have FMR i.e. 12-20 time higher than equalized ectothermic reptiles.

$$\text{FMR} = aM_B^{\ b}$$

FMR - Field metabolic rate (KJday^{-1}): a - intercept, MB body mass in gram:b - is the slope of the equation.

Endotherm FMR = 8.53 $M_B^{0.676}$ (N, 174; $P<0.001$; $r^2 = 0.91$),

Ectothrem FMR = $0.196M_B^{0.889}$ (N, 55; $P<0.001$; $r^2 = 0.945$),

Mammals FMR = $4.82M_B^{0.734}$ (N, 79; $P<0.001$; $r^2 = 0.95$) and

Birds FMR = 10.5 $M_B^{0.681}$ (N, 95; $P<0.0001$; $r^2 = 0.938$).

It appears that the variation in FMR among terrestrial vertebrates is influenced more strongly by thermal physiology than taxonomic class.

Digestible energy requirement of roe deer for maintenance was 144 kcal/kgW$^{0.75}$ and 202.8 kcal/kgW$^{0.75}$ in captivity and free ranging conditions, respectively (Papageorgiou *et al.*, 1981). Such variation could be attributed to energy expenditures during locomotion. Monthly energy requirement for fetal growth (kcal retention/kg fetus) was calculated for white tailed deer by using the formula $e^{0.0501x-0.8393}$, where x is stage of gestation from 0-100% (Robbins *et al.*, 1974). Monthly energy requirement of lactation can be determined using milk production (ml/d) and composition (kcal/ml) for black tailed deer (Sadleir, 1980). The energetic cost of deer for both up slope and down slope locomotion is greater than horizontal movements (Parker *et al.*, 1984 and Kie *et al.*, 1991). Enright *et al.* (2001) reported that prepubertal fallow deer fed with high energy (HE) diet gave birth to a higher proportion of male offsprings, whereas female deer fed with low energy (LE) diet produced predominantly female offspring (Luna-Estrada *et al.*, 2006). Similar reports have also been documented in red deer, fallow deer and mule deer (Kucera, 1997; Flint *et al.*, 1997).

Fawns fed with diets higher in energy had greater gain in body weight and skeletal size, larger internal organs and accumulated heavier fat depots, compared to those given less energy diet. Proportion of dietary proteins in itself had very little effect on the relative health of fawns, although protein and energy interaction were common (Verme and Ozoga, 1980).

An adult tigress weighing 123 kg requires 5171 Kcal/day, whereas a male tiger weighing 160 kg requires 6300 k cal/day (Dierrenfeld, 1987). Energy requirement for rhinoceros is not known. However, energy consumption of 109 KJ/Kg BW is sufficient for maintenance (Frape *et al.*, 1982).

Energy requirement for many a wildlife species is not known. As a thumb rule, an adult eutharian mammal's ME requirement is two times BMR, it is six times for growth and eight times for lactation.

Requirement of Protein

In cervids, maintenance rations should contain at least 10-12% crude protein, whereas rations for lactation or antler growth should provide 14-18% crude protein. Growing rations should contain 16-20% crude protein for elk. Fawns require 22-25 % CP in diet for maximum growth (Ramirez *et al.*, 1996). If a single diet is fed to all age groups, a diet containing 16-17% crude protein level is optimal. DCP requirement of deer for maintenance was found to be 4.1g/kg$W^{0.75}$ and 5.7g/kg$W^{0.75}$ in captivity and free ranging deer, respectively (Papageorgiou, *et al.*, 1981; Deerfarmer, 2003).

Like other ruminants, elk and other deer can make use of non-protein nitrogen sources to satisfy part of their protein requirements. Rumen microbes transform non-protein nitrogen into microbial protein. The microbial protein passes out of the rumen with the digesta and becomes available for digestion in the lower gastro-intestinal tract. Urea may be used to replace a portion of true protein nitrogen in an elk ration with no adverse results (Deerfarmer, 2003). The proportion of dietary nitrogen lost in urine increases as dietary protein level is increased. When serum protein level decreases, deer recycle nitrogen (Robbins, 1992; Asleson *et al.*, 1996). Amount of urea nitrogen recycled is found to be 0.66-1.98gN/kg$W^{0.75}$, 0.43-1.38gN/kg$W^{0.75}$ for elk and white tailed deer, respectively (Robbins *et al.*, 1974).

During winter, dietary protein intake was moderate. But, diets contained highly digestible new growth of grasses and browses. Deer utilized browses as protein source, because browses are rich in protein. Pregnancy increased requirement of protein slightly, particularly in the first 2 trimesters. Lactation placed the greatest protein demands on a deer. The milk of white-tailed deer contained about 8.2 per cent protein on a wet basis or 36.4 percent on a dry matter basis. Hinds without adequate protein during lactation will probably, not produce poor quality milk, but simply less milk. Hinds with twins had an even higher protein requirement, around 18 per cent in the diet (MSU, 2001).

With the exception of Cebus monkey, protein requirement as % of ME will decrease as the age advances in most of the primates. NRC recommends protein requirement of 12.5 and 10% during pregnancy and lactation, respectively (NRC, 2003).The precise requirement of protein in captive big cats is not known; however, it is generally high and diet must supply at least 19% CP. One of the striking features is the requirement of taurine in case of felids. The taurine requirement has been reported to be 0.04-0.20% of diet. The normal concentration of taurine is 80-120 nmol/ml plasma and 300-600 nmol/ml whole blood (Hedberg *et al.*, 2007).

Nutrition and Health

Nutritional status is intimately linked to health and reproductive output in numerous species. All nutrient categories - energy and protein, fatty acid, fat-soluble vitamin, and mineral imbalances - have been shown directly, as well as indirectly to affect conservation goals of captive breeding.

Energy

Over-nutrition, with accompanying obesity, is a health issue for many captive psittacines, and may negatively impact reproduction in these species. Over condition can also be problematic for health of zoo primates, carnivores, and hoof stock leading to problems with diabetes, respiratory and cardiac distress, hypertension, hypercholesteremia, foot/hoof problems, and reduced reproduction (Taylor and Poole, 1998; Von Houwald and Flach, 1998; Schwitzer and Kaumanns, 2001; Kenny *et al.*, 2003). We need to develop a series of species-specific body condition indices, similar to those developed for domestic livestock and pet species and for captive species (Videon *et al.*, 2007). These standardized scores can then be used to establish guidelines for amount of diet to be fed

Protein Malnutrition and It's Impact on Health of Captive Animals

Excess protein can also prove detrimental to animal health. Within weeks of switching from a high (>40% crude protein on a dry matter (DM) basis) to a low (<10%) protein nectar diet that better duplicated native diet composition, humming birds successfully reproduced (Brice and Grau, 1989).

A wide variability exists in commercial nectar product composition (Frederick *et al.*, 2003), with protein ranging from 2 to >20% of DM; these ranges appear to encompass levels that can prove harmful to captive populations of nectarivores (Frederick *et al.*, 2003). Similarly, the vulturine parrot (*Psittrichas fulgidus*), a fig specialist, experienced health problems associated with excessive dietary protein (kidney disease, poor reproduction and growth) on diets containing approximately 20% crude protein (DM basis). Nitrogen balance trials confirmed that adults of this species can maintain protein balance on diets containing only 2% protein (Pryor *et al.*, 2001). A similar trend regarding a link between diet and disease in the Goeldi's monkey, or callimico (*Callimico goeldii*) has also been observed. Diets containing more than 25% crude protein (DM basis), have been linked with kidney disease, poor growth and reproduction. These problems have not been reported in animals, where diets contained approximately, 15% protein in accordance with the newly updated National Research Council recommendations for non-human primates (NRC, 2003).

Health Problems of Zoo Animals Associate with Fatty Acid Deficiency

Imbalanced omega-6: omega-3 fatty acid ratios have been associated with immune system, neurologic disorders and abnormalities of carbohydrate metabolism in the black rhinoceros (Miller, 1995). Freshly-harvested browses contained about 15 times higher concentrations of α-linolenic acid (an omega-3) than linoleic acid (an omega-6 FA). However, when fed in captivity, diets for this species showed the opposite proportions, with linoleic acid levels about 5 fold higher than seen in nature, and linolenic acid, about 1/3 that in native browsers (Grant *et al.*, 2002). Clinical investigations with zoo rhinos showed a health response to dietary FA supplementation with a flax-based product that favourably altered circulating omega-3: omega-6 ratios; the typical zoo diet had the opposite effect on plasma FA ratios (Suedmeyer and Dierenfeld, 1998). Zoo diets themselves may predispose to FA deficiency/imbalances, as the most common sources of linoleic acid (the omega-6 eicosanoids) include typical ingredients in formulated rations: corn, safflower, cottonseed, soybean and sunflower oils. The omega-6 FA are prinflammatory, associated with allergies, psoriasis, arthritis and colitis. Linolenic acids (including the omega-3 eicosanoids) are found in green leafy plants, canola, flax, walnut, fish and seafood oils and have the opposite effects on immune function.

Fatty Acids and Reproduction

Fatty acids also have effects upon animal reproduction. Sperm morphology and motility is positively correlated with polyunsaturated fatty acid (PUFA) concentrations, and avian sperm has been shown to contain lower levels of PUFA, compared with mammalian sperm. We know that dietary FA supplements can alter the n-3: n-6 PUFA ratios; increased fertility has been demonstrated and implemented in livestock breeding programs, as well as in reptiles (alligators). Fatty acid concentrations and amounts also impact gonadotrophic hormone production. An area yet to be investigated thoroughly is the effect of varying dietary FA concentrations on elephant sperm quality (and ultimately, reproduction). African elephant sperm has been demonstrated to have viability following freeze-thaw cycles, hence can be used successfully in artificial insemination programs. Asiatic elephant sperm, however, is not as viable following freezing (Swain and Miller, 2003). Dietary FA effects on semen membrane characteristics need to be investigated in more detail to better understand the links between nutrition and reproduction in a variety of species.

Health Problems of Captive Animals Associated with Mineral Deficiency

Mineral imbalances have long been recognized in zoo species – the first documented nutrition problems in large carnivores fed meat-based diets, and primates and birds raised primarily on fruits – were reported from the London Zoo. Unfortunately many kinds of foods are low in calcium and have Ca: P ratio less than 1. Excessive use of fruits, seeds or grains, muscle meat and insects can have severe consequences for zoo animals. Demineralization of bone, tetany and eventual death may occur as animals deplete skeletal store of Ca. Grain and plant protein source contain more P than Ca, but much of the P may be unavailable if it is bound to phytate. P deficiency may well be the most critical mineral deficiency in grazing mammals (Underwood and Suttle, 1999).

Deficiency of Mg, Na, Cl and S are generally, not seen in zoo animals. However, Na deficiency may result from excessive perspiration during extreme hot climate. Although iron deficiency is rare in healthy animals receiving solid foods, dietary iron may be important for animals that has become anemic as a consequence of blood loss. Many mammalian milk, including cow's milk, contain low concentration of iron. Use of cow's milk in hand rearing program may lead to iron deficiency if iron supplements are not added. Deficiency of copper usually unseen in zoo animals, may result from licking of metallic cages, due to excessive zinc, as has been reported in a monkey. Deficiency of iodine may occur in areas deficient in iodine and or presence of excessive goitrogenic substances in the diet. In such case, iodine salt @ 0.05 to 0.1 ppm is to be supplemented. In normal feeding situation, zoo animals may not experience deficiency of manganese and cobalt. However, captive birds fed largely on maize may develop Mn deficiency symptoms, which may be reversed by supplementation of Mn @ 40ppm. The relatively high cobalt (0.1ppm) requirement of wild ruminant is due to the inefficiency of absorption in the small intestine. The zinc content of feedstuff varies greatly. Plants that are high in zinc may also be high in phytate, so that the availability of the zinc is low. Zinc deficiency is more likely, when diets do not contain animal feed sources. Selenium deficiency becomes more probable as dietary concentration drops below 0.05 ppm, although white tailed deer consuming a diet of 0.04 ppm of Se was not pathologically deficient. Chlorinated hydrocarbons may raise the requirement, since they apparently interfere in selenium metabolism (Robbins, 1992).

Large herbivores often retain excess of iron (Smith *et al.*, 1995). The natural forage contains more chelator and less iron than those cultivated ones fed to zoo animals. Superoxides are converted to hydroxyl radicals under the catalytic effect of iron. Limiting dietary iron or increasing its chelator will increase the antioxidant activity. Feeding of tannin rich feed, which acts as a chelator, increased the anti-oxidant activity in mule deer and rhinoceros (Clauss *et al.*, 2003).

Apart from these health aspects, mineral nutrition also has direct and indirect effects on animal reproduction. Lesser adjutant stork (*Leptoptilos javanicus*) chicks fed whole prey containing 2% Ca (DM basis) developed beak and leg deformities indicative of calcium deficiency/imbalance - even though their diet appeared adequate in both Ca and P (Dierenfeld and Fidget, 2003). Further, comparisons of semen characteristics in cats fed a nutritionally-complete commercial feline diet compared to chicken necks or red meat revealed improved motility (40 to 56%), % normal sperm (9 to 20%), and an increase in the amount of sperm per ejaculate (up to 10 times more; Swanson *et al.*, 1994).

Vitamin Deficiencies and Their Impact on Captive Animals Health

Vitamin A deficiencies are far common in captive than in free ranging wildlife because of feeding of inadequate diets. For examples, captive carnivores fed exclusively on carcass meat without liver, cod liver oil or synthetic sources of vitamin A and granivorous birds are prone to deficiencies. Coupled with the inadequacy of a pure meat diet, a higher requirement may exist for cats, polar bears and other specialized carnivores. Hand reared armadillos and polar bear cubs developed several clinical signs suggestive of vitamin A deficiency. Similarly a captive white tailed deer being fed winter browse very low in carotene became blind.

One must be very careful in supplementing diets of captive animals with vitamin A because it can be toxic if fed in excess. Laboratory-reared whole rodents have been found to contain vitamin A concentrations more than 10-fold those measured in free-ranging rodents (Thomas *et al.*, 2004), and may result in spondylysis. Typical signs of hypervitaminosis A include internal haemorrhage, yellow discolouration of the liver and fat deposits, weight loss, deformed embryos, bone fracture and reduced reproduction. Because of very high liver storage capabilities of marine mammals for vitamin A, some of the classical cases of hypervitaminosis- A have occurred when human have consumed polar bear liver (Robbins, 1992).

Vitamin A is also linked with reproduction, both directly and indirectly. Deficiency leads to impaired sperm production, birth defects and reduced immunity, whereas excess has been associated with teratogenicity (Olson, 1984). Additionally, β-carotene added to diets of domestic cats has been shown to increase progesterone, estradiol and uterine protein content (Chew *et al.*, 2001). Deficiency symptoms can occur within several days to weeks if dietary or irradiation sources are inadequate. Ring necked pheasant without dietary vitamin D_3 or sunlight developed rickets starting the fifth day after hatching. Non-supplemented domestic cow's milk and perhaps, the milk of many other species whose youngs normally experience sun light shortly after birth are severely deficient in vitamin D and hence, require either dietary supplementation if the animal is bottle raised, or exposure of the young animal to sunlight. For example, captive maternal nursed snow-leopard and cape hunting dog developed rickets when not allowed exercising outside. Among the largest naturally occurring sources of vitamin D_3 available for dietary supplementation is fish oil, particularly liver oils. Supplementation from such sources is unusual, since few animal products contain any significant quantity of vitamin D_3, purified vitamin D_2 and D_3 are also commercially available. Thus, supplementation of the diet of captive animals can be achieved easily, although overdose should be avoided since they are quite detrimental (Robbin, 1992).

By comparison, vitamin E nutrition has been evaluated in much more detail in zoo species (Dierenfeld and Traber, 1992, Dierenfeld, 1994). Clinical signs of deficiency vary by species, but can include: skeletal/cardiac myopathies (in any species, but particularly in hoofstock), equine degenerative myoencephalopathy (in equids), microangiopathy (noted in swine and elephant species), erythrocyte hemolysis (primates including humans), exudative diathesis (avian species) and steatisis in carnivores (Dierenfeld and Traber, 1992). Although vitamin E occurs in many common foods and feeds, numerous deficiencies in captive wildlife fed diets based on frozen fish have been reported. Relatively high concentration of poly-unsaturated fatty acids in marine fish, the frozen storage of the fish for several months before being fed, and the evisceration of the fish before freezing contribute to the deficiency.

As vitamin K is widespread in food of plant and animal origin, it's deficiency in captive wildlife is rare. Thiamin has been studied far more frequently, than all other water-soluble vitamins needed by wildlife. Thiamin deficiency has been reported in captive Atlantic bottle nose dolphin, herring gull, seals, polar bear cubs, mink, falcon and sea lion, which in most cases were consuming diets composed of raw, dead fish, such as, herring, mackerel, blue runner, alewives and carp. Many species of fresh water fish of the species cyprinidae, contain a thiaminase that destroys thiamin in the fish or in other foods fed during the same meal. Thiaminase is not found in the muscle, but is confined in relatively large concentration in the viscera and trimming, including the head, skin, fins and skeleton. Thiaminase is also found in heart and spleen of warm-blooded animals, newly hatched chicks and bracken fern. Thiamin deficiency can usually be rapidly and easily cured even in near terminally sick animals by the addition of adequate thiamin to the diet or by injecting thiamin hydrochloride. Although, the average thiamin requirement of animals consuming diet devoid of thiaminase 1-2 mg/kg of diet, the effective thiamin requirement of animals consuming diet devoid of thiaminase is 17 mg/kg of diet, the effective thiamin requirement of seals and foxes consuming thiaminase containing fish would be as high as 25-35 and 147 mg/kg diet, respectively (Robbins, 1992). Riboflavin, niacin, pantothanic acid, choline, folacin and pyridoxine metabolism and requirement have been studied in pheasants, quail, mink, guinea pig, primates and virtually, all common laboratory animals (Robbin, 1992). Riboflavin deficiency may occur in captive animals if the diet is contaminated with toxicants interfering in riboflavin metabolism. Biotin deficiency can occur if the diet is high in raw egg white.

Vitamin C is dietary essential for primates, bats, guinea pigs and some fruit eating birds like bulbul, as already mentioned. However, vitamin C should not be ignored even if those species able to synthesize it, since rapid early growth, stress or organochloride pesticides may increase the ascorbic acid requirement beyond the capabilities of endogenous synthesis. Vitamin C is not as widespread, as many of the other water soluble vitamins. The richest sources are green plants and fleshy fruits, such as citrus fruits, but is virtually absent in eggs, seeds, grains, most bacteria and protozoa. Animal tissues are in general poor source of the vitamin (Mc Dowell, 1989).

References

Arora, B.M. (2001). Dietary Husbandry of Wild Mammalia. Central Zoo Authority, New Delhi, India.

Asano, S. Ikeda, S. Kurokawa, Y., Kand, S. and Itabashi, H. (2005) . *Anim. Sci.J.*, 76:447-451.

Asleson, M.A, Hellgren, E.C. and Varner, L.W. (1996). and maintenance in white tailed deer. *J. Wildl. Management.*, 60:744-752.

Bass Pro Outdoors Online. (2006-2007). Deer Nutrition for a Healthier Herd. Bass Pro.com.

Brice, A.T. and Grau. C.R. (1989). *Zoo Biol.*, 8:223-237.

Chew, B.P., Weng, B.C., Kim, H.W., Wong, T.S., Park, J.S. and Lepine, A.J. (2001). *Vet. Res.*, 62A:1063-1067.

Clauss, M., Polster, C., Keinzle, E. and Wiesner, H. (2003). Studies on feed digestibility in captive Asiatic elephant (*Elaphus Maximus*). *J. Anim. Physiol. Anim. Nutr.*, 87: 160-173.

Clauss, M., Polster, C., Keinzle, E., Wiesner, H., Katrin, B., Van Houwald, F., Streich, W.J. and Dierrenfeld, E. (2005). *Zoo Biol.* 24: 1-14.

Deerfarmer.com. (2003). Nutrition requirements for deer and elk. 21:14, Jul. 25.

Dempsey, J., Brit, A., Lambano, B., Sohmidt, D. and Kerley, M. (2002). *Am. J. Primatol.*, 57: 31-38.

Dierenfeld, E.S. (1987). Nutritional considerations in captive tiger management. In:Tiger of the World. R.L. Tilson and U.S. Seal, Eds. Noyes Publications: Park Ridge, NJ. pp-149-160.

Dierenfeld, E.S. (1994). Vitamin E in exotics: effects, evaluation, and ecology. *J. Nutr.*, 124:2579S-2581S.

Dierenfeld, E.S. and Fidget, A.L. (2003). Investigating calcium requirements of growing stork chicks. Proc. AZA Regional Stork Workshop. Columbia, SC.

Dierenfeld, E.S. and Traber, M.G. (1992). Vitamin E status of exotic animals compared with livestock and domestics. In: Vitamin E in health and disease. L. Packer and J. Fuchs, eds. Marcel Decker, Inc, New York. pp. 345-360.

Douglas, T.C., Pennino, M. and Dierenfeld, E.S. (1994). *J. Comp. Biochem. Physiol.*, 107A: 419-424.

Edwards, M.S. (1999). Nutritional management of acute and chronic bloat in eastern giant eland. Proc. 4th Nutr. Advis. Group Conf. pp. 25-29. Columbus, OH.

Enright, W.J., Spicer, L.J., Kelly, M., Culletonn, N. and Prendiville, D.J. (2001). *Small Rumin. Res.*, 39:253-259.

Flint, A.P.E., Albon, S.D. and Jafar, S.I. (1997). Gen. Comp. *Endocrinol.*, 106, 374-383.

Frape, D.L., Tuck, M.G., Sutcliffe, N.H. and Jones, D.E. (1982). *Comp. Biochem. Physiol.*, 72A: 77-83.

Frederick, H., Irlbeck, N. and Dierenfeld, E.S. (2003). Proc. 5th Nutr. Advis. Group Conf. 38-43. Minneapolis, MN.

Fowler, M.E. (1986). Principles of zoo mammal nutrition. Zoo and Wild animal medicine, 2nd edition, pp 516-532.

Garg, A.K. (1996). Nutritional trials in deer. *Wild Inf. Bull.*, 2:6.

Grant, J.B., Brown, D.L. and Dierenfeld, E.S. (2002). *J. Wildl. Dis.*, 38:132-142.

Heusner, A.A. (1982). *Resp. Physiol.,* 48:1.

Hedberg, G.E., Dierenfeld, E.S. and Rogers Q.R. (2007). *Zoo Biol.,* 26:517-531.

Holdo, R.M., Dudley, J.P. and McDowell, L.R. (2002). Elephant. *J. Mammal.,* 83: 652-664.

Howard, J., Roger, Q.R., Koch, S.A., Goodrowe, K.L. Montali, R.J. and Bush, M. (1987). Diet Proc. Am. Meeting Am. Assoc Zoo Vet. Philadelphia. pp. 496-498.

Jenson, B.B. (1986). Environmental Monitoring and Assessment. 42: 99-112.

Kenny, D.E., Knightly, F. Haas B., Hergott, L. Kutinsky, I. and Eller, J.L. (2003). *J. Zoo Wildl. Med.,* 34:394-399.

Kie, J.G., Evans, C.J. and Menke, J.W. (1991). *J. Wildl. Manage.,* 55:665-674.

Knott, C.D. (1999). Reproductive, physiological and behavioral response in Orangutan in Borneo to fluctuation in food availability. Cambridge University Press.

Kucera, T.E. (1997). *J.Mammaol.,* 72:745-749.

Kusmartono, Shimada, A. and Barry, T.N. (1997). *J. Agric. Sci. Camb.,* 128:87-94.

Li, S. and Qin, R. (1991). In: The Biology of Deer, Brown, R.D. (Ed.), Springer-Verlag, London pp-450-455.

Luna-Estrada, A.A., Avila, H.R.V., Mora, O., Serrano, B.A., Carlos, C., Pelaez, V. and Shimada, A. (2006). Small Rumin. Res. 65:154-160.

Mc Dowell, L.R. (1989). Vitamin in Animal Nutrition, Academic Press, San Diego, CA.

McBece, R.H., Johnson, J.L. and Bryont, M. (1969). *J. Wildlife Management.,* 33: 181-186.

Miller, R.E. (1995). Verh. Ber. Erkrg. Zootiere., 37:47.

Milton, K. (1981). Food choice and digestive strategies of two sympatric primate species. *The American Naturalist.,* 117, 496-505.

MSU. (2001). Extension Service. Dept. Wildlife & Fisheries. MSU cares.com.

Nagy, K.A. (2001). *Austr. J. Zool.,* 42: 43-53.

Nagy, K.A. (2005). Field metabolic rate and body size. *J. Exp. Biol.,* 208: 1621-1625.

NRC. (2003). Nutrient Requirements of Non-Human Primates, 2nd revised edition. National Academy of Sciences, Washington, DC.

Oftedal, O.T. and Allen, M.E. (1997). Nutrition and dietary evaluation in Zoos. In: Wild mammals in captivity: principles and technique: Eds. Kloman, D.G., Allen, M.E., Thompson, K.V. and Lumpkin, S. Chicago University Press Chicago, USA.

Olson, J.A. (1984). Vitamin A In: Handbook of vitamins:nutritional, biochemical, and clinical aspects. L.J. Macklin, editor. Marcel Decker, Inc.: New York. pp. 1-44.

Papageorgiou, N.; Neophytou, C.; Spais, A. and Vavalekas, C. (1981) J. *Wildl. Manage.,* 45:728-732.

Parker.K.L., Robbins, C.T. and Hanley, T.A. (1984). *J.Wildl.Manage.*, 48:474-488.

Pathak, N.N., Pattanaik, A.K., Patra, R.C. and Arora, B.M. (2001). *Small Rumin. Res.*, 42: 61-65.

Pryor, G.S., Levey, D.J. and Dierenfeld. E.S. (2001). *The Auk* 118:1080-1088.

Ramirez, R.G., Haenlein, G.F.W., Trevino, A. and Reyna, J. (1996). *Small Rumin. Res.*, 23: 7-16.

Robbins, C.T. (1992), Wildlife Feeding and Nutrition, Academic Pres, New York.

Robbins, C.T., Moen R.L. and Visek, W.J. (1974). *J.Anim.Sci.*, 38:186-191.

Rode, K.D., Chiyo, P.I., Chapman, A. and McDowell, L.R. (2006). *J. Tropical Ecol.*, 22: 441-449.

Roger, M.E., Maiseh, F., Williumson, E.A., Fernandez, M. and Tutin, C.E.G. (1990). *A Oecologia.*, 84: 326-339.

Sadlier, R.M.F.S. (1980). Can.J.Zool., 58: 1347-1354.

Sanyal, R.H. (1892). A handbook of the management of wild animals in captivity in Lower Bengal, Bengal Secretariat Press, Calcutta.

Schmidt, D.A., Kerley, M.S., Poster, J.H. and Dempsey, J.L. (2005). *Zoo Biol.*, 24: 359-373.

Schwitzer, C. and Kaumanns, W. (2001). *Zoo Biol.*, 20:61-269.

Smith, S.H., Holter, J.B., Hayes, H.H. and Silver. H. (1995). *J.Wildl. Manage.*, 39:582-589.

Suedmeyer, W.K. and Dierenfeld, E.S. (1998). Clinical experience with fatty acid supplementation in a group of black rhinoceros (*Diceros bicornis*). Proc. AAZV, Omaha, NE. pp. 113-115.

Suresh, C. (2008). Study on effect of feeding two different levels of energy on nutrient utilization in captive spotted deer. M.V.Sc. Thesis, IVRI (Deemed University), Izatnagar, India.

Swain, J.E. and Miller, R.R. (2003). *Zoo Biol.*, 19: 461-473.

Swanson, W.F., Howard J., Roth, T., Kaemmerer, K., Alvarado, T., Burton, M., Starnes, D., Sims, L. and Collins. L. (1994). Felid Taxon Advisory Group Action Plan.

Taylor, V.J. and Poole, T.B. (1998). *Zoo Biol.*, 17:311-332.

Thomas, J., Glatt, B. and Dierenfeld. E.S. (2004). *Zoo Biol.*, 23:253 - 261.

Underwood, E.J. and Suttle, N.F. (1999). The mineral nutrition of livestock 3rd ed., CABI, Publishing, Farnham, UK

Van Hoven, W., Prins, R.A. and Lankhorst, A. (1981). *S. Afr. J. Wild Res.*, 11:78-86.

Van Soest, P. J., Robertson, J. B. and Lewis, B. A. (1991). *J. Dairy Sci.*, 74:3583-3587.

VanSoest, P.J. (1994). Nutritional ecology of the ruminants, 2nd ed., Cornell University Press, 9th Academy.

Verme, L.J. and Ozoga, J.J. (1980). *J.Wildl.Manage.*, 44:305-314.

Videon, E.N., Fritz, J. and Murphy, J. (2007).development of guidelines for assessing obesity in captive chimpanzee. *Zoo Biol.*, 26:93-104.

Von Houwald, F. and Flach, E.J. (1998). Prevalence of chronic foot disease in captive greater one-horned rhinoceros (*Rhinoceros unicornis*). *Proc. Eur. Assoc. Zoo Wildl. Vet.*, 2: 323-327.

Yeager, C.P., Silver, S.C. and Dierrenfeld, E.S. (1997). *Am. J. Primatol.*, 41: 117-128.

□□□

Animal Nutrition, 2012
eds. Dr. (Mrs.) Usha R. Mehra et al., pp. 329-350
Satish Serial Publishing House e-mail : info@satishserial.com; website : www.satishserial.com

Chapter 15

Feeding and Nutrition of Animals at High Altitude

A. SAHOO

High altitude regions in India are mostly confined to Himalayan mountains. The area is characterized with considerably large area under rangelands which are uncultivated areas or abandoned cultivated areas and occasionally, fallow lands that harbour natural or seeded/planted vegetation of herbaceous and woody species and that serves as habitats of a variety of wild and domesticated animals and provide unique products and ecosystem services, especially vital for the livelihoods of livestock-dependent communities. Animals living at high altitude encounter several environmentally induced challenges including increased wind speeds, severe cold temperatures, intermittent and inconsistent rain and thunderstorms and decreased partial pressures of oxygen. Several animals have adapted to these conditions and are thus capable of living at high altitude. High altitude presents an adverse environment that challenges the physiological processes in the body. At high altitude (1700–2600m), alpine cattle had higher respiration rates, body temperatures, higher resting heart rates and greater blood volume than the valley cattle. In addition to strategic general (housing, environment) and health management practices, nutritional intervention warrants meeting the challenges of stressful conditions for sustaining livestock production in this region.

Animals at High Altitude

One third of the country's land mass is covered under hills. The hill regions, spread out in most of the states and notably in Himachal, Uttarakhand, J&K and NE region, represent unique agricultural and livestock production system largely rain-fed, bereft of defined bovine breeds, but having excellent breeds of sheep, goat, horse (pony), yak and mithun. The typical environment of sub-Himalayan region with natural grasslands support livestock breeds (e.g. Gaddi sheep) and defined populations (e.g. Terai buffalo). Besides, a large number of undefined breeds and populations abound in all the species *viz.* cattle (e.g. Kumauni, Motu, Ladakhi, Thotho), buffalo (e.g. Terai, Assamese, Sikamese, Ching Iroi), sheep (e.g. Biangi, Ghurpala, Monpa), goat (e.g. Assam-Hill, Baltistani, Chogerkha, Kel), pony (e.g. Sakawar), pig (e.g. Doom, Ponree, Zovawk), and poultry (e.g. Dumsi, Nangey). Such lesser known breeds are well adapted in respective geographical tracts, utilize the local fodder resources and also provide valuable nutrition and livelihood opportunities.

Hill Ecology and Livestock Production

The mountain ecosystems tend to be relatively unstable, non-resilient, and of low inherent productivity. Thus, a typical family's livelihood is based mainly on the farm, various livestock, common pasture and forest, and economic activities unrelated to the farm. The common features of livestock production systems of rural underprivileged families are i) mixed farming system and diversified crop and livestock activities ii) low external input-low output and highly internalised system making maximum use of available resources like crop residues, feed, labour, animal waste etc., iii) extensive grazing with limited supplementary feeding in semi-arid/arid areas and limited grazing/semi-stall feeding in other areas, iv) local breeds of livestock/poultry preferred over 'improved' stock as part of risk management, except in areas where there is organisational support, v) traditional systems of livestock management and feeding are preferred and adoption of scientific recommendations or technologies is very low, vi) livestock output is low, but represents major share of daily cash income to family and vii) women plays major role in livestock production and sale of produce (Sahoo *et al.,* 2008).

Livestock production processes have both positive and negative effects on environment. The positive effects include i) managed grazing improves species (flora) wealth, ii) mixed farming (crop cultivation and livestock keeping) enhances water infiltration and recharges groundwater reserves, iii) mixed farming sustains the resource base and iv) mixed farming effects resource enhancement and supports resource sparing. The negative effects are i) land degradation, ii) deforestation (loss of bio-diversity), iii) waste production, iv) pollution–land, water and air. The other major role of livestock is the transfer of basic plant nutrients from the forest and grasslands to cultivated lands, in the form of manure. This cycle of transfer obliges the farmer to keep large numbers of animals, which has resulted in having the greatest number of livestock in the hill regions of the country. But, with increasing human population, dependency on traditional agricultural systems that exerts pressure upon the land that is unsupportable and hill farmers' efforts to increase agricultural production to meet their requirements for basic survival, have exacerbated an already critical situation, leading to further intensification of the downward spiral of decline in soil fertility and environmental degradation, as more marginal areas are brought into cultivation, and forests are overexploited to support livestock and humans alike. Thus, the major limitation faced in hill livestock production is a deficit in feed, which has placed the whole region into ecological imbalance. The critical time of fodder/forage shortage is during the dry winter period (November - April), and forest serves as the major supplier during this period. Although the contribution of forest to fodder production varies from place to place (Table 1), the forests in the hills are generally exploited for fodder collection, and are utilized for free grazing and browsing. Forest biomass and livestock are crucial components in this process, both to exploit and cycle the nutrients available in the region. Depletion of forest resources through foraging and use as bedding material by the livestock sector and for farmland use and composting by the agricultural sector is a continuous process and this needs to be sustained. Otherwise, this may result into a vicious cycle of low productive soil-crop-livestock-forest sub-sectors (Fig. 1).

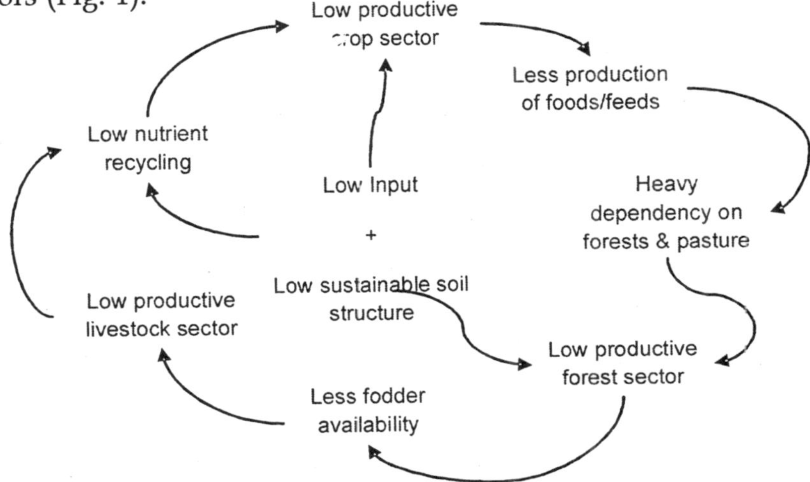

Fig. 1 : Vicious cycle of crop-livestock-forest sub-sectors

Table 1 : Forest dependent population in different regions of India (in proportion to thousand)

Agro-ecological region	Timber	Fuel wood	Fodder	Other leaves	others
Western Himalaya	338	880	741	704	28
Eastern Himalaya & Brahmaputra Valley	294	704	346	360	160
Central plateu & Hills	366	756	342	349	204
Eastern plateu & Hills	156	492	346	189	134
Western plateu & Hills	100	643	322	315	61
Southern plateu & Hills	151	573	283	314	103

Feed and Fodder Resources

Crop by-products and grasses from forests and cultivated land, and fodder from the forest constitute the main forage source for animals. The major feed resources are pasture, and fodder in summer and crop residues, particularly maize stover, grass hay and tree lopping during winter. There are basically three feed resources, such as crop residues, rangeland biomass and grazing on the side of water channel and fallow lands. Because of the small landholdings and the limited irrigation facility, only a relatively small area is planted for fodder. Farmers employ a variety of strategies to meet fodder requirements, but crop residues and stubble grazing remains the mainstay of winter nutritional support. Because the hill agriculture production system has a multidisciplinary approach, without which no sustainable agriculture can be conducted, some farmers have adopted an agro-forestry system, planting fodder/fuelwood trees and cereal crops together on the terrace risers of 'Bariland', and on the bunds of 'Khetland'. Though, the actual loss in crop yield from competition from the trees has yet to be fully quantified, farmers do report an adverse effect on crop yields. However, the need for trees to supply fodder to the livestock has obliged the retention of trees in and around cultivated land, and the losses in crop yield are accepted as part of the price to be paid to sustain the system. The vegetable crops grown in the hills can also provide a source of fodder. Though, their contribution as livestock feed has been neglected by many researchers, considerable amounts are used by farmers as an animal feed. Data on the amounts of fodder available from green vegetables after utilization for human consumption are not available, but one rough estimate shows that various vegetables, such as cabbage, cauliflower, radish, peas, can give at times nearly 50% of feed/fodder of the total mass of vegetable grown (Sahoo, 2005). Many people having orchards also fed animals on damaged/waste apple, pears and other fruits. The traditional feed resources and feeding practices are summarized below.

- Summer grazing in high altitude, alpine pastures are exploited to the maximum
- Local grasses at fallow and forest land, people used to preserve as hay to feed during lean season.
- Excluding alpine/forest grazing, livestock feed resources are derived mostly from maize stover, vegetable crop residues, straws (millet, rice, wheat, etc.) and leaves from trees and shrubs.
- Farmers deliberately select tall growing wheat and maize varieties, which produce relatively low grain yields, but large amounts of straws and stovers. The crop residues are carefully conserved and stored, often on roofs or in trees.
- Multi-purpose trees like willow (*Salix spp.*), mulberry (*Morus spp.*), poplar (*Populus spp.*), oaks (*Quercus spp.*), etc. are planted on field edges and marginal land. Their leaves and shoots provide supplementary fodder in winter and woods serve as fuel. In some areas, leaves are dried and stored for winter use. Some other fodder species at relatively lower altitude are Biul (*Grewia spp.*), Kachanar, *Acacia spp., Ficus spp., Dendrocalamus spp., Robinia spp. etc.*

Out of the total geographical area of 328 m ha in the country, pastures are spread over 12 m ha (3.9%) and sustain a livestock population of 406 million. Analyzing the estimates of availability (500 MT) to requirements (800 MT) a gap of around 300 MT of feed and fodder from all sources green fodder from arable area, forests & wastelands, top feeds and agrowastes commulates to the problems of insufficiency. There is a need to evaluate the existing resources of the sub-Himalayan pastures to meet the production potential of the native animals and for the up keep of the improved germplasm. With the exception of some farmers in the double-cropped areas, who may have access to fodder produced elsewhere, most farmers do not procure additional feed supplies. The shortfall is made up almost entirely by summer grazing. However, many animals are poorly fed during the summer months and enter the winter in poor condition and thus, experience a nutritional shortfall throughout the year. Winter feed derived from mature maize stover and dried grass is high in fibre, but low in digestible energy and protein. Maize and grass are harvested late, when fibre content and quantity are at their highest. This deliberate strategy links to the scarcity of forage and the long tradition of under-feeding. Farmers know that fibrous feed slows down digestion, thus enabling livestock on less fodder over the winter. Many animals, however, are physically unable to consume sufficient quantities to satisfy their needs and lose considerable bodyweight during the course of winter. Thus, a significant proportion of the livestock- particularly, lactating cows and goats are deficient in protein, energy, trace elements and vitamins. The estimates indicated that there is a severe deficiency of digestible protein and total digestible nutrients to the tune of 50 and 40 per cent, respectively (calculated figures based on availability and requirement). This deficiency has resulted into low production performance of both small and large ruminants. The nutrient composition of different feed resources available at high altitude regions is presented in Tables 2 and 3.

Table 2 : Chemical composition of some important tree forages

Species	OM	CP	EE	CF	NFE	NDF	ADF	Lignin	Ash	Tannin
Acacia catechu	94.7	23.4	2.5	12.1	56.8	58.0	28.5	14.7	5.3	2.8
Albizzia stipulata	93.4	22.3	3.6	30.5	37.0	68.1	47.1	20.5	6.6	4.2
Albizzia chiinensis	92.4	19.8	I.9	10.3	6.5	-	42.4	22.3	7.6	1.9
Artocarpus lakoocha	86.9	15.8	I.8	19.8	49.5	49.9	36.7	8.9	13.1	0.6
Bauhinia variagata	93.5	14.7	1.8	31.6	50.6	62.7	46.8	-	6.5	-
Bahuinia retusa	94.2	5.8	6.0	-	-	39.7	31.6	11.7	5.8	6.7
Bridela retusa	94.0	16.9	2.4	19.4	55.4	43.5	26.0	7.6	6.0	12.8
Carissa spinarum	91.8	10.2	4.2	15.4	62.0	30.7	23.1	13.2	8.2	5.4
Celtis australis	89.8	16.8	2.5	13.8	56.7	39.8	21.2	8.1	10.2	1.7
Dendrocalamus hookeri	89.5	16.8	2.1	25.9	44.8	66.8	38.4	-	10.5	-
Dendrocalamus hamiltonii	84.4	19.8	2.3	25.2	37.1	78.4	47.7	8.6	15.6	0.6
Ficus roxburghii	86.6	16.7	1.7	18.1	50.1	52.9	41.6	7.8	13.4	-
Garuga pinnata	88.8	13.7	3.4	15.4	58.3	45.2	27.1	8.7	11.2	2.7
Grewia optiva	88.7	24.4	3.8	15.3	45.2	48.4	25.9	4.3	11.3	1.8
Grewia opositifolia	88.6	12.5	1.9	21.0	53.1	46.7	33.6	6.8	11.4	1.3
Hipophae rhamnoides	92.1	21.8	4.5	13.8	52.0	43.2	19. 1	8.6	7.9	10.3
Leucaena leucocephala	90.4	19.1	2.1	18.6	50.7	46.0	28.2	15.2	9.6	0.6
Melia azedarach	90.4	28.0	1.6	1 0.0	50.8	31.1	22.1	3.9	9.6	0.6
Morus alba	86.6	20.2	3.8	17.8	44.8	43.3	28.0	4.2	13.4	15.1
Morus multicaulis	84.4	16.6	7.4	15.5	44.9	33.1	23.0	9.1	15.6	-
Populus ciliata	93.0	14.6	6.9	-	-	55.7	27.9	6.7	7.0	4.86
Populus deltoids	86.8	14.1	3.5	20.5	48.7	52.1	39.3	10.3	13.2	-
Quercus incana	96.2	8.4	3.5	34.1	50.3	62.1	47.0	20.1	3.8	4.6
Quercus semicaprifolia	95.6	10.1	6.0	-	-	63.1	49.1	21.6	4.4	6.4
Quercus leucotricofora	96.3	9.4	6.3	-	-	55.4	41.6	17.2	3.7	7.7
Robinia pseudoacacia	91.1	24.4	2.5	20.6	43.6	67.1	44.8	27.2	8.9	1.0
Zizyphus jujuba	91.0	20.2	1.9	20.5	48.4	41.4	26.1	14.1	9.0	5.4
Zizyphus nummularia	91.0	17.7	1.8	22.8	48.8	44.1	27.8	10.8	9.0	4.8

Table 3 : Nutrient composition of high-altitude pasture and some promising fodder of the Himalayan region

Plant species	CP%	TDN%	ME (Mcal/kg DM)
Anaphalis contarta	9.4	-	-
Anaphalis triplensis	15.2	-	-
Chrysopogon echinulatus	8.3-11.1	55.0	1.98
Chrysopogon montanus	5.1-9.3	-	-
Cyananthus microphyllus	14.3	60.0	2.16
Fescue alpinum	15.0-22.0	60.0-72.0	2.16-2.59
Geramium donainum	10.2	-	-
Geranium aconitofolium	13.4	-	-
Heictotrichon pretense	7.1	-	-
Hemiphroma heterophylls	11.3	-	-
Heteropogon contortus	6.1-8.0	40.0-50.0	1.44-1.80
Hippophae rhamnoides	17.5-20.0	45.0-60.0	1.62-2.16
Hippophae salicifolia	21.6	52.0	1.87
Hippophae tibetana	20.5	-	-
Iris clarkei	8.7	-	-
Juncus membranaceous	8.7	-	-
Pennisetum orientale	20.9	65.0-72.0	2.34-2.59
Penesetum clandestinum	10.9	50.0-60.0	1.80-2.16
Phacelurus spaciosa	11.0	48.0-550.	1.73-1.98
Pimpuella trifoliata	11.3	-	-
Pipanthus nepalensis	19.4	65.0-70.0	2.34-2.52
Polygonum alatum	13.4	55.0-58.0	1.98-2.09
Polygonum amplexicoule	13.6	60.0	2.16
Polygonum polystachyon	18.4	62.0-70.0	2.23-2.52
Populus ciliata	18.0	-	-
Populus euphratica	14.0-18.1	50.0	1.80
Populus grandidentata	7.0-10.0	45.0-52.0	1.62-1.87
Populus nigra	15.0-21.0	30.0-45.0	1.08-1.62
Populus tremula	12.8	68.0	2.45
Populus tremuloides	12.0-21.0	55.0-70.0	1.98-2.52
Potentilla argycophyl!a	11.1-15.2	-	-
Potentilla leschanaultiana	12.9	-	-
Potentilla penduncularis	9.5	55.0	1.98
Potentilla polyphylla	13.2	-	-
Selenium veginatume	21.2	>60.0	>2.16

Contd...

Senecio alatus	10.6	-	-
Tanecetum longifolium	10.6-11.0	50.0-58.0	1.80-2.09
Thuja occidentalis	8.0-13.0	55.0-65.0	1.98-2.34
Tritoliunt repens	19.1	55.0-70.0	1.98-2.52
Trigonella foenum-graecum	13.1	-	-

N.B. Nutritive value of some of the pasture/fodder species.

Nutrient Requirements

Interaction with altitude and cold climate

The food requirement of animals can be estimated by calculating the amount of food needed to provide the requisite amount of ME for maintaining its state of production. The values on fasting heat production (FHP) are similar to the results of most previous studies on cattle at similar altitude, but different from cattle when yaks are kept at higher altitudes (Sahoo and Singh, 2004). FHP is measured at three different altitudes of 2260, 3250 and 4270 m on the Tibetan plateau in both summer and winter, after a 90 d adaptation period at each experimental site. Increasing altitude at similar ambient temperature (Ta) does not affect (P>0·10) FHP in the summer, but decreases (P<0·05) it at different Ta in the winter. The decrease of FHP in the winter is attributed to the decrease of Ta, rather than the increase of altitude. At all altitudes for all groups, the daily FHP is higher (P<0·05) in the summer (Ta 6–24°C) than in the winter (Ta 0 to -30°C), and the Ta-corrected FHP becomes on 920 kJ/kg $BW^{0·52}$ at Ta 8–14°C and 704 kJ/kg $BW^{0·52}$ at Ta -15°C, respectively. This suggests that high altitude has no effect on the energy metabolism in yak, whereas the cold ambient temperature has significant depressing effect. An estimate of daily food intake depends primarily, on data obtained from practical feeding trials. However, the recorded data needs scientific validation based on information from the local people, chemical composition of available pasture/fodder species, *in vitro* and *in sacco* study trials. Nutritional adequacy, on the other hand, needs assessment of the availability of feed and nutrients and sustainability for a particular state of production without affecting the productive life cycle of the animal. The time spent on grazing is dependent on the amount of forage consumed, and the relative availability of herbage. Therefore, free ranging animals pay relatively higher costs of foraging for dispersed foods, avoiding or battling predators and parasites, dealing with more extreme climatic conditions, and interacting socially with other species competing for the same pasture or fodder resources (Sahoo, 2005). The additional supply of nutrients in terms of energy (TDN) thus, ranges from 11-22% higher than that by lactating cattle reared in plains. The energy and protein requirements in Table 3 emphasize a proportional supply of DM to have 60-70% TDN and 7-13% CP at different intake and production levels.

The data on feed intake and digestibility (Table 5), many a times fails to meet the major nutrient requirements (CP and TDN), even for maintenance.

Metabolism and feed intake

Animals at high altitude exhibit various adoptive and behavioural changes when environmental temperature lowers which include variation in terrain or other topographical features, such as windbreaks, huddling in groups or changes in pasture to minimize heat loss. Physiological adoptions include changes in basal metabolism, respiration rate, and distribution of blood flow to skin and lungs, feed and water consumption, rate of passage of feed through the digestive tract, hair coat and body composition or distribution of fat. Subcutaneous fat provides insulation and reduces the heat loss for maintaining the body warm. Shivering also helps in heat production. There is a need for documentation of data from practical experimental feeding trial to validate nutritive value of different feeds and fodder as per seasonal availability for feeding the livestock. Nutritional husbandry of captive wild ruminants often requires feeding these animals a supplemental diet to enhance their health, reproductive performance, and productivity. Voluntary intake of dry matter, energy, and nitrogen was similar between mountain goats and mountain sheep (Baker *et al.*, 1998). Differences in digestive efficiency among species are inversely related to dry matter intake rates, and species comparisons are seemed to be inconclusive because of the confounding effects of season and ambient temperature on voluntary intake and digestion (Sahoo, 2005).

Seasonality of metabolism

The most remarkable adaptation of cervids is well-developed seasonality of metabolism and productive functions, but debate on whether appetite, metabolic demand or productive functions drive the circannual bioenergetic cycle is still on, because these cycles are adaptations to meager winter (northern and temporate regions) or summer (tropical regions) feed supplies. Energy expenditures also show seasonal cycles although, the cycle is strongly influenced by feed intake, thermoregulation, and activity. The differences between metabolic rates measured in captivity and those in the field are largely hypothetical. The size of the animal, expressed as body mass (or metabolic body size), explains most of the difference in whole-animal fasting metabolic rate (FMR) between species, with larger animals generally (but, not always) using more total energy each day than do smaller ones. The food requirement of an animal can thus be estimated from its energy requirement by calculating the amount of food needed to provide that amount of metabolisable energy (ME). Animals that are held captive will probably, but not necessarily have lower daily food need than those due to lower activity levels and more benign microclimates than those they experience in nature. The FMR for a species, in units of kcal/d, is divided by the ME content of its diet, either in units of Mcal/kg dry or fresh matter, to calculate feeding rates in units of g dry matter intake (DMI)/d or in units of g fresh matter intake (FMI)/d. The conversion factor for mammalian herbivores is 3.87Mcal/kg DMI or 1.06 Mcal/kg FMI (Nagy, 2001). Free-living animals that are growing or reproducing or storing fat for winter or migration will have feeding rates that are higher than estimated for the steady-state situation. Similarly, animal uses body stores of energy during migration will have actual feeding rate that is lower than calculated. Generally, herbivorous mammals have higher food needs during the lactation period for nursing mothers and the migration period for many migratory species (buffalo, sheep and goat, yak, mithun, etc.). Further, the foods given to captive animals are usually of higher quality (more ME per kg of dry or fresh matter), so less biomass needs to be consumed, and this reduces food requirements. Also, animals spent less time, as well as energy for mastication and regurgitation and a reduced metabolic cost of food processing due to its greater digestibility.

Rumen ecology

The enhanced ability of some ruminants (North American buffalo, Asian water buffalo), to digest poor quality feeds results from a change in rumen retention time, rate of passage of digesta and recycling of nitrogen to the rumen, rather than superior rumen bacteria. Browsing ruminants have been shown to tolerate a certain amount of tannins in their natural diet, and studies with feral goats have suggested an active selection for a low dose of hydrolysable tannins (Brooker *et al.*, 1994). *Streptococcus gallolyticus* appears to be widely distributed in ruminants fed tannin-rich diets, but their ecological role in digestion of these forages is yet to be defined (Miller *et al.*, 1996).

Feeding behavior, digestive and metabolic adaptation

On the basis of digestive anatomy, the ruminants are classified as concentrate selectors (browsers; e.g. goat), roughage feeders (grazers; e.g. cattle, yak, mithun, sheep) and intermediate feeders (e.g. deer, goats). Browsers are best adapted to forage with rapid initial fermentation, but low asymptotic digestibility. They skim readily digestible nutrients and propel refractory particles rapidly through the digestive tract so that distension does not limit intake. Grazers, on the other hand, do best on forages that ferment slowly, but more completely. Mixed feeders probably, use each feed type less well, but benefit from greater nutritional flexibility.

Nutritional Requirements of Major Nutrients for Large Ruminants

Examination of the relationships between cold environmental temperature and animal production is usually based on the premise of a zone of thermoneutrality for an animal within which its heat production is constant and independent of the thermal environment (Fig. 2; Kleiber, 1961). The effectiveness of various insulative and behavioral responses to cold stress is maximal at the lower boundary of the thermoneutral zone, a point referred to as the lower critical temperature (LCT). Maintenance requirements increase during periods when temperature falls below the animal's LCT (Ames, 1986, Fig. 3). Although, Holsteins have some advantages during hot conditions due to their thinner skin, less subcutaneous fat, and reduced hair coat density, this becomes a distinct disadvantage during periods of severe cold conditions. Early research has suggested the LCT for dairy cattle to be estimated at 7°F (NRC, 1981), which is dependent on housing, pen conditions, age, nutrition, time after feeding, thermal acclimation, hair coat etc. This estimate assumes that the animal is standing outside with no effects of wind, snow, or mud. In comparison, the LCT for beef breeds is estimated at -32 °F and is lower than for dairy breeds due to greater internal and external insulation (NRC, 1981). Figure 4 depicts the maintenance requirements for a 600 kg cow over a temperature range of -15 to +40°C. NRC (1996) prediction equations indicate that maintenance requirement adjustments occur at higher temperatures. A 450 kg body weight, Holstein steer i.e. fed outside with no wind, it feed intake increases 0.4 lb as air temperature drops from 40 to 20 °F. A further increase in feed intake of 1.7 lb occurs when air temperature continues to fall to 0 °F. If we take the same animal and the coat is wet from rain or wet snow, feed

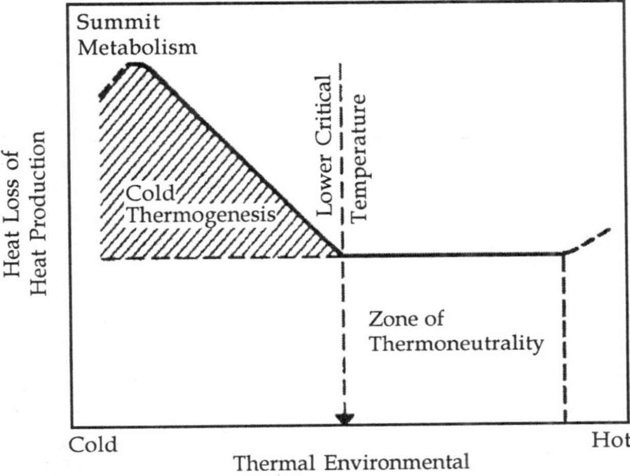

Fig. 2 : Relationship between the thermal environment and rate of heat loss or production of animals.

intake at 20°F becomes 3.1 lbs lower than for a dry animal. In addition, as air temperature falls to 0°F, feed intake increase 1.5 lbs, but is still 3.3 lbs lower than a dry animal. Similarly, maintenance requirement increases and gain decreases as the animal is exposed to lower air temperatures, greater wind speeds and wetter coats. The reductions in gain become more severe as the air temperature decreases and wind speed increases.

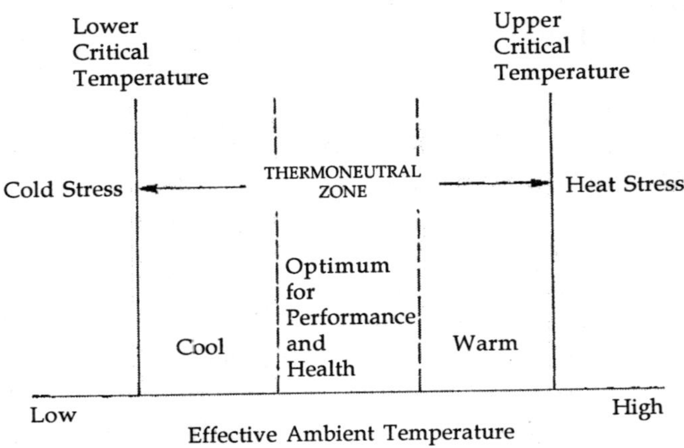

Fig. 3 : Schematic representation showing relationship of thermal zones and temperatures

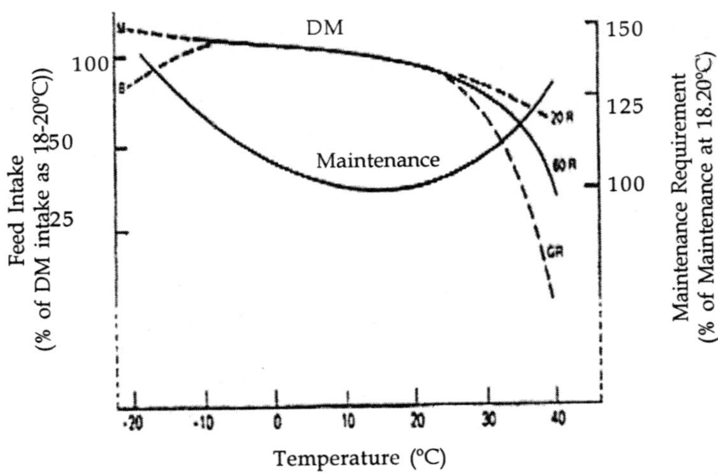

Fig. 4 : Estimated maintenance requirements for a 600-kg cow over a temperature range of -15 to +40 °C; percentage changes in intake of DM under low and high temperatures expressed as percentage of level at 18-20 °C for cows consuming ration of 60% roughage and 40% concentrates (60 R); and percent decline from 20°C for cows on 20% roughage, 80% concentrates (20 R) or on grazing alone (GR); "M' , depicts estimated need at -15 to -20 °C with "B" indicating most likely intake level due to changes in behavior to conserve body heat

Table 4 : Effects of coat condition and wind speed on DMI (kg/d) of Holstein steers (450 kg)

Air Temp. (°C)	Clean and dry coat		Some mud on lower body		With wet snow or mud	
	0 wind	10 wind	0 wind	10 wind	0 wind	10 wind
40	9.03	9.03	9.03	9.03	7.67	7.67
30	9.03	9.03	9.03	9.03	7.67	7.67
20	9.21	9.21	9.21	9.21	7.80	7.80
10	9.21	9.21	9.21	9.21	7.80	7.80
0	9.98	9.98	9.98	9.98	8.48	8.48
-10	9.98	9.98	9.98	9.98	8.48	8.48
-20	9.98	9.98	9.98	9.98	8.48	8.48

Heat production by animals depends on feed intake, body condition, physiological condition, genotype and sex of the animals. Amongst the multitude of factors encompassing both physical and psychological aspects of the animal's surroundings, thermal environment provides a strong influence on farm animals with air temperature having the primary effect but affected by wind, precipitation, humidity and radiation. Ultimately, there is altered energetic efficiency which demands a change in nutrient to energy ratios in the diet. The incremental costs of free existence appear greater in summer than in winter because, animals that are fed supplemental feed are inactive during cold and snowy weather choosing to bed around the premises (Jiang and Hudson 1994). Further, within thermoneutral zone body temperature is controlled by regulation of heat dissipation and when effective ambient temperature decreases below the LCT, heat increment from normal body tissue mobilization fails to maintain body temperature and it needs to increase its metabolic rate referred to as cold thermogenesis (CSIRO, 1990). Amongst animals at cold-temperate zone, yak, the migratory type high altitude animal requires extra for sustaining against cold, high altitude grazing and adverse windy climate. Grazing animals are generally susceptible to parasitism and they demand supplemental nutrition to fight against infection as well as to replenish the loss of nutrients due to parasitism (Louvandini *et al.*, 2006; Sahoo and Ram, 2007). There is also requirement for pregnancy and reproduction, since seasonality of reproduction exists in species like migratory buffalo, some goat species and yak. Grazing activity was estimated to increase energy requirements relative to maintenance by 20% on flat and as much as 50% on hilly terrain (CSIRO, 1990). NRC (2001) suggested the following equation for the calculation of extra energy spent in grazing on a hill terrain.

NE for grazing on hill terrain = $(0.00045 \times BW \times D) + (0.0012 \times BW) + (0.03 \times VD \times BW)$

(BW, body weight in kg; D, distance travelled in km; VD, vertical distance in km)

The metabolic rates increase by 70% above resting in severely cold stressed animals resulting an increase in maintenance digestible energy (DE) intake by 2.5% for adult horses and 1.3% for growing horses fed for moderate gain per 1°C decrease in ambient temperature below LCT (-15°C for adult and 0°C for growing horses; Cymbaluk, 1994). The protein content in the ration needs to be proportioned to the increase in food intake so as to maintain the absolute intake. For cattle fed restricted diet in a cold climate, an increase in roughage may at times be advantageous. However, if feed is not restricted in cold conditions substituting roughage for concentrate feeds may limit the total available energy intake and reduce rate of productivity. The energy and protein requirement of cattle/yak heifers and cow reared at high altitude is presented in Tables 5 and 6 for some ready reference. There is an increase in maintenance requirement of about 10-30% for grazing animals in hill terrain depending on the vertical distance travelled and total distance covered by the animal. There is also need to supplement energy for environmental temperature below the LCT (<5°C). In milch animals, as milk yield increases, appetite and the amount of energy spent gathering food would increase. A similar allowance would also be required for migratory population depending on the proximity of pasture land and the distance travelled in hilly terrain in a day.

Requirements of Minor Nutrients for large Ruminants

The role of hormones in the normal fluid metabolism at higher altitudes is not clear, but various hormones play a role in retention of salt and water in pathologic states like acute and sub acute mountain sickness in human at extreme altitudes. Besides cold, induced diuresis at high altitude and hyper ventilation along with the dry environment at high altitudes make individuals more prone to hypohydration (Rose *et al.*, 1988). Increased urinary excretion of Na^+ and K^+ is reported at high altitude. It is also recommended that antioxidant nutrients such as vitamin A (β-carotene), C and E, as well as Se, Cu, Zn and Mn are required in greater amounts in cold and high altitude environments to reduce lipid peroxidation. These antioxidants act in a concerted manner to combat the oxidative stresses arising from different sources. Vitamins C and E provide help in combating oxidative stresses and concomitant effects on cell membrane integrity. Cold exposure did not consistently affect apparent digestibility of Mg, P, or S in gastrointestinal tract of sheep. Apparent digestibility of Ca was consistently depressed due to an increased endogenous secretion in the gut.

Table 5 : Energy and protein requirement of growing heifers* reared at high altitude

BW (kg)	Gain (kg)	Nutrient requirement/d				% Extra requirement	
		Energy		CP	DCP		
		ME (Mcal/d)	TDN (kg)	(g/d)	(g/d)	ME/TDN	CP/DCP
100	0	5.64	1.57	140	70	11.29	10.00
	0.1	5.97	1.66	264	145	10.61	11.65
	0.2	6.26	1.74	320	192	10.07	13.18
	0.3	6.61	1.84	372	242	9.49	10.83
	0.4	6.94	1.93	418	293	9.00	10.99
	0.5	7.29	2.02	465	349	8.53	9.61
150	0	7.73	2.15	200	98	12.50	7.80
	0.1	8.21	2.28	295	159	11.69	9.52
	0.2	8.60	2.39	375	221	11.10	10.63
	0.3	9.02	2.51	440	282	10.52	10.63
	0.4	9.49	2.64	492	339	9.95	9.83
	0.5	9.96	2.77	530	392	9.44	10.62
200	0	9.68	2.69	240	115	13.43	10.19
	0.1	10.26	2.85	350	186	12.56	10.30
	0.2	10.77	2.99	440	255	11.90	10.09
	0.3	11.34	3.15	515	324	11.23	9.81
	0.4	11.91	3.31	566	385	10.64	10.64
	0.5	12.49	3.47	602	439	10.09	10.09
250	0	11.52	3.20	280	132	14.20	14.20
	0.1	12.22	3.39	400	208	13.28	13.28
	0.2	12.80	3.55	490	279	12.60	12.60
	0.3	13.42	3.73	575	357	11.94	11.94
	0.4	14.16	3.93	630	422	11.25	11.25
300	0	13.28	3.69	310	143	14.86	14.86
	0.1	14.09	3.91	340	173	13.89	13.89
	0.2	14.77	4.10	560	314	13.16	13.16
	0.3	15.54	4.32	636	388	12.43	12.43
	0.4	16.30	4.53	697	460	11.79	11.79
400	0	16.64	4.62	380	171	15.97	15.97
	0.1	17.59	4.89	500	250	14.97	14.97
	0.2	18.51	5.14	600	330	14.13	14.13
	0.3	19.67	5.46	681	409	13.18	13.18

NRC (1989, 2001); BW - body weight, TDN - total digestible nutrients; CP - crude protein
*A heifer (cattle, yak or mithun), grazing on hill terrain is supposed to travel 1.0 km with 50m height.

Table 6 : Nutrient requirements of lactating cattle* at high altitude and exposed to cold (<5°C) stress.

BW (kg)	Milk[1] yield(kg)	Nutrient requirements/d			Nutritive value(%)		% Extra requirements	
		DM(kg)	TDN(kg)	CP(g)	TDN	CP	ME/TDN	CP
200	2	5.5	3.33	450	60.55	8.18	32.91	21.84
	3	6.0	3.66	550	61.00	9.17	29.45	19.74
	4	6.5	3.98	650	61.23	10.00	26.37	18.33
	5	7.0	4.30	700	61.43	10.00	23.87	9.49
	6	7.5	4.62	800	61.60	10.67	21.79	9.69
250	2	6.2	3.87	500	62.42	8.06	36.05	23.82
	3	6.7	4.19	600	62.54	8.96	32.32	21.50
	4	7.2	4.51	650	62.64	9.03	29.28	11.34
	5	7.7	4.83	780	62.73	10.13	26.75	15.76
	6	8.2	5.15	920	62.80	11.22	24.62	20.45
300	2	7.0	4.33	540	61.86	7.71	36.72	23.68
	3	7.5	4.66	640	62.13	8.53	33.56	21.53
	4	8.0	4.98	750	62.25	9.38	30.68	21.63
	5	8.5	5.30	870	62.35	10.24	28.24	23.12
	6	9.0	5.95	980	66.11	10.89	33.56	23.02
	8	10.0	6.59	1200	65.90	12.00	29.24	22.87
400	3	9.5	5.59	700	58.84	7.37	36.46	18.96
	4	10.0	5.91	800	59.10	8.00	33.76	17.92
	5	10.5	6.23	920	59.33	8.76	31.42	19.73
	6	11.0	6.55	1020	59.55	9.27	29.38	18.82
	8	12.0	7.20	1200	60.00	10.00	26.17	15.56
	10	13.0	7.84	1400	60.31	10.77	23.45	14.90

NRC (1989, 2001) [1]Milk with 4% fat

BW - Body weight; TDN - Total digestible nutrients; CP - Crude protein

*A cow (cattle, yak or mithun), grazing on hill terrain is supposed to travel 1.0 km with 50 m height.

Free Ranging and Requirement of Small Ruminants

In free ranging, if the food availability is scarce, the animals are forced to travel long distances to meet their energy requirements and this extra energy drain can be an important contributor to ME for maintenance. Both sheep and goats adapt well to environmental conditions prevailing in arid lands, being able to obtain and adequate diet even when forage is scarce and they can feed over rugged and inaccessible terrain. Thus, ME requirements in open range may increase several fold over values assessed for restrained animals. The NRC (1981) considers that in goats the increased muscular activity of the animal under grazing conditions accounts for increment of 25% in the case of light activity, 50% on semi-arid rangeland pasture and on slightly hilly land and 75% in case of long-distance travel on sparsely vegetated grassland or on mountainous transhumance pasture. Both the increased energy expenditure of eating and the energy spent in walking would account to this higher maintenance requirement. There has been considerable review on assessment of nutritional standards since the publication of NRC (1981) for goats and NRC (1985) for sheep. Estimates of the energy cost of walking were 3.35, 31.7 and -13.2 J kg^{-1} BW^{m-1} for horizontal, ascending and descending movement, respectively (Lachica and Aguilera, 2003; 2005). The heat production (HP) attained 401 kJ $kg^{-0.75}$ per day for restrained goats. The increase in HP for unrestrained over restrained goats was 43.1% and daily distance traveled (say 2km) accounted for 9% of the extra HP. AFRC (1998) suggested that energy used in activity (MEa) for stall-fed goats was 10% of fasting heat production (10% of 315 kJ/$kgBW^{0.75}$), with additional costs for grazing based on $BW^{1.0}$ for horizontal movement (3.5 J/(kgBW×m)), vertical movement (28 J/(kgBW × m)), standing (0.417 kJ/(kgBW×h)) and change in position (0.26 kJ/(kg BW × number of changes)), and then application of the efficiency of ME for maintenance. In this line, there is a strong need to assess the nutrient requirements of migratory flock of sheep and goats which followed an annual cycle of upward (4000-5000 m above msl) and downward migration (plains) and exposed to a variable degree of undernutrition. NRC (2007) revised many concepts in small ruminant nutrition and came out with guiding principles for formulating rations based on nutritional requirement for different levels of activity (Table 7) and state and type of production. The time spent grazing, is dependent on the amount of forage consumed and the relative availability of herbage. Therefore, free ranging animals pay relatively higher costs of foraging for dispersed foods, avoiding or battling predators and parasites, dealing with more extreme climatic conditions, and interacting socially with other species competing for the same pasture or fodder resources (Sahoo, 2010).

Poultry Rearing at High Altitude

In hilly states like Himachal Pradesh, North Eastern region and Uttarakhand the poultry sector has witnessed rapid growth rate during the last few decades. However, such farming activities are mostly confined to the lower altitude areas of the hilly regions where the climate is conducive for poultry rearing. Efforts are being made to develop and improve poultry production system at Ladakh situated at an average altitude of 4000 m with about 35,000 poultry birds and similarly, under NATP (Jai Vigyan) efforts were made to popularize the commercial poultry production in the NEH region. Concerted efforts by CARI, Izatnagar in collaboration with Temperate Animal Husbandry Division, IVRI, Mukteswar are in practice for popularizing poultry rearing at high altitude. Besides the problem of asphyxia and related ascites problem, no convincing evidence suggests that supplementation has an advantage, provided that energy intake is adequate for birds at high altitude. However, antioxidants especially vitamin E and the energy releasing B vitamins (thiamine, riboflavin and niacin) have received some attention, which support energy metabolism at low oxygen pressure and increased energy demand during cold stress. High altitude is associated with inadequate supplies of oxygen and poor ventilation, which may lead to ascites and supplementation of additional vitamin C (ascorbic acid) and E helps in alleviating the problem. It is also advocated to use L-arginine and salts in drinking water for the prevention and/or treatment of pulmonary hypertension syndrome (ascites) in avians. Formulation of balanced feed using locally available ingredients and strategic feeding and most importantly, the housing management during stress in inclement weather will hold promise for future poultry production at high altitude.

Table 7 : Nutrient requirements of goats at hilly and mountainous pasture.

BW (kg)	Feed Energy				Crude Protein		Minerals		Feed DM per Animal			
									1 kg=2.0 Mcal ME		1kg=2.4 Mcal ME	
	TDN (g)	DE (Mcal)	ME (Mcal)	NE (Mcal)	TP (g)	DP (g)	Ca (g)	P (g)	Total (kg)	% of BW	Total (kg)	% of BW
***Maintenance plus medium activity* (=50% increment, semiarid rangeland, slightly hilly pastures, & early pregnancy)**												
10	239	1.05	0.86	0.48	33	23	1	0.7	0.43	4.3	0.36	3.6
20	400	1.77	1.44	0.81	55	38	2	1.4	0.72	3.6	0.60	3.0
30	543	2.38	1.95	1.10	74	52	3	2.1	0.98	3.3	0.81	2.7
40	672	2.97	2.42	1.36	93	64	4	2.8	1.21	3.0	1.01	2.5
50	795	3.51	2.86	1.62	110	76	4	2.8	1.43	2.9	1.19	2.4
60	912	4.02	3.28	1.84	126	87	5	3.5	1.64	2.7	1.37	2.3
70	1023	4.52	3.68	2.07	141	98	6	4.2	1.84	2.6	1.53	2.2
80	1131	4.98	4.06	2.30	156	108	6	4.2	2.03	2.5	1.69	2.1
90	1236	5.44	4.44	2.50	170	118	7	4.9	2.22	2.5	1.85	2.0
100`	1336	5.90	4.82	2.72	184	128	7	4.9	2.41	2.4	2.01	2.0

Contd...

Maintenance plus high activity **(=75% increment, arid rangeland, sparse vegetation, mountainous pastures, & early pregnancy)**

10	278	1.22	1.00	0.56	38	26	2	1.4	0.50	5.0	0.42	4.2
20	467	2.06	1.68	0.94	64	45	2	1.4	0.84	4.2	0.70	3.5
30	634	2.78	2.28	1.28	87	60	3	2.1	1.14	3.8	0.95	3.2
40	784	3.46	2.82	1.59	108	75	4	2.8	1.41	3.5	1.18	3.0
50	928	4.10	3.34	1.89	128	89	5	3.5	1.67	3.3	1.39	2.7
60	1064	4.69	3.83	2.15	146	102	6	4.2	1.92	3.2	1.60	2.7
70	1194	5.27	4.29	2.42	165	114	6	4.2	2.14	3.0	1.79	2.6
80	1320	5.81	4.74	2.68	182	126	7	4.9	2.37	3.0	1.98	2.5
90	1442	6.35	5.18	2.92	198	138	8	5.6	2.59	2.9	2.16	2.4
100	1559	6.88	5.62	3.17	215	150	8	5.6	2.81	2.8	2.34	2.3

NRC, (2007); Sahoo, (2010)

Nutritional Adequacy and Feeding Management

Nutritional inadequacy has been identified as a principal limiting factor for low livestock productivity in these areas (IFAD, 2003). Nutritional adequacy needs assessment of the availability of feed and nutrients and sustainability for a particular state of production without affecting the productive life cycle of the animal. Lack of sufficient feed resources particularly the quality fodder during the winter season is mainly responsible for reduction in body weight of adult animals and death losses in newly born lambs and kids. Feeding management and delivery schedules are another strategy used to reduce the impact of cold conditions on feedlot cattle. It is focused on restricting intake of high energy diets as an alternative management practice to full feeding high roughage diets during the growing phase (Loerch, 1990). Further, altering the feeding time for limit-fed cattle in the winter can help to maintain body temperature (Holt and Pritchard, 2005).

Grazing, Nutrition and Forage Management

The mountain areas exhibit a great diversity in climate, landforms, resource availability and agricultural practices. Remunerative agriculture in the form of double cropping is practiced up to an elevation of 1000 m only, and beyond this altitude, the uncertainty of climate and steep slopes have restricted the agricultural activity, mainly to livestock husbandry. The forage resources are limited to grasslands, cultivable wastelands, fodder trees and crop residues. About 40.0% of the total geographical area is under natural grasslands, which get shrunken in the period of long winter due to snow coverage. The rapid changes in political boundaries and policies that have led to restricted livestock mobility and the marginalization of pastoral people, pointing out that such changes need to be understood in order to identify realistic strategies for livestock and rangeland development. Limbach *et al.*, (2000) studied adaptability of forage grasses at higher altitudes and graded *Poa compressa, Poa pratensis var. alpinum, Dactylis glomerata, Festuca ovina, Agrostis alba, Phleum pratense, Deschampsia caespitosa, Trisetum flavescens, Elymus trachycaulus,* Tibetan mixture, and two varieties of *Medicago sativa* as best varieties. Grasses and fodder trees like *Dactylis glomerata,* oats (var. Kent), *Salyx humboldtiana* and *S. babolicana* are proved successful in the mid-altitude. Doyoddorj (2000) has investigated twenty-five species of plants edible by yak, and found 3.8 to 27.9% of selections with excellent edibility, such as *Trifolium repens, Medicago falcata, Festuca supina sehur, Festuca lenesis, Phleum phlecites, Stipa glareosa* and *Poa pratensis* and 4.5 to 26.3% with good edibilities such as *Stipa sibirica, Alopecurus brachystakyus, Alopecurus venticosus, Cleistogenes uguakroca, Poa tibetica Trifollum bupinastek, Melilotus entatus, Melilotus suaveolens, Vicia amoona fisch, Biomus inermus leyss, Carex capiliformis, Carex melanthea fermis lint.*

Managing livestock during periods of inclement weather remains a challenge. Management strategies are aimed at alleviating rather than eliminating climatic challenges on these animals. The animals in this ecology and the existing housing and management systems are unable to utilize their normal behavioral activities to maintain heat balance. Although in the confinement, there are opportunities for altering the environment by using shade structures, shelters, and windbreaks, or via management such as changing feeding times to improve conditions. High altitude rangelands, tree forages and some agricultural by-products constitute the main and ultimate feed resources of the livestock. The nomadic people usually travel long distances with their animals in search of nutritious alpine pastures up to an altitude of 3000-5000 m above msl during summer and down to mid altitude (1000-2000 m above msl) or plains during winter. The principal factors that govern the nutritional adequacy of native and migratory livestock are 'relative availability of herbage' for different state of production and 'pasture utilization capacity' of the available rangelands in competition with the migratory flock and wild ruminants. The animals at high altitudes spend a lot of energy in walking up/down the hills for grazing, maintaining body temperature during adverse climatic conditions (chill and windy weather, rain, frost bite etc.) and partial starvation during inclement weathers. A detailed survey of the highland Himalayan region, identification of edible plant species and their chemical and nutritional characteristics, selection and improvement of the species with potential of good pasture component, efficient management of the existing grasslands by adjusting the stocking rate, cultivation of promising fodder crops, trees and grasses, supplementation of concentrates are some of the measures to upgrade the potential of livestock productivity for sustaining economic livelihood of hill farmers. Continuing research in animal responses to varying altitude and cold climatic conditions and strategic nutritional interventions is providing a better understanding of the way in which animals cope with these stresses.

References

AFRC. (1998). CAB Internat, Wallingford, UK.

Ames, C. (1986). Effective motivation: The contribution of the learning environment. In R.Feeeldman (Ed) pp235-236. Cambridge University Press.

Baker, D.L., Stout, G.W. and Miller, M.W. (1998). *J. Zoo Wildlife Med.*, 29: 150-156.

Brooker, J.D., O'Donovan, L.A., Skene, I., Clarke, K., Blackall, L. and Muslera, P. (1994). *Lett. Appl. Microbiol.*, 18: 313-318.

CSIRO. (1990). Ruminants Subcommittee. CSIRO. Publications. East Melbourne. Australia.

Cymbaluk, N.F. (1994). *Liv. Prod. Sci.*, 40: 65-71.

Doyoddorj, D. (2000). Proceedings of the Third International Congress on Yak. Zhao (Ed). Publisher: International veterinary information service, Ithaca, New York, USA.

Holt, S.M.and Psitchard, R.H. (2005). *J. Anim. Sci.*, 83 (suppl): 174.

IFAD (2003). International Fund for Agricultural Development.

Jiang, Z. and Hudson, R.J. (1994). *Can. J. Anim. Sci.*, 74: 97-102.

Kleiber, M. (1961). John Willey and Sons, New York.

Lachica M. and Aguilera J.F. (2003). *Small Rumin. Res.*, 49: 303–318.

Lachica, M., Aguilera, J.F. (2005). *Small Rumin. Res.*, 59: 105–121.

Loerch, S.C. (1990). *J. Anim. Sci.*, 73: 55-62.

Louvandini, H., Veloso, C.F.M., Paludo, G.R., Dell'Porto, A., Gennari, S.M. and McManus, C.M. (2006). *Vet. Para.*, 137: 103-111.

Miller, S.M., Brooker, J.D., Phillips, A. and Blackall, L.L. (1996). *Austral. J. Agric. Res.*, 47: 1323-1331.

Nagy, KA. (2001). *Nutr. Abst. and Rev.* (Series B), 71: 1R-12R.

NRC (1981, 1985, 1989, 1996, 2001, 2007). National Academy of Science, Washington, DC.

Rose, M.S., Houston, C.S., Fulco, C.S., Coates, G., Carlson, D., Sutton, J.R. and Cymerman, A. (1988). *J. Appl. Physiol.*, 65: 2545- 2551.

Sahoo, A. (2005). In: *Procceedings, National Symposium on "Wildlife Health and Husbandry Constraints"*, 4th Annual Convention of Association of Indian Zoo and Wildlife Veterinarians. 25-26 Oct., 2005, College of Veterinary Science, AAU, Khanapara, Guwahati, Assam.

Sahoo, A. 2010. Feeding management of small ruminants in cold climates of temperate region. *In Sheep and Goat Production* (S.A. Karim, A. Joshi, S.K. Sankhyan, A.K. Shinde, D.B. Shakyawar, S.M.K. Naqvi, B.N. Tripathi) Satish Serial Publ. House, Delhi. pp 125-138.

Sahoo, A. and Ram, Hira. (2007). XVIII Nat. Cong. of Vet. Parasit. and Nat. Sym. Sept. 7-9, 2007, Faculty of Vet. Sci. and Anim. Hus., Sher-e- Kashmir Univ. of Agri. Sci. & Tech., Jammu, India, pp. 102-112.

Sahoo, A. and Singh, B. (2004). Proceeding, Conference on Sustainable Yak Husbandry in India. 24-25 Dec., 2004, NRC on Yak, Dirang, India, pp. 23-31.

Sahoo, A., Meena, H.R., Mahapatra, R.K. and Ram, Hira. (2008). In: Souvenir cum Abstracts, "Integrated Livestock Farming Systems in the Foot-Hills of Himalayas (HILF-2008)" May 17-18, 2008, IVRI, Mukteswar Campus, Uttarakhand, India.

□□□

Animal Nutrition, 2012
eds. Dr. (Mrs.) Usha R. Mehra et al., pp. 351-377
Satish Serial Publishing House e-mail : info@satishserial.com; website : www.satishserial.com

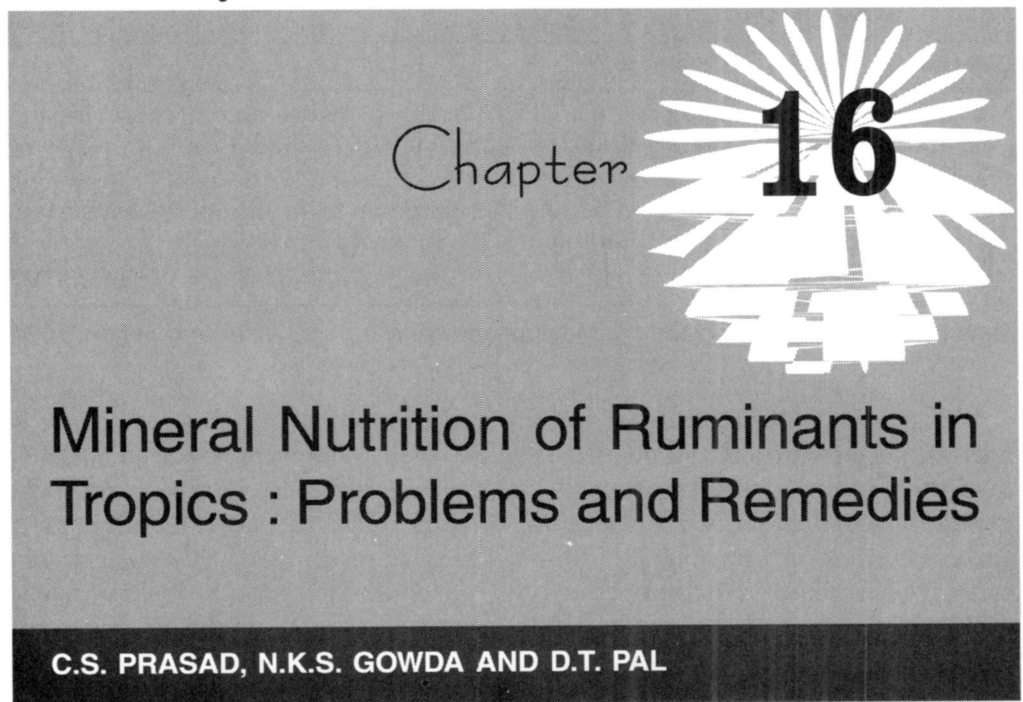

Chapter 16

Mineral Nutrition of Ruminants in Tropics : Problems and Remedies

C.S. PRASAD, N.K.S. GOWDA AND D.T. PAL

Minerals are an integral part of the total nutrient management system as they are essential for growth and reproduction and are also involved in a large number of digestive, physiological and biosynthetic processes within the body. The most obvious function is as components of body organs and tissues and to provide structural support. In addition, they act as electrolytes, as constituents of body fluids and as catalysts in both enzymes and hormones. Therefore, they fulfill several important functions for the maintenance, growth and reproduction as well as health status (Carlisle, 1986; Mc Dowell, 1992, 1997). The mineral elements that are of particular importance are categorized as calcium, phosphorous, potassium, sodium, chlorine, sulfur and magnesium and trace elements viz. iron, iodine, copper, zinc, manganese, cobalt, selenium, fluoride and molybdenum (Table 1).

Table 1 : Classification of minerals

Category	Element
Macro minerals	Calcium (Ca), Phosphorus (P), Magnesium (Mg), Potassium (K), Sodium (Na), Chlorine (Cl), Sulfur (S)
Trace minerals	Copper (Cu)[a], Zinc (Zn)[a], Cobalt (Co)[a], Iodine (I)[a], Iron (Fe)[a], Manganese (Mn), Selenium (Se)[a], Chromium (Cr), Molybdenum (Mo)[a], Cadmium (Cd)[b], Arsenic (AS)[b], Lead (pb)[b]
Newer trace elements	Nickel (Ni), Boron (B)[b], Lithium (Li)[b], Tin (Sn)[b], Vanadium (V)[b].

[a] Important under grazing systems (Masters and White, 1996; O' Dell and Sunde, 1997)
[b] Inconclusive evidence of essentiality.

Based on identification of one or more metabolic function, at least 15 minerals are regarded as essential (Spears, 1999). They are required in small quantities as compared to other major nutrients like protein and energy and generally are considered to have less immediate impact on overall performance and economic efficiency but should never be underestimated as their deficiency can have a marked effect on productivity, particularly reproduction and health (Table 2).

There is an apparent increase in mineral requirements and simultaneous deficiencies in ruminants of tropical countries, and the reasons could be 1. Improved genetic selection of livestock for better growth rates and higher production, 2. Changes in traditional cropping practices with poor soil management, higher fertilization and plant breeding for higher crop yield, 3. Modification of traditional feeding programs to improve production and use of feed additives. In recent years, number of mineral disorders in livestock which may be characterized as chronic or marginal have been reported (Suttle, 2000). In tropical countries, animals are mostly fed on crop residues, natural grasses, tree leaves and shrubs. In such diets the mineral content is generally low and their availability to the host is not known. Intensive cultivation of pastures, changes in agricultural practices and differences in agro-climatic conditions and infusion of superior germplasm for upgrading the production traits of cattle and the changes in techniques used for feed processing and manufacturing have greatly altered the mineral requirement of animals. The plants derive the minerals from soil, and the animals from the plants/feed they consume and there is a direct interrelationship between soil, plant and animals (Fig 1), which may not be linear always (Reid and Horvath, 1980). Several factors regulate the transfer of minerals from soils to plants and from plants to animals. Soil characteristics (pH, moisture), the type of plant (green fodder, legume and mature straws etc.), the physiological status of the animal (lactating, growing, pregnant) and the accompanying feed, all of these collectively or individually contribute to the mineral uptake and utilization.

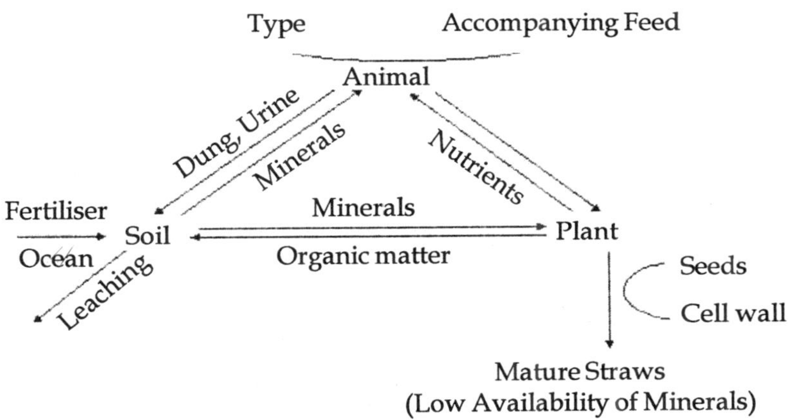

Fig. 1 : Soil, plant, animal inter-relationship

Soil and its Effect on Mineral Deficiency in Animals

The mineral content of soils depends not only on the parent material but on a complex of pedogenic factors like laterization, calcification and salinization (Kumar *et al.*, 2002). Translocation further occurs by processes of surface erosion, leaching, evaporation and redeposition of minerals on the surface. Of the total mineral concentration in soils, only a fraction is taken up by the plants. The "availability" of minerals in soils depends upon their effective concentration in soil solution. Several factors influence the uptake of minerals by crops and pastures from the soil. These include soil acidity, soil moisture, soil temperature, plant variety, fertilization, organic matter and microbial activity of soil. For trace mineral absorption, the pH has the most marked effect on the availability. Alkaline soils lead to an increased biological availability of some trace elements such as Se and Mo. With decreasing soil pH, Se is less available, but the uptake of some cationic metals like Cu is increased. Soil leaching, erosion and long term cropping, lead to depletion of trace minerals. Crop management and climatic conditions also influence the eventual trace minerals level in feeds. Fertilization and/or heavy rainfall can result in lush pasture growth and the dilution of some trace minerals (Reid and Horvath, 1980).

With increased soil pH, there is drastic decrease in Manganese (Mn) content. Water logging of a soil results in conversion of an aerobic to an anaerobic environment in the root zone area. The concentration of nitrogen in the plant tends to decrease and that of phosphorus increases with increasing moisture level, but no definite trends are seen for other minerals. The soil temperature and season can influence the uptake of minerals with respect to the growth of the pastures. At low temperature, the mineral uptake is slower possibly because of depressed root extension and membrane permeability.

With the advent of green revolution, deficiencies of micronutrients have been observed widely in several Indian soils and crops. The soil in tropical climate is mostly deficient in P. Zn deficiency is widely observed in rice, wheat, maize, groundnut, cotton and their residues in the intensively cultivated and irrigated areas. In India, Bihar, Andhra Pradesh, Tamil Nadu, Madhya Pradesh and Haryana as well as all Indo-Gangetic Alluvial plains showed extensive deficiency of Zn in soil (Prasad *et al.*, 1995).

Plant and Its Effect on Mineral Deficiency in Animals

Feeds/fodders are the main source of minerals for livestock. Grazing animals receive certain level of minerals from water and soil ingestion. Of the minerals present in soil only a fraction is taken up by plants depending on geophysical/chemical conditions as explained above. Plant mineral content is dependent on other factors like type of soil, plant species and stage of maturity, pasture management and agro-climatic conditions (Cardose *et al.*, 1999).

Mineral concentrations and availability are mainly affected by four interdependent factors:

1. The genus, species, or variety of plants
2. Type and mineral concentration of soil
3. Climatic or seasonal conditions
4. Stage of plant maturity

Genus, Species, or Varietal Effects

Plant varieties growing on the same soil under the same environmental conditions show marked differences in mineral uptake. Legumes are superior in mineral efficiency to the grasses particularly in terms of Ca and Mg uptake. In general, legumes are higher in calcium, copper, zinc, iron, and cobalt than grasses. In contrast, grasses tend to be higher in manganese and molybdenum than legumes when grown on the same soil. Most of the trace mineral concentration is higher in pasture legume species than other grasses. Research has shown that even variety within a species affects mineral composition. Straws and stovers are deficient in most of the minerals. They contain excess of silica, oxalate and tannins, which may interfere in the utilization of other minerals/nutrients. Plant requirement of certain minerals (Mn, Zn, K) may exceed animal requirements and certain minerals may be required at higher levels in animals (Na, Cl, I, Co and Se). Mature plants are low in minerals as most of the minerals may get accumulated in seeds due to translocation(Reid and Horvath, 1980).

Mineral Needs of Animal

The mineral needs of animals depend on the requirement and the availability of minerals. The mineral requirement is related to animal output and therefore providing minerals in the diet is particularly important for high producing animals (Table 2). For calculating the mineral requirements, it is necessary to know the type of feed ingredients that are used in the ration along with the accompanying roughage source (grass/straws/stovers). The requirement of minerals for different classes of livestock is discussed subsequently. Several factors govern the uptake of minerals from soil to plants and plants to animals and existence of soil-plant-animal interrelationship for some trace elements has been reported. The status of micronutrients in soil, plant and animals would be a useful tool in understanding the severity of the deficiency for providing cost effective supplementation for improving production, reproduction, and profitability of livestock owners (Corah, 1996).

The surveys conducted under All India Coordinated Research Project in different agro-climatic zones of the country suggest that nearly all forages are deficient in one or more minerals and that there is a widespread occurrence of the deficient levels of calcium, phosphorus, copper and zinc for ruminants grazing forages (Table 5). This is further complicated by the fact that the availability of minerals may be affected by the distribution and form of minerals in the feedstuff, as well as interactions with other minerals or dietary components like fiber, that inhibit absorption or utilization of a given mineral. The mineral deficiencies in ruminants fed forages often result from low availability rather than low concentration of a given mineral.

Mineral Distribution in Animal Body

The minerals are generally stored in bones, muscles and other soft tissues which are primary storage sites (Table 3). Most minerals are distributed more evenly in the body and exist in accordance with their function. Based on their tissue concentration, the minerals have been classified as major and micro minerals.

Mineral Interaction

Minerals often interact with other minerals, vitamins and proteins. These interactions can take place in the feed, in the digestive tract and also during the tissue and cell metabolism. (Phillippo *et al.*, 1987). Example of synergistic effect of interaction are between Ca & P, Na & Cl, Zn & Mo and those of antagonistic effect are Mg & P, Cu - Mo - S and Se & S. Presence of vitamin D has synergistic effects on Ca & P absorption while vitamin E and Selenium has synergistic action.

Table 2 : Functions of minerals

Element	Function	*Manifestation of deficiency* Severe	Marginal	Likely occurence of deficiency
Ca	Mineralization of bone and teeth, nerve conduction, muscle contraction, blood clotting	Lameness, milk fever, tremors	Reduced growth and milk production	Prolonged feeding on fodder grown in acidic soil, high grain feeding, peak lactation
P	Bone formation, energy metabolism and component of DNA/RNA, acid-base balance	Lameness, reduced appetite, pica	Reduced growth and fertility	Prolonged feeding on dry fodders alone
Mg	Energy metabolism and cofactor of many enzymes, nerve conduction and muscle contraction	Tetany, convulsions	Loss of appetite and production	Feeding on lush pasture high in potassium, heavy nitrogen fertilization of fodder
S	Component of methionine, cysteine, biotin, thiamine, heteropolysaccharides, detoxification process in liver	Reduced feed intake and digestibility, weight loss	Reduced feed intake, reduced wool growth	Prolonged feeding of dry fodders alone
Na	Maintenance of acid-base balance and osmotic pressure	Depressed appetite, licking of soil	Reduced growth and milk production	Feeding of high grain diets during growing or peak lactation period
Fe	Oxygen transport, electron transport, activation of oxidases, oxygenases, component of catalase, aconitase, peroxidase, constituent of haemoglobin, myoglobin, transferrin, ferritin	Anaemia, reduced appetite	Reduced appetite and growth rate	Parasitic infestation, raw cotton seed meal feeding

Contd ..

Cu	Mobilization and transport of iron in body, synthesis of collagen, pigmentation of hair and wool, myelin sheath formation, keratinization, component of cytochrome oxidase, lysyl oxidase, superoxidase dismutase, tyrosinase, ceruloplasmin, provide stability to RNA / DNA	Anzootic ataxia, fragile bones, anaemia, depigmentation of wool, loss of crimp, depressed growth, delayed ovulation, reduced conception rate, embryonic mortality, rough hair coat, cessation of estrus activity	Anaemia, loss of appetite, reduced immunity	Low copper in soil, soil high in Mo, Cu and Mo ratio below 3:1, continuous feeding of poor quality straw
Zn	Component of over 70 enzymes like, alcohol dehydrogenase, carbonic anhydrase, carboxy peptidase,DNA/ RNA polymerase etc., keratinization, spermatogenesis, regulation of hormone production, DNA and protein synthesis, cell replication, integrity of immune system, helps in vitamin A utilization, prostaglandin metabolism	Reduced feed intake and growth rate, loss of crimp, alopecia, parakeratosis, rough hair coat, inflammation of nose and mouth, male and female infertility, low semen quality and infertility	Reduced growth rate, and reproductive performance, reduced feed efficiency, decreased resistance to infection and stress, delayed puberty	Low zinc in soil, dry pasture, over cultivation of soil.
Mn	Constituent of arginase, carboxylase, superoxidase dismutase, activator of hydrolases, kinases,	Muscular weakness, fatty syndrome, weak bones, delayed and irregular estrus,	Loss of appetite; reduced growth and feed efficiency. Loss	Prolonged feeding of dry fodder, in poultry Mn deficiency is caused due to high Ca, P and phytate intakes

Contd...

	decarboxylases and transferases, mucopolysaccharide synthesis, glycoprotein and steroid hormone synthesis, regulate corpus luteum function, maintains membrane integrity, immune functions	foetal deformities, slipped tendon in chicks, abortion in animals	of hair colour, cystic ovaries, silent heat	
I	Component of thyroid hormones that are necessary for energy and protein metabolism and for foetal growth and development	Enlarged thyroid gland, cold stress, reduced basal metabolism, reduced foetal size and brain development, loss of wool, still birth, irregular estrus cycle, low sperm count	General weakness, loss of appetite, retention of placenta, weak and blind calves	Low soil iodine, hilly areas with high rainfall, goitrogenic substances, high dietary arsenic, fluoride and calcium
Co	Component of vitamin B_{12}, propionic acid metabolism, recycling of methionine, purine and pyrimidine synthesis	Loss of appetite, loss of weight, anaemia, rough hair coat, fatty liver, reproductive disorders, emaciation	Unthriftiness, reduced growth, low conception rate, abortion, weak calves	Grazing on dry pasture and feeding of dry fodders for prolonged period
Mo	Component of xanthine oxidase, aldehyde oxidase, sulfite oxidase, metabolism of purine and pyramidines, uric acid metabolism in poultry	Low performance of animals, gout in poultry, swollen joints due to uric acid accumulation	-	Deficiency is quite uncommon, generally toxicity is observed

Contd...

Se	Detoxification of peroxides, activation of thyroid hormones, component of glutathione peroxidase, type 1 iodothyronine deiodinase, preserves the integrity of pancreas, cell membranes, acts synergistically with Vit E., Se has a role in prostaglandin synthesis and immune response, complex with heavy metals like Pb, Cd, Hg and exert protective effect	Muscular dystrophy, lesions in heart and skeletal muscles (white muscle disease), liver necrosis, retention of placenta, mastitis, induced thyroid hormone deficiency, infertility	Reduced growth, ill thrift, reduced wool growth, poor feathering in chicken, cystic ovaries, reduced immunity	Green pasture, low Se soil, high rainfall, low vitamin E intake. Relatively toxic if the pasture / forage are high in Se
F	Essentiality is not confirmed. But evidence of improving Fe utilization and preventing dental caries at very low levels has been reported	Natural deficiency has not been reported, mostly toxicity is observed in endemic areas	-	Toxicity is observed due to excess fluoride in soil and water, fluorosis causes bone deformities
Cr	Act as glucose tolerance factor and increases the uptake of glucose by cells, plays an important role in secretion of pregnancy specific proteins for preventing early embryonic mortality. It potentiates insulin action. Chromium supplementation helps in lean meat production and improves reproduction and immunity	Deficiency generally not encountered, but supplementation either in organic or inorganic form is found to be beneficial	-	-

Hannam and Reuter, 1987; Hosking *et al.*, 1986; Masters, 1996; Mc Dowell *et al.*, 1993, 1997; Mc Dowell, 1996; Regius *et al.*, 1993; Sharma and Sharma, 1997; Smart *et al.*, 1981

Requirements

The mineral requirements can be expressed in amounts per day or per unit of the product or as percentage of the dietary dry matter intake (Table 4). The former is more accurate but the later is simpler and practical as long as there is no variation in the feed intake. Where the dry matter intake varies considerably (particularly when straws and stovers are fed), the expression in absolute amount may be more appropriate. Feeding low quality roughages results in increased faecal endogenous losses of Ca and P leading to increased requirements of these minerals. Presence of certain antinutritional factors like oxalates, silicates and phytates beyond a particular level may affect the utilization of certain minerals like Ca, P, Zn, Mn and Fe. Also the need to supplement minerals may be more in animals with parasitic infestation. Mineral requirements are highly dependent on the level of productivity. Increased growth rates and milk production will greatly increase mineral requirements. Marginal mineral deficiencies, under low levels of production become more severe with increased levels of production. Dairy animals producing more than 10 litters of milk have a greater requirement of Ca & P as compared to low yielder as milk contains high concentration (0.11-0.13%) of these two minerals.

Table 3 : Mineral distribution in animal body

Element	% in body	Primary storage
Calcium	1.3 - 1.5	Bones and soft tissues
Phosphorus	0.74	Bones and soft tissues
Magnesium	0.04	Bones, muscles
Sodium	0.16 - 0.20	Extra cellular fluids
Chlorine	0.11	Intracellular / extracellar fluids
Potasium	0.20 - 0.30	Skin, muscles and intra cellular fluids
Sulphur	0.15	Liver, muscles, skin
Iron	0.007 (70 ppm)	Haemoglobin
Copper	0.0002 (2 ppm)	Liver
Molybdenum	Traces	All tissues
Cobalt	Traces	Liver, bone, kidney
Iodine	Traces	Thyroid
Manganese	Traces	Liver, bone, pancreas, kidney
Zinc	30 ppm	Skin, hair, wool and other tissues

(Underwood, 1981)

Similarly the requirement for zinc for spermatogenesis and testicular development in male sheep are higher than for growth. Manganese requirement is also lesser for growth than for fertility in sheep. Important difference in mineral utilization can occur due to breed variation and also the nutritional status of the animals. The variation in the efficiency of mineral absorption within breeds could be as high as 5-30 % for magnesium, 40-80 % for phosphorus and 2-10 % for copper. When the energy and protein supplies are adequate there is a higher requirement for minerals with better utilization with improved livestock performance. The micronutrient requirement can be influenced by metabolic or nutritional factors that result in other elements complexing specific microelements rendering them nutritionally unavailable to animals. Most of the nutrient requirements have not accounted for relatives' new information that describes the effect of nutrition on immune function, and many of the requirements have not been evaluated in terms of optimal reproduction. There is reason to suggest that optimal immune responsiveness and decrease resistance and cobalt deficiencies have been shown to alter various components of the immune system.

Requirements for copper can vary from 4 to 15 mg/kg depending largely on the concentration of dietary molybdenum and sulfur. The recommended concentration of copper in cattle diets is 10 mg Cu/kg diet. This amount provides adequate copper if the diet does not exceed 0.25 percent sulfur and 2 mg Mo/kg diet. Less than 10 mg Cu/kg diet may meet requirements of feedlot a cattle as copper is more available in concentrate diets than in forage diets. Copper is believed to react with thiomolybdates in the rumen to form poorly absorbed insoluble complexes. Thiomolybdates can result in copper becoming tightly bound to plasma albumin and unavailable for biochemical functions. They also may directly inhibit certain copper-dependent enzymes. Sulfur reduces copper absorption, perhaps via formation of copper sulfide in the rumen. High concentrations of iron and zinc also reduce copper status, which may increase copper requirements.

Sulfur in feedstuffs is largely a component of protein. Dietary sulfur requirements may be higher when diets high in rumen bypass protein are fed because of sulfur's limitation for optimal ruminal fermentation. Sulfur supplementation may be needed when urea or other nonprotein nitrogen sources replace natural preformed protein. Mature forages, forages grown in sulfur-deficient soils, corn silage and sorghum x sudangrass are low in sulfur. Sorghum forages seem inherently low in sulfur relative to other forages.

Minerals in Production and Reproduction of Ruminants

The mechanism of mineral-reproduction interactions is not fully understood because of the complexity of neuro-hormonal dialogue. Some minerals act directly on the gonads, while others act through hypophyseal - pituitary - gonadal axis. Elements like Se once considered toxic, is known to improve both male and female fertility when supplemented in organic form as selenomethionine. During reproductive events reactive metabolites of oxygen are produced and are removed through antioxidant process by Se and vitamin E and provide a convenient environment for reproduction. Similarly other trace elements like Cu, Zn, Mn, Cr and I also act as co-factors or activate enzymes and helps in hormone synthesis and hence influence biochemical functions associated with reproduction (Smith and Akinbamijo, 2000 ; Chhabra *et al.,* 1991). Because of their role in the endocrine system and in tissue integrity, minerals have a beneficial role to play in resumption of follicular growth and fertility in dairy cows and buffaloes. The potential for minerals to play a significant role in herd fertility is indisputable. The minerals that affect reproduction in ruminants are generally found within the trace element group, although deficiencies of calcium and phosphorous can also affect the fertility. Reproductive problems are frequently reported in association with trace mineral deficiencies, particularly copper, zinc, selenium and manganese.

Deficiency of Ca may delay uterine involution and increase incidence of dystocia, retained placenta and prolapse of uterus. Excess Ca may impair reproductive function by causing secondary deficiency of P,K Mg, Zn, Cu and other trace minerals by inhibiting their absorption in the intestine. Calcium-dependent mechanisms are involved in steroid biosynthesis in the tests, adrenal glands and ovaries. Calcium plays a role in the utilization of cholesterol by mitochondria or by stimulating the conversion of pregnenolone to progesterone. Phosphorus is often associated with reproductive abnormalities in cattle although infertility due to P deficiency is usually manifested after other signs are readily apparent. Phosphorus deficiency induces lowered conception rate, irregular estrus, anestrus, decreased ovarian activity, increased incidence of cystic follicles and generally depressed fertility. The involvement of P in Phospholipid and c-AMP synthesis may be a key to its effect on reproduction (Hurley and Doane, 1989).

Zinc deficiency in ruminants has been postulated to weaken the skin and other stratified epithelia as well as reducing the basal metabolic rate following infectious challenge. Zinc is a co-factor for many proteins and enzymes involved in acute phase response to infection and inflammation. Because the mammary gland is a skin gland, it is likely that zinc will have a positive role in its protection. Skin integrity of the teat has been shown to be specially linked with mastitis prevention. Zinc activates several enzyme systems and is a component of many metalloenzymes. It plays a vital role in hormone secretion, especially related to growth, reproduction, immunocompetence and stress. Zinc is also involved in the generation of keratin and in skin nucleic acid and collagen synthesis as well as in the maintenance of normal vitamin A concentration in plasma and in ovarian function. Many animals therefore require supplemental zinc in the diet for normal body function because of either low levels in the dietary ingredients or the presence of antagonistic factors, which decrease the bioavailability of the element. Antagonism might be due to metals ion interactions such as iron or copper. Source of fibre has also been reported to decrease the availability of zinc.

The need for iodine for the thyroid activity and for the prevention of goiter has been well recognized. Reproductive failure often is a secondary manifestation of thyroid dysfunction resulting from iodine deficiency in cattle. Fetal development during iodine deficiency may be arrested at any stage and lead to early embryonic death, fetal resorption, stillbirth or birth of goitrous, weak or dead fetus. Hypothyroidism also can reduce gonadotrophin output by the pituitary. Iodine deficiency in bulls is associated with depressed libido and deterioration of semen quality-several studies have revealed that supplementation of iodine has improved fertility, reduced stillbirths, abortions and incidence of retained placenta. Infertility in dairy cattle resulting from irregular or suppressed estrus is often responsive to iodine therapy. Iodine supplementation is necessary in many areas of deficiency but toxic amounts of iodine are not favourable. Manganese is involved in the activities of several enzyme systems including hydrolases, kinases, decarboxylases and transferases as well as Fe-containing enzymes which require Mn in their activity. It is therefore involved in carbohydrate, lipid and protein metabolism. It is also needed for bone growth and maintenance of connective and skeletal tissue. Mn also plays a role in reproduction and in immunological function. Mn deficiency results in abnormal skeletal growth, increased fat deposition, reproductive problems and reduced milk production. Selenium (Se) is a semi-metal that is very similar to sulfur in its chemical properties. It is an essential component of glutathione enzyme system, and a deficiency of selenium will leave the cell vulnerable to oxidation and increase the requirement of vitamin E. It has therefore been usual to supplement in the diets of all classes of animals, because of its antioxidant properties (Gutteridge and Halliwel, 1994). Cobalt is an essential trace element in ruminant diets for the production of vitamin B_{12}, which has 4% cobalt in its chemical structure, by the rumen microbes to meet the vitamin B_{12} requirements of both the ruminal bacteria and the host animal. This means that a cobalt deficiency is really a vitamin B_{12} deficiency, which would lead to anaemia.

Table 4 : Requirement of minerals (NRC, 2001)

Macro element (% of diet)	Young stock	Lactating animal	Sheep and goat
Ca	0.50	0.70	0.50
P	0.31	0.48	0.27
Mg	0.16	0.20	0.15
K	0.65	1.00	0.70
Na	0.10	0.18	0.18
S	0.16	0.25	0.26
Micro element (mg/kg dry matter intake)			
Co	0.10	0.10	0.10
Cu	10.0	10.0	10.0
I	0.25	0.6	0.50
Fe	50.0	50.0	50.0
Mn	40.0	40.0	40.0
Mo	-	4.0	-
Se	0.30	0.30	0.20
Zn	40.0	40.0	30.0

Mineral Deficiency

Mineral deficiencies occur more often when animals are confined within a given area and are closely dependent on soil profile and plant grown in that limited area. Deficiencies of minerals are more common in tropical countries where poor quality straws/stovers are the major roughages (Prasad *et al.*, 1995). Calcium deficiency can occur in soil in humid regions under conditions in which rainfall exceeds evapotranspiration and where bases have been depleted and soil acidity has developed. Calcium deficiency has been widely reported from many parts of the world and in India. However, the lower incidence of calcium than phosphorus disorders is attributable to three major factors (a) higher concentration of Ca than of P in the leaves and stems of most plant species; P is concentrated in seeds, (b) a wider distribution of P-deficient than Ca-deficient soils and (c) a lesser decline in the concentration of Ca than of P with advancing maturation of the plant. Further, inclusion of bran and oil cakes in ruminant diets at higher levels impairs the Ca :P ratio, thus affecting the mineral utilization. Most naturally occurring mineral deficiencies in ruminants are associated with specific geographic regions.

Tropical animal husbandry is mostly semi-intensive. The small holding livestock system is dependent mainly on grazing and crop residues as source of dry matter. Mineral imbalances are quite common in this system and there have been evidences of trace mineral deficiency/excess in different regions of the country (Garg *et al.*, 1999, 2002). Many recent studies have indicated the deficiency of Cu and Zn in most fodders available in different regions and the level of Fe and Mn in most feeds and fodders was quite high (Gowda *et al.*, 2001, 2004; Samantha and Samantha, 2002; Yadav *et al.*, 2002). There are incidences of low reproductive efficiency in livestock in most regions (Baruah *et al.*, 2000; Das *et al.*, 2002), which is often attributed to the deficiency of Cu, Zn, or Mn. The trace mineral deficiency in livestock in industrial areas due to more lead and cadmium also has been reported (Dey *et al.*, 1997). The areas of high rainfall and hilly regions are likely to be deficient in iodine and selenium, which needs much investigation.

Table 5 : Major limiting minerals in some states of India

State	Mineral deficiency
Andhra Pradesh	Ca, P, Cu, Zn, Mn
Arunachal Pradesh	Na, K, Mg, Cu, Mn
Assam	Ca, P, Mg, Cu
Bihar	P, Cu, Zn, Co, Mn
Gujarat	Ca, P, Zn
Haryana	Ca, P, Cu, Zn, Mn
Himachal Pradesh	Ca, P, Zn, Cu, K
Karnataka	Ca, P, Cu, Zn, Mg
Kerala	Ca, P, Cu, Zn, Mn, Mg
Madhya Pradesh	P, Zn, Fe, Mn
Maharashtra	Ca, P, Mg, Cu, Fe, Zn
Punjab	Ca, P, Cu, Zn
Rajasthan	Ca, P, Z, Cu
Tamil Nadu	Ca, P, Cu, Zn, Mn
Uttar Pradesh	Ca, P, Cu, Zn, Mn, Co
Uttaranchal	Ca, P, Cu, Co
West Bengal	Ca, P, Cu, Zn, Mn

Source : AICRP on feed resources

Diagnosis and Assessment of Mineral Deficiency

The diagnosis, assessment and the prevention of trace mineral deficiency need a thorough understanding of the factors like age of animal, season, clinical signs, soil profile, plant mineral content and feeding practices. Based on this preliminary information, further biological diagnostic tests can be followed for confirmation. In general mineral deficiency is diagnosed by observing the clinical symptoms. But mineral deficiency signs are often confusing as the observed symptoms can be associated with more than one mineral and can be combined with the effects of protein and/or energy inadequacy, various types of parasitism, toxic plants, infectious diseases or with deficiency of other micronutrients. Except for characteristic signs like goiter in iodine deficiency or white muscle disease in selenium deficiency, most trace element deficiencies produce non-specific signs such as loss of appetite, retarded growth, unthriftiness or reproductive problems, and hence clinical/pathological examination of biological materials is required (Pattanaik, 2001a). Some mineral like Ca, Mg and P are stored in body tissues and their deficiency symptoms are exhibited only after a period of time. Calcium and phosphorous deficiency can be observed more quickly, particularly in high producing animals and fast growing calves. Critical values of certain minerals in soil, plant and animals are provided in Table 6, which will be of much use in ascertaining the mineral deficiency. Certain naturally occurring mineral deficiency/toxicity is directly related to soil characteristics as in case of fluoride, Se and Mo, but the level of mineral in soil does not necessarily indicate its availability to plants growing on the soil. Other limitation of plant mineral analysis is the biological availability and factors influencing the utilization like chelating agents, mineral antagonism etc. Analysis of mineral content in body tissues is a better indicator of the mineral adequacy because mineral deficiency results in subnormal concentration of the element and will usually be associated with clinical signs, however for certain minerals due to homeostatic mechanisms the levels may remain normal even during deficiency, but will respond positively to supplementation. Research is being conducted for using biochemical markers like specific enzymes/tissues to assess the mineral status more precisely.

Commonly Used Indices of Mineral Element Status in Animals

There are numerous measures of essential mineral element status, including growth rate, tissue and physiological fluids concentrations, enzyme concentrations and activities, chemical balance and mobilizable stores. Blood and its specific nutrient concentrations provide a useful but frequently inadequate index. The first limiting biochemical system should provide the most valid index, but in many cases it is not known or not readily measured. Chemical balance and mobilizable stores provide valid measures but are difficult to determine. Two indices are infinitely more valuable than one and should be determined if possible. Commonly used indices of mineral element adequacy are:a) Growth rate, b) Blood and plasma concentrations, c) Hair concentrations, d) Biopsy tissue concentration, e) Enzyme concentrations and activities, f) Physiological functions, g) Chemical balance, h) Mobilizable stores, i) Immune competence and j) Behaviour and appearance.

Table 6 : Critical values of trace minerals for assessment of status

Element	Soil	Feed / Fodder	Animal body	
			Normal level	Deficient
Ca	0.1%	0.3 %	8-12 mg %	< 8 mg % (plasma)
P	45-130 ppm	0.25 %	4-6 mg %	< 4 mg % (plasma)
Mg	0.01 %	0.20%	1.9-3.2 mg %	< 1.9 mg % (plasma)
Fe	2.5 ppm	50 ppm	1-2 ppm (serum)	< 1 ppm (serum)
Cu	0.3 ppm	8 ppm	0.65-1.2 ppm (serum)	< 0.6 ppm (serum)
Zn	1 ppm	30 ppm	1-2 ppm (serum)	< 0.6-0.8 ppm (serum)
Mn	5 ppm	40 ppm	0.3-0.5 ppm (serum)	< 6 ppm (liver)
I	-	0.1-0.2 ppm	-	< 5-10 Microgram/dl iodine (serum) Plasma-protein bound iodine < 0.8 mg/dl
Co	-	0.08-0.1 ppm	-	< 0.5 ng/ml (rumen fluid) < 0.05 ppm (liver) Vit B_{12} < 200 pg/ml (plasma)
Mo	-	0.5 ppm	-	-
Se	-	0.1 ppm	-	< 0.2 ppm (liver) < 0.05 ppm (blood) < 0.03 ppm (serum)

Kincaid (1999)

Subclinical mineral deficiencies are thought to be very widespread and are likely to be of more economic significance than are easily recognized cases. With inadequate mineral intakes, animals may have lower milk production, growth and reproductive efficiency without recognizable signs. So, it is utmost important to diagnose the mineral inadequate animals at marginal or sub optimum levels. Evolving strategies of considerable potential include use of biochemical markers such as ceruloplasmin for Cu, ferrtin/transferrin for Fe and superoxide dismutase for Zn/Cu, and molecular techniques like metallothionein mRNA in lymphocytes for Zn.

Amelioration of Mineral Deficiency

Strategic Approach for Mineral Supplementation

Performance of livestock in the tropics is mainly governed by the quality and quantity of nutrients provided in the diet. In most of the developed countries, the principal means by which cattle producers try to meet the requirement is through use of free - choice dietary minerals. This is neither practical nor cost effective in developing countries where the livestock are fed on crop residues and concentrate by-products. Where compounded concentrate diets are not fed, it is necessary to rely on both indirect and direct methods of providing minerals.

Table 7 : Catagorization of common feeds and fodders based on mineral content

Mineral	Good sources	Moderate sources
Ca	Fodder / Grass : Lucerne, cowpea, rice bean,dolichos lab-lab, stylosanthus, velvet bean,green panic,dinanath grass Top feeds:Glyrecidia leaves,mulberry leaves,erythrina leaves,neem leaves,jack leaves,Carrot tops Unconventional feeds:Sunflower heads,horse gram pods,groundnut haulms	Fodder / Grasses:Maize fodder, sorghum fodder,guinea grass,anjan grass,green panic,mixed local grasses Oil seed cakes: Rapeseed cake sunflower cake, castor bean cake,rubber seed cake Top feeds: Banana leaves,rain tree leaves Unconventional feeds: Finger millet pods gram husk,silk worm pupae meal,meat meal
P	Oil Seed Cakes: Groundnut cake,coconut cake,cotton seed cake,soyabean cake,sunflower cake,rape seed cake By Products :Rice polish,wheat bran,rice bran Unconventional feeds:Soya husk,meat meal	Fodder / Grasses :Lucerne,velvet bean,para grass,blue panic, guinea grass Oil seed cakes:Sunflower cake,neem seed cake,karanj cake,castor cake,rubber seed cake,guar meal Unconventional feeds,Maize husk,rain tree pods
Mg	Fodder / Grasses:Cow pea fodder,dinanath grass Oil cakes:Cotton seed cake,sunflower cake By Products :Rice polish ,rice bran Top feeds:Glyrecidia Unconventional feeds :Cocoa seed husk, groundnut haulms, sea weed	Dry roughage:Ragi straw Fodder / Grasses: Rice bean fodder,cow pea fodder,hybrid napier,guinea grass,maize fodder,soybean fodder Oil seed cakes:Rapeseed cake,castor cake,coconut cake,groundnut cake Top feeds: Subabul leaves,mulberry leaves

Contd...

S	Protein sources: Mustard cake, soyabean meal, groundnut cake, meat meal	By- Products: Wheat bran, rice bran, rice polish
Cu	Fodder / Grasses:Cow pea,dolichos lab lab,soybean fodder,NB - 21 fodder, guinea grass,maize fodder Top feeds:Banana leaves,carrot tops,glyrecidia Unconventional:Subabul pods,castor cake rubber seed cake,bamboo leaves,groundnut haulms	Fodder / Grass:Guinea grass,hybrid napier,Co-I fodder,para grass,local grasses Oil seed cakes:Groundnut cake,coconut cake,sunflower cake,soya meal,neem seed cake,copra cake By-products : Rice polish Top feeds:Mulberry leaves,erythrina leaves,glyrecidia leaves,subabul leaves,Rain tree leaves
Zn	Fodder / Grasses:Stylosanthus,velvet bean fodder,anjan grass,guinea grass,NB - 21 fodder,Co-I fodder, soybean fodder Oil seed cakes: Copra cake,neem seed cake karanj seed cake By-products :Wheat bran Unconventional feeds :Tapioca meal,ginger waste,coffee husk, silk worm pupae meal,meat meal	Fodder / Grasses:Rice bean, fodder,dinanath grass,green panic,para grass,sorghum fodder Oil seed cakes:Groundnut cake,cotton seed cake,sunflower cake,safflower cake By-products:Rice Polish Top feeds:Banana leaves,jack leaves,glyrecidia leaves,neem leaves Unconventional :Tapioca meal sugarcane bagasse,subabul pods
Fe	Fodder / Grass:Cowpea,Rice bean fodder dinanath fodder,anjan grass,signal grass,NB - 21 fodder,Co - I fodder,para grass,mixed local grasses,weeds Oil seed cakes: Cotton seed cake,sunflower cake,rubber seed cake Top feeds: Glyrecidia leaves,erythrina leaves,subabul leaves Unconventional Feeds:Spent coffee,cocoa seed husk, meat meal,groundnut haulms	Dry fodder:Ragi Straw,paddy straw,bajra straw,maize kadbi,jowar kadbi Fodder / Grasses:Dolichos lab lab guinea grass,maize fodder,jowar fodder,sorghum fodder Oil seed cakes:Groundnut cake By-products :Rice polish,rice bran Grains:Maize,rice

Contd...

		Top feeds:Banana leaves,mulberry leaves,neem leaves,sugarcane tops
Mn	By-products: Wheat bran, rice bran Crop residues: Paddy and ragi straw Green fodder: Lucerne, cow pea	Green fodders, leafy vegetation.
I	Marine products, oil seed cakes, iodized common salt, yeast.	Green fodders
Co	Legume fodders, animal proteins, fermented products.	Green fodders, tree leaves
Mo	Legumes, green grasses.	Fodder tree leaves
Se	Marine products, meat meal, Se-Yeast	Cultivated green fodders, legumes

Indirect Methods of Mineral Supplementation

Enrichment of Soil with Essential Minerals through Fertilization

Indirect provision of minerals to grazing livestock includes; mineral fertilization of pasture and altering soil pH, however this may not be always feasible due to complex soil – plant - animal interrelationship. In the indirect approach, soil treatment of deficient minerals would make these elements accumulate in plants. For instance soil treatment of cobalt and selenium will improve their concentration in plants without having any effect on plant yield. This effect may be neutralized in high alkaline or calcareous soils, as the uptake of cobalt by plants in such soils would be affected. Copper application makes it more available to plants in soils low in molybdenum content, but will not be effective when soils contain high molybdenum. High application of NPK fertilizers reduces the calcium, magnesium and sodium availability to plants. So the approach to enrich the soil through micronutrient supplementation may not be very cost effective and also may not yield the desired results due to the variation in soil profile in different zones. Trace element intakes that can be improved by fertilization include selenium, cobalt, copper, zinc, boron, and possibly nickel.

Direct Methods of Mineral Supplementation

In India the livestock farmers provide some quantity of cakes, bran, rice polish and husk as concentrate supplement to productive animals. Unproductive animals are generally allowed to graze. Except in some parts of Punjab, Haryana and Uttar Pradesh green fodder is not fed to the animals. Some quantity of greens are offered during rainy season which are grown on the bunds in the field. The animals do not receive any mineral supplement and even salt is not being fed. The possible reasons would be the high cost involved and lack of awareness. The direct approach of supplementing micronutrients in the diet of cattle depending on the severity of deficiency may be a more practical method. The most efficient method of providing trace minerals is through mineral mixture mixed with concentrate feed ingredients. This assures an adequate intake of mineral elements by each animal (Lall *et al.*, 2002). This procedure represents an ideal system for providing supplemental minerals but it cannot be used with grazing cattle, which receive little concentrates and depend on forages or where concentrates are not fed. Use of mineral supplements in the form of mineral mixture or mineral licks and premixes are most commonly used methods. Supplementation can also be achieved through feeding compound feeds, oral drenching or dosing or by administering slow releasing mineral boluses which are retained in the gut and in the form of injectable preparations. Heavy pellets of the mineral or soluble glass which has the specific mineral impregnated into it are lodged in reticulo-rumen are useful in steady supply of specific minerals continuously for long periods. This approach is useful during peak period of milk production to overcome certain metabolic disorders like milk fever and grass tetany (Ellis *et al.*, 1988).

Supplementation of Area-Specific Mineral Mixture

Feeding of 'free-choice' mineral supplements could be the easiest way of supplementing minerals. Alternatively providing area-specific mineral mixture based on the deficiency of minerals in soil, plant and animals in different agro-climatic zones are most appropriate and cost effective method of mineral supplementation. The former approach could sometimes lead to deleterious effect, as some of the minerals may be available in excess than requirements affecting utilization of other minerals. For example, excess of calcium disturbing the Ca - P ratio, excess of selenium affecting sulphur utilization, excess of molybdenium and sulphur reducing copper absorption and excess of iron disturbing copper metabolism. More practical method is of supplementing only the most deficient minerals through area specific mineral mixture by assessing the mineral content in soil, feeds and fodders and in animals in different agro-climatic zones. This approach has been found to improve the reproductive efficiency in crossbred cattle under field conditions and this technology has been a success (Gowda and Prasad, 2005).

Supplementation through Locally Available Mineral Rich Natural Feed Resources

One of the other cost effective method of mineral supplementation is to provide feed and plant sources rich in the specific micronutrient, which are commonly being fed/grown in that particular region (Gowda *et al.*, 2004a). For example cakes, brans and rice polish are rich sources of phosphorus. Similarly top feeds/tree leaves and legumes are good sources of calcium, copper and zinc. Some of the unconventional feed resources are also rich in certain minerals (Table 7). In general legume fodders, cultivated green fodders and tree leaves are good sources of Ca, Fe, Zn, Cu, Co and Mn and oil cakes and bran are good sources of P, Zn, Cu and Mn (Gowda *et al.*, 2004b).

Bioavailability of Minerals

Several factors influence the bioavailability of minerals like the chemical form of mineral salt, physiological status of animal, species and mineral interaction with other constituents of feed. Bioavailability; hence is the proportion of the ingested element that is absorbed, transported to target site for performing its function. Physiological status like growth, bone development, pregnancy, lactation or stress may increase the requirement of mineral. Animals deprived of an essential trace element become more efficient in absorbing when supplemented due to adaptive mechanism. Intrinsic factors like solubility of chemical salt, adsorption to large molecules of fibre, silica and other compounds, competitive antagonism amongst metal ions e.g. Cu-Zn, Cd-Zn, Fe-Zn, Mn-Fe will determine the ultimate availability of mineral elements. Anti-nutritional factors like tannins, phytates, oxalates and excess sulfates will depress the absorption of trace minerals, whereas peptides, amino acids, ionophores and lactose may enhance the bioavailability of certain minerals. The mineral release from the feed/fodder on digestion also varies depending on their distribution within the plant cell and the form in which they exist (Ibrahim *et al.*, 1998). Some minerals when they are supplemented in inorganic form are better utilized than through natural green fodders, probably due to the interference of fibre. Similarly the paddy straw which contains more ADF has less bioavailable minerals than finger millet straw (Gowda and Prasad, 2005; Gowda *et al.*, 2003b). Several legumes though rich in Fe and Zn, their bioavailability is limited due to phytate. Among the individual inorganic salts the mineral availability depends on their chemical form and elemental proportion. Among the better bioavailable salts Ferrous sulfate, Cupric chloride, Copper sulfate, Zinc oxide, Zinc sulfate, Zinc carbonate, Manganese oxide, Potassium iodide, Cuprous iodide and Sodium selenite have higher proportion of Fe, Cu, Zn, Mn, I and Se, respectively (Ammerman *et al.*, 1995).

Supplementation Chelated Minerals

Of late there is a growing interest in the use of organic or chelated minerals due to better bioavailability, improved reproductive performance, immune response, decrease in the incidences of mastitis and carcass quality (Spears, 1996). Organic forms of Zn and Cu as Zn-methionine or Cu-lysine bypass the rumen and are available at intestine, thus protecting the essential amino acids from degradation and make them available for absorption in the gut

(Sundberg, 2002; Spears, 2003). Zn-methionine supplementation in cattle has improved disease resistance and prevented foot rot and hoof problems. Copper in chelated form would have an advantage over an inorganic form when Mo level is high, as it may escape the complexing. A mixture of Zn, Mn, Cu, Co, Se in organic forms may stimulate feed intake and growth during stress period. The association of Se was known only to glutathione peroxidase. But recently it has been known that Se is a part of at least 25 selenoproteins and Se research and its practical applications are fast developing and are very promising. The use of Se- enriched yeast appears to become a reality in dairy cattle nutrition replacing the traditional inorganic Se (Lyons *et al.*, 2007). The organic form of these minerals also has an antioxidant property, thereby improving the feed efficiency and immunity of animals. These chelated minerals can be of much use in areas of severe deficiency of trace minerals like tropical feeding systems, but the cost benefit ratio need to be established. However, this approach is more environment's friendly as there is less faecal excretion of minerals.

Mineral Biofortification of Plants

One sustainable agricultural approach for reducing the mineral deficiencies in livestock animals is to enrich major staple food crops (rice, wheat, maize) with minerals through plant breeding strategies. Biofortification of plants with minerals may be a promising and cost-effective intervention. The idea is to breed food crops for higher micronutrient content, which can be done through crossbreeding or genetic engineering. It is time to move forward with a strong program to develop micronutrient-rich crop varieties, demonstrate their impact on human and animal nutrition. So, finding the appropriate answers on future mineral research requires the coordinated efforts of soil scientists, plant scientists and animal nutritionists.

Newer Trace Elements

There are few trace elements which are present in very low concentrations and their beneficial functions have been studied in monogastric animals (Anke *et al.*, 1983; 1990). Chromium (Cr) is known to influence glucose utilization and is termed as glucose tolerance factor. Practical diets of livestock appear to contain enough Cr to meet the requirement inspite of its low availability from feed stuffs. Supplementation of Cr as Cr-picolinate to pigs (Amoikon *et al.*, 1995) and Cr-yeast to broilers (Hussain *et al.*, 1998) has increased the feed efficiency. Boran (B) supplementation has shown to improve bone strength and increased Ca and Mg retention (Brown *et al.*, 1989). Lithium (Li) is suggested to be essential in several species of animals. Lithium supplementation improved weight gain and reproductive efficiency in ewes and Li is found to be an effective mineral in the recovery of bovine spastic paresis. Experimentally induced Nickel (Ni) deficiency reduced growth rate in rats, pigs and goats and feeding diet low in Ni produced skin and skeletal lesions, abortion and lower testicular weight in goats. Bacterial urease in rumen also require Ni for maximum activity but may not provide absolute advantage in terms of urea metabolism. Silicon (Si) is essential for growth and bone development in rats and chicks and believed to be associated with glycosamine and collagen synthesis. Studies in ruminants showed better growth and wool quality after supplementing Si at 580 and 1430 ppm. Induced Vanadium (V) deficiency in rats and chicks resulted in reduced feather growth, iron metabolism and impaired bone development. Supplementation of vanadium at 0.1 ppm level increased growth rate, RBC and haemoglobin levels in calves and also helped in bone formation in surgically induced jaw defect of rabbits. Further detailed research is required to confirm the essentiality and supplementary value of these newer trace elements (Pattanaik, 2001b).

Minerals play a significant role in production and reproduction either singly or in combination. Ameliorating the deficiency or imbalance of minerals improves the productive efficiency of ruminants to great extent. Hence minerals are to be considered in tropical feeding system not in isolation but as a part of total nutrient management system. The emphasis should be on ways of mineral supplementation cost-effectively based on prevailing livestock farming system and available resources. Bioavailability of minerals should be given emphasis while supplementing and better bioavailable inorganic salts or organic/chelated form of trace minerals are to be used for enhancing the efficiency of utilization. While suggesting the mineral requirement for livestock, the level of dry matter intake, physiological status and mineral content of feed/fodder are to be considered. Though trace elements have not received much attention in formulating diets, their long term practical impact on production, reproduction and immunity must be considered. Further research efforts are required in understanding the complex interaction of different minerals to improve bioavailability, antioxidant/prooxidant potential of minerals and evolving biochemical/molecular markers for easy detection of mineral status of animals.

References

Ammerman, C.B., Baker, H.D. and Lewis, A.J. (1995). *Bioavailability of nutrients for animals*, Academic press, Inc., California.

Amoikon, E.K., Fernandez, J.M., Southern, L.L., Thompson, D.L., Ward, T.L. and Olcott, B.M. (1995). *J. Anim. Sci.*, 73 : 1123-30.

Anke, M., Groppel, B. and Krause, U. (1990). In: Seventh International symposium on trace elements in man and animals (TEMA 7), Dubrovnik, Yugoslavia, p. 36.

Anke, M., Groppel, B., Kronemann, H. and Fuhrer, E. (1983). In : Spuren element symposium. Abteilung wissenschaftliche publikationen, Friderich Schiller Universistat, Jena, Germany, p. 135.

Arnault G A. (1983). C F. (Pattanaik 2001a).

Baruah, K.K., Newar, S., Baruah, A. and Bhuyan, D. (2000). *Ind. J. Dairy Sci.*, 53 (6): 424-427.

Brown, T.F., Mc Cormick, M.E., Morris, D.R. and Zeringue, L.K. (1989). *Nutr. Res.* 9: 503-12.

Cardose, E.C., Mc Dowell, L.R., Vale, W.G., Viega, J.B. and Neto, S. (1999). *Intl. J. Anim. Sci.*, 14 : 1-7.

Carlisle E M. (1986). In : Trace elements in human and animal nutrition, 5th Ed., Vol. 1, Academic press, New York, p. 373.

Chang, X., Mowat, D.N. and Bateman, K.G. (1991). (C.F. Pattanaik 2001b).

Chhabra, A., Prasad, T. and Arora, S.P. (1991). In : *Proceedings of First International Animal Nutrition Workers Conference for Asia and Pacific*, held at Bangalore, 23-28 September 1991, pp. 185-189.

Corah L. (1996). *Anim. Feed Sci. and Tech.*, 59 : 61-70.

Das, P., Biswas, S., Ghosh, T.K. and Haldar, S. (2002). *Anim. Nutr. and Feed Technol.*, 2: 19-26.

Dey, S., Dwivedi, S.K. and Swarup, D. (1997). *Ind. J. Anim. Sci.*, 67(9): 780-81.

Ellis, G.L., Mc Dowell, L.R. and Conrad, J.H. (1988). *Nut. Rep. Intl.*, 38 : 1137-47.

Garg, M.R., Bhanderi, B.M. and Sherasia, P.L. (1999). *Ind. J. Dairy Sci.*, 52 (2): 69-77.

Garg M.R., Bhanderi, B.M. and Sherasia, P.L. (2002). *Ind. J. Dairy Sci.*, 55 (3) : 154-58.

Gowda, N.K.S. and Prasad, C.S. (2005). *Asian -Australasian J. Anim. Sci.*, 18 (1) : 48-53.

Gowda, N.K.S., Prasad, C.S. and Ramana, J.V. (2004a). *Ind. J. Anim. Sci.*, 74 (6) : 653-58.

Gowda, N.K.S., Prasad, C.S., Ashok, L.B. and Ramana, J.V. (2003b). *Asian- Australasian J. Anim. Sci.*, 17 (2): 221-27.

Gowda, N.K.S., Prasad, C.S., Ramana, J.V. and Ramachandra, K.S. (2001). *Ind. J. Anim. Sci.*, 71(2):150-54.

Gowda, N.K.S., Ramana, J.V., Prasad, C.S. and Singh, K. (2004b). *Trop. Anim. Health and Prod.*, 36: 77-94.

Gutteridge, J..M.C. and Halliwel, B. (1994). Antioxidants in Nutrition, Health and disease. Oxford University Press, Oxford.

Hannam, R.J. and Reuter, D.J. (1987). Trace element nutrition of pastures. In : Wheeler J L, Pearson C J and Robards G E (Ed), Temperate Pastures – Their production, use and management. Melbourne, Australia Wool Corporation/CSIRO, 175-90.

Hopkins, L.Jr. and Mohr, H.E. (1974). (CF Pattanaiak 2001b).

Hosking, W.J., Caple, I.W., Halpin, C.G., Brown, A.J., Paynter, D.I., Conley, D.N. and North Coombes, P.L. (1986). Trace elements in pasture and animals in Victoria (C F Masters and White, 1996).

Hussain, S.M., Barrento, S.L. and Silva, C.G. (1998). *Anim. Feed Sci. & Technol.*, 71: 217-228.

Hurley, W.L. and Doane, R.M (1989). *J. Dairy Sci.*, 72: 784-804.

Ibrahim, M.N.M., Zemmelink, G. and Tamminga, S. (1998). *Asian Australasian J. Anim. Sci.*, 11 (5): 530-37.

Kincaid, R.L. (1999). *Proc. Am. Soc. Anim. Sci.* 1-8.

Kumar B., Pachauri, S.P. and Kumar, N. (2002). *Ind. J. Anim. Sci.*, 72(4): 332-336.

Lall, D., Dahiya, S.S., Lailer, P.C., Chauhan, T.R. and Punia, B.S. (2002). *Ind. J. Anim. Nutr.*, 19 (3) : 204-209.

Lyons, M.P., Papazyan, T.T. and Surai, P.F. (2007). *Asian. Aust. J. Anim. Sci.*, 20 (7) : 1135.

Masters, D.G. (1996). Mineral deficiency problems in grazing sheep-an overview. In: Detection and treatment of mineral nutrition problems in grazing sheep (Eds. Masters D G and White C L), ACIAR Monograph No. 37, pp. 1-14.

Mc Dowell, LR. (1992). *Minerals in Animal and Human Nutrition*, Academic press, Inc., California.

Mc Dowell, L.R. (1996). *Anim. Feed Sci. and Technol.*, 69 : 247-71.

Mc Dowell, L.R.(1997). *Minerals for grazing ruminants in tropical regions* (3rd ed), University of Florida Cooperative Extension Service.

Masters, D.G. and White, C.L. (1996). Detection and treatment of mineral nutrition problems in grazing sheep, ACIAR monograph No. 37, Canbera, Australia.

Mc Dowell. L.R., Conrad, J.H. and Glen Hembry, F. (1993). Minerals for grazing ruminants in tropical regions, 2nd Edn., University of Florida, Gainesville.

Milne, J.S., Whitelaw, F.G., Price, J. and Shand, W.J. (1990). (CF Pattanaik 2001b).

N.R.C. (2001). *Nat. Res. Coun.*, Washington, D.C.

Nelson, J. (1988). Review of trace mineral chelates complexes available to the feed industry (C F. Mc Dowell 1996).

O' Dell, B. and Sunde, R.A. (1997). Introduction. In : *Hand book of nutritionally essential mineral elements*. Marcel Dekker Inc., New York, pp. 1-12.

Pattanaik A K. (2001). Diagnosis of trace element deficiencies of livestock. In : *Short course on Nutrition and Dietetics under clinico–therapeutic conditions of pet and farm animals* held at IVRI, Izatnagar, March 20 – April 18, pp. 171-79.

Pattanaik A K. (2001a). Diagnosis of trace element deficiencies of livestock. In : *Short course on Nutrition and Dietetics under clinico–therapeutic conditions of pet and farm animals* held at IVRI, Izatnagar, March 20 – April 18, pp. 171-79.

Pattanaik A K. (2001b). Essentiality of newer trace elements. Recent developments. In : *Short course on Nutrition and dietetics under clinico-therapeutic conditions of pet and farm animals* held at IVRI, Izatnagar, March 20 – April 18, PP 197-203.

Phillippo, M., Humphries, W.R. Atkinson, T. Henderson, G.D. and Gaythwaite, P.H. (1987). *J. Agri Sci. (Camb.)* 09: 326-336.

Prasad, C.S., Arora, S.P., Prasad, T., Chhabra, A. and Ibrahim, M.N.M. (1995). In : *Hand book for straw feeding systems* (Ed. Kiran Singh and J B Schiere), ICAR, New Delhi, PP 225-38.

Ramana, J.V., Prasad, C.S., Gowda, N.K.S. and Ramachandra, K.S. (2001). *Ind. J. Dairy Sci.*, 54 (1): 40-46.

Regius, A., Anke, M., Sardi, J. and Mucsy, I. (1993). In : *Trace elements in man and animals.* TEMA 8 : 603-04.

Reid, R.L. and Horvath, D.J. (1980). *Anim. Feed Sci. and Technol.*, 5 : 95-167.

Samanta, A. and Samanta, G. (2002). *Ind. J. Anim. Sci.*, 19 (3): 278-281.

Sharma, R.K. and Sharma, Manju. (1997). *Ind. J. Expt. Biol.* 35: 696-713.

Smart, M.E., budmunson, J. and Christensen, D.A. (1981). *A Rev. Canad. Vet. J.*, 22: 372-376.

Smith, O.B. and Akinnbamijo, O.O. (2000). *Anim. Reprod. Sci.*, 60-61: 549-560.

Spears, J.W. (1996). *Anim. Feed Sci. and Technol.*, 58 : 151-63.

Spears, J.W. (1999). *Asian -Australasian J. Anim. Sci.*, 12 (6) : 1002-08.

Spears, J.W. (2003). *J. Nutr.* 133 (suppl) : 1506-1509.

Sundberg, A S. (2002). *Bri. J. of Nutri.*, 88 (3): 281-286.

Suttle, N.F. (2000). *Asian –Austral. J. Anim. Sci.*, 13 (Supplement) : 1-9.

Underwood, E.J. (1981). The Mineral Nutrition of Livestock, Commonwealth Agriculture Bureaux, Slough, U.K.

Van, Niekerk, B.D.H. and Jacobs, G.A. (1985). Protein, energy and phosphorus supplementation of cattle fed low quality forage (C.F. Mc Dowell 1996).

Yadav, P.S., Mandal, A.B. and Dahiya, D.V. (2002). *Animal Nutr. and Feed Tech.*, 2:127-38.

□□□

Animal Nutrition, 2012
eds. Dr. (Mrs.) Usha R. Mehra et al., pp. 379-393
Satish Serial Publishing House e-mail : info@satishserial.com; website : www.satishserial.com

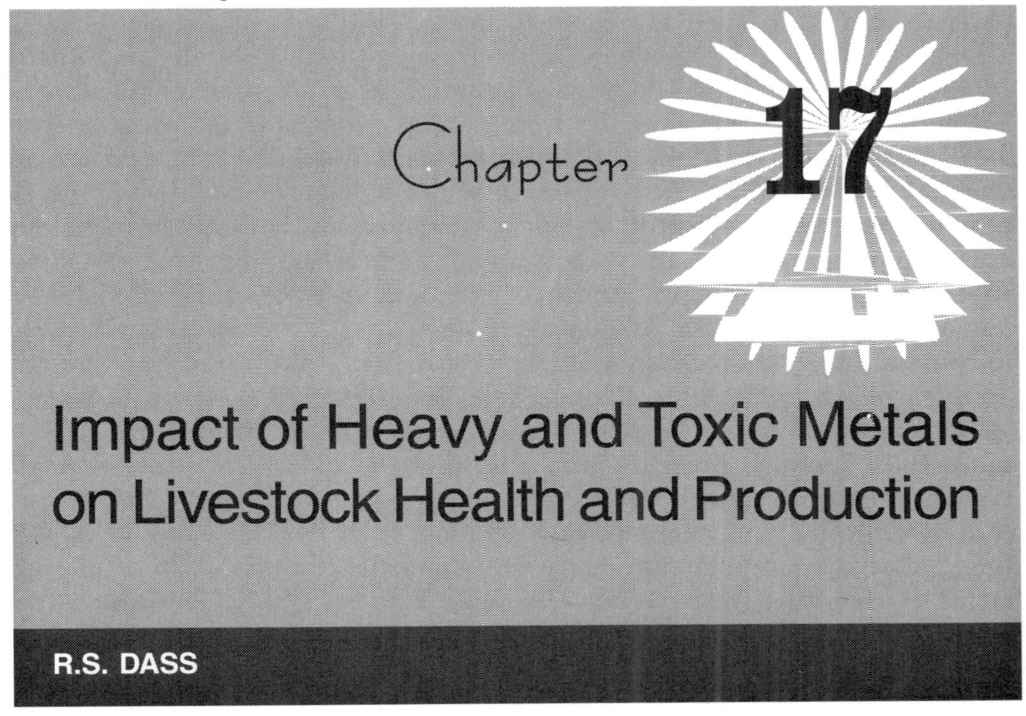

Impact of Heavy and Toxic Metals on Livestock Health and Production

R.S. DASS

Heavy metals are widely prevalent in nature owing to their abundance in earth's crust, and constitute an important fraction of the biosphere. Many of these heavy metals such as copper, iron, cobalt, selenium, zinc etc., are essential for life, as they play a vital role in number of biological processes; whereas heavy metals like arsenic, cadmium, lead and mercury have little or no known beneficial biological function though observed to be present in animal body, and detrimental to them at even low concentration. A special quality of heavy metals is their strong affinity and long persistence in biological system. Once in biological system their excretion from the body is very slow; these are stable in the environment and are not degradable rapidly. Similarly, fluorine is known more for its toxicity rather than its usefulness in the body of animals. These heavy metals and toxic metal fluorine are discussed in brief in this chapter.

Arsenic

Arsenic (As) is a metalloid, which is odourless and tasteless. It exists in three common valance states: As (0) (metalloid arsenic, 0 oxidation state), As

(III) (trivalent state, such as arsenites), and As (V) (pentavalent state, such as arsenates). Arsenic is present in the environment both naturally and due to certain human activities. The principal natural reservoirs of arsenic are rocks. It enters drinking water supplies from natural deposits in the earth or from agricultural and industrial practices. Release and mobilization of arsenic from these sources constitute the availability of this element in soil, water and air in various forms. As a result, arsenic is ubiquitous in our environment, and animals and humans are always unavoidably exposed to this toxic metalloid. It occurs in ground water in the form of arsenites, arsenate, and methyl arsenic and dimethyl arsenic acid. Arsenites and arsenate compounds are highly toxic to human beings as well as animals (Singh *et al.*, 2005). Soil may contain arsenic levels between 0.1 to 40 ppm (Yan Chu, 1994). The range of As concentrations found in natural waters is large, ranging from less than 0.5 µg/l to more than 5 mg/l (Smedley and Kinniburgh, 2002). Sometimes, much higher concentrations are found, particularly in ground water.Chakaraborti *et al.* (2003) analyzed the arsenic content in water of 206 tube wells, and found that 56.8% water sample exceeded arsenic concentration of 50 µg/l and 19.9% samples were having >300 µg/l; whereas (WHO, 2004) has given a provisional guideline value of 10 µg/l arsenic in drinking water. Well known high-As groundwater areas have been found in Argentina, Chile, México, China and Hungary, and more recently in India (West Bengal), Bangladesh and Vietnam.

Metabolism of Arsenic

Arsenic mainly enters the body by ingestion or inhalation. Arsenic has no nutritional requirement to the biological world, yet the metabolic processes of this element in animal and humans have been evolved. The dietary soluble arsenic compounds in the gut are rapidly absorbed into the blood stream and initially accumulates in the liver, spleen, kidneys, lungs and gastrointestinal tract. It is likely that metabolism of arsenic , like other toxic metals, is associated with the conversion of the most potentially toxic forms of this element to the less toxic form, followed by accumulation in or excretion from the body. Biomethylation of As is considered as the primary detoxification mechanism; inorganic As is methylated to monomethylarsonic acid (MMA) and finally to dimethylarsenic acid (DMA) by the methyl donor,S-adenosylmethionine (SAM) catalyzed by methyltransferase in the presence of glutathione(Styblo and Thomas, 1997). The trivalent arsenicals are preferred substrates for methylation reactions and hence the reduction of arsenic from pentavalent to trivalent may be a critical step in the control of the rate of metabolism of arsenic (Styblo *et al.*, 1995). Clearance of As from the tissues is rapid, and two to four weeks after exposure ceases, most of the arsenic remaining in the body is found in keratin rich tissues such as skin, hair, and nails, and to a lesser extent in bones and teeth. Tissue accretion of arsenic is slow as the absorbed arsenic is excreted extensively through urine.

Arsenic Toxicity

The mechanism of arsenic toxicity is due to the ability of arsenites (As (III) to bind protein thiol. Glutathione (GSH) is the most abundant cellular thiol, and both GSH and GSH-related enzymes are important antioxidants that play an important role in the detoxification of arsenic and other carcinogens. Arsenic is a pro-oxidant and thus may cause lipid per oxidation, protein and enzyme oxidation, DNA oxidation and GSH depletion. Further, As generates reactive oxygen species like nitric oxide; which are known to induce poly ADP-ribosylation which is implicated in DNA repair, signal transduction and apoptosis. Arsenic binds to sulphydryl groups of proteins and interferes with their function. The symptoms of arsenic toxicity vary with the rate and duration of exposures and source of arsenic involved (Bahri and Romdane, 1991).Accidental exposure to large oral doses of inorganic arsenic cause acute toxicity, with major effects on the gastrointestinal tract and cardiovascular system. Arsenic has a direct effect on the capillaries, causing damage to micro vascular integrity and loss of blood. Acute and per acute episode of poisoning by inorganic arsenic are usually explosives with high morbidity and moderate mortality over a period of 2-3 days. Symptoms are manifested by intense abdominal pain, staggering gait, extreme weakness, trembling, salivation, diarrhea, feeble pulse, prostration, and rumen atony, normal to subnormal temperature, collapse and death. Water soluble inorganic salts, (arsenites and arsenates) in the trivalent form are more toxic than organic arsenicals.

Prevention and Alleviation of Arsenic Toxicity

In animal studies, dimercaprol has been found to reduce the deposition of arsenic in rabbit (Snider *et al.*, 1990). Oral agents such as 2, 3 dimercaptosuccinic acid (DMSA) and D-penicillamine have been used as alternatives to British antilevisite (BAL). DMSA appears to be effective chelators of arsenic in experimental animals and humans, which form complexes with arsenic to both neutralize the toxic action and to facilitate its excretion. Concomitant oral supplementation of *Aloe vera* (Gupta and Flora,2005) *or Centella asiatica* (Gupta and Flora,2006) to arsenic exposed rats had remarkable protective effects on blood delta-aminolevulinic acid dehydratase activity and restored blood GSH level while most of the other biochemical parameters remain unchanged.

Tolerable level: The maximum tolerable level of arsenic was set at 30 mg/ kg diet DM (NRC, 2005).

Lead

Lead (Pb) is one of the most ubiquitous heavy metals that have been detected virtually in almost all phases of environmental and biological systems. The quantity of lead used in the 20th century far exceeds the total lead consumed in all previous eras. The two products which have added massive amounts of lead contamination to the environment are lead-based paints and lead additives to gasoline (Nriagu, 1990). There are no known physiological requirements of lead. In fact, exposure to lead either by acute or chronic exposure, often results in severe and debilitating toxicological problems (Ekong *et al.*, 2006). Anthropogenic activities such as mining, smelting and use of automobile fuels have substantially altered the natural ecological distribution of lead in the environment leading to globally elevated levels of lead in air, water and soil. Lead levels in ground and river water ranged from 1-60 µg/litre and 1-10 µg/litre, respectively, and the earth crust normally contains 13 mgPb/kg.

Lead Metabolism

Lead may be absorbed into the body via gastrointestinal tract, lungs and skin. Many factors have been reported to affect the absorption of lead, among which age is the most important that influences the retention of ingested lead. There is a higher rate of absorption in younger animals than older animals (Quarterman and Morrison, 1978). In children, the retention levels are ~30-40% of the total ingested lead; whereas in the adult lead retention is ~8-10%. However, these levels can be greatly increased during fasting or between meals (James *et al.*, 1985). In these cases, stomach pH is considered to play an important role in at least solubilizing the lead compounds, as stomach pH is presumed to be lower in the fasting individual. Certain dietary factors have been shown to influence the amount of lead absorbed, which have been enumerated and discussed (NRC, 1980). Dietary amounts of calcium, iron and zinc can influence the amount of lead absorption; presumably by competition for the same carrier or transport mechanism (Watson *et al.*, 1980).Lead is transported in blood as an aggregate of lead phosphate, which is adsorbed to the surface of red blood cells. Lead accumulates in the bone, blood, liver and kidney. Accumulation reaches plateaus in the blood and liver but increase linearly in the kidney at higher levels of intake (Fick, *et al.*, 1976).Increased levels of lead in newborns and milk suggest placental and mammary transport (Suttle *et al.*, 1997). Major routes of lead excretion are the gastrointestinal tract and kidneys. Whatever is lost through the gastrointestinal tract is excreted largely via the bile. Urinary lead output is proportional to blood lead concentration.

Lead Toxicity

Plumbism or saturinism is popular name given to toxicity caused by lead. It is a cumulative tissue poison and get stored in different parts of the body especially in bones, liver, kidneys and brain. Clinical intoxicosis interfere with normal metal dependent enzyme functions. Smith *et al.* (2008) demonstrated a significant dose dependent increase in tissue lead concentration in bone, liver and kidney of rats given different dietary lead levels. Besides, direct ingestion of lead leading to increased blood lead levels, accumulated lead in the body also acts as a significant source of blood lead burden. Lead toxicity affects several organs and tissues. Microcytic, hypochromic anemia is produced in lead toxicity as a result of a decrease in survival time of red blood cells (excessive hemolysis) and a decrease in red cell formation due to blockage in heme synthesis. In the kidney, pathological changes occur, resulting in amino aciduria, glycosuria, and hyperphosphaturia. Necrosis, hemorrhage and ulceration of the stomach and small intestine are common in lead toxicity in animals. Lead also affects the nervous system leading to loss of myelin from nerve sheaths in the brain, accompanied by cerebrocortical softening after prolonged exposure to lead. Lead toxicity also affects the skeleton, causing osteoporosis and reduced bone matrix formation and excess resorption of mineralized bone. Enlarged joints of long bones are common in swine and equine. Chronic exposure to low levels of lead is not associated with clinical symptoms in cattle because bones sequester lead and release it gradually to the blood for excretion. Acute toxicity is characterized by gastrointestinal hemorrhage and anemia together with liver necrosis and kidney damage. Lead toxicity also causes intestinal pain, colic and abortion. Lead accumulates in the kidney cortex and impairs renal function.

Prevention and Alleviation of Lead Toxicity

Calcium and phosphorus supplementation may reduce lead poisoning by capturing and diluting lead in newly formed bone (Underwood and Suttle, 1999). Absorption of lead from gastrointestinal tract as well as the partitioning of the lead in various body compartments is suggested to be regulated by the same physiological mechanisms, which control the metabolism of calcium and phosphorus. It has been speculated that lead and calcium compete for the common transport mechanism. As such, adequate dietary level of Ca and P in a correct ratio could prevent lead from accumulating in body tissues. Further, interaction between lead and zinc is also considered to influence the lead toxicity. Zinc and lead compete for the similar binding sites on the metallothionein-like transport protein in the gastrointestinal tract. The competition between lead and zinc might decrease the absorption of lead, thus reducing lead toxicity. Further, interaction between iron and lead and between calcium and zinc is also considered to influence the lead toxicity.

Klauder and Petering (1977) have shown that the toxic effects and the body uptake of Pb are greatly minimized when dietary Cu, Fe and Zn are adequate and they suggested a complex interaction of Pb with these essential elements. Rastogi *et al.* (1976) reported that low dietary intake of Se was effective in checking the tissue uptake of Pb, while excess Se exaggerate the toxic effects of lead. Similarly, injection vitamins like thiamine hydrochloride, niacin, vitamin B_{12} and ascorbic acids are used with chelators in treatment and prevention of lead intoxication. Thiamine hydrochloride reduces the deposition of lead in most tissues, especially in liver, kidney and central and peripheral nervous system. Ascorbic acid is more effective than thiamine and their combination is more effective than either of them individually in both prevention and treatment of Pb intoxication in animals. Protective role of vitamin C against lead may be due to its property to act as a chelator like EDTA (Goyer and Cherion, 1979). Alpha tocopherol, the most predominant and active form of vitamin E is the most important free radical scavenger with in the cell membranes. This free radical scavenging vitamin showed marked potential in mitigating toxic effects of lead. Sulphur containing amino acids like cysteine and methionine are also capable of reducing lead level from bone, soft tissues and visceral organs like liver. The protective action of these amino acids has been attributed due to the sulphur moiety of these amino acids. It is proposed that amino acids chelate the Pb in gut to form non-absorbable complex. Ancient Indian system of medicine -Ayurveda, mentions number of plants and herbs for the amelioration of metal toxicity and many of them including garlic (*Allium sativum*) have been evaluated scientifically and found beneficial in alleviating the toxic effects of lead (Patra *et al.*, 2001), who reported that garlic juice given at the rate of 100,200 and 400mg/kg body weight prevented the accumulation and toxicity of lead in rats. The efficacy of garlic in heavy metal toxicity is attributed to sulphur containing amino acids and compound having free carboxyl and amino groups in their structure. These biologically active substances are speculated to chelate Pb and enhance its excretion through urinary route.

Tolerable level: The maximum tolerable level of Pb for cattle and sheep was set at 100mg/kg diet DM (NRC, 2005).

Cadmium

Cadmium (Cd) is an environmental pollutant and constitutes 0.000011 per cent of the earth crust. In the lithosphere cadmium is present as sulphide and carbonate ores in association with zinc ores. Cadmium is a ubiquitous pollutant with intractable nature of intoxication in relation to other metals. It is widely distributed in the environment with no known biological activities, posing potential threat to human and animals (Friberg *et al.*, 1974).

Anthropogenic sources of cadmium are related to mining operations, incinerators, combustion of coal and oil, sludge based fertilizer and phosphate fertilizer. In heavily polluted soil, its concentration may reach up to 69 mg per kg (Friberg *et al.*, 1979). Fresh water contains varying concentration (0.0002-0.15mg/litre)of Cd (Ryan *et al.*, 1982).

Metabolism of Cadmium

Farm animals may have access to cadmium from water, soil and vegetation contaminated by industrial and automobile emissions. Oral route is the major route of Cd exposure to human and animal population, but acute toxicity occurs in highly polluted working environment mainly by inhalation of dust and fumes. Cadmium is poorly absorbed but can accumulate in the muscle and can disturb the balance of other minerals in the body (Phillip *et al.*, 2004).Cadmium is poorly absorbed from solid diets by all species, particularly ruminants, which usually take up less than 1% of the cadmium ingested as inorganic salts (Neathery *et al.*, 1974). In contrast, pulmonary absorption is 15-30%, thus making the respiratory tract a predominant route of cadmium intake (IARC, 1993). Intestinal metallothionein binds cadmium tightly and limits the absorption of cadmium. Absorption is enhanced by dietary deficiencies of calcium and iron, and by low protein diets. Low dietary Ca stimulates synthesis of calcium binding protein, which enhances cadmium absorption. Absorbed Cd is excreted through urine; gastrointestinal excretion is possible, particularly in bile as glutathione complex. Cadmium excretion in urine increases proportionately with its level in the body (ATSDR, 1999). Little cadmium is secreted into milk, but the mammary gland limits cadmium transport and the concentration of cadmium in the milk is not increased by high dietary concentration of cadmium. Cadmium is transported through blood after binding to red blood cells and high molecular weight plasma proteins, particularly, albumin. In liver, cadmium induces synthesis of metallothionein and then stored either in liver as Cd-MT complex or transported via blood to kidney, where it accumulates and induce renal toxicity.

Cadmium Toxicity

Cadmium is a heavy metal that accumulates with in the body, particularly the kidney, to cause renal damage, and once absorbed by animals or human beings, it is poorly excreted. The principal sites of cadmium retention are the gastrointestinal tract, liver and kidney (Houpert *et al.*, 1995). It has been found that in acute exposure, the relatively more soluble cadmium chloride, cadmium oxide fumes and cadmium carbonate compounds are more toxic than the relatively less soluble cadmium sulphide (Klimiisch, 1993). Specific adverse effects of Cd, when fed to experimental animals, include kidney damage and hypertension, as well as microcytic, hypochromic anemia. Powell *et al.* (1964) reported that in ruminants fed high dietary cadmium concentration (>40 mg Cd/kg OM) the symptoms of cadmium toxicity were loss of appetite, poor growth, retarded testicular development and parakeratosis. Recently, Sethy *et al.* (2011) observed depressed growth in kids given cadmium at a dietary level of 4.5 ppm and further reported decreased immune status of kids even at low level such as 1.5 ppm. Because cadmium is a cumulative poison, chronic toxicity is more likely to occur in aged breeding stock than in young stock slaughtered for meat consumption.

Prevention and Alleviation of Cadmium Toxicity

Experiments have also shown that excess dietary levels of essential elements like selenium, iron and zinc can reduce cadmium toxicity. Cadmium toxicity can be alleviated partially by high dietaey Zn, Fe and Ca; a complex interaction has been observed between levels of dietary Ca, Fe and Zn in protecting against Cd toxicity. Prior injection of zinc prevented cadmium induced testicular necrosis and hypertension in animals. Experiments have also shown that excess dietary levels of essential elements like selenium, iron and zinc can reduce cadmium toxicity. It is opined that selenium protects against cadmium toxicity by changing tissue cadmium concentration and by shifting cadmium to a less critical selenium containing protein. Glycine is another conditionally essential amino acid found in plant and animal protein. It combines with many toxic substances and converts them to harmless forms, which are then excreted from the body. Glycine appeared to reduce the oxidative stress of chronic cadmium toxicity. Shaikh and Tang (1999) reported a protective effect of glycine against chronic Cd toxicity by reducing oxidative stress. Alpha-lipoic acid also appears to have positive effects for cadmium toxicity, providing a protective effect for cadmium-induced cell dysfunction and membrane damage in hepatocytes (the most basic liver cells that perform all functions of the liver).

Tolerable level: Maximum tolerable level for cattle and sheep was set at 2mg/kg diet DM (NRC, 2005).

Mercury

Mercury(Hg) is a toxic heavy metal which poses a challenge to livestock and human population; though do not originate in the farm environment, as the soils contain little mercury. Mercury is a naturally occurring element existing in multiple forms and in various oxidation states. The toxicity of mercury has been recognized for many years; it is a hazardous environmental contaminant because of its use in industry and agriculture.

Mercury is a heavy metal of increasing concern as a global pollutant and occurs in the environment naturally and also as a result of anthropogenic sources. Atmospheric mercury enters aquatic system primarily in the inorganic form and is methylated to the more toxic methyl mercury (MeHg) in some aquatic system by sulphate reducing bacteria (Fitzergerald *et al.*, 1991).Nearly all mercury (approximately 95-99 %) in fresh water fish is MeHg, which readily bioconcentrates from water or diet. This is a matter of great concern for human beings as the fish is a part of human food chain.

Metabolism of Mercury

Absorption, distribution, metabolism, and excretion of mercury are dependent upon its form and oxidation state. Mercury is a poisonous heavy metal that is poorly absorbed in its inorganic form (1-15%) and highly absorbable in its organic form (59 percent as methyl mercury chloride and 90 per cent as phenyl derivatives) in the body. Organic mercurials are fat soluble and therefore, much more absorbable and tend to cross the blood-brain barrier easily and cause neurological problems. Young mammals absorb mercury very efficiently even from inorganic sources. The majority of mercury absorbed in its organic form is retained in the muscles and very little is excreted through urine and milk (1.1 percent, 0.17 percent, respectively; Neathery *et al.*, 1974).An oxidation-reduction cycle is involved in the metabolism of mercury and mercury compounds in both animals and humans.

Mercury Toxicity

All forms of mercury are toxic and methyl mercury (MeHg) is neurotoxic. MeHg in sufficient exposure causes damage to the central nervous system. Toxicity resulting from sub chronic and chronic exposure to mercury and mercury compounds usually involves the kidneys and/or nervous system. Ingestion of inorganic salts may cause severe gastrointestinal irritation, renal failure, and death. Mercuric (divalent) salts are usually more toxic than are mercurous (monovalent) salts. Inhalation of mercury vapour may cause irritation of the respiratory tract, renal disorders, central nervous system effects characterized by neurobehavioural changes, peripheral nervous system toxicity, renal toxicity (immunologic glomerular disease), and death. Methyl mercury irreversibly destroys the neurons of the central nervous system, and toxicity in mammals is primarily manifested as central nervous system damage, including sensory and motor deficits and behavioural impairment. Symptoms of methyl mercury exposure include anorexia, inability to drink, blindness, ataxia, recumbence and death. Generally, any form of mercury in high acute doses may cause tissue damage resulting from the ability of mercury to denature proteins, thereby disrupting cellular processes. Ingestion of inorganic salts of mercury such as mercury dichloride may cause gastrointestinal disorders including pain, vomiting, diarrhea and hemorrhage, and renal failure resulting in death. Additional effects of acute mercury poisoning include shock and cardiovascular collapse. The effects of acute exposure to organic mercury compounds are not well documented. The acute toxicity of inorganic mercury in animals is similar to that observed in humans. The toxicity of inorganic mercury has been suppressed by administration of various thiol compounds because inorganic mercury has high affinity for sulphydryl groups. Neurological effects and death have been reported for various animal species receiving inorganic mercury orally. The LD_{50} values in animals for elemental mercury range from 10 to 40 mg/kg. The suggested maximum tolerable concentration of dietary mercury in organic or inorganic form is 2mg/kg for cattle (NRC, 1989).

Prevention and Alleviation of Mercury Toxicity

The organic mercury species with greatest toxicity are methyl mercury compounds, which have a high affinity for the brain and nervous system. DMSA (2, 3 Dimercaptosuccinic acid) has been shown to cross the blood-brain-barrier and remove mercury from these organs. DMSA may be considered as the treatment of first choice in cases of acute or sub acute methyl mercury poisoning. Mercury creates an oxidative stress at the cell membrane level and addition of Se or vitamin E provides some protection against mercury toxicity.

Tolerable level:Maximum tolerable level for cattle and sheep was set at 2mg/kg diet DM (NRC, 2005).

Fluorine

Fluorine is a highly reactive, electronegative, non-metallic halogen element. It exists in nature in diatomic molecular form fluoride (F), and is known to be the 13th most abundant element in the earth crust and is the strongest oxidizing agent known. Biologically, F has strong affinity to positive ions like Ca^{++} and is reported to be essential as well as toxic. Natural as well industrial sources contribute to higher concentration of F in the environmental media leading to exposure of man and animals to excess F. The condition is endemic in those areas where F content is high in drinking water or soil. In addition, livestock may receive excess F from phosphate supplements in mineral mixtures and from pasture and forages contaminated due to top dressing with phosphate fertilizers. Long-term intake of excess F by animals induces F toxicity, which is commonly termed as 'Fluorosis'.

Metabolism of Fluoride

Approximately 75-90 percent of the ingested fluoride is absorbed in the stomach and small intestine as well as rumen of animals. The efficiency of fluoride absorption depends upon the solubility of the fluoride compound and presence of other dietary component. In the stomach, low pH conditions favour the formation of highly diffusible hydrogen fluoride. Therefore, the conditions that promote gastric acidity increase the rate of F absorption and it is impaired by alkalinity. Absorption from the small intestine occurs as fluoride ions by non-pH dependent diffusion. Soluble fluoride sources such as sodium fluoride are 100 percent absorbed, whereas less soluble sources like bone meal are relatively poorly absorbed. Absorption of fluoride is reduced by the presence of calcium, magnesium, aluminum, sodium chloride and high level of fat in the diet. After absorption fluoride is removed from the circulation principally through two mechanisms: renal excretion and calcified tissue deposition. After absorption the concentration of ionic fluoride increases in plasma, where it reacts with calcium to form calcium fluoride. It has been reported that about 50 percent of the fluoride absorbed each day is deposited in the calcified tissues. Urine is the major route of fluoride excretion, which accounts to the tune of 90 percent.

Toxicity of Fluoride

Fluoride is largely a cumulative poison and clinical signs of toxicity may not appear for many months in animals ingesting moderate amount of fluoride. The severity and course of clinical fluorosis depend on species, age and nutritional status of animal and the extent of fluoride contamination. In cattle, between the age of a few months and five years, 20-30 ppm of F in diet causes mild dental lesions, 30-40 ppm causes osteofluorosis, 40-50 ppm lameness, and >50 ppm causes decreased milk yield (Wheeler and Fell, 1983). The effects are enhanced by short-term increases in dietary F. Sheep are more tolerant to F than cattle and 50-160 ppm is considered to be limit of tolerance in them (Suttie, 1980). If the F intake is constant, pathological changes develop in bone and teeth with rise in F level in blood and urine. General signs to toxicity thus appear in other organs at the same time as bone lesions develop. The effects of fluorosis in cattle are mainly manifested by lameness, bone and dental lesions. The bone lesions have been described as osteosclerosis (increase in bone density), osteophytosis (presence of bony outgrowth), hyperostosis (increase in size of the cartilage capped protuberance at the end of the bone), osteoporosis (decreased density of the bones) and osteomalacia (failure of ossification due to decreased availability of calcium). These signs may appear singularly or in combination depending upon animal species, age of the animals and duration and level of intake. Small doses of F cause osteosclerosis, while larger doses induce osteoporosis and osteomalacia, especially with animals with high calcium demand. Young animals and lactating cows suffer from marginal calcium deficiency, and when it is coupled with lack of vitamin D and excess F, signs of osteomalacia appear. In cattle, first clinically palpable bone lesions occur bilaterally on the medical aspects of the proximal third of metatarsal bones. Later the lesions appear on mandible, metacarpal and ribs. The pelvis, vertebrae and other bones are also affected, but the most severe lesions are found on ribs, mandible and metaphyseal areas of metacarpal and metatarsal bones. Although exostosis often develops at sites of tendinous or fascial insertion, this may not be the rule. Spurring and bridging of joints, stiffness and lameness are some of the important clinical manifestations, particularly in advanced cases of fluorosis. Spurring and bridging of joints occur due to periosteal hyperostosis. Intermittent of lameness, stiffness, hip arthritis and fracture of third distal phalanx are important implications of osteofluorosis and calcification of periarticular structures and tendon insertion. Animals with fractured third phalanx may be unable to rise and would crawl on knee when forced to do so (Swarup and Dwivedi, 2002).

Lesions in developing permanent teeth are the most obvious and distinctive primary signs of fluorosis. Developing teeth are extremely sensitive to F. As the period of incisor development in cattle extends from age of few months to 30 months, the animals not exposed to F until they are 2.5-3 yr old will not show F-induced typical lesions (Bunce, 1985). The dental lesions can, therefore, be used to differentiate industrial and endemic fluorosis. In the former case, the teeth lesions may or may not be present and may be of variable grade; whereas in endemic fluorosis, affected adult animals will show dental lesions of almost similar grade. Lacks of luster, excessive wearing, mottling, discoloration of enamel, gingival bulging due to alveolar recession are common dental lesions in fluorotic animals. Teeth lesions are often used for diagnosis of fluorosis. The general effects of fluorosis include impaired appetite eventually resulting in diminished milk production, decreased weight gain, cachexia and wasting of main masses of muscles. Animals become anemic and more or less unproductive. The calving interval is increased, and the fertility and growth rate of young animals are reduced. There may be high neonatal mortality. Affected animals die after a prolonged course of illness.

Prevention and Amelioration of Fluoride Toxicity

Prevention of F intoxication in animals depends on the removal of excess F from potential sources like water, feed-fodder, rock phosphate, industrial contamination, etc. Water offered to the animal should not contain more than 0.7-1.7 mg fluoride/liter water. In F rich endemic areas, animals may be provided defluorinated water or potable water from the other safe places. One of the important methods of deflourination of water is Nalgonda process. In this process high F containing water is defluorinated by adding freshly slaked lime @ 0.5-1.0 gm/liter and water is allowed to settle at least for 6 days before its use. Rock phosphate having high F content can be defluorinated by wet digestion by phosphoric acid. Feed and fodder contaminated with high F could be defluorinated by processing of feed/fodder by dipping in 2% limewater at least for 4-6 hrs. The F emitting industries must be equipped with smelting technology, which is being controlled by Pollution Control Board. Provision should be made so that fumes from the industry are released above a particular height recommended by Pollution Control Board.

It is difficult to remove F from 'fluoroapatite' crystals in bone. As such, amelioration of Fluorosis is a big challenge, especially, after the onset of osteofluorosis. However, limited success has been achieved by using boron, vitamin C and aluminum sulfate. The prevention and control remain the main strategies to reduce incidence of fluorosis. Various F alleviating agents have been tried to ameliorate fluorosis. Calcium, phosphorus, aluminum sulphate and chloride, diethylstilbestrol and oxytetracyline have been examined as possible alleviator (NAS, 1974). Recently, vitamin C, molybdenum, copper, iron, boron, glutamine and cysteine have been added to the list. Perhaps most promising new alleviator is boron. Boron does not mobilize the skeletal or visceral fluoride, but it forms a complex- boron tetra fluoride with F at metabolic or digestive level. Aluminum salt is effective as neutralizer of the hydrofluoric acid produced in the stomach. Doses of 30-50gm aluminum sulphate daily have been used in prevention of chronic fluorosis. In acute toxicity intravenous administration of calcium salts is effective to replace the precipitated calcium.

Usefulness of Fluoride

As an essential trace element, F is required for four main functions; (i) calcification of mineralized tissue, (ii) maintenance of fertility, (iii) haematopoiesis and (iv) activation of certain enzyme systems such as adenyl cyclase, isocitric dehydrogenase, and acid and alkaline phosphatase. However, several research workers doubt the essentially of F in the diet of animals. Perhaps, requirement of F for the normal physiological functions of the body is so less, that the deficiency can not be produced under most careful experimental conditions (Wheeler and Fell, 1983). It is now well established that beyond a tolerance limit, F is a toxic element.

Tolerable level: The maximum tolerable level is 60mg/kg diet for sheep and 40mg/kg diet DM for cattle (NRC, 2005).

References

ASTDR (1999). Toxicological Profiles of Cadmium. Agency for Toxic Substances and Drug Registrar, US Department of Health and Human Services, Atlanta, GA.

Bahri, K.E. and Romdane, S.B. (1991). *Vet. Human Toxicol.*, 33:259-264.

Bunce, H.W. F. (1985). *J. Dairy Sci.*, 68: 1706-11.

Chakaraborti, D., Mukherjee, S.C., Pati, S., Sengupta, M.K., Rahman, M.M., Chowdhury, U.K., Lodh, D., Chanda, C.R., Chakaraborti, A.K. and Basu, G.K. (2003). *Environ. Health Perspect.*, 111(9):1194-1201.

Ekong, E.B., Jaar, B.G. and Weaver, W.M. (2006). *Kidney Internat.*, 70: 2074-2084.

Fick, K.R., Ammerman, C.B., Miller, S.M., Simpson, C.F. and Loggins, P.E. (1976). *J. Anim. Sci.*, 42:515-523.

Fitzergerald, W.F., Mason, R.P. and Vandal, G.M. (1991). *Water, Air, Soil Pollut.*, 56: 745-767.

Friberg, L., Kjellostorm, T. and Nodberg, G.E. (1979). Cadmium: Handbook on the Toxicology of Metals. Elsevier-Amsterdam, pp. 355-381.

Friberg, L., Piscator, M., Nodberg, G.E. and Kjellostorm, T. (1974). Cadmium in the Environment, CRC Press, Cleveland, Ohio, USA.

Goyer, R.A. and Cherion, M.G. (1979). *Life Sci.*, 24:433-38.

Gupta, R. and Flora, S.J. (2006). *J. Applied Toxicol.*, 26:213-222.

Gupta, R. and Flora, S.J. (2005). *Phytother Res.*, 19:23-28.

Houpert, P., Mehennaoni, S., Joseph-Enriquez, Bfederspiel, B. and Milhaud, G. (1995). *Vet. Res.*, 26:145-154.

IARC (1993). In IARC Monogram Evaluating the Carcinogenic Risks of the Human 58: 119-237.

James, H.M., Hilburn, M.E. and Blair, J.A. (1985). *Human Toxicol.*. 4: 401-407.

Klauder, D.S. and Petering, H.G. (1977). *J. Nutr.* 107:1779-1785.

Klimiisch, H.J. (1993). *Toxicology*, 84:103-124.

NAS (1974). National Academy of Sciences. NRC, Washington, DC.

Neathery, M.W., Miller, W.J., Gentry, R.P., Stake, P.E. and Blackmon, D.M. (1974). *J. Dairy Sci.*, 57:1177-83.

NRC. (1980). Nutrient Requirement of Dairy Cattle. National Academy Press, Washington, DC.

NRC. (1989). Nutrient Requirement of Dairy Cattle. National Academy Press Washington.

NRC. (2005). Mineral Tolerance of Animals, 2nd revised edition, The National Academy Press, Washington.

Nriagu, J.O. (1990). *Science Total Environment* 92:13-28.

Patra, R.C., Swarup, D. and Dwivedi, S.K. (2001). *Toxicology*, 162: 81-88.

Phillip, C.J.C., Chiy, P.C. and Omed, H.M. (2004). *J. Anim. Sci.*, 82: 2489-2502.

Powell, G.W., Miller, W.I., Morton, J.D. and Clifton, C.M. (1964). *J. Nutrition*, 84:205-211.

Quarterman, J. and Morrison, J.N. (1978). *Br. J. Nutr.*, 34:351-362.

Rastogi, S.C., Clausen, J. and Srivastava, K.C. (1976). *Toxicol.*, 6:377-388.

Ryan, J.A., Pahren, H.R. and Lucas, J.B. (1982). *Environ. Res.*, 28:251.

Sethy, K., Dass, R.S., Garg, A.K. and Badhane, K.P. (2011). *Indian J. Anim. Nutr.* (In Press)

Shaikh, Z.A and Tang, W. (1999). *Toxicol.*, 133: 139-146.

Singh, R.B., Saha, R.C. and Mishra, R.K. (2005). Arsenic profile of livestock feeds and Livestock products in West Bengal. A report of NDRI, Kalyani, Nadia, West Bengal, India.

Smedley, P.L. and Kinniburgh, D.G. (2002). *Applied Geochem.*, 17:517-568.

Smith, D.M., Mielke, H.W. and Heneghan, J.B. (2008). *Arch. Environ. Contam. Toxicol.* 55: 518-528.

Snider, T.H., Wientjes, M.G., Joiner, R.L. and Fisher, G.L. (1990). *Funda. Appl. Toxicol.*, 14: 262-272.

Styblo, M. and Thomas, D.G. (1997). In Arsenic: Exposure and Health Effects (Abernathy, C.O., Calderon, R.L. and Chappel, W.R. Eds). Chapman and Hall, UK.

Styblo, M., Yamayuchi, H. and Thomas, D.G. (1995). *Toxicol. Appl. Pharmacol.*, 135: 172-178.

Suttie, J.L. (1980). *J. Anim. Sci.*, 51: 759-66.

Suttle, N.F., Brebner, J., Stark, B., Sweet, N. and Hall , J.W. (1997). In: Proc.9th Symposium on Trace Elements in Man and Animals, Fischer, P.W.F., Labbe, M.R., Cockell, K.A. and Gibson, R.S., eds. Ottawa, NRC Press, pp. 168-170.

Swarup, D. and Dwivedi, S.K. (2002). Environmental Pollution and Effects of Lead and Fluoride on Animal Health. ICAR, New Delhi, p.160.

Underwood, E.J. and Suttle, N. (1999). The Mineral Nutrition of Livestock, 3rd edition, New York, CAB, International.

Watson, W.S., Hume, R. and Moore, M.R. (1980). *Lancet*, 2:236-237.

Wheeler, S.M. and Fell, F.R. (1983). *Nut. Abst. Rev.* (Series B) 53: 741-767.

WHO (2004). Guidelines for drinking water quality 3rd edition, Chapter 12, Chemical fact sheet, p. 306.

Yan Chu, H. (1994). In: Arsenic in Environment. Part 1: Cycling and Characterization (Ed. Nriagu, J.O.), John Wiley and Sons Inc., pp.17-49.

□□□

Animal Nutrition, 2012
eds. Dr. (Mrs.) Usha R. Mehra et al., pp. 395-417
Satish Serial Publishing House e-mail : info@satishserial.com; website : www.satishserial.com

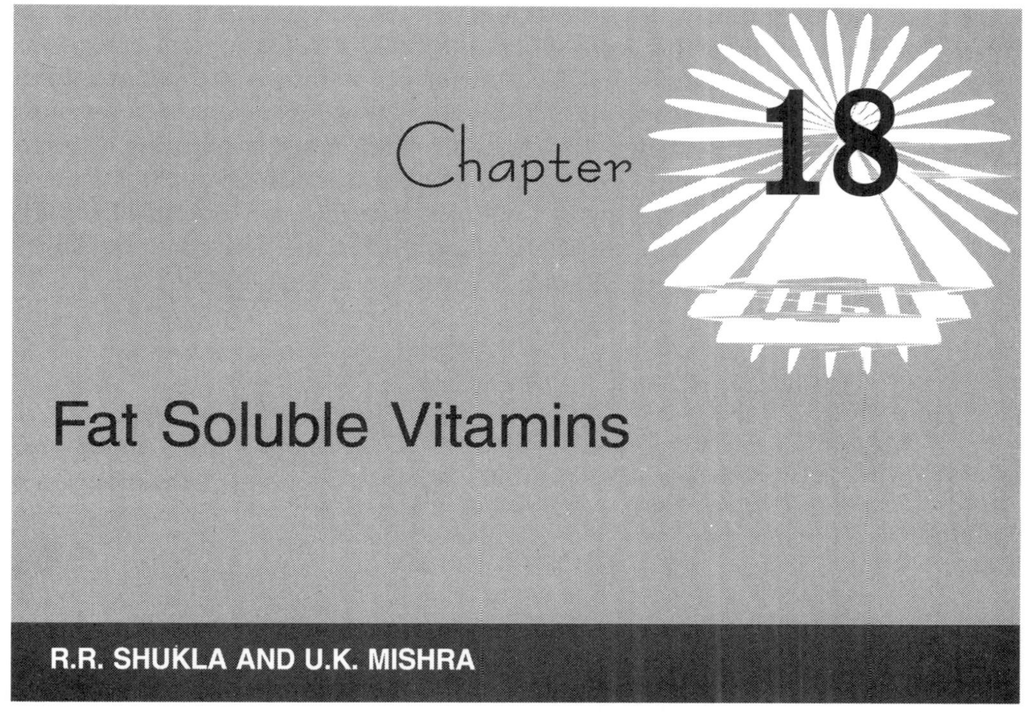

Chapter 18

Fat Soluble Vitamins

R.R. SHUKLA AND U.K. MISHRA

The term 'vitamine' was used by Funk in 1912 for an amine, the active factor from rice polishing which was necessary for existence of life (vital + amine). Later on the terminal 'e' was omitted, leaving 'vitamin' and vitamins were classified as fat soluble and water soluble, based on their properties. A vitamin may be defined as an organic substance of nutri tional nature present in low concentration, as a natural component of enzyme systems, catalyzes required reactions and may be derived externally to the tissues or by intrinsic biosynthesis (Mortan, 1974).

The present chapter describes in brief various aspects of nutrition and metabolism of fat soluble vitamins *viz.* A, D, E and K.

Vitamin A

Chemistry

Vitamin A was discovered as the fat soluble growth promoting compound in egg yolk, cod liver oil and butter fat and was first called 'Fat Soluble A'. Since then it has been found to be necessary for vision, reproduction and development in animals. Vitamin A is a generic term used for all compounds, other than carotenoids, that exhibit qualitatively' the biological activity of retinol. The alcohol, aldehyde and acid forms of vitamin A are called retinol, retinal and retinoic acid respectively. Retinol is a polyisoprenoid compound containing a cyclohexenyl ring with a long aliphatic chain, containing termihal $-CH_2OH$. The terminal $-CH_2OH$ of the aliphatic chain in retinol, can be converted to other functional groups without harming the biological activity of the parent compound. Modifications elsewhere in the molecule abolish the activity, only exception bring the 3- dehydroretinol (Pitt, 1983) (Fig. 1).

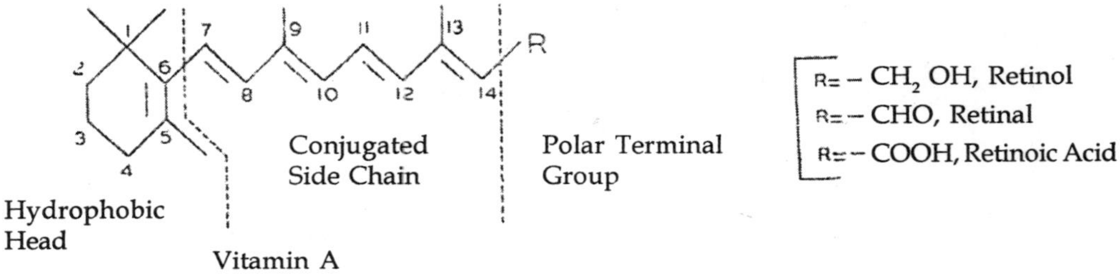

Hydrophobic Head

Conjugated Side Chain

Polar Terminal Group

Vitamin A

R= $-CH_2OH$, Retinol
R= $-CHO$, Retinal
R= $-COOH$, Retinoic Acid

Fig. 1 : Structure of vitamin D forms and precursors

Natural sources and dietary requirements

The major sources of vitamin A in the diet of animals are certain plant carotenoids and long chain retinyl esters found in animals tissues. Of about 400 naturally occuring carotenoids only eleven have vitamin A activity, of which beta-carotene has the maximum activity (about I million units per gram). One molecule of beta-carotene produces two molecules of vitamin A. The biological value of vitamin A is expressed in terms of International Units (I.U.) which is equivalent to *0.3* microgram of pure beta-carotene or 12 mg of mixed carotenoids. The biological potency of carotenes in animals depends on their capability to convert the carotene to vitamin A. In case of cattle feeds the method of hay preparation and storage considerably affects its vitamin A value. Addition of an antioxidant is beneficial in protecting feeds and vitamin concentrates from vitamin A destruction. Actively growing green plants, legume hay, carrot, sweet potatoes are rich in carotene whereas mature weathered pasture, grass, hay, cereal grains and roots are low in carotene content (Morrison, 1956).

Vitamin A in milk is present predominantly in ester forms while only about 2-6% is present in alcohol form. In addition carotenoids are also present in the milk and may contribute up to 11 to *50%* of the total vitamin A activity of wl1ich beta-carotene makes up the largest fraction. Vitamin A content of milk depends on a variety of factors viz., diet season, breed etc., e.g., summer milk contains 1.5 to 15 times more vitamin A than the winter milk. Milk vitamin A can be increased by feeding cattle with concentrates, vitamin A supplements or fodder rich in carotenes. In human milk vitamin A is present as retinol, retinyl esters and beta-carotene. Colostrum contains higher vitamin A levels than the normal milk. Under conditions of good maternal health and nutritional status, human milk provides 400-600 I.U. of retinol per litre. Human beings depend heavily for their nutrient requirements on farm and domestic animals. Animal products e.g. milk, milk products, hen eggs, or meat products are affected by the vitamin A supply of the animal (Hartman and Dryden, 1974.).

Intestinal absorption, transport, storage and metabolism

After ingestion dietary carotenoids and vitamin A are liberated into fat globules in the stomach, dispersed by bile salts, hydrolysed and trapped into mixed micelles in the intestinal lumen and finally absorbed into mucosal cells. Here beta-carotene is converted into retinol, by the stepwise action of two soluble enzymes, beta-carotene -15, 15-dioxy genases and retinaldehyde reductase. The absorbea retinol is re-esterified with long chain fatty acids and then transported with low density lipoproteins of the lymph. The absorption of vitamin A and carotenoids is affected by the dietary status of proteins, fat and luminal concentration of bile salts. Of the absorbed vitamin A, about *60%* is stored in the liver while *40%* is rapidly metabolized and excreted in the faeces and urine. The major excretable forms of vitamin A are glucuronoids of retinol, retinaldehyde and retinoic acid in bile.

The low density lipoproteins containing retinyl esters in the plasma are taken up by the liver cells and stored in fat storing cells or 'ITO CELLS'. Vitamin A stored in liver is secreted in the blood when needed and transported to target tissues in the form of a carrier protein bound complex. The binding carrier protein for retinol is a single polypeptide chain, with a molecular weight of 20,000 daltons and contains single binding site for one molecule of retinol. This protein is known as serum retinol binding protein (s-RBP). The s-RBP-retinol complex is transported in the blood bound to prealbumin containing 4 binding sites for complex in a 1:1 molar ratio. This RBP-retinol-prealbumin complex binds to specific cell surface receptors on target cells, where retinol is supposed to cross the membrane while RBP is metabolized and excreted in the urine. After its uptake retinol is transported intracellularly by cellular retinol binding protein (C-RBP).

Metabolic functions and systemic mode of action

Essentiality of vitamin A has been observed for a number of metabolic processes *viz.* epithelial differentiation, reproduction, growth and development, vision, immunity etc. However, its exact mechanism of action is known only *in* vision (Wolf, 1984).

Vitamin A acts in the visual process in the form of retinal and change in its isomeric forms cis and trans. The first step is catalyzed by retinol dehydrogenase where retinol is converted into retinal while retinal isomerase causes the change from. all-trans-retinal to 11-cis retinal. The 11-cis-retinal is bound to rod cell membrane protein called opsin by schiff base linkage and the whole complex is called rhodopsin due to excitation by light the ll-cis-retinal changes to all-trans-retinal *causing* the movement of schiff base linkage and during this process a photon is converted *into* atomic motion. Ultimately the schiff base is hydrolyzed and a nerve impulse is generated. It is believed that during *this* process light hyperpolarizes the plasma membrane by decreasing its permeability to Na^{++}. These processes are highly amplified responses, however, exact sequence of events and *mechanism* involved is not understood. Involvement of Ca^{++} and/or cyclic GMP (cGMP) as transmitter of signals has also been proposed. A diagramatic hypothetical outline of the process is shown in the Fig. 2 (Wald, 1960; Fung and Stryer, 1980; Stryer, 1981).

Involvement of *vitamin* A as a sugar carrier molecule (retinyl phosphate) during the glycosylation of membrane proteins is believed to be responsible for, the role of vitamin A *in* the *maintenance* of epithelium. Vitamin A is also necessary for the maintenance of testicular germinal epithelium, placental and fetal development, growth and differentiation of the mammalian embryo. *Vitamin* A also shows antitumor activity which varies in its various natural forms and str.uctural analogs. The mechanism of the antitumor properties of vitamin A is yet nuclear, however, it is believed that it might inhibit the enhanced cell proliferation and DNA *synthesis* induced by carcinogens (Deluca, 1977; Shukla *et al.*, 1983; Zile and Cullum, 1983; Shukla *et al.*, 1984, 1984a).

Deficiency and toxicity

Vitamin A status of an individual is defined in terms of his total body pool. On this basis, vitamin A deficiency can be defined where the individual has subnormal vitamin A status while the reverse is true for hypervitaminosis A. The plasma concentration. gives an indication of vitamin A status, while liver content defines the total body reserve of the subject. The signs and symptoms of vitamin A deficiency can be broadly classified into (1) occular and (2) non occular lesions. The most studied example of eye lesions is xerophthalmia which may be characterized by conjunctival xerosis, conjunctival thickness, wrinkling and pigmentation of the retina etc. Other occular lesions include bitot spot, corneal xerosis, corneal ulceration, defective dark adaptation etc. Non occular signs of vitamin A deficiency extend from ceased growth, reduced food intake, keratinization of epithelium, impairment of vestibular balance, changed taste and smell sense, anaemia, anoxia, diminished water intake and decreased resistance to infection. In pregnant animals under extreme conditions abortion/resorption of fetus, fetal malformations of bone, followed by xerophthalmia and other symptoms in the progeny may result.

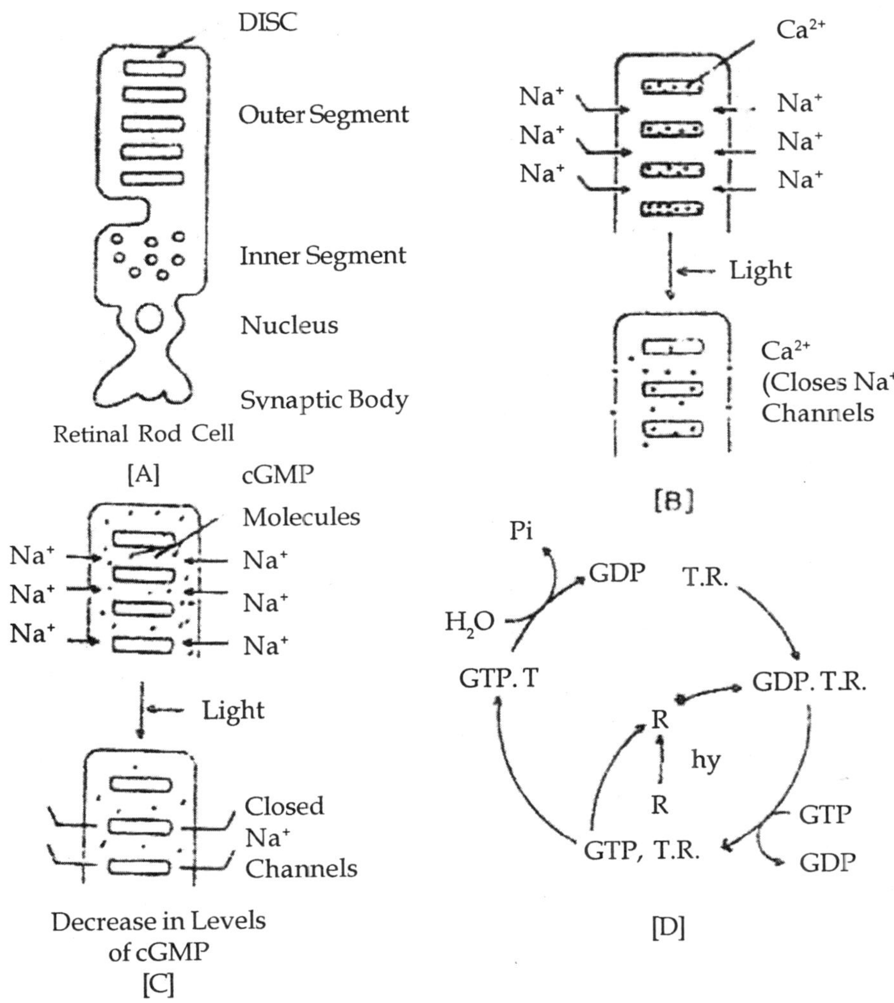

Fig. 2 : Role of vitamin A in vision : Hypothetical schemes of possible mechanism. (a) Rod cell (b) Mechanism involving calcium as the transmitter (c) Mechanism involving cGMP as the transmitter (d) Photolyzed rhodopsin catalyzes the formation of the GTP complex of transducin, which in turn activates the cGMP phosphodiesterase.

The symptoms of vitamin A toxicity or hypervitaminosis A resemble those of its deficiency. Teratogenic effects of maternal hypervitaminosis have been reported in offsprings of humans as well as experimental animals. Various abnormalities as a result of maternal toxicity range from that of skull and brain to encephaly, cleft palate, spina bifida etc. However, susceptibility varies from species' to species (Ong and Chytil, 1983).

Vitamin B

The eight recognized B vitamins are: B_1 (thiamin), B_2 (riboflavin), B_3 (niacin), B_5 (pantothenic acid), B_6 (pyridoxine), B_7 (biotin), B_9 (folic acid) and B_{12} (cobalamin). Each of the B vitamin plays a key role as either an enzymatic cofactor or metabolic constituent in many facets of intermediary metabolism, e.g. about half of the propionate that reaches the ruminant liver is converted to glucose by a series of enzymatic reactions (Brockman, 1993) which require biotin, B_{12}, niacin, pantothenic acid, and riboflavin. Since glucose is included as part of the lactose molecule in the mammary cells, all of these five B vitamins are also essential to the production of milk. These B vitamins also play key roles in the metabolism of carbohydrates, fats, and proteins.

Ruminal synthesis of B-vitamins

The specialized bacteria that live only in the rumen, synthesize all the eight B vitamins, as well as vitamin K, inside their cells. Ruminants obtain these B vitamins when the rumen bacteria are passed to the abomasum along with the digested feed. Ruminants are unique in that they produce an enzyme which digests bacteria releasing their B vitamin store. In the rumen, hundreds to thousands times more B vitamins are found inside the bacterial cells than in the free fluid. The wall of the rumen absorbs only a minimal amount of some B vitamins and in normal conditions is completely impermeable to others such as thiamin. B vitamins found in the feed or supplied as a supplement are either used by the microbes or changed by them into a different form, or may be absorbed across the rumen membrane. There is little information on just how much of the dietary B vitamins are degraded in the rumen or manage to be available to the ruminant further on in the intestine. In studies where the entire rumen has been completely emptied, there is some indication that all B vitamins are absorbed through the rumen wall. When large quantities of B vitamins are introduced to the rumen, most of them including thiamin do appear to be absorbed across the rumen, although the process is slow.

Large, single-cell rumen protozoa have a requirement for many B vitamins and do not make their own vitamins. They probably get most of what they require when they eat bacteria, but may use up some of those vitamins free in rumen fluid. This could account for some of the ruminal loss of supplemented vitamins. It is known that in normal conditions, rumen protozoa use biotin that is available in the diet and seem to have some negative effect on bacterial use or synthesis of biotin under certain conditions. Current focus is on producing B vitamin supplements that are ruminally potected which may help improve the overall health and productivity of goats, cows, sheep and other ruminants.

Need to supplement B-vitamins

It has been accepted that ruminants do not require B vitamin supplements since the bacteria supply all that they need. Such observations were made about half a century ago on the basis of criterion of minimum amount of B-vitamins required to prevent deficiency conditions in ruminants. But, the concept of animal nutrition has drastically changed during the recent past. Some new studies have shown that supplementation of some of the B vitamins have positive effects on hoof health, milk production, as well as other health benefits in ruminants. High producing crossbred cows have been developed with the advent of crossbreeding techniques. Such animals need to be fed sufficient amounts of all the nutrients to fully exploit their genetic potential. It has been observed recently that B-vitamins supplied through diet and that synthesized by ruminal microbes are not always sufficient for maximising productive performance of high producing dairy cows. The B vitamins are of importance in the young calf which has not yet developed a functional rumen. Some of the B-vitamins which need supplementation in ruminants are discussed.

Thiamin

Thiamin, or vitamin B_1, acts as a coenzyme in producing a neurotransmitter molecule which is critical to proper functioning of the nervous system. A deficiency of thiamin causes the disease seen in goats called polioencephalomalacia (PEM) or what is commonly called goat polio. If thiamin levels are low, this neurotransmitter cannot be formed and communication between nerves is interrupted. The reason for this deficiency in ruminants is thought to happen due to the presence of an enzyme called thiaminase which destroys or alters thiamin. It is known that the production of thiaminase is related to rumen bacteria, but it is not known exactly under what condition or which species produces thiaminase. It is suspected that diets high in concentrates which causes a more acidic environment in the rumen may either promote the growth of thiaminase-producing species or in some way increases the activity of the enzyme. Another possibility is that for some reason, one or more species of rumen bacteria may produce a thiamin "look-a-like" molecule which competes for the uptake of normal thiamin. There is also evidence that high levels of sulfur in the diet produce PEM in beef cattle. Sulfur in the rumen produces hydrogen sulfide gas which is toxic to the rumen bacteria. In addition, some plant species contain thiaminase which may cause a thiamin deficiency if ingested.

Thiamin is not stored in the body and is quickly depleted under high energy requirements. It is one B vitamin which must be continuously supplied. Therefore, if conditions in the rumen cause a destruction of thiamin, animals rapidly become deficient. When a ruminant develops PEM, any thiamin given orally will be degraded by the presence or high activity of thiaminase in the rumen. To correct a thiamine deficiency, B_1 must, therefore, be given as an injection.

Niacin

Niacin exists in two dietary forms known as nicotinic acid and nicotinamide. It can also be synthesized in the intestine of animals from an amino acid, tryptophan. In ruminants, microorganisms present in the rumen can synthesize all the B-vitamins. Therefore, NRC has not given any recommendation for the supplementation of niacin as well as other B-vitamins for cows because of the assumption that niacin present in the feed and that produced by rumen microbes is adequate to fulfill their requirements. Niacin requirements vary with the dietary composition. Requirement of niacin is increased when there is excess of energy or amino acids content (leucine, arginine and glycine) in the diet. High content of dietary tryptophan reduces niacin requirement because of its conversion to niacin in the body. However, niacin synthesis from tryptophan decreases in early lactating cows because of its diversion towards milk synthesis in the mammary gland. Dietary niacin needs of high producing dairy cows can not be met from dietary intake and microbial synthesis alone. A high producing cow in her early lactation has difficulty meeting her energy needs for milk production. In order to fulfill the energy demands, such cows undergo mobilization of body reserves resulting in increased circulatory levels of non-esterified fatty acids (NEFA) which get converted into acetyl CoA and produce energy via TCA cycle. However, all acetyl CoA produced cannot enter TCA cycle due to non-availability of oxaloacetate. Therefore, it gets converted into acetoacetate and b-OH butyrate (ketone bodies). Acetoacetate breaks down to another ketone body known as acetone. These ketone bodies are toxic in nature and reduce the appetite of the animals and hence feed intake. The already existing energy deficit situation therefore gets further aggravated and results in still greater tissue mobilisation. Thus, a chain of events starts ending in even greater accumulation of ketone bodies in the blood, known as ketosis.

Niacin helps prevent ketosis and associated disorders by slowing down the process of lipolysis and improving feed intake. Niacin supplementation increases microbial protein synthesis and affects the pattern of rumen fermentation as well resulting in increased propionate production and decreased butyrare production. Propionate is used as a precursor for glucose synthesis and elevates blood glucose level resulting in reduction of ketosis. Decrease in butyrate production also helps in combating ketosis due to decreased production of ketone bodies from butyrate. Supplementation of 12 g niacin/cow/d in early lactation has been found to be effective in reducing the incidence of clinical ketosis. Greater milk yield and milk fat percentage are also observed due to niacin supplementation. Improvement in milk production from nil to 17.4% has been recorded with niacin addition from 3-12 g/cow/d. Feeding 6g niacin/d to cows from 2 weeks before parturition to 60-100d after parturition is considered as the effective dose for optimum milk yield response. Supplemented cows also show less number of days and required less services per conception. Niacin should be fed only with natural protein diets and not with urea containing diets. Over conditioned cows benefit from niacin, because they are more likely to develop ketosis, and other disorders which may induce ketosis. Even though niacin has been determined to completely disappear in the rumen, suggesting that the microbes destroy it when supplemented, it seems to wind up getting into the system to help where needed.

Biotin

Due to ruminal and intestinal synthesis of biotin, a need for supplemental sources was at one time not expected for ruminants. Nevertheless, promising preliminary results in preventing lameness in dairy cattle with biotin supplementation have been reported (Frigg *et al.*, 1993). Hoof disorders occur in both confinement and pasture-based considerable economic loss to the dairy industry. In biotin-deficient dairy cows, the hoof horn is of poor quality, soft, and crumbling, with no distinct separation of keratinizing and cornified cells. This results in the omission of the granular layer at the epidermis of the bulb of the heel. Decreased stabilizing filaments in the upper spiny layer of the hoof corium in biotin-deficient cows reveal the depressed hormone-like activity of biotin in the synthesis of protein. Increased plasma biotin levels have been associated with hardness and conformational changes in the bovine hoof (Higuchi and Nagahata, 2000, 2001).

Need to supplement biotin have also been felt in peripartum and lactating animals because of their high demand of gluconeogenesis. Biocytin, the coenzyme form of biotin, acts as a cofactor for various enzymes involved in carboxylation reactions, e.g. pyruvate carboxylase, acetyl CoA carboxylase and propionyl CoA carboxylase. All these three enzymes are important for early lactating cows because of their high energy demands at that time. Biotin helps to improve the energy status of animals through increased gluconeogenesis. Biotin is also essential for maintaining the cellulolytic activity of ruminal microbes. Numerous studies have shown that supplementing biotin in the feed of cows improves the health of the hoof wall and decreases the occurrence of several common hoof problems especially those seen in wet conditions. At the same time, it also has a positive effect on milk production and conception rates in cows. There are no consistent reports towards the beneficial effects of biotin supplementation in cows. More work is still required to establish the need for the supplementation of biotin in ruminants.

Folic acid

The coenzyme form of folic acid is tetrahydrofolacin (FH_4). It is mainly involved in the transfer and interconversion of one-carbon units in different processes of metabolic pathways. FH_4 combines with 1-C unit to form methyl derivatives which are used to synthesize methionine (from homocysteine), choline (from ethanolamine) and serine (from glycine) during amino acid metabolism which are required in purine and pyrimidine biosynthesis. Thus, folic acid is essential for cell division and protein synthesis e.g. during gestation and lactation period. It is also required in the synthesis of niacin from tryptophan. Folic acid synthesis by rumen microorganisms increases in the presence of highly fermentable carbohydrates, like the diet consisting of barley as compared to fibrous diet. On the other hand, utilisation of fibrous material increases the requirement of folic acid. The requirement increases during pregnancy and lactation. It has been observed that serum folate concentration decreases by 40% in cows during pregnancy which indicates that folic acid available from diet and that synthesised by rumen microbes is not sufficient during that period.

Folic acid supplementation @ 4 mg/kg body weight increases milk production in multiparous cows, but, not in primiparous cows. Feed intake does not increase which shows that nutrient utilisation improves due to folic acid supplementation. Both serum and ruminal folate concentrations increase due to supplementation. There is also an increase in propionate production in the rumen of supplemented animals. Folacin supplementation during lactation increases milk folate content which is of great value from human nutrition point of view as it helps in reducing cancer and cardiovascular diseases. An increase in milk production due to folate supplementation suggests that dietary folacin alone is not sufficient for lactating animals.

Cobalamin

B_{12} or cobalamin is the largest B vitamin molecule and has the most complex structure of all vitamins. Unlike other B vitamins which can be synthesized in plants, it is only synthesized by bacteria and they require an atom of cobalt in order to make a molecule of B_{12}. Unlike other B vitamins, B_{12} can be stored in the liver for a long period of time. Beside assisting in the metabolism of fats, carbohydrates, and proteins, B_{12} has the very important role in helping to produce all the red blood cells in the body. It also helps to maintain the protective sheaths around nerves and to repair DNA. B_{12} works with folic acid in the production of an essential amino acid called methionine. In order for folic acid to be used by cells, it has to be altered by B_{12}. A deficiency of B_{12} therefore, results in a deficiency of available folic acid.

Rumen bacteria use B_{12} during the fermentation process of forming propionate. B_{12} is used in the liver in the chain of chemical reactions which convert propionate to glucose. Ruminants, however, have a higher requirement for B_{12} than monogastric animals because the rumen microbes produce a large amount of propionate which requires B_{12} to convert it into usable molecules. Propionate can build up in the blood stream if there is a deficiency of B_{12}.

Several factors can lead to a B_{12} deficiency. Since each molecule of B_{12} requires one atom of cobalt, a diet deficient in cobalt results in a B_{12} deficiency since the rumen bacteria cannot synthesize it. Diets high in concentrates lead to a high level of propionate production and therefore a high demand for B_{12}. These diets also promote the synthesis of molecules that are similar to B_{12} but are not beneficial. Therefore, a high concentrate diet causes a higher demand for B_{12} but at the same time has a negative influence on the amount produced by rumen bacteria. Severe parasite infections can damage the lining of the intestinal wall, reducing the amount of B_{12} that is absorbed. At the same time, chronic bleeding from the actions of these parasites causes an anemia which requires B_{12} to help restore lost red blood cells. Symptoms of B_{12} deficiency include depressed appetite, and poor growth in young ruminants. B_{12} supplied in the feed is not well absorbed through the wall of the rumen and most will be used by the microbes since they have a high requirement. B_{12} is most useful as an injected supplement when required until the underlying cause of deficiency is corrected.

The existing literature indicates that there is a great need to review the B-vitamin requirements in ruminants as their supplementation has shown beneficial effects in dairy cows.

Vitamin D

Chemistry

Vitamin D was discovered as the antirachitic factor of cod liver oil in 1921. Later on similar beneficial effects of UV light were also noticed. Compounds showing vitamin D activity are a family of sterols containing 3 (b)-hydroxy groups with different chains at the C-17 carbon a:om. Modification of the 3-hydroxyl group results in complete loss of antirachitic activity (Sebrel and Harris, 1971, pp. 156; Deluca and Schnoes, 1983).

B. Natural Sources and Dietary Requirements

Vitamin D is practically absent from all common foods except for egg yolk, butter and some fish species. One International Unit of vitamin D is defined as the activity of 0.025 μg of cholecalciferol contained in the U.S.P. vitamin D reference standard. In fishes, vitamin D amounts range from 100 to 500 I.U. per 100 g weight. In the skin vitamin D is produced primarily in the malpighian layer of the epidermis, by a nonenzymic photolysis reaction in presence of U.V. light. Fig. 3 shows the structure of sterols and the reaction taking place in the skin when U.V. light falls on it (Holick aDd Clark, 1978).

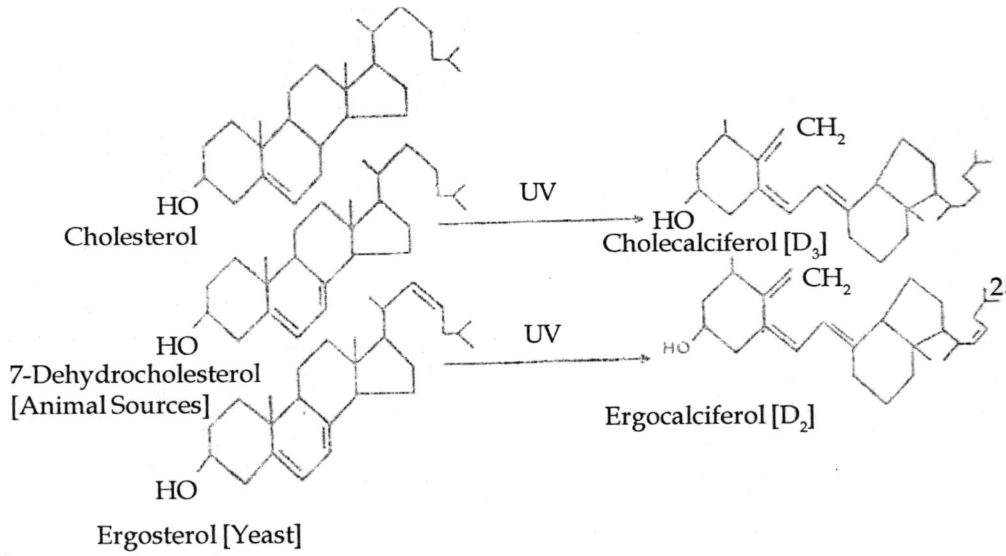

HO
Cholesterol
UV
HO
Cholecalciferol [D_3]
CH_2
HO
7-Dehydrocholesterol
[Animal Sources]
UV
HO
CH_2
25
Ergocalciferol [D_2]
HO
Ergosterol [Yeast]

Fig. 3 : Structure of vitamin D forms and precursors

Among the common cattle feeds, the vitamin D sources are sun cured or exposed hay and roughages, wilted grass silage and cocoa shells (Morrison, 1956).

Vitamin D may appear both as ergocalciferol and cholecalciferol in milk. Cholecalciferol is formed by solar radiation acting on the skin exposed to sunlight and then translocated to mammary gland and then secreted in the milk. Average vitamin D content of unfortified cattle milk is quite low and ranges from 3-23 I.U./liter during winter and 12-23 I.U./liter during summer. Vitamin D content of colostrum is about 3-10 times that of normal milk. For human milk following values have been given: Vitamin D_2: 338 ng/l and vitamin D_3: 41 ng/l. Vitamin D content of milk can be increased either by feeding substances rich in vitamn 0 and or by adding vitamin D concentrates directly to the milk. Vitamin D in milk is very stable and is not affected by pasturization, boiling or sterilization (Hartman and Dryden, 1974).

Vitamin D requirement of the animals is affected by a variety of factors *viz.* exposure to sunlight, dietary supply of calcium and phosphorus and the acidity of the diet. Increasing the acidity of diet lessens the vitamin D supply externally.

Intestinal absorption, transport, storage and metabolism

Vitamin D_3 is absorbed in the mall intestine like other fat soluble vitamins through the lacteal system into the chylomicrons. Bile salts are required for optimal absorption. After its absorption vitamin D is transported to liver like other fats where in the endoplasmic reticulum it undergoes hydroxylation at 25°C position in the presence of magnesium, NADPH, molecular oxygen and cytoplasmic factor. Hydroxylated vitamin S is transported in the plasma bound to a transport protein. In kidney, further hydroxylation takes place at C-I and 24-R positions of which the hydroxylation at C-l position is most important. The product thus formed i.e. 1 a, $25(OH)_2$ D_3 is the metabolite responsible for the cellular actions of vitamin D. The hydroxylation reaction is catalyzed by a three component mixed-function monoxygenase system (renal ferredoxin, renal ferredoxin reductase and cytochrome P-450). Recently, it has been reported that placenta also has C-l, hydroxylation activity. 1 α, $25(OH)_2D_3$ is metabolically degraded by side chain oxidative cleavage leading to the formation of C-23 carboxylic acid, calcitroic acid (Deluca and Schnoes, 1976, 1983; Henry and Norman, 1984; Kumar, 1984).

Metabolic functions and systemic mode of action

1 α, 25 $(OH)_2$ D_3, the active metabolite of vitamin D is taken up by the target tissues from the plasma. In the target tissues it is reported to be primarily localized in the nucleus and is translocated to the nucleus bound to a receptor protein. The receptor protein is present in the highest concentrations during the log phase growth period of cells and in lower concentration after the cells reach confluency.

The vitamin D regulated calcium homeostasis in the body is shown in the Fig. 4. The effect of 1 α, $25(OH)_2$ D_3 has been most extensively studied in intestine, where it acts in a biphasic way. Initial response is nuclear mediated action on the villi cells followed by response in the cryptic cells. However, the exact sequence of events is not well understood. One of the sites of vitamin D action is brush border membrane where calcium entry is stimulated by its active metabolite, which is believed to be as a result to change in the ratio of phosphatidyl choline phosphatidyl ethanolamine and free to esterified cholesterol due to the action of 1 α, $25(OH)_2$ D_3. Other effects are on the endoplasmic reticulum, golgi-apparatus, calcium uptake, nuclear events involving chromatic template activity and DNA dependent RNA polymerase activity and calcium dependent ATP and alkaline phosphatase activity. However, the exact mechanism is not known in the above mentioned processes (Fraser, 1980; Chaney, 1982; Henry and Norman, 1984; Kumar, 1984).

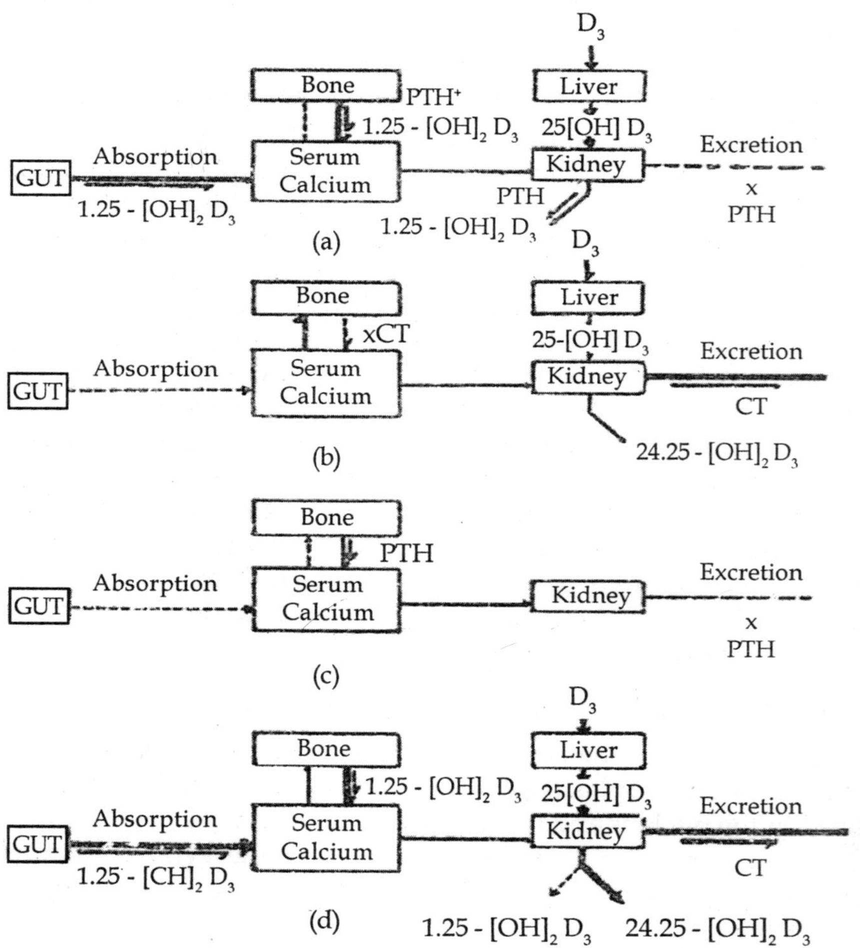

Fig. 4 : Vitamin D mediated calcium homeostatis : (a) When serum calcium level is low (b) Low vitamin D (c) Excess vitamin D show stimulation ; (d) white x, shows repression; PTH, Parathyroid hormone ; CT, Calcitonin ; D_3, Cholecalciferol; 25-(OH) D_3, 25-Hydroxycholicalciferol; 1, 25 $(OH)_2$ D_3 ; 1, 25-Dihydroxycholicalciferol.

Deficiency and toxicity

Vitamin D was discovered as an antirachitic agent. Rickets is a disease of growing bones in the absence of deficiency of vitamin D. It is characterized by depressed deposition of inorganic bone minerals calcium and phosphate in the bone matrix, deformation of calcification zone, bow legs, knock-knee, rachitic rosary (a beaded appearance of the ribs) and 'pigeon breast' in the rachitic children. Other malfunctions observed in the absence of vitamin D are diminished intestinal absorption of calcium and phosphate, decreased calcium concentration in the extracellular fluid, neuromuscular irritability, tetany and seizures, retarded growth and altered muscular tone. Serum calcium and phosphorus concentrations are decreased while serum alkaline phosphatase activity is increased. In the X-ray bones are visualized as less impervious due to the failure of depositing calcium salts in the skeleton. A lack of vitamin D in diet, not severe enough to cause visible symptoms of rickets, may retard growth and result in a weak skeleton, impaired joints and poor teeth.

Excessive quantities of vitamin D given over a prolonged period, either to children or adults, produces demineralization of bone-arid multiple fracture. Serum calcium and phosphorus levels are markedly elevated, resulting in the metastatic calcification of many soft tissues and formation of renal calculi, leading to the blockage of renal tubules (Deluca and Schnoes, 1976, 1983; Fraser, 1980; Chaney, 1982; Henry and Norman, 1984; Kumar, 1984).

Vitamin E

Chemistry

Vitamin E was discovered as the dietary factor whose absence in the diet caused fetal resorption in rats. Vitamin E belongs to a family of compounds called tocopherols and the tocotrieno1s. Tocopherols are derived from cyclic compounds called Tocols. According to the number of methyl groups present, various tocopherols are named as alpha-tocopherol (5,7,8-trimethyltocol), beta-tocopherol (5,8-dimethyltocol) and gamma-tocopherol (7,8-dimethyltocol). The structure of tocol, tocopherol and other forms of vitamin E are shown in Fig. 5 one international unit (I.U.) of vitamin E is defined as the activity of 1 mg of di-alpha-tocopheryl acetate (sebrell and Horris, 1972 pp. 166).

Natural sources and dietary requirements

Tocopherol is a plant product. Although it is also found in the meat, fish, eggs etc., various foods of animal origin, there is no evidence suggesting its synthesis in any animal tissue. All higher plants have alphatocopherol in leaves *or* at other places where photosynthesis takes place. Intracellularly it occurs in the chloroplast while in the non-photosynthetic tissues it occurs in the various plastids and chromoplasts. Tocopherols are present in highest concentration in cereals, wheat germ, corn, cotton seed, sunflower seed, rapeseed, soybean oil, lettuce and alfalfa. Vitamin E is also widely distributed in the livestock feed and is destroyed by rancid fat or other substances favouring oxidation. Alpha-tocopherol is the major form of vitamin E present in milk, where it is associated with the fat mainly concentrated in the fat globule membrane as compared to innerside. The average milk vitamin E content during summer is higher than during winter season. Supplementation of the diet with the tocopherol concentrate increases the milk vitamin E content. Colostrum vitamin E content averages from, 2.5-7.0 times that of normal milk. Heat and other processing treatments do not bring about significant loss of milk vitamin E content. Several dietary factors particularly fat, polyunsaturated fatty acids, selenium amino acids and antioxidants markedly affect the vitamin E requirement of the individual. A high fat diet increases the need for vitamin E while polyunsaturated fatty acids (PUFA) accentuate the deficiency symptoms. Synthetic antioxidants appear to have sparing action on the vitamin E requirements (Bieri and Farrel, 1976; Janiszowsk and Pennok, 1976; Machin, 1980).

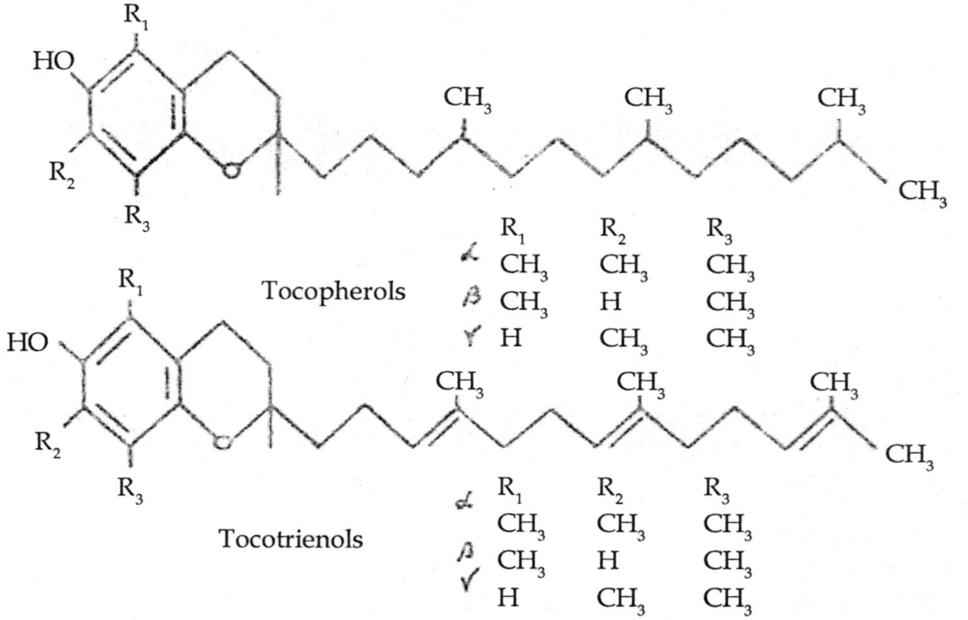
HO
R1
R2
R3
CH3
CH3
CH3
CH3
Tocopherols
R1 R2 R3
CH3 CH3 CH3
CH3 H CH3
H CH3 CH3
HO
R1
R2
R3
CH3
CH3
CH3
CH3
Tocotrienols
R1 R2 R3
CH3 CH3 CH3
CH3 H CH3
H CH3 CH3

Fig. 5 : Structure of vitamin E and related compounds.

Intestinal absorption, transport, storage and metabolism

Like other fat soluble vitamins, vitamin E is also absorbed into the intestinal lacteals along with other dietary fats, requiring bile and pancreatic juice for optimal absorption and is completely hydrolyzed prior to absorption. In Birds, vitamin E and its esters are entirely absorbed by portal route. Presence of PUF A in the diet considerably decreases the tocopherol absorption but other dietary lipids/like triglycerides and phospholipids facilitate the absorption. Tocopherol present in lymph on entering the blood rapidly equilibrates with plasma lipoproteins. In blood it is associated with two lipoprotein fractions with densities of 1.00-1.035 and 1.063-1.21. Plasma levels of tocopherol are affected by a variety of factors like nutritional status of individual, pregnancy, diseases, age etc., most important being the plasma lipid concentration.

Circulating tocopherols are rapidly taken up by most tissues especially adipose tissue where it accumulates. Presence of metabolites e.g. quinones, hydro-quinones, dimers, trimers and some more polar metabolitles of tocopherol have been reported. Major route of vitamin E excretion is faeces though minor part is excreted in bile and urine as tocopheronic acid and tocopheronic lactone (Bieri and Farrel, 1976; Machin, 1980).

Metabolic functions and systemic mode of action

Although many biochemical abnormalities have been found as sequel of vitamin E deficiency, the exact mechanism whereby vitamin E prevents these metabolic lesions is not understood. The principal function attributed to vitamin E is its role as an antioxidant in the biological system. It is believed that vitamin E acts as a biological lipid antioxidant that scavanges free radical intermediates arising during the peroxidation of unsaturated fatty acids, both in foods during storage and within the gastrointestinal tract, as well as in the tissues. The mechanism of its action as an antioxidant may be depicted as shown in Fig. 6.

Role of vitamin E beyond as an antioxidant is controversial. Structural role for vitamin E in biological membranes has also been put forth. Traces of dietary selenium has been found to improve the degeneration of necrotic liver in vitamin E deficient rats. However, the exact relationship of the two is not known.

Vitamin E appears to playa role in cellular respiration either by stabilizing coenzyme Q or by helping in the transfer of electrons to coenzyme Q. It also appears to enhance heme synthesis by increasing synthesis of α-amino levulinic acid (ALA) and ALA-dehydratase. A number of metabolic functions are impaired in vitamin E deficiency like protein and nucleic acid biosynthesis, activities of creatine kinase and xanthine oxidase. Supplementation of normal diets of experimental animals with vitamin E results in increased humoral antibody production and also increased protection againt infections. However, most of these functions are perhaps an indirect effect of its antioxidant potential rather than its actual participation in biological reactions (Scott *et al.*, 1974; Diplock, 1974; Machin, 1980).

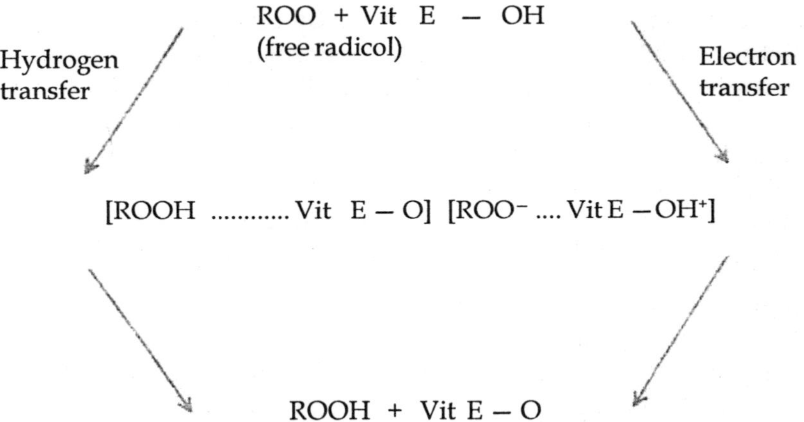

Fig. 6 : Action of vitamin E as an antioxidant

Deficiency and toxicity

In animals vitamin E deficiency symptoms range from sterility, muscular dystrophy, central nervous system changes and megaloblastic anemia. In humans, however, the symptoms are limited to increased fragility of the red blood cell membrane, presumably due to peroxidation membrane components. Premature infants fed on formulas low in vitamin E often develop a form of hemolytic anemia that can be correct by vitamin E supplementation. Fat malabsorption in adults also causes decreased red blood cell survival time but seldom leading to anaemia itself, though respond to vitamin E supplementation.

Recent emphasis on high PUFA diets to reduce serum cholesterol be of benefit in controlling heart diseases. The property of PUFA form free radicals on exposure to oxygen may lead to an increased cancer risk. Thus it might be beneficial to increase vitamin E intake along with PUFA diets.

Vitamin E toxicity commonly does not occur upto doses of 300 mg/day in humans. However, its excess dose may cause toxicity eg. consuming doses of 800 mg/da:o may result in malaise and frequent fatigueability (Machin, 1980).

Vitamin K

Chemistry

Vitamin K was discovered as the anti-hemorrhagic factor. The group of natural compounds showing vitamin K activity comprise a series of naphthoquinone derivatives that contain an unsaturated side chain four to thirteen isoprene units linked together head to tail. The import natural forms of vitamin K are K_1 and K_2. Vitamin K_1 (phyllohone) occurs in alfalfa meal while vitamin K_2 (menaquinone) is formed fish meal. A synthetic compound menadione has even greater potency In vitamin K itself. Structural formulae of vitamin K and menodione shown in Fig. 7 (Sebrell and Harris, 1971 pp. 99, 417).

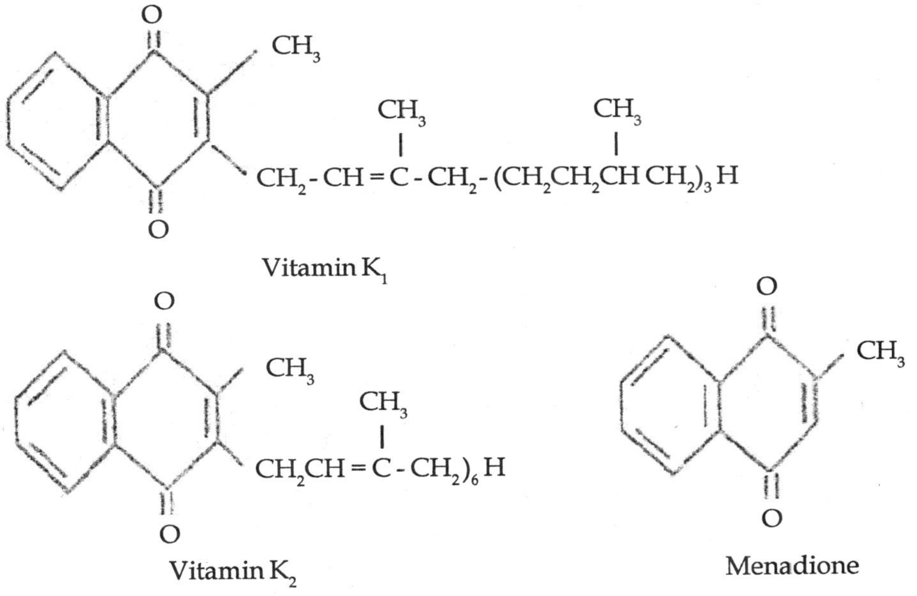

O
CH$_3$
CH$_3$ CH$_3$
$CH_2\text{-}CH=C\text{-}CH_2\text{-}(CH_2CH_2CH\,CH_2)_3H$
O

Vitamin K_1

O
CH$_3$
CH$_3$
$CH_2CH=C\text{-}CH_2)_6H$
O

Vitamin K_2

O
CH$_3$
O

Menadione

Fig. 7 : Structure of various forms of vitamin K.

Natural sources and dietary requirements

Different forms of vitamin K are found in plants, microorganisms and animals. Green leaf vegetables viz. carrot top, cabbage outer leaves spinach, cauliflower, nettle and chest nut leaves are rich sources of vitamin K.

The form of vitamin K in milk depends upon the form available to animal. However, large quantities of vitamin K are synthesized in the rumen of cattle by bacteria. The concentration of vitamin K is very low in milk and milk products. The vitamin K content of mature human milk has been estimated to be 2.0 μg/liter and for colostrum it is 2.3 μg/liter.

Though vitamin K is needed for the maintenance of normal physiological functions in all the species, any dietary supply may not be needed except in birds because of their smaller gut, where bacterial synthesis of vitamin K in the gut is low. In human beings, about half of the vitamin K requirement is met from plant sources while the remainder is supplied by bacterial biosynthesis. On this basis the vitamin K requirement for normal healthy human subject has been estimated to be 1-2 μg/kg body weight/day (Hartman and Dryden, 1974; Sebrell and Harris, 1971).

Intestinal absorption, transport, storage and metabolism

Dietary vitamin K is absorbed in the small intestine and requires bile and pancreatic juice for maximum absorption. Absorbed vitamin K is then incorporated into chylomicrons and transported to liver through lymph. In the liver it is incorporated into very low density lipoproteins (VLDL) and ultimately distributed to target tissues via blood. Liver represents the primary uptake site for vitamin K followed by skin and muscle. Its turnover is very high and thus total body pool size is very small. From approximate daily intake of vitamin K, its body pool size has been estimated to be 50-100 mg in human beings.

Operation of vitamin K-2,3 epoxide cycle in the liver has been shown which not only helps in the vitamin K mediated functions but also in its intermediary metabolism. In this cycle vitamin K is converted into vitamin K-2,3 epoxide by the action of enzyme vitamin K-2,3 epoxidase. This epoxide can be converted back to vitamin K by the action of another enzyme vitamin K-2,3 epoxide reductase (Fig. 8). The lactone of the glucuronides of the oxidative metabolites of vitamin K epoxide and vitamin K quinone represent the major metabolites of vitamin K present in urine (Sebrell and Harris, 1971; Bell, 1982; Olson, 1984).

Metabolic functions and systemic mode of action

Vitamin K was discovered as the missing factor in the diet of chicks with hemorrhage caused due to the delayed coagulation. Later this was found to be due to the absence of prothrombin whose biosynthesis was in turn dependent upon the vitamin K supply of the birds. Various functions attributed to vitamin K include a role in mitochondrial electron transport, a possible function as an inducer of protein synthesis and as an agent for post translational precursor for proteins. Eight coagulation proenzymes viz. proenzymes II, VII and X, proteins C,S,M and Z depend on vitamin K for their activity. It has been established that vitamin K is involved in the γ-carboxylation of glutamate in the precursors of prothrombin and other vitamin K dependent coagulation proenzymes leading to formation of γ-carboxy glutamic acid, though the precise mechanism of its involvement is not clear. The possible postulations are (a) the activation of oxygen (b) activation of carbon dioxide and (c) activation of glutamic acid, of which the activation of γ-methylene group of the glutamyl residues to a γ-methylene carbonion or γ-methylene radical is the most accepted. During this process, oxidation of vitamin K hydroquinone to vitamin K 1-3-epoxide has been proposed as intermediate step. Fig. 9 shows the recent hypothesis for the action of vitamin K dependent carboxylation (Bjorusson *et al.,* 1980; Shearer *et al.,* 1980; Suttie, 1980; Bell, 1982).

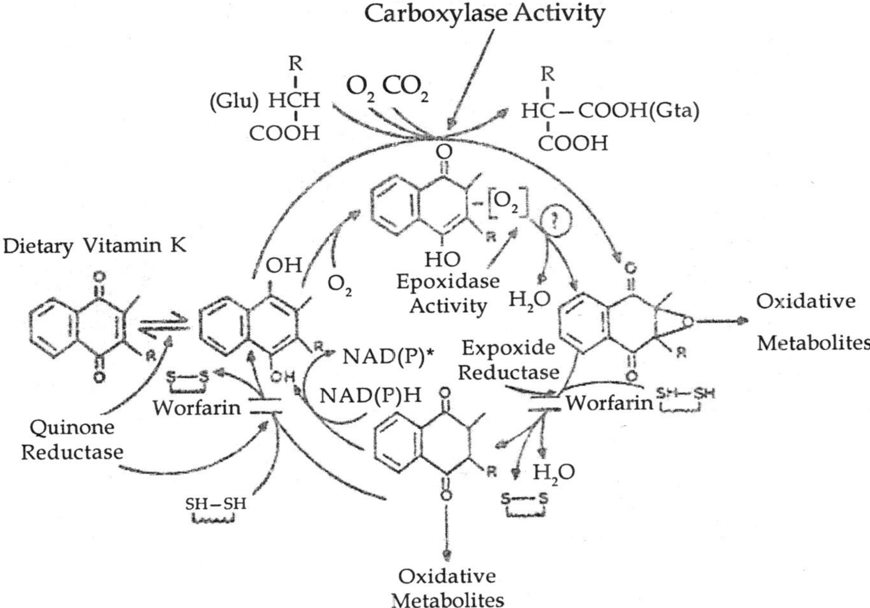

Fig. 8 : Vitamin K-vitamin K-2, 3-Epoxide cycle.

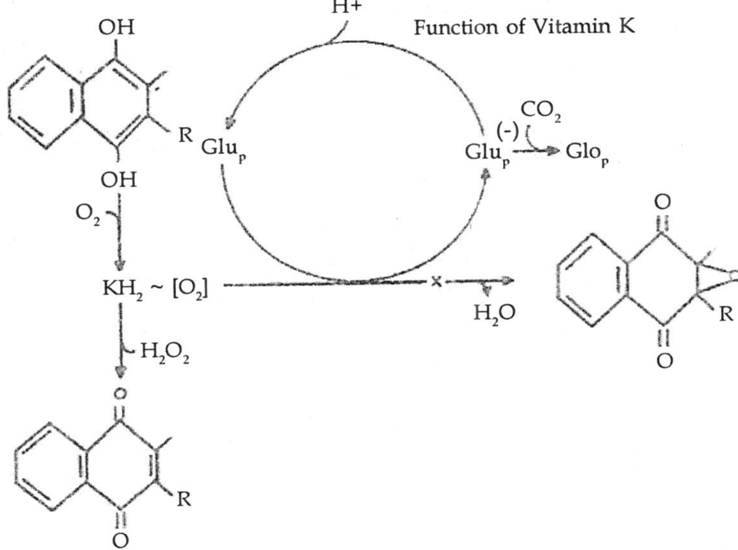

Fig. 9 : Mechanism of action of vitamin K dependent. Y-carboxylation. KH2 = Vitamin K Hydroquincne, X = Chemical intermediate of KH2 and O_2, Glu_P = Glutmiic acid containing peptide substrate, Glu_P (-) = Activated form of glup, Gla_P = Y - Carboxyglutamate containing peptide substrate.

Deficiency and toxicity

Primary vitamin K deficiency is uncommon in humans and animals because of its wide occurence in plant and animal sources and also because of its synthesis in the intestine. Thus the deficiency of vitamin K is usually secondary-due to a number of factors like (1) hemorrhagic disease of the newborn due to sterile gut and/or due to restricted placental transfer from mother, (2) dietary inadequacy in poor sections of society getting low fat diet or in protein calorie malnutrition, (3) biliary obstruction and malabsorption and some diseases like cystic fibrosis, sprue, celiac disease, ulcerative colitis, ascaris infection and short bowl syndrome. Another important secondary reason leading to vitamin K deficiency is drug therapy with coumarin and other related anticoagulants and broad spectrum antibiotics. Fat soluble vitamins A and E also antagonize vitamin K. Feeding high vitamin A diets (hypervitaminosis A) results in increased vitamin K requirements in rats. Similarly consumption of large doses of vitamin E by experimental animals or human subjects results in vitamin K deficiency. Vitamin A is believed to decrease the absorptions of vitamin K but mechanism of "vitamin E related antagonism is not clear. No report of vitamin K toxicity are available (Matschiner and Doisy, 1982; Olson, 1984).

References

Bell, R.G. (1982). *J. Nutr.*, 112, 287-292.

Bleri, J.G. and Farrel, P.M. (1976). *Vitam and Horm*, 34, 31.

Bjornsson, T.D., Meffln, P.J., Swezey, S.E. and Blaschke, T.F. (1980). In: Vitamin K Metabolism and Vitamin K dependent Proteins. (Ed. Suttie, J.W.), pp. 328. Baltimore, U.S.A., University Park Press.

Chaney, S.G. (1982). Fat Soluble Vitramlns. In *I* Text Book of Biochemistry with Clinical Correlations (Ed. DevUn, T.M.) John Wlley- & Sons, New York, pp. 1200.

Deluca, H.F. and Schnoes, H.K. (1976). Annu Rev Biochem, 45, 631-666.

Deluca, H.F. and Schnees, H.K. (1983). Annu Rev Biochem, 52, 411-439.

Deluca, L.M. (1977). *Vitam and Horm.*, 35, 1-57.

Diplock, A.T. (1974). *Vitam and Horm*, 32, 445-449.

Fraser, D.R. (1980). *Physiol Revs*, 60, 551-613.

Frigg, M., Stuarb, D. and Harmann, D. (1993). *Int. J. Vitam. Nutr. Res.*, 63 : 122-128.

Fung, B.K.K. and Stryer. (1980). *Proceedings of National Academy of Sci.* (USA) 77:1500.

Funk, (1912). Cited from "Water Soluble Vitamine" In Biochemistry (By White, A., Handler, P. and Smith, E.L.) V edition (1973). McGraw Hill Kogakusha ltd., Tokyo, Japan.

Hartman, A.M. and Dryden, L.P. (1974). The vitamins In milk and milk products. In: Funda mentals .of Dairy Chemistry (Ed. Webbe, B.H., Johnson, Mi. and Alford, J.A.) 2nd edition. The AVI Publishing Co., Inc., Westport.

Henry, L.M. and Norman, A.W. (1984). *Ann. Rev. of Nutr.*, 4, 493-520.

Higuchi, H. and Nagahata, N. (2000). Relationship between serum bioten serum biotin concentration and moisture content of sole horn in cows with clinical laminitis and in cows with sound hooves. Report Animal Health Laboratory Faculty of C. Calbius, 1999. *Veterinary Medicine*, Rakomo Gabuen University.

Higuchi, H. and Nagaliata, H. (2001). Vet. Rec. 148 : 201-210.

Hollck, M.F. and Clark, M.B. (1978). *Fed. Proc.*, 37, 2567-2574.

Janiszowsk, W. and Pemnck, J.F. (1976). *Vitam and Horm*, 34, 77-105.

Kumar, R. (1984). *Physiol. Rev.*, 64, 478-564.

Machin, J.L. (1980). Vitamin E: A comprehensive treatise. Marcel and Dekker, New Yon.

Mabehiner, J.T. and Dalay, Jr..E.A. (1982). *Proc. Socie Exp. Bio. and Med.*, 109, 139-142.

Morrlecm, F.B. (1956). Feeds and Feeding. 22nd edition. The Morrison Publishing Co., New York.

Mortan, R.A. (1974). *Vitam and Horm.* 32, 155-166-337.

Olson, R.E. (1984). *Annu Rev of Nut.*, 4, 281-337.

Ong, O.E. and Chytil, F. (1983). *Vitam and Horm* 40, 105-144.

Pitt, G.A.J. (1983). *Proc Nutr. Soc.*, 42, 43-51.

Scott, M.L., Noguchl, T. and Cobs, Jr.. G.F. (1974). *Vitam and Horm*, 32, 429-444.

Sebrell, Jr., W.H. and Harris, R.S. (1971). Vitamin D group. In The Vitamins : Chemistry, Physiology, Pathology, Method.. 2nd edition. Academic Press New York, pp. 156.

Sabrell, Jr., W.H. and Harrl. RS. (1972). TocopheroL In: The Vitamins: Chemistry, Physiology, Pethology, Method. Vol. V. 2nd edition. Academic Pru, New York, pp. 166.

Shearer, M.J., Allan, V. Haroon, Y. and Barkhan, P. (1980). In: Vitamin K Metabolism.

and Vitamin K dependent Proteins. (Ed. Suttle, J.W.), pp. 317, Baltimore, USA, University Park Press.

Shukla, R.R., Joshi, H.C., Srivastava, N. and Misra, U.K. (1984). *Biol of Neonate*, 46: 291-295.

Shukla, R.R., Joshi, H.C. and Misra, U.K. (1983). *Biol of Neonate*, 44, 243-250.

Shukla, R.R. Srivastava, N. and Misra, U.K. (1984a). *Biology of the Neonate, 46 : 285-290.*

Stryer, J. (1981). In: Biochemistry. W.H. Freemaan and Co., San Francisco, pp. 883.

Suttle, J.W. (1980). *CRC Critical Reviews in Biochemistry*, 8: 191.

Wald, G. (1960). *Vitam and Horm*, 18, 417.

Wolf, G. (1984). *Physio. Rev.*, 64, 873-937.

□□□

Animal Nutrition, 2012
eds. Dr. (Mrs.) Usha R. Mehra et al., pp. 419-437
Satish Serial Publishing House e-mail : info@satishserial.com; website : www.satishserial.com

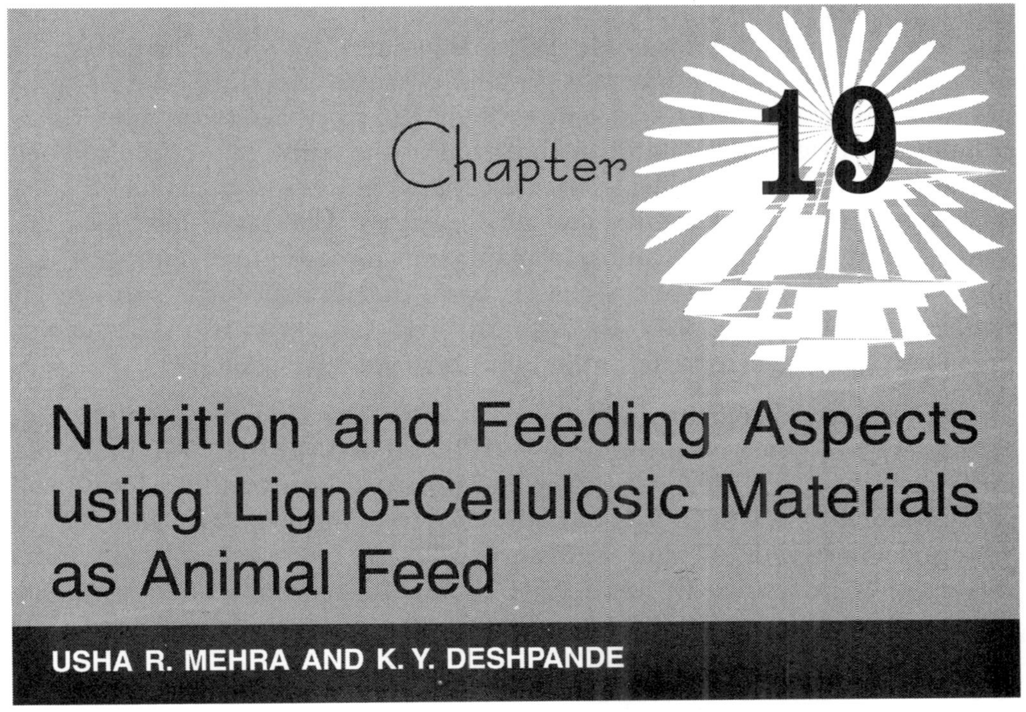

Chapter 19

Nutrition and Feeding Aspects using Ligno-Cellulosic Materials as Animal Feed

USHA R. MEHRA AND K. Y. DESHPANDE

The amount of lignocellulosic material in nature is enormous and in the Indian sub-continent it is common practice to feed ruminants on poor quality roughages like native grasses, weeds and cereal crop residues. Most of these feeds are generally deficient in nitrogen and many mineral elements. Complexes of hemicellulose and cellulose with lignin are highly resistant to cellulolysis by microbial enzymes. Thus, lignin and silica hinders intake and digestibility of crop residues posing questions to their inclusion in ration of high yielding animals. It so becomes imminent to deal these deficiencies on the whole while feeding fibrous crop residues. Nevertheless, along with all these disadvantages the crop residues also have some beneficial properties, which make their inclusion inevitable to feeding ruminants in developing countries. They are produced in large quantum (India produces 388 Tg crop residues, Sarkar, 2007). They can substantially reduce the feed cost and can satisfy the maintenance requirement of animal with a due care of energy and protein supplement as well as optimum N:S ratio.

Apart from feed constraints, animal factors also need to be dealt to improve utilization of lignocellulosics. For production of meat, milk, work and wool ruminants depend on a sufficient intake of absorbable nutrients. Only when this intake exceeds the needs for their maintenance (in the widest sense, i.e. including locomotion), there is a possibility for production: own or faetal growth, milk yield, work and hair growth. Intake depends on abundance, palatability, extent and rate of degradation of the feeds in the forestomach, properties on which certainly in the case of forages climate has a great influence. Furthermore, intake depends on production level, heat load and health of the animal. The animal's maintenance requirement in the widest sense may include not only needs for basal metabolism but also those for walking to collect the feed, for fighting high temperatures, deficiencies, parasites (internal & external), thirst and high mineral intake, etc.

In the second half of the dry season the warm and dry weather may negatively influence both the feed and the animal. In that case these two influences may intensify each other and so may lower fertility, completely stop production, result in loss of body weight or in the worst cases, loss of young stock or even of older animals too. In the next sections the various factors that influence utilization of lignocellulosic has been materials discussed.

General

Digestibility and N content of stems and leaves of forages decrease with stage of maturity. Moreover, under poor growth conditions plants may synthesize substances e.g. lignin, tannins etc or grow thorns, which make them less palatable and nutritious or less approachable for insects and higher animals. Plants produce compounds that provide, among other things, a degree of protection against microbial invasion. Included in these protective compounds are lignin, the phenyl propanoids associated with lignin structure, tannins, cutin and silica. The structure and function of these compounds and their relationship to nutrients digestion in the rumen were considered by Van Soest (1982) and reviews on effects of tannins (Kumar and Singh, 1984) and phenolic monomers and lignin (Jung and Fahey, 1984) on nutrition were published.

The negative relationship between degree of lignification and cell wall digestion in forages is well recognized (Van Soest, 1982). In addition to this limitation on fibre digestion by microbes appears that the presence of the phenyl propanoid units, P. Coumaric and Ferulic acids or their complexes with hemicellulose and cellulose also reduce ruminal digestion (Burritt *et al.*, 1984). The combination of low N & high tannin content is especially detrimental to the value of the plant as a feed for ruminants.

Silica has a negative effect on digestibility of grasses (Van Soest and Jones, 1968) causing a 3% decrease *in vitro* digestible DM per unit increase in silica. Most of the decrease is in digestion of cell wall carbohydrate. A reciprocal relationship between silica and lignin content of forages has also been noted and digestibility depressions are more closely associated with the sum of lignin and silica than with either single component (Van Soest, 1970).

Cutin content has been shown to vary markedly among fibre sources; seed hulls have particularly high amounts (Van soest, 1982). Monson *et al.* (1972) reported that intact cuticle could cause a 6 to 48 h lag time in initiation of digestion of plant particles, which varied with plant species and genotype. They reported that no digestion took place as long as the cuticle remained intact. These observations suggest that plant components can alter cell wall degradation through physical barriers including lignin, cutin and silica and these may be expressed as a lag time phenomenon.

It is well known that forages grown at higher environmental temperatures usually have a lower digestibility for ruminants (Van Soest, 1985 and Minson, 1985). Long droughts and dry seasons will kill much herbage and so leave dead material of low digestibility and N content. The effect of short droughts appears to be less detrimental, they of course reduce plant growth, but plant digestibility is not much affected (Wilson, 1983).

Plant Limitation of Fibre Digestion and Utilization Effect on Intake by Ruminants

Plant cell walls are the major sources of dietary fibre for animals. Polysaccharides in cell walls can not be degraded by mammalian enzymes. Instead, animals depend on microbial fermentation and ruminants are especially well adapted for using plant fibre for satisfying energy needs. Fibre, measured as neutral detergent fibre (NDF), usually accounts for 30-80% of the organic matter in forage crops. The remaining organic matter, cell solubles, is almost completely digestible. The nutritional availability of fibre to livestock, however varies greatly, depending on its composition and structure. Lignin has been identified as primarily responsible for limiting digestibility of fibre, but fibre utilization is also limited by physical constraints at the cellular organization level (Dwayne *et al.*, 1997).

Amount of Fibre in Plants

Stems of most plant species have a greater fibre concentration than do leaf blades and grasses usually contain more fibre than legumes. Fibre concentrations also increase as plants mature, which is the most important factor affecting dry matter digestibility. Neutral detergent fibre accounts for about 25 percent of legumes leaf blade mass in alfalfa (*Medicago sativa L.*) and red clover (*Trifolium prtense L.*); when these species are at the mid-flowering stage of maturity (Buxton *et al.*, 1995a).

Differences in digestibility between leaves and stems are normally less in grasses than in legumes. Stems decline in digestibility more rapidly with increasing plant maturation than do leaf blades. Digestibility also declines in alfalfa and birdsfoot treefoil (*Lotus corniculatus L.*) about 20g kg per node (Buxton *et al.*, 1995a). In addition to fibre concentration increasing within stems and most leaves with plant maturity, fibre concentration is also increased in total forage because the leaf:stem ratio decreases as plants mature. Albrecht *et al.* (1987) reported that the leaf:stem ratio of alfalfa decreased from 1.5 at the early vegetative stage to 0.5 by the late flowering stage.

Type of Plant

One of the most obvious difference in fibre digestibility and utilization among forage species is between legumes and grasses. Legumes are typically more digestible than grasses because they contain less fibre, not because legume fibre is more digestible. In fact, legume fibre is more lignified and less digestible than that of grasses. Similarly, the major factor lowering digestibility of forages is the higher fibre and lower cell soluble concentrations as they mature. Small particles are digested at faster rates than large particles because they have more surface area exposed for volume of tissues. In ruminants forage particles are regurgitated and chewed (ruminated) after eating to reduce their size (Wilson and Kennedy, 1996). Ruminants spend more time for regurgitating and chewing grasses than legumes and more time chewing mature than immature forage. Legume particles in the rumen are often cuboidal, whereas grass particles are elongated and slender (Buxton *et al.*, 1996). Filamentous grass particles are usually slower to pass from the rumen than the cuboidal fragments of legumes.

Lignin is necessary to provide mechanical support for stems and leaf blades and to impart strength and rigidity to plant walls. Also much evidence shows that lignin and lignin like compounds along with other cell wall components provide resistance to diseases, insects, cold temperatures and other biotic and abiotic stresses. Thus practical limits exist as to how much lignin and other cell wall constituents can be reduced in forages to grow and survive under field environments. Alfalfa selected for low lignin concentration grew less vigorously and had lower field survival than alfalfa selected for high lignin concentration (Buxton and Casler, 1993). Likewise, switch grasses selected for three cycles of high digestibility had lower field survival than the base population (Buxton *et al.*, 1995b).

For the past three decades, a growing awareness has developed that plant anatomy at the cellular level also influences fibre digestibility and that cell types differ in digestibility (Akin and Burdick, 1975). Sclerenchyma, vascular tissues and sometimes stem parenchyma and stem epidermis are digested very slowly and contain a substantial indigestible component. These tissues are the most lignified.

Leaf blades of C_3 grasses are usually more digestible than that of C_4 grasses because they have more mesophyll cells. In C_3 species, mesophyll, phloem, epidermal and parenchyma bundle sheath cells are all totally degraded. In contrast the epidermal and parenchyma bundle sheath cells of C_4 grasses may be slowly or only partially degraded (Akin and Chesson, 1989). The greater fibre concentration in C_4 compared with C_3 grasses is primarily due to larger amount of vascular tissues and parenchyma bundle sheath cells (Akin and Burdick, 1975).

Antinutritional factors

In various parts of the world (particularly where animals are reared on natural range grazing in the tropics) it is customary to feed low quantity non conventional feeds such as agricultural byproducts. These feed usually contain high fibre and unbalanced minerals and vitamins. They may also contain secondary plant compounds, such polyphenols (including condensed tannins) and saponins that may have antinutritional effect (Kumar, 2000). Tannins which protect plant from degradation in the rumen are reported to form insoluble complex with plant protein rendering them unavailable for digestion and consequently increasing their output in faeces (Robins and Brooker, 2005). In non-ruminants they interfere with nutrient digestion and promote excretion of endogenous nitrogen through formation of tannin-enzyme complexes (Longstaff and Mc Nab, 1991). There are some reports that they might also cause physical damage to the digestive system (Walton *et al.*, 2001). Antinutritional factors may also affect the lipid metabolism by promoting the excretion of bile acids and decreasing the activity of lipase (Longstaff and Mc Nab, 1991).

Feeding nonconventional (NCF) feeds to animals may not only reduce body weight, growth rate but may also affect their health status and ability to withstand diseases. Macro (energy and protein) and micro (vitamins and minerals) malnutrition negatively affects the immune system rendering animals more prone to diseases (Huges and Kelly, 2006). Feeding animals for extended period on same rangelands containing high level of antinutritional compounds was reported to produce detrimental effects on animal health (Tobosa *et al.*, 2000; Adedapo *et al.*, 2005). A study was carried out to investigate the effects of feeding low quality NCF containing phenols and condensed tannins on the clinical profiles of sheep (Mahgule *et al.*, 2008). This experiment implied that feeding low quality NCF containing antinutritional factors for relatively longer periods might produce subtle negative effects on the physiology and chemistry of digestive systems and blood parameters, which might negatively affect sheep health and makes them more susceptible to the diseases.

Environmental Factors

Thermoregulation

Homoeothermic animals such as cattle, buffaloes sheep, goats and in most circumstances, camels maintain a nearly constant body temperature by balancing the own heat production and heat absorbed from the environment against their heat loss by radiation, conduction, convection and evaporation (Thomson, 1973; Monteith and Mount, 1974).

Adaptation to environmental fluctuations

Most ruminants live under conditions where periods of abundance were interspersed with periods of deficit. In the temperate regions the growing season is summer and frost prevents growth in winter. In other areas, wet seasons alternated with dry seasons, which allow little growth especially of grasses that were of very low quality and vulnerable to fire. The ruminants adapt to these conditions by accumulating large quantities of fat stores during the good season. This is let down in different parts of the body as subcutaneous fat in hump, tails or as internal kidney and mesenteric fat. Grazers probably have better greater capacity to deposit fat than browsers. Goats generally deposit less fat than cattle. Goats seem to be able like camels to find and select some nutritious feeds even when forage is poor and scare (Lechner-Doll *et al.*, 1991). The ability to restore fat and subsequently use it for maintenance, pregnancy and lactation was a strategy essential for survival. Energetics of this strategy need to be further exploited. Much has been learnt for the utilization of fat for pregnancy and lactation and more recently it was demonstrated that animals can utilize fat depots not only to support pregnancy and lactation but also growth of sufficient dietary protein is made available to them (Ørskov and Tyler, 1990). In fact Ørskov and Chowdhury (1993) demonstrated that lambs could retain an equivalent to a growth rate of 400-500g/d and cattle at more than 1 Kg/d when no exogenous energy was supplied other than the protein, being infused into the abomasum. It was further stressed by authors, that for both the economic and environmental reasons, ruminants should be fed as far as possible on fibrous roughages and other feed that are not in competition with human food. New feed evalution systems are needed that is especially suitable for roughages including feed intake as an integral part of the system. A system has been suggested and some evidence provided for the development of an expression of feed potential that gives an estimate of the intake of digestible energy, and the performance that can be achieved; if the feeds are offered *ad libitum*.

Requirements and Feed Quality

Energy

Our knowledge of energy requirements of ruminants especially cattle, is as given in ARC (1980), Ranjhan (1993a,b) NRC (2000). Nevertheless there exist some serious gaps. Most of the information obtained comes from balance experiments with ruminants which received diets of moderate to good quality. Hardly any results of such studies are available in which low quality diets were fed. So, it has not yet been proved that the 0.4-0.5% decrease of the net energy value of ME for maintenance and milk production, mentioned above, may be extrapolated to low quality diets or feeds with energy digestibility of 45 percent and lower. Also the equation to predict K or K from content of ME was not derived in experiment with such feeds (Van Es, 1980). Low quality feeds, when fed alone, hardly allow the animal to be in positive energy balance so that reliable K or K values for such feeds can not be obtained because this would require at least results of two experiments; one with a small positive and one with a moderate to high positive energy balance.

Some information on the energy requirements comes from feeding trials. Only experiments of 6 weeks and larger with careful weighing, sampling and analysis of feeds offered and refused, in which the diets digestibility is determined and in which energy is the only limiting factor are of value for such studies of energy requirements. Such experiments have hardly been performed. Because lignocellulosic feeds are nearly always fed as (part of) rations allowing low to moderate production levels and thus are mainly utilized for maintenance, it is very important to know whether or not decrease in net energy value of ME for maintenance with decreasing ME content derived from feeds of moderate to high quality holds true for low quality feeds.

System has been suggested (Ørskov, 1998) and some evidence proved for the development of an expression of feed potential that gives an estimate the intake of digestible energy and the performance that can be achieved if the feeds are offered *ad libitum*. It is suggested by Ørskov (1998) that it may be possible to select ruminant with greater gut volume and thus, greater capacity to digest and utilize roughages. Further, it is sometimes forgotten that ruminants fed lesser low quality feeds often have a greater gastrointestinal fill (Vn Engelhardt, 1985) and thus a higher weight and slaughter loss. It is still not known how much maintenance energy this extra fill asks from the animal.

Protein and Nitrogen

Our knowledge of protein or N requirements of ruminants is seriously hampered by lack of sufficient quantitative insight in N conversions in the forestomachs (Tamminga, 1980, 1983; Waldo and Glenn, 1984). There exist several new theories on the subject. In their general approach they do not differ much. It is not very probable that requirements for absorbed amino acids between ruminant and simple stomached animals of similar size will differ much, but it is the translation of these quantities into actual feed requirements regarding necessary N, amino acids and other properties of the ration which up till now can not be done very reliably. The responses obtained from varying digestible crude protein (DCP) intakes are influenced by the source of protein and energy supply besides other factors (Walli *et al.*, 1993; Sampath *et al.*, 1993).

It was recognized that the biological value (BV) of protein in ruminant feeding varies with the nature of the feed. The BV is determined by the extent to which the amino acids from microbial protein formed in the rumen are supplemented by those from undegraded protein. In ruminants, the need for the tissues are met by amino acids absorbed from the dietary protein which has escaped fermentation (Rumen undegradable protein or bypass protein) and partly from the microbial protein formed in the rumen. The microbial protein is the most important; it contributes some $2/3^{rd}$ of the total under many circumstances. In Europe, Alderman (1984) showed that more and more research workers are of the opinion that most attention therefore should be paid to this microbial contribution. Microbial protein synthesis in the forestomachs depends on the conditions for microbial growth; continuous supply of ATP, ammonia and some peptides or amino acids, S, minerals, rate of passage, pH (Ben-Ghedalia and Miron, 1984; Mould and Ørskov, 1983, 1984). On an average, under ordinary conditions, 20g microbial N is produced per Kg organic matter apparently digested (Waldo and Glenn, 1984). Only a small number of such determinations have been performed with low quality diets. Efficiency of bacterial protein synthesis in the rumen was not limited by the supply of peptides and amino acids, and that protein supplements do not consistently stimulate intake of low quality roughages when requirements for rumen degradable N have been met (Sriskandarajah *et al.*, 1982). Higher flows of N to the intestines when HCHO-casein, and to a lesser extent casein given were associated with a shift from negative to positive live-weight changes. These live-weight changes were not significantly correlated with DM intakes from which it appears that effects of casein supplements on live-weight may have been attributed to effects of absorbed amino acids on efficiency of tissue protein synthesis either directly or through gluconeogenesis.

Glucogenic Precursors

There existed considerable disagreement on the requirements for glucogenic precursors of ruminants. MacRae (1983) concluded, from studies with glucose infusions in abomasum or blood that even during lactation shortage occurs. Nolan (1983) had a similar view, but is not so sure when it concerns milk production from low quality rations. Preston and Leng (1984) stated that the need for glucogenic precursors is highest during high levels of milk production and during early growth and low for maintenance, work, late growth and gestation. In the case of diets with high contents of low quality feeds they recommend supplementations with a by-pass a -carbohydrate, even in growing ruminants.

Above we have seen that the ruminant brain needs little glucose, so the maintenance requirements for glucogenic precursors will be small. Also theoretically the amount of glucose required for growth is small. Thus one would expect that the propionic acid of the volatile fatty acids (VFA) absorbed from forestomach and large intestine would supply sufficient glucogenic precursor except may be at high milk yield. Bergman (1983) stated that during absorption in the rumen epithelium about 50% of propionic acid is converted into CO_2 and lactic acid, raises some caution although lactic acid is also glucogenic.

Indeed, there are quite a number of observations which do not support the theory of shortages of glucogenic precursors; many cows in early lactation can produce 40 kg of milk per day and more despite low feed intake. Growth hormone does increase milk yield although initially feed intake hardly changes (Tyrrell *et al.*, 1982). Replacing half of the starch and sugars of the concentrate mixture by hemicellulose raised milk yield and concentrate intake of high-yielding dairy cows in early lactation, but the gap between intake and requirement remained unchanged (Visser, 1982).

The positive effect of bypass α-carbohydrate in the experiments mentioned by Preston and Leng (1984) might have been caused by an escape from forestomach fermentation. Part of such by-pass a -carbohydrate - corn starch, rice starch is degraded in the forestomach. This occurs so slowly that a steady supply of easily available carbohydrate for the microbes is guaranteed without the risk of short periods after intake with great supply leading to low pH of the rumen fluid.

Optimal Use of Lignocellosic Feeds by Ruminants

Use of Lignocelullosic Materials as the Main Feed

From what has been said above it will be clear that everything possible should be done to maximize the rate of fermentation. Of course, the measures to be taken should be economically feasible. While deciding on this, all costs and all benefits - higher intake, higher nutrient supply and higher production to maintenance ratio should be taken into account.

Easily fermentable CHO, NPN or protein, S and mineral supplemented to lignocellulosic diet speeds up rate of fermentation. Sahoo *et al.* (2004) investigated that catalytic supplementation of fish meal over liquid diet and semisolid urea molasses liquid diet improved nutritional performance of male buffalo (*Bubalus bubalis*) significantly by higher intake of basal roughage i.e. the wheat straw. Diet and such additions preferably should be available at every moment during the 24 hours of the day and in the mixed form; anyway, excessive intake of additions should be prevented. Intake can be further stimulated by treatment of the lignocellulosic material or by offering large quantities of such materials if heterogeneous to permit selective uptake of the better parts (Zammelink, 1980).

The Use of Lignocellulosic / Materials as Part of the Ration

When the lignocellulosic material is of so low quality that despite additions, treatment and other measures mentioned above, it gives too low intake and too low absorption of nutrients, its use in a mixed ration with feed of better quality might be possible. To obtain most profit from such feeds under these circumstances, attention be paid to way of feeding as well as type of the better quality feed offered in whole diet in a well mixed form prevents the animals from selective feeding. Feed blocks (FB) also called as multinutrient blocks, were being used in about 60 countries. The benefits from FB depend upon the appropriate formulation. Examples of formula reported in the literature are given by Mehra *et al.* (2002). Solidification of ingredients with a binder will ensure that animal consumes small amount of FB over the day. This intake regulation will result in a controlled supply of nutrients (energy, nitrogen and minerals) to the animal necessary to stimulate optimum rumen fermentation, thereby improving digestion of low quality diets (Leng, 1990). Seasonal crop residues, such as straws (wheat, *Triticum vulgare*/ paddy, *Oryza sativa L.*) and stovers (maize, *Zea mays L.*, sorghum, *Sorghum vulgare* etc.) form staple part of ruminant diet in developing countries (Jayasuriya, 1987). But handling storage and transportation of these low density (65-70 Kgm^{-3}) residues (Yadav *et al.*, 1990) became a major constraint in the feeding of livestock. Compressed complete feed block was prepared (Verma *et al.*, 1996) with the help of indigenously designed and fabricated feed block machine operable on compression technology. Because of a decrease in the bulk density, the handling storage and transportation becomes easy and economical. Further, they can be a part of famine feed banks for drought prone regions of developing countries as evolved technology is easy to adapt requirements of milch animals.

Such compressed feed block will not meet the requirements of high yielding dairy cows as intake and absorption of nutrients will be too low because of the slow degradation of low quality feed which also leads to high fill of the gastrointestinal tract. Some good quality green fodder and concentrates need to be added in such blocks. The mixed rations might be fortified with fat. For the microbes in forestomach and hindgut fat has hardly any value as an energy source because it has a very high H to O ratio, when the fat particles cover the lignocellulosic materials. Moreover, the fatty acids resulting from lipolysis in the forestomach, especially the unsaturated ones have some antimicrobial activity. For the animal fat is excellent energy source, however, unsaturated fat, probably through their effect on fermentation, may lower milk fat content. Fats that have not been preserved well may depress the animal appetite.

Fate of Cellulose in Rumen: Molecular Aspects

Cellulose, hemicellulose and lignin form the plant cell wall. Cellulose is found embedded in the matrix of hemicellulose and lignin. In its most pure form in nature cellulose is found in cotton ball. Cellulose (35-50%), hemicellulose (20-35%) and lignin (5-30%) limit the degradation of plant tissue in rumen. Lynd *et al.* (2002) described in details the structure of cellulose, cellulase enzyme systems, molecular aspects of enzymatic degradation and physiology of cellulolytic microorganisms. Out of these a few topics focusing anaerobic microbes and cellulose degradation are discussed hereunder.

Structure of Cellulose

Cellulose is crystalline in nature, but may occur in purely amorphous form. Around 30 molecules of cellulose aggregate to form protofibrils or elementary fibrils. Elementary fibrils aggregate into microfibrils and eventually microfibrils aggregate to form cellulose fibre. The cellulose microfibrils are bound with intra and interchain 'hydrogen (H)' bonds; which render cellulose resistant to action of enzymes. Cellulose due to kinks, twists and pits in its structural unit i.e. microfibril possess more surface area than a smooth fibre of same dimension.

Two major complexities may hinder cellulose degradation by rumen microbes. Different plants have different size and make up of cellulose. Thin cell wall (mesophylls) get degraded even by polysaccharide degrading enzymes, in case the middle lamella (separating cells of sclerenchyma) is highly lignified, an inside out attack approach is inevitable; rather than an outside attack in pure cellulose substrate. This hindrance is further complicated by difficulties in transport and diffusion of cellulolytic agent (Wilson and Mertens, 1995).

Microbial Diversity in Rumen and Cellulolysis

Rumen is the primary site for degradation of complex carbohydrates such as cellulose and hemicellulose. This is accomplished by variety of microflora i.e. bacteria and fungi, which degrade cellulose and hemicellulose to convert it into VFA, CO_2, H_2 and organic acids.

Table : List of microbes along with their substrate in domestic and wild animals reviewed by Kamra (2005).

Substrate	Bacteria/Fungi
Cellulose degraders	*Fibrobacter succinogenes (Bacteroids succinogenes)*
	Ruminococcus flavefaciens
	Ruminococcus albus
	Clostridium cellobioparum
	Clostridium longisporum
	Clostridium lochheadii
	Eubacterium cellulosolvens (Cillobacterium cellulosolvens)
Hemicellulose	*Butyrivibrio fibrisolvens*
	Prevotella ruminicola (Bacteroides ruminicola)
	Eubacterium xylanophilum
	Eubacterium uniformis
Lignocellulose bond	*Neocallimastix frontalis*
	Neocallimastix patriciarum
	Neocallimastix hurleyensis
	Sphaeromonas communis (Caecomyces communis)
	Caecomyces equi
	Orpinomyces bovis
	Anaeromyces mucronatus (Ruminomyces mucronatus)
	Ruminomyces elegans
	Piromyces mae
	Piromyces dumbonica

Most of the bacteria and fungi enlisted in table are obligate anaerobes. The bacterial species have been isolated by various workers from cattle and buffalo rumen, while fungus *N. patriciarum* from sheep, *C. equi* from horse, *P. communis, P. mae* and *P. dumbonica* from horse and elephant. Rest all fungi in table have been observed in cattle rumen (Kamra, 2005). Other than ruminants, some animal species like termites and crayfish have also found to produce cellulases (Lynd *et al.,* 2002).

Microbial Mechanisms of Cellulolysis

Microbes differ in their tools and schemes to hydrolyze cellulose. Aerobic bacteria and fungi through their hyphal extensions penetrate the cellulose and release cellulase in liquid phase or on the surface to efficiently degrade the substrate. They do not form the stable complex leading to non-complexed enzyme system. However, the focus of upcoming discussion will be on anaerobic ruminal bacteria and fungi which lack in above ability and thus may have developed complexed/cellulosome enzyme system. Complexed cellulase system is a general feature of ruminal microbial degradation of cellulose; whereas non-complexed systems are used for wine production from cellulosic biomass.

Types of enzyme activities in cellulase systems

Based on structural differences they are classified as follows (Henrissat *et al.*, 1998):

a. Endoglucanases / 1,4-β-D-glucan-4-glucanohydrolases
b. Exoglucanases / 1,4-β-D-glucan-4-glucanohydrolases (Cellulo-dextrinases) and 1,4-β-D-glucan cellobiohydrolase (cellobiohydrolases)
c. β-glucosidases or β-glucoside glucohydrolases

Endoglucanase action yield odd length oligosaccheride fragments by attacking at random on internal amorphous sites of cellulose. Glucose and cellobiose are the hydrolytic products obtained due to action of glucanohydrolase and cellobiohydrolases. These exoglucanases systematically cut cellulose at reducing and non-reducing ends. Microcrystalline cellulose can also be a substrate for exoglucanases. Glucose is the ultimate product of action of β-glucosidase on soluble cellulodextrins and cellobiose. Affinity towards β-1,4-glucosidic linkage and its cleavage followed by an acid hydrolysis involving a proton donor and a nucleophile base differentiates cellulase from glycoside hydrolases. Carbohydrate binding modules (CBM) bring cellulase catalytic domain opposite to cellulose; which specially enhance efficiency of exoglucanases. (Teeri *et al.*, 1998).

Complementary actions or synergism are the quintessential characteristics of cellulase enzyme system which are as follows:

i. Endo-exo (between endo and exo glucanases)
ii. Exo-exo (between exoglucanase attacking on reducing or non-reducing ends of cellulose chains)
iii. Exoglucanase and β-glucosidase
iv. Intra-molecular synergy between catalytic domains and CBMs

It was essential to learn enzyme actions and synergism (Lynd *et al.*, 2002) before we go for enzyme system.

Complexed Cellulase System for Efficient Cellulolysis

The cellulase mechanism of rumen microbes is also viable against hemicellulose. In rumen cellulolysis occurs at redox potential lower than -350mV, with pH 6.0-6.9 and optimum temperature 39°C. Rumen of animals fed on fibrous crop residues harbor a mixed population of cellulolytic and noncellulolytic microorganisms. When cellulolytic organisms attach to feed particle many enzymes described earlier attack synergistically either at the sloughed off places of cellulose or make a definitive enzyme attack to break up particle. These myriad of enzymes are stored in the protuberances called cellulosome that occur on cell wall of cellulolytic bacteria. They enhance the attachment to substrate, thus making it susceptible to microbial attack. Schwarz (2001) studied the cellulosome and cellulose degradation by anaerobic bacteria and found that architecture of cellulosome is quiet similar, though there occur considerable difference in enzyme composition/activity amongst various species of rumen microbes. Two rumen bacteria i.e. *R. flavefaciens* and *R. albus* have been found to develop cellulosomes of 1.5 MDa and 250 Kda scafoldin respectively in presence of cellulose, cellobiose and organic acid (Ding *et al.*, 2001). *F. succinogenes* does not possess cellulosome but has efficient cellulolytic activity.

Factors Affecting Cellulase Production

The β-glycosidase and cellulase production in part may be affected by presence or absence of certain substances. Easily digested (simple) sugars such as glucose depress the production of cellulase. Modulation of cellulase production at molecular level can be achieved by expression or deletion of certain genes that govern the production of inducer of enzyme or directly enzyme itself. Some inducers of cellulase production are sophorose, cellobiose, δ-cellobiose -1,5-lactone and oxidized products of cellulose hydrolysis (Lynd *et al.*, 2002). Most of the rumen microbes are cellulotrophs, i.e. they prefer cellulose or its products (cellobiose) to that of glucose or other sugars; probably to ensure its expeditious access to the fermentation products of cellulose.

Microbial Adhesion of Feed Particles

The enzymatic attack by rumen anaerobes in complexed systems has a prerequisite of proximity of cellulosome to the feed particle. This occurs in rumen mainly through cellulose binding proteins and glycocalyx protein resulting in strong cohesion as seen in *F. succinogenes* (Lynd *et al.*, 2002). They further reviewed that in F. succinogenes and ruminococci, cellulose utilization has major setback on inhibition of adhesion or detachment. Thus the cellulose-enzyme-microbe ternary complex appears to be most important step of cellulolysis in rumen. This mechanism has an obvious upper hand over the cellulolysis by cell free cellulases in a mixed culture; possibly due to masking of feed particle surface by glycocalyses and ultimately depriving adsorption of cell free enzymes.

Czerkawski and Cheng (1988) partitioned ruminal microbes into three compartments i.e. 1) those associated with rumen fluid 2) those loosely attached to feed particle 3) those firmly attached to feed particle. The last two of these account for 70 to 80 percent of microbial matter and cellulose degradation.

Adhesion is pronounced in slow growing ruminal fungi and bacteria. The longer retention time of digesta increases maintenance energy requirement, but on the contrary also enhances the cellulose degradation by aforesaid efficient microbes. Attachment (glycocalyces) in complexed systems facilitates the concentrated enzyme attack, preferred access to cellulolytic end products, shield against protozoal grazing; bacteriophages and protection to hydrolytic enzymes from proteases in rumen. The mechanisms for apposition of enzymes to substrate may be rounded up as a) cellulosome b) non-catalytic cellulose binding proteins c) glycosylated moieties of bacterial glycocalyx or of specific binding protein d) fimbriae or pilus like structure e) involvement of specific molecules.

Cellulose Utilization

A vivid description of biofilm development has been discussed by Mc Allister *et al.* (1994). The structural carbohydrates of plant cells are degraded simultaneously by complementary bacteria. The primary consortium colonizes the feed particle with glycocalyces and associated binding protein and initiate cell division to produce sister cells as well as a potentiated enzymatic attack to release nutrients. The secondary consortia utilize soluble nutrients to produce their microbial protein. These colonies form biofilm around the feed particles, which contain nutrients, substrates (succinate, isobutyrate and hydrogen) to be exchanged amongst the colonies. The glycocalyces sustain chances of subsistence of microbes in changing niche e.g. pH (from roughage to concentrate diet), osmolarity (fine particle size), and high energy. The chemoattractants (product of mastication) act as driving force for adhesion of fungal zoospores as well as protozoa to feed particles. Isotricha (special domain on cell) and dystricha (oral cavity) use special mechanisms for adhesion. The schemes of fungi are similar to that of cellulolytic bacteria as evidenced by the inability of either to attach substrate in presence of methylcellulose. Moreover the notion is strengthened by the common attachment site on cellulose fibre as blocked by cellulolytic ruminococci and ruminal fungi (Mc Allister *et al.*, 1994).

Salient Features of Cellulose Utilization

The juxtaposition of enzymes and substrates (cellulose, cellobiose, cellodextrin or glucose) is accompanied by intracellular or extracellular cleavage. These substrates are hydrolyzed by ATP dependent systems. ATP binding cassette protein (ABC protein) and Na^+ ion gradient are the major tools used for substrate transport. Phosphorolysis by cellobiose and cellodextrin phosphorolyases (CbP and CdP) and hydrolysis by extracytoplasmic cellodextrinase and intracellular β-glucosidase of cellulolytic bacteria form the major basis of cleavage of cellobiose and cellodextrins. The possible way of uptake of substrate in presence of mixture of above enzymes may include: i) extracytoplasmic hydrolysis with subsequent uptake and catabolism ii) direct uptake followed by intracellular phosphorolytic cleavage and catabolism iii) direct uptake followed by intracellular hydrolytic cleavage and catabolism.

The phosphorolytic cleavage has advantage of greater ATP generation. Thus enzymatic or microbial breakdown of cellulose proceeds through formation of soluble oligomers (slow process) like cellodextrins and further degradation to cellobiose (fast process). These intermediate sugars are converted to their ultimate end products via various pathways. Most of the ruminal cellulolytic bacteria convert substrate to CO_2 and acetate. The G-1-phosphate produced by their enzymatic action is changed to G-6-phosphate leading them to enter into EM pathway (Lynd *et al.*, 2002). Clostridium and *R. albus* produce ethanol and H_2 through acetyl Co-A formation. A shift towards glucose via succinate pathway is observed in *F. succinogenes* and *R. flavefaciens*.

The ruminal fungi e.g. *N. frontalis* bear special device, the hydrogenosome containing pyruvate:ferredoxin oxidoreductase and hydrogenase that convert the substrate to pyruvate and eventually yield ethanol, acetate, lactate, formate, H_2 and CO_2 etc. Other reduced products of cellulolysis in rumen include methane, acetate and H_2S. The fermentation products of cellulolysis (Lynd *et al.*, 2002) hardly vary with change of microbial species or growth stage and the equilibrium or similar pattern of terminal products is maintained by concentrations of intermediates, electron carriers, products and enzyme activity.

References

Adedapo A.A., Adegbayibi, A.J., Emikee, B.O. (2005). *Phytother. Res.*, 19: 971-976.

Akin, D. E. & Burdick, D. (1975). *Crop Sci.*, 15: 661–668.

Akin, D. E. & Chesson, A. (1989). In: Proc. 16th Int. Grassl. Congr., 4–11 October 1989, Nice, France (Desroches, R., ed.), pp. 1753–1760. Assoc. Francaise pour la Production Fourragere, Nice, France.

Albrecht, K.A., Wedin, W.F. & Buxton, D.R. (1987). *Crop Sci.*, 27: 735–741.

Alderman, G. 1984. Summary of replies to questionnaire. 35th Ann. Meeting EAAP, Commission on Animal Nutrition, paper N5.

ARC (Agricultural Research Council) (1980). Unwin, Surrey, 351 pp.

Ben-Ghedalia, D. and Miron, J. (1984). *J. of Nutri.*, 114, 880-887.

Bergman, E.N. (1983). In: Dynamic tiochemistry of animal production (P.M. Riis, ed.) World Animal Science A3, Elsevier, Amsterdam, p. 186.

Burritt, E.A., Bittner, A.S., Street, J.C. and Anderson, M.J. (1984). *J. Dairy Sci.*, 67:1209-1213.

Buxton, D.R. & Casler, M.D. (1993). In: Forage Cell Wall Structure and Digestibility (Jung, H. G., Buxton, D. R., Hatfield, R. D. & Ralph, J., eds.), pp. 685–714. American Society of Agronomy, Madison, WI.

Buxton, D.R., Mertens, D.R. & Fisher, D.S. (1996). In: Cool-Season Forage Grasses (Moser, L.E., Buxton, D.R. & Casler, M.D., eds.), pp. 229–266. American Society of Agronomy, Madison, WI.

Buxton, D.R., Mertens, D.R. & Moore, K.J. (1995a). *Prof. Anim. Sci.*, 11: 121–131.

Buxton, D.R., Vogel, K.P., Casler, M.D. & Moore, K.J. (1995b). In: Agronomy Abstracts, p. 163. American Society of Agronomy, Madison, WI.

Czerkawski, J.W. and Cheng, K.J. 1988. Compartmentation in the rumen, pp. 25. In : P.N. Hobson, Editor, the Rumen Microbial Ecosystem. Elsevior Publication.

Ding, S.Y., Rincon, M.T., Lamed, R. Martin, J. C., McCrae, S. I. , Aurilia, V., Shoham, Y. Bayer, E.A. and Flint, H.J. (2001). *J. Bacteriol.*, 183:1945–1953.

Dwayne R., Buxton and Redfearn, D.D. (1997). *J. Nutr.*, 127: 814S–818S.

Fields, M.W., Mallik, S. and Russell, J.B. (2000). *Appl. Microbiol. Biotechnol.*, 54:570–574.

Henrissat, B., Teeri, T.T., and Warren, R.A.J. (1998). *FEBS Lett.*, 425:352–354.

Huges S., Kelly, P., (2006). *Par. Immun.*, 28: 577-588.

Jayasuriya (1987). In: U.B. Singh (Editor), Advances in Animal Nutrition for developing countries. Indo Vision Private Ltd. Ghaziabad, pp. 236-259.

Jung, H.G. and Fahey Jr., G.C. (1984). *Can. J. Anim. Sci.*, 64 (Suppl.): 50.

Kamra, D.N. (2005). Current Science, 89 : 124-135.

Kumar, R. (2000). FAO 102. *Anim. Prod. and Health paper,* pp: 145-160.

Kumar, R., and Singh, M. (1984). *J. Agric. Food Chem.*, 32:447-453.

Lechner-Doll, M., Kaske, M., Engelhardt, W. (1991). In: Tsuda, T., Sasaki, Y., Kawashima, R. (Eds.). Physiological aspects of digestion and metabolism in ruminants. Proceedings of 7th International Symposium on ruminant physiology. Academic press, New york, London.

Leng, R.A. (1990). *Nutr. Res. Rev.*, 3: 277-303.

Longstaff, M. and McNab, J.M. (1991). *Br. J. Nutr.* 65: 199-216.

Lovitt, R.W., Kim, B.H., Shen, G.J. and Zeikus, J.G. (1989). *Crit. Rev. Biotechnol.* 7:107–186.

Lynd L.R., Weimer, P.J., Willem H. van Zyl and Pretorius, I.S. (2002). *Microbiol. Molecular Biol. Rev.*, Vol. 66, No. 3, p. 506–577.

MacRae, J.E. (1983). In: Recent advances in animal nutrition in Australia (DJ. Farrell, and P. Vohra eds.), Unlv. New England, Publ. Unit, Armldale, p. 23-24.

Mc Allister, T.A., Bal, H.D., Yanke, L.J., Cheng, K.J. and Muir, A. (1994). *Can. J. Microbial,* 40: 298-305.

Mahgule, O., Kadirss, I.T., Tageldin, M.H., Al-Manjooqu, W.S., Khalaf, S.Q., Ambu Ali, A. (2008). *J. Anim. Vet. Advances (In Press).*

Mehra, U.R., Dass, R.S., Pathak, N.N. (2002). Patent No. 210528 (944/DEL/2002).

Minson, D.J. (1985). Proc. 3rd AAAP Animal Science Congress, Seoul, May, P, 105.

Mitchell, W.J. (1998). *Adv. Microbiol. Physiol.* 39:31–130.

Monson, W.G., Powell, J.B. and Burton, G.W. (1972). *Agron. J.*, 64:231-233.

Monteith, J.L. and Mount, L.E. (1974). *Butterworth & London,* 457 pp.

Mould, F.L. and Ørskov, E.R. (1983/4). *Anim. Feed Sci. and. Technol.*, 10: 1.

Nolan, J.V. (1983). In: Recent advances in animal nutrition in Australia (DJ. Farrell and P. Vohra eds.), Univ. New England Publ Unti, Armidale, p. 1-12.

NRC (2000). 8th ed. National Academy Press, Washington.

Ørskov, E.R. (1998). Small Rumin. Res., 28, 1-8.

Ørskov, E.R., and Chowdhury, S.A. (1993). In: Feeding strategies for improving ruminal productivity in areas of fluctuating nutrient supply. FAO/IAEA coordinated research programme. IAEA, Vienna, Austria.

Ørskov, E.R., and Tyler, M. (1990). Elsevier Ames, Amsterdam.

Preston, T.R. and Lang, R.A. (1984). In : Straw and other fibrous by-products as feed (F. Sundstol and Eo Owen eds.), Elsevier, Amsterdam, p. 373-413.

Ranjhan (1993b). ICAR-Bulletin 26. Indian Council of Agriculture Research.

Ranjhan, S.K. and Singh Kiran (1993a). Proc. of an International Workshop held at National dairy Research Institute, Karnal (Haryana, India) Feb. 4-8, 1991.

Robins, C. and Brooker (2005). *Anim. Feed Sci. Technol.*, 121: 205-215.

Rogers, P.and Gottschalk, G. (1993). p. 25–50. In D. R. Woods (ed.), The clostridia and biotechnology. Butterworth-Heinemann, Stoneham, Mass.

Sahoo, A., Elangovan, A.V., Mehra, U.R. and Singh, U.B. (2004). *Asian Aust. J. Anim.*, 17: 621-628.

Sampath, K.T., Prasad, C.S., Walli, T.K. and Shivaramaiah, M.T. (1993). Proceedings of an international workshop held at the National dairy Research Institute, Karnal (Haryana, India), Feb. 4-8, 1993.

Sarkar A. (2007). *International J. Global Energy Issues*, 28: (2/3). pp. 181-194

Schwarz, W. H. 2001. *Appl. Microbiol. Biotechnol.*, 56:634–649.

Sriskandarajah, N., Kellaway, R.C. and Jane Laibholz (1982). British J. Nutr. 47: 553-563.

Tamminga (1983). Proceedings 4th Symposium on protein metabolism and nutrition, EAAP Publ. 311, p.263-287.

Tamminga, S. (1980). Proceedings 3rd symposium on protein metabolism and nutrition, EAAP Publ. 2711, p.

Teeri, T.T., Koivula, A., Linder, M., Wohlfahrt, G. Divne, C. and Jones, T.A. (1998). *Biochem. Soc. Trans.*, 26:173–178.

Thompson, G.E. (1973). *J. Dairy Res.*, 40: 441-473.

Tobosa, I.M., Souza, J.C., Graca, D.L., Barbosa-Filho, J.M., Almeida, R.N., Rie Correa, F., 2000. *Vet. Hum. Toxicol.*, 42: 155-158.

Tyrrell, H.F'., Brown, A.C.G., Reynolds, P.J., Haaland, G.L., Peel, C.J., Bauman, D.E. and Stelnhour, W.C. (1982). Proceedings 9th Symposium on Energy MetaboUsrn, EAAP publ 29, p. 46-49.

Van Engelhandt, W. (1985). Contribution to ACSAD/AOAD conference on Animal Production in Arid Zones Damaxus.

Van Es, A.J.H. (1980). Anim. zootech, 29: 73.

Van Soest, P. J. (1970). pp. 103 in Proc. Cornell Nutr. Conf.

Van Soest, P.J. (1985). Proceedings pre-congress I of 3rd AAAP Animal Science Congress, Seoul, May, p. 24.

Van Soest, P.J. (1982). Durham and Downey, Portland, 374 pp

Van Soest, P.J., and Jones, L.H.P. (1968). *J. Dairy Sci.*, 51: 1644.

Verma, A.K., Mehra, U.R., Dass, R.S. and Singh, A. (1996). *Anim. Feed. Sci. Technol.*, 59: 255-263.

Visser, H. de (1982). Proceedings 12th World Conference Animal Diseases, p. 415-420.

Waldo, D.R. and Glenn, B.P. (1984). *J. Dairy Sci.*, 67: 115-123.

Walli, T.K., Sampath, K.T., Rai, S.N. and Tamminga, S. (1993). Proceedings of on international workshop held at the National dairy Research Institute, Karnal (Haryana, India), Feb. 4-8, 1993.

Walton, J.P., Waghorn, G. C., Plaizier, J.C., Birtles, M., McBridge, B. W., (2001). *Can. J. Anim. Sci.*, 81: 605-607.

Wilson, J.R. & Kennedy, P.M. (1996). *Aust. J. Agric. Res.*, 47: 199–225.

Wilson, J.R. (1983). *Austral. J. Agricul. Res.*, 34, 377-390.

Wilson, J.R., and Mertens D.R. (1995). *Crop Sci.*, 35:251–259.

Yadav, K.K., Rathee, C.S. and Lohan, O.P. (1990). *Ind. J. Anim. Nutr.*, 7: 27-30.

Zammelink, G. (1980). Thesis, Wagenlngen, Pudoc, Wagenlngen, 100 pp.

□□□

Animal Nutrition, 2012
eds. Dr. (Mrs.) Usha R. Mehra et al., pp. 439-458
Satish Serial Publishing House e-mail : info@satishserial.com; website : www.satishserial.com

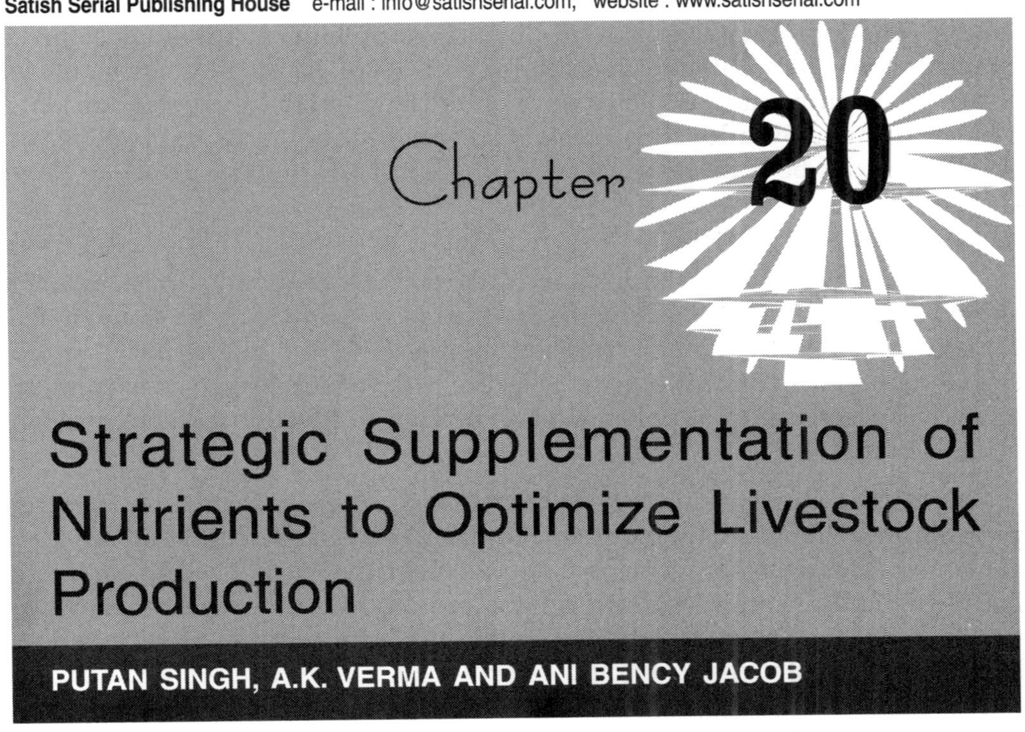

Chapter 20

Strategic Supplementation of Nutrients to Optimize Livestock Production

PUTAN SINGH, A.K. VERMA AND ANI BENCY JACOB

The Indian livestock sector accounts for a large share of the livestock resources in the global market. India contributes about 500 million tonnes (mt) of livestock with buffalo, goat and sheep ranking as first, second and third, respectively to the global market. The country's milk production in the year 2008 stood at about 104 mt, which was the highest in the world. Even though the scenario of livestock sector is encouraging, the production potential of majority of superior livestock remains unexploited. The feed available for these elite animals consists of cereal crop residues, supplemented with grazing and/or cut grasses and tree leaves. Good quality forage is often scarce, limiting productivity because of imbalance of nutrients and low digestibility of the available feed. Therefore, the primary constraint to productivity is an inefficient utilization of the feed because of deficiencies of critical nutrients in the diet. The deficient nutrients may be those critical to the growth of rumen microbes which ferment the feed as well as those required to balance the protein to energy ratio absorbed.

The major strategies for improving productivity in animals fed crop residues or mature pastures are: (1) to supplement nutrients to ensure efficient rumen function and (2) to provide bypass supplements to balance those available from fermentative digestion (Leng, 1986). These strategies aim to ensure maximum intake and efficiency of utilisation of the absorbed nutrients by the animal. By adopting these strategies, highly acceptable level of production can be achieved.

Supplementation Priorities

If supplementation is the goal for cattle grazing low quality forage, priority should first be placed on meeting the protein requirement in order to maximize forage intake and digestion. It is inconsistently proven that protein supplementation for cattle grazing protein deficient forage is extremely effective. In fact, energy supplementation will not be effective if dietary protein is deficient.

Once the producer ensures that the supplementation or feeding programme will meet the protein requirement, energy intake should be evaluated. The decision must be made whether the cattle need to maintain body weight and condition, gain weight and condition, or whether they can be allowed to lose some weight and condition. This decision will dictate how much supplemental energy should be provided. Lastly, vitamin and mineral requirements should be compared to expected intake, potential deficiencies identified, and supplemental alternatives evaluated. This is not to say that vitamins and minerals are not important. Priority is given to protein and energy nutrition first because these items are needed in much greater quantities and they have the potential to have much greater impact on animal performance and efficiency of forage utilization.

Protein Supplementation

Supplemental protein is extremely important for grazing cattle when forages fail to provide enough protein to meet their nutrient needs. The response to supplementation is high when the CP content of the basal forage is less than 6 to 8% (Kartchner, 1981). Moreover, other factors that necessitate the protein supplements are:

i) Digestibility and availability of forage : as the digestibility of the forage decreases, the availability of the CP to the microbial population and the host animal also decreases (Allden, 1981).

ii) Availability of other essential nutrients like energy, vitamins, and minerals, sulfur: nitrogen ratios.

iii) Stage of production and growth requirements : Young, growing animals and adults at high production levels are more likely to respond with increased intake and gain when provided protein supplements.

Therefore, all the above factors must be considered when predicting performance responses to supplemental protein.

Supplemental Protein

Many protein feed stuffs are available as supplement to roughage diet. The "ideal supplement" is one that best fits the target animal's nutritional needs, easier to handle and present to the target animal and is most economical. They are categorized as follows:

Oil Cakes

The most common supplemental protein is derived from oilseed by-products such as soybean meal, cottonseed meal, groundnut cake, sunflower cake, rapeseed meal and copra meal. Although we usually consider these as supplemental protein sources, they also provide significant energy to the diet. However, these feed sources can be expensive at times, and identifying inexpensive alternative native feed sources that provide supplemental protein would be beneficial to ruminant livestock producers. Protein supplementation in the form of groudnut cake, soyabean meal, fish meal (Prakash et al., 1996) or cotton seed cake (Ocen, 1992) increase the DM intake, nutrient utilization, N retention, and thus improves the performance of ruminants fed on rice straw. Among the protein meals, fish meal has been found to be superior in view of greater efficiency of N utilization. The supplemental value of rapeseed and sunflower meals for growing sheep grazing low quality grass pastures was evaluated (Coombe *et al.*, 1987). Sheep receiving no supplement or a urea supplement lost weight, whereas sheep receiving sunflower meal gained weight. Intake of rapeseed meal was low and variable, and resultant sheep performance was also variable and intermediate compared to the performance of control and sunflower meal-supplemented sheep.

Tree Foliage

Forage shrubs and trees can be one of the best options to intensify tropical animal production by supplementing traditional low quality crop residues. The legumes species belonging to the genera of Albizzia, *Callandra, Gliricidia, Mimosa, Leucaena, Samanea, Erythrina, Desmanthus, Morus* and *Acacia* are considered as good supplements in ruminant ration. Strategic supplementation of tree legumes is inevitable in small farms because of regular feed shortages. These tree legumes play significant role in ruminant nutrition because they

i) Provide high quality and high digestibility biomass resource which is easily available in and around the farm.

ii) Supplement the nutrients deficient in the diet resulting in enhancement of microbial growth and digestion of cellulosic biomass in the rumen.

iii) Act as a source of undegradable protein (Table 1).

iv) Act as a source of vitamins and minerals to complement deficiencies in the basal fed resource.

Table 1 : Rumen degradable nitrogen (RDN), rumen undegradable nitrogen (UDN) and rumen undegradable but available post ruminally (DUN) of some tree forages calculated at a passage rate of 0.05/hours (g/kg DM)

Forage	RDN	UDN	DUN
Acacia catechu	4.8	28.7	16.0
Albizzia stipulata	7.3	28.4	11.6
Artocarpus lakoocha	19.7	11.4	4.6
Bauhinia variegata	16.9	16.1	9.45
Dendrocalamus hamiltonii	11.1	20.6	11.2
Ficus roxburghii	13.2	8.9	2.6
Leucaena leucocephala	14.6	19.1	5.8
Morus alba (mature)	16.3	12.2	5.8

Source : (Singh and Makkar, 2000)

The leaves of *Leuceana, Erythrina , Desmanthus* and *Morus* are reported to produce beneficial responses like higher average daily gain (ADG) and better milk production in ruminants. Majority of tree leaves are rich in nitrogen, sulphur and minerals their supplementation can increase the efficiency of utilization of crop residues by enhancing microbial protein synthesis in the rumen. Tropical legumes generally are richer in tannins than temperate legumes and therefore should function better as sources of bypass protein. It must be emphasized that when legumes contain a high proportion of protected protein, some other source of rumen fermentable nitrogen is required, usually urea.

Apart from fresh foliage, the scope of supplementation of dried leaves and hay is under research. Intake and rumen degradation of maize stover in sheep could be improved by supplementing the animals with *Leucaena* hay up to 6 g DM/kg live weight per day (Kimambo et al., 1991). Cassava hay is also palatable to ruminants and is proved to be an excellent feed either as the sole diet or as a supplement in diets based on crop residues eg. urea-treated straws/sugarcane tops (Wanapat et al., 1997). Supplementation of cassava hay upto 400g/day in the diet of goats resulted in increased milk yield, probably due to a higher intake of protein as well as possible effects of bypass protein from the cassava hay (Wanapat *et al.*, 1997). Supplementation with cassava hay can lower use of concentrate and improve milk yield and milk composition.

NPN

Nonprotein nitrogen (NPN) and readily available sources of energy optimize rumen function resulting in increased DMI and improved performance in animals fed diets based on low-quality roughages (Winter and Pigden, 1971). NPN in the form of urea is generally a cheap source of protein. Urea is used directly by rumen microorganisms as a source of nitrogen and is completely ruminally degradable. However, this source of nitrogen is very unpalatable and should be used in moderation. Urea can be used to reduce cost of protein supplement without causing negative effects on performance as long as not more than 25% of the RDP in the diet is supplied by urea (Woods, 1997). Including higher concentration of urea in protein supplements reduces the supplement palatability and ultimately suppresses intake and animal performance. Moreover, feeding high levels is not cost-effective because much of the urea is not utilized due to the rapid ammonia release rate of urea. This rapid release of ammonia from urea exceeds the rumen microbe's ability to use the ammonia and results in more ammonia being converted back into urea by the liver and excreted. Rapid ammonia release also causes ammonia toxicity, which can lead to death.

Slow-Release NPN

The rate of ammonia release from NPN sources can be influenced both by the physical form of the NPN-containing feed and the specific ammonia-releasing molecule. Various heat and chemical treatment are popular to combine urea with starch from grains and molasses. Biuret is a very safe source of NPN and has an ammonia release curve very similar to soybean meal. The slower release of ammonia also improves the synchronization of nitrogen availability with the slow release of fermentable energy from forages and, potentially yields more efficient microbial growth in the rumen. Biuret can be utilized at very high levels with forage-based diets and is more cost-effective than feeding natural proteins sources or urea.

The Indian Veterinary Research Institute and National Dairy Development Board of India has successfully developed and introduced pashy chocolate (UMMB) and multinutrient blocks respectively based on molasses and urea for dairy buffaloes kept by village smallholders. These blocks-provide micro-organisms rich in sources of fermentable nitrogen, minerals, vitamins, amino-acids and peptides. Rates of consumption of blocks are of the order of 300-500 g/animal/day for adult animals fed on rice and wheat straw under conditions of complete confinement. UMMB supplementation of straw based diet increases digestibility, feed intake, live weight gain and milk production. Various micro and macrominerals can be incorporated in the blocks to correct the respective deficiencies of the ruminants in developing countries.

Bypass Protein

For high producing animals the feeding strategy should also be aimed at supplementation with bypass protein of dietary origin in addition to creating an efficient ecosystem. The source of bypass protein should be an oilseed meal or an animal byproduct meal (supplying protein and fat) and should be given maximum 30% of the total diet dry matter. The 30% limit is to prevent depression/substitution of the digestible energy of the basal diet. The optimum level and the degree of response to the supplement depend upon the fermentability of the basal diet.

Supplementation stretigies and Livestock Productivity

Feeding supplemental protein improves the amount of forage intake in cattle, plus it can improve the digestibility of the forages consumed. Protein supplementation (185 g/day) in the diet of crossbred calves improves intake of low quality roughages and reduces rate of live mass loss under dry winter condition. Protein supplementation of forages containing more than 9% crude protein has little effect on digestibility and intake in cattle. When the limiting nutrients are supplied through available supplements, the nutrient digestibility of basal straw has been improved dramatically. This improvement in forage utilization can lead to improved body condition scores, which can in turn lead to improved profit potential of a cattle operation. Table 2 estimates the daily dry matter intake for dry and lactating cows with or without protein supplementation. The value of protein supplementation was slightly enhanced by combining the protein supplement with energy and phosphorus (Van Niekerk and Jacobs, 1985).

Supplementation with CP usually improves weight gain and body condition score. An average daily gain of 500 g/day was observed through the supplementation of 500 g cottonseed cake in the ration of HF calves maintained on maize stover (Ocen, 1992). Supplementation of locally available concentrate ingredients and tree foliage has beneficial effect on growth rate of small ruminants. The highest live weight gain and cost benefit ratio was recorded due to *Leucaena* supplementation followed by groundnut cake, stylo and concentrate. Thus, the supplementation of locally available feed resources to ruminants have wider future application because the technology has ability to improve the production by slight modification of their existing traditional system of management. In addition, nutrient supplementation offers solution to reduce calf mortality during the period of nutritional shortage and may also increase calf performance.

Table 2 : Estimated intake of forage with and without supplementation

	Forage intake (% BW, DM basis) of brood cows	
	Dry bred cows	Lactating cows
Low-Quality Forage (<7% CP)		
No supplement	1.5	2.0
Protein Supplement	1.8	2.2
Average-Quality Forage (7-9% CP)		
No supplement	2.0	2.3
Protein Supplement	2.2	2.5
High-Quality Forage (>9% CP)		
No supplement	2.5	2.7
Protein Supplement	2.5	2.7

Source : (Hibbard and Thrift, 1992)

Strategic supplementation through locally available feed ingredients is an effective method for improving milk production and digestibility of cereal straws in the crossbred cows. Sutton (1989) mentioned possible beneficial effects on milk yield when supplementing diets with extra C.P. Sharma *et al.*, (2004) also reported positive effect on milk production and growth when diets were supplemented with oil cakasie protein supplements.

Supplementation Strategies

Although some researchers have suggested that synchrony of release of nitrogen from protein supplements is an important factor for obtaining optimal ruminal digestion of low-quality roughages (Orskov, 1982), most studies conducted under practical conditions do not support this contention. Alternate-day, once-weekly, and daily feeding of protein supplements have yielded similar responses (Huston *et al.*, 1999). Daily CP supplementation is not advantageous over infrequent supplementation. Cows grazing on low quality forage perform equally on daily or infrequent supplementation (Schauer, 2005). Moreover, infrequent supplementation of CP is a managemental alternative to reduce labour costs. In a study by Huston *et al.* (1999), variation in animal weight change was decreased with less-frequent supplementation. This effect was presumably due to less competition for the supplement when greater quantities were provided in a single setting. Research has also suggested that timing of supplementation may influence response to supplementation. Limited data are available, however, relative to timing of supplementation and the performance of cattle grazing low-quality forages.

One strategy of supplementation should be to use the most efficient delivery system to minimize costs and variation of animal intake within a group of cattle. The intake of self fed supplements is dependent on trough space, supplement allowance, supplement form and supplement formulation. Limited trough space generally increases the proportion of non feeders, whereas low levels of competition, as with self-fed supplements, generally increases variation in individual supplement intake (Bowman and Sowell, 1997). By providing a supplement delivery system that optimizes uniformity of consumption and minimizes economic inputs, we can effectively improve beef cattle production systems.

Strategic Energy Supplementation

Although protein supplements provide some energy and may stimulate additional energy intake, generally the term "energy supplement" refers to either cereal grains or by-products of the milling industry. In recent years, energy supplements have been classified into either those high in soluble carbohydrate (high in starches and sugars; cereal grains) or those high in structural carbohydrates (high in fibre; soybean hulls, ground nut husk, etc.). Carbohydrates are the main energy yielding substrates for ruminal microbes, however the type of carbohydrate may have a major effect on the rate and extent of fibre digestion.

Energy supply to the rumen can be most efficient when there is a fast NH_3 production. The slower degradation of the fibre may enable better synchrony between energy and NH_3 release. However, the high fibre can lead to substitution effects and use of these feeds as supplements may be more suitable for low fibre basal diets (Poppi and McLennan, 1995). Soluble carbohydrates such as starch or sugar may impede cellulose digestion due to factors such as lowered pH, competition between cellulolytic and non-cellulolytic bacteria for essential nutrients other than energy, or use of alternative energy sources by certain cellulolytic bacteria (Fahey and Berger, 1988). Orskov (1986) found that a small amount of grain (20 to 30% of the diet) produces little or no depression of intake and digestibility of roughages, but a higher level can depress intake to an extent that it is no longer a supplement, but becomes a substitute. In most cases, it is important to insure that the supplement complements the basal diet and does not substitute for it.

When choosing an energy supplement, it is important to consider the effect the supplement on the basal diet. The type of carbohydrate has a major effect on the rate and extent of forage digestion (Bowman and Sanson, 1996). Intake and digestibility are often depressed when cattle consuming low-quality forages are supplemented with nonstructural carbohydrates such as cereal grains, but low-quality forage intake and utilization has been shown to increase when cattle have been supplemented with fibrous by-product feedstuffs that contain high levels of structural carbohydrates. Some studies have shown an increase in intake when supplementing with structural carbohydrates. However, it was noted that intake does not continue to increase beyond certain levels of supplementation.

Average hay dry matter digestibility for lambs fed supplemental beet pulp was 3.7% greater than for lambs fed supplemental corn. It was concluded that the difference arise as a result of an improved ruminal environment for fibre digestion when beet pulp was fed, which was higher in digestible fibre. However, other studies with corn as a supplement have shown a decrease in forage digestibility. Chase and Hibberd (1987) observed that digestibility of hemicellulose and cellulose decreased linearly as the amount of supplemental corn increased. Additionally, hay and fibre digestibility also decreased as the amount of supplemental corn increased. Supplementation with corn or other concentrate feeds can negatively affect fibre digestion.

Soybean hull based energy supplement was better for body weight gain in pregnant cows compared to soybean meal based protein supplement (Marston *et al.*, 1995). Energy supplemented cows looses less body condition score before calving than protein-supplemented cows, with this advantage continuing throughout the breeding season and until weaning.

Energy supplementation has been shown to improve reproductive performance. However, the response appear to be dependent on the timing (pre or postpartum) of supplementation. An early return to estrus following parturition is commonly observed phenomena in high level energy supplemented cows. Pre or post-partum supplements affect different reproductive variables (Wiltbank *et al.*, 1962). The level of energy intake in mature cows pre-calving influenced the length of interval from calving to first estrus and the level of energy intake post-calving influenced the conception rate. The postpartum level of energy intake is probably more critical than prepartum level when considering total reproductive performance. However, cows fed energy during gestation had greater pregnancy rates than cows fed protein, but the pregnancy rate was not influenced by postpartum supplementation (Marston *et al.*, 1995).

Supplemental Feeding for Small Ruminants

When forage or browse is limited or of low quality for lactating does, does in the last 30 days of gestation and developing/breeding bucks should be fed nearly 500 g/day of a 16% protein commercial feed or homemade mixture (77:20:2.5:0.5, cereal: oilcakes/meal: mineral mixture: limestone). As a general recommendation a complete goat mineral mixture should be offered free choice throughout the year. Low to medium quality forage (> 10% protein) will meet requirements of dry does and non breeding bucks.

In goats nutritional stress appears to be a prime cause of acyclicity (Ndlovu, 1992). It is, therefore, beneficial to supplement the goats maintained on poor nutritional status with those nutrients which have an impact on reproductive performance at the time of stress. Additional nutrient allowance is not needed for pregnant goats grazed on good quality pasture for the purpose of improving kid birth weight. However, during lactation it would be advisable to supplement to improve growth and survival rates of kids especially when rain is below the long-term average for the area. Therefore, supplementation throughout the reproductive cycle would not be beneficial (Madibela et al., 2002) for well grazed goats.

Rapid rate of foetal growth during the final six weeks of pregnancy imposes a metabolic challenge to the doe, which is met by the mobilization of maternal body tissue and this may result in weight loss of doe, if the dietary supply of nutrients is inadequate (Sibanda *et al.,* 1997). Strategic supplementation of pregnancy allowance during the last month of gestation may be adopted to economize goat production and to minimize reproductive wastage. Optimum period for pregnancy allowance supplementation may depend on intrauterine growth pattern of goat breed; the last month of pregnancy appears to be the most nutritionally sensitive period of gestation for non-descriptive goats found in northern plains of India (Rastogi *et al.,* 2006).

Strategic Supplementation of Minerals

Cattle will generally obtain enough minerals and vitamins from available forages and grain to survive. But, they do not receive enough minerals and vitamins from forages or grains to optimize digestion and performance. This is because mineral and vitamin content of forages and grains is deficient in certain minerals and varies tremendously depending upon the soil type, weather conditions, time of year, fertilization levels, stage of maturity and storage conditions. Over time, soils can also become depleted in mineral content, resulting in lower mineral levels in forages. Hence, it is needed to provide supplemental minerals and vitamins.

Mineral Supplementation Strategy

Mineral supplementation for livestock is considered to be the least cost insurance for a better productivity and hence, can be recommended in all types of livestock farming cutting across the economic barrier. The best means of providing minerals to ruminants receiving concentrates would be to combine the minerals with the concentrate diet, including Ca, P, and a trace mineralized salt. Iron may be included if condition deserves for. Sulphur may be added to the premix if non-protein nitrogen is added to the concentrate.

The balance of individual minerals is important in this regard to ensure proper absorption and utilization of the minerals.

Animals that primarily depend on pasture have different supplementation needs, compared to those receiving concentrates. Free choice mineral mixture or a mineral lick is the preferred option to supplement these animals. A good free choice mineral supplement should have the following characteristic features (McDowell, 1985).

1. Contains a minimum of 6-8% total P. In areas where forages are consistently lower than 0.2% P, mineral supplements with P range 8-10% are preferred.
2. Has a Ca: P ratio not substantially over 2:1
3. Provides a significant proportion (i.e., about 50%) of the trace elements for Co, Cu, I, Mn, Zn and Se if required. Fe is not needed in most circumstances.
4. Sufficiently palatable to allow adequate consumption in relation to requirements.
5. Has an acceptable particle size that will allow adequate mixing without smaller size practice settling out.

Trace mineralized salt is prevalent in organized farming sector. Customized trace mineral premixtures are becoming more common because they are formulated to balance mineral profiles and meet mineral needs depending on the farm condition. Forage testing is recommended for Zn, Cu, Mn and Fe an annual basis to establish herd micro mineral profiles and avoid/correct mineral imbalance.

Organic Minerals

Organic minerals are the supplementation strategy for modern age livestock. The source of minerals in the diet can affect the performance of the animals and the cost-effectiveness of the supplementation programme. Organic mineral sources are characterized by the presence of an amino acid or a carbohydrate carrier for the trace mineral that is to be fed to cattle. In a process termed chelation or proteination, the organic carrier molecule is chemically bound to the trace mineral of interest. Organic mineral sources have higher bioavailabilities than inorganic sources of minerals; however, chelated minerals are usually more expensive than inorganic sources.

Requirement

Cattle require different levels of minerals, depending on age, size, sex, physiological state, and level of performance. Nutrient requirements of cattle at different stages of maturity and production are provided in Table 3.

Table 3 : Mineral requirements and maximum tolerable levels for beef cattle

Mineral units	Growing and finishing cattle	Gestating and dry cows	Lactating cows	Maximum tolerable level
Calcium, percent	0.31	0.18	0.27	
Chlorine, percent				
Chromium, ppm				1000.00
Cobalt, ppm	0.10	0.10	0.10	10.00
Copper, ppm	10.00	10.00	10.00	100.00
Iodine, ppm	0.50	0.50	0.50	50.00
Iron, ppm	50.00	50.00	50.00	1000.00
Magnesium, ppm	0.10	0.12	0.20	0.40
Manganese, percent	20.00	40.00	40.00	1000.00
Molybdenum, ppm				5.00
Nickel, ppm				50.00
Phosphorus, percent	0.27	0.18	0.27	
Potassium, percent	0.60	0.60	0.70	3.00
Selenium, ppm	0.10	0.10	0.10	2.00
Sodium, percent	0.07	0.07	0.10	
Sulfur, percent	0.15	0.15	0.15	0.40
Zinc, ppm	30.00	30.00	30.00	500.00

Source : NRC, 1996.

A brief account of the essentiality of individual mineral supplementation is furnished below.

Calcium : Calcium is usually not deficient in grass forages fed to cattle. In addition, legumes such as alfalfa and clover are high in calcium. Grains and by-product feeds are low in calcium, and diets high in these feed ingredients need to be supplemented, usually with feed grade limestone or calcium carbonate. Like phosphorus, calcium is a structural part of bone, so temporary shortfalls in the diet can be overcome by the animal mobilizing some of the calcium in bone.

Phosphorus : Phosphorus is often deficient in forages for lactating cows with superior milking ability. In addition, mature forages are often deficient in phosphorus for most cattle. Phosphorus is high in oilseed meals and also fairly high in grains; so when diets contain substantial amounts of these ingredients, supplementation is usually not needed. Phosphorus is one of the structural components of the skeletal system, and levels build up when cows are grazing lush forages that contain phosphorus at levels above requirements. Some of the phosphorus in bone can be mobilized during early lactation to overcome shortfalls in intake, but prolonged dietary deficiency has been reported to result in depressed reproductive efficiency and milk production.

Salt (sodium chloride) : Salt supplementation is always required in ruminates unless the water salinity is very high. Sodium and chlorine are major electrolytes found in body fluids, and there is very little storage. Because of this, cattle will develop deficiencies rapidly and should have constant access to salt or a supplement containing salt.

Magnesium : Forages contain adequate magnesium during most of the year, but levels can be very low during times of rapid growth, especially in well-fertilized pastures. The magnesium deficiency may occur during calving seasons and the onset of lactation and when the forage contains high levels of potassium which can interfere with the absorption of magnesium. Supplementation with magnesium oxide is recommended for 30 days prior to calving and during the first three months of lactation.

Sulfur : Sulfur is a component of several amino acids that are the building blocks of protein. Sulfur, other than that fed in the form of protein, is usually needed only when diets contain substantial amounts of nonprotein nitrogen (NPN). In these situations, the ratio of nitrogen to sulfur should be maintained between 10:1 and 15:1. High sulfur levels can interact with copper and molybdenum, which can result in a copper deficiency. It has been shown that the supplementation of poor quality fibre diets with sulphur improved ruminal fibre degradation as well as apparent organic matter digestibility.

Trace Minerals

Zinc : Zinc is a part of many important enzyme systems in the body, and its deficiency leads to depressed feed intake and growth rate, an abnormal hair coat and skin lesions. Zinc is important for male reproduction and immunity. Storage of zinc is minimal, and deficiencies occur rapidly following introduction of animals to a diet severely deficient in zinc. Zinc methionine, an organic form of zinc, has proven to improve performance in cattle.

Copper : Copper is important for adequate growth, reproduction, immunity and enzyme function. Unlike zinc, copper is stored in the liver, and levels build up rapidly when animals are fed high levels of copper. Copper oxide should be avoided as a copper source because of its poor bioavailability, which will affect the level of copper required in supplements. High levels of molybdenum, sulfur, iron or zinc in the diet interfere with normal copper absorption and metabolism.

Selenium : The activity of selenium is related to vitamin E, and supplementation with either will help in preventing white muscle disease. Marginal selenium deficiency can result in retained placenta, impaired fertility, silent heats and unthrifty weak calves with poor immune response (resulting in high preweaning death losses). Selenium can be provided in mineral mixes or in an injectable form. The maximum level of selenium that can be legally added to a supplement is 3 mg per head per day at its highest intake.

Manganese : Manganese levels in forages vary considerably, depending on the soils on which they are produced. Manganese is a part of several important enzyme systems. A deficiency may result in impaired reproductive performance in both cows and bulls and in the birth of deformed calves.

Cobalt : Cobalt is needed only for the ruminal synthesis of vitamin B_{12}. Cobalt requirements are higher when cattle are fed high-grain diets, because more B_{12} is required to metabolize the end products of rumen fermentation. Cobalt may be very deficient in some soils, so including it in trace mineral supplements is a sound practice.

Iron : Iron is a part of haemoglobin which transports oxygen to body tissues. Since most forages contain high levels of iron and because substantial amounts of soil are consumed during grazing, iron is almost never deficient in cattle fed forage-based diets. A more common problem with iron is that it may be excessively high in forages or in drinking water, which can interfere with the absorption of copper and zinc.

Iodine : Iodine makes up part of the thyroid hormones. Iodine is normally included in trace mineral supplements. Added iodine compounds should provide no more than 10 mg of iodine per day.

Mineral Supplementation- Effect on Animal Productivity

The supplementation of minerals can be recommended for augmenting the productive performance of grazing ruminants. The common reproductive failures in cattle can be successfully managed with mineral supplements. They exert beneficial effects on reproductive performance of indigenous cattle maintained on cereal straw where nutrient imbalances and deficiencies are common. The importance of proper mineral supplementation was demonstrated in the work of Prabowo et al. (1984). Lambs fed only chopped napier grass, napier grass plus 100 g/d rice bran, or napier plus rice bran and a complete mineral supplement, gained 8, 37 and 69 g/d, respectively. Feeding mineral increases the rumen microbe population, which is critical to increasing forage digestion. In a study it is demonstrated cattle fed hay had only 39% of the microbial population of cattle fed a full supplement package, while cattle fed minerals and vitamins had 69% of the rumen microbe population.

Increased rumen microbe populations can lead to improved forage digestion, which leads to improved body condition scores.

Vitamins

Ruminants are able to meet most of their vitamin requirements through rumen microbial synthesis and dietary supply. Even though, calves are born with minimal stores of vitamins, colostrum feeding satisfy their requirement. The ability to synthesize B vitamins and vitamin K in the rumen develops rapidly when solid feed is introduced into the diet. In ruminants, five classes of vitamins are important. Vitamin A is the most important. Vitamins D, E, K, and some of the B vitamins also are known to be essential. High-quality forages contain large amounts of vitamin A precursors and vitamin E. Vitamin D is synthesized by animal exposure to sunlight and is found in large amounts in sun-cured forages. Supplemental vitamins can be added to the trace mineral salt mixture, if needed.

Vitamin A

Liver stores of vitamin A can be depleted when cattle consume a diet of low-quality, mature forage. In that case, supplementation is recommended to prevent potential problems on productive ability of cattle. Supplementing brood cows with vitamin A before (16,000 IU/day) and after (40,000 IU/day) the calving season can increase conception rates by 10% and decrease calf morbidity by as much as 50% as compared to a deficient state. Typically, 2 to 4 months of protection can be expected from stored vitamin A. Increasing dietary vitamin A by 5,000 IU per day can double the amount of vitamin A stored in the liver. Supplemental vitamin A is not required when cattle are grazing dormant rangelands, or if the cattle are fed properly cured and stored hay.

Vitamin E

Supplementation is recommended for brood cows consuming poor quality forage during late pregnancy through early lactation. During the late stages of pregnancy, vitamin E concentration in the blood tends to decrease below marginal levels. Feeding supplemental vitamin E is an effective method of maintaining proper levels during this period. Neonatal calves must receive dietary vitamin E since placental transfer is very limited. However, it may not be necessary to supply supplemental vitamin E directly to the calf. Feeding an additional 1,000 IU of α-tocopherol (vitamin E) to cattle during the last trimester of pregnancy can increase antibody production and sequestration in the colostrum and increase vitamin E concentration in the colostrum by up to 30 percent. Plasma concentrations of vitamin E in the calf can be maintained above the minimal level by continuing maternal supplementation into the early stages of lactation.

Vitamin D

Sunlight typically stimulates sufficient production of vitamin D in grazing cattle. Vitamin D status is improved more effectively by increasing the animal's exposure to sunlight than by dietary supplementation.

Vitamin K

Ruminal microorganisms generally synthesize and supply vitamin K in amounts adeaquate to meet the ruminant's requirements. Supplemental vitamin K usually is justified only when cattle are suspected to have been exposed to vitamin K antagonists. Consumption of a natural vitamin K antagonist (dicumarol) can be a problem if cattle ingest moldy sweet clover forage. Therefore, prevention (avoid feeding moldy sweet clover hay) is a better alternative to supplemental treatments.

B vitamins

Microbial synthesis of the B vitamins in the rumen usually satisfies the ruminant's requirements. Supplementation with B vitamins should not be necessary under normal production situations, especially if cattle consume high-quality forage or are fed supplemental protein and/or energy that improve ruminal digestibility and subsequent microbial synthesis. Injections of B vitamins seem to be beneficial only to combat over stress and disease.

Mineral and vitamin supplementation is critical for cattle to achieve the most economical gains possible from the forage and grain they consume. Minerals and vitamins are needed in very small quantities, yet they are a critical part of the overall nutritional package fed to cattle and are the backbone of a successful range cattle programme. They play a vital role in nutrient digestion, reproductive performance, the immune system, and in the development of muscle, bones, and teeth. Typically, inadequate intake of essential minerals and vitamins may result in reduced forage intake, inefficient feed utilization, decreased average daily gains, lower reproductive efficiency and poor disease immunity. Supplementing with a balanced mineral and vitamin programme enables cattle to obtain more of their needed nutrients from the forages consumed rather than getting needed nutrients from grains or additional supplements.

Multinutrient Blocks

The type of supplement is important to minimize wastage and to maximize its impact on productivity. Multi-nutrient supplements as blocks, in contrast to liquid or mash supplements hold several advantages, namely, simplicity for transport and management, a more homogeneous intake among animals, reduced need for salt as an intake regulator and less risk in the use of urea as a source of non-protein nitrogen (Ben Salem and Nefzaoui, 2003; Kawas, 2010). Multi-nutrient blocks based on molasses and urea can be hand-crafted by livestock owners. This type of block consist of molasses (25-50%), urea (5-10%), cereal byproducts such as wheat bran or rice bran (15-25%), oil seed meals (10-20%), salt (4-10%), lime (5-10%), and a mixture of a phosphorous source, trace minerals and feed additives (1-5%). The lime will provide more hardness than cement, which has been frequently used to produce blocks in developing countries, and lime is generally 30–40% cheaper (Kawas, 2010). Vitamin A supplement should be added to the protein–mineral mixture during the dry or winter seasons, when low quality forage is available. Two different types of multinutrient lick-blocks can be prepared for wet and dry seasons, respectively, with the following characteristics.

Mineral-protein blocks : This is a low intake block (approximately 0.2–0.3% of body weight) with 30% crude protein or more. The purpose of offering this block is to supplement protein, macro-minerals (calcium, phosphorous, and magnesium), trace minerals (iron, manganese, zinc, copper, iodine, cobalt and selenium), and vitamin A. This supplement can be offered during dry or wet seasons as a reproductive management tool for goats. It is important to consider that during the wet season, forages contain more protein and energy, so it is important to emphasise in mineral supplementation, so that these nutrients can be better utilized. Protein supplementation produces a greater response on DM intake with forages of lower protein content as compared to forages with relatively high protein content.

Protein-energy blocks: These blocks contain minerals, but more energy and less protein (20–25% crude protein) than a mineral-protein block. Intake of this block should be greater (approximately 0.4–0.5% of body weight). This supplement is recommended for the dry season, when availability and quality of forages limit energy intake by goats (Kawas, 2010).

The per unit production potential of Indian livestock is very low. The most important extraneous factor accounting for this is the poor quality feed resources. Forage availability from sources other than crop residues is often scarce, limiting productivity because of imbalance of nutrients and low digestibility of the available feed. Therefore, supplemental feeding strategies are inevitable to supply deficient critical nutrients and complement the nutritional attributes of the poor quality roughages. The basic supplemental nutrients are energy from cereals and cereal byproducts, protein from oilseed meals and legume trees, minerals and vitamins. However, nutrient supply should be prioritized according to the physiological stages of the animals. A supplemental feeding programme can reduce total cost of production by increasing forage digestion and optimizing the performance. Multinutrient blocks are getting popularized in tropical countries by reducing feed wastage and increasing the intake. All he supplemental strategies are reported to maximize rumen fermentation and microbial protein synthesis, which in turn contributes to higher milk production, growth rate and profit.

References

Allden, W. G. (1981). Energy and protein supplements for grazing livestock. In: F.H.W. Morley (Ed.) Grazing Ruminants. Elsevier Scientific Publishing Co., Amsterdam. pp 289-307.

Ben Salem, H. and Nefzaoui, A. (2003). *Small Rumin. Res.*, 49: 275–288.

Bowman, J.P., and Sowell. B.F. (1997). *J. Anim. Sci.*, 75:543-550.

Bowman, J.G.P. and Sanson, D.W. (1996). Starch- or fiber based energy supplements of grazing ruminants. *Proc. West. Sec. Amer. Soc. Anim. Sci.*, 47:118- 135.

Chase, C.C., Jr. and Hibberd, C.A. (1987). *J. Anim. Sci.*, 65:557-566.

Coombe, J. B., Axelsen, A. and Dove, H. (1987). *Aust. J. Exp. Agric.*, 27:513-523.

Fahey, G.C.and Berger, L.L. (1988). Carbohydrate nutrition of ruminants. In: D.C. Church (ed.). The Ruminant Animal: Digestive Physiology and Nutrition. Prentice-Hall, Englewood Cliffs, NJ. p. 269.

Hibberd, C.A. and Thrift, T.A. (1992). Supplementations of forage-based diets: Are results predictable? *J. Anim. Sci.*, 70:181. (Abstr.).

Huston, F.E., Lippke, H. Forbes, T.D.A., Holloway, J.W. and Machen, R.V. (1999). *J. Anim. Sci.*, 77:3057-3067.

Kartchner, R.J. (1981). *J. Anim. Sci.*, 51:432-438.

Kawas, J.R., Andrade-Montemayor, H. Lu, C.D. (2010). *Small Rumin. Res.*, 89: 234-243.

Kimambo, A.E., Makiwa, A.M., Shem, M.N. (1991). The use of Leucaena leucocephala supplementation to improve the utilisation of maize stover by sheep. Joint Feed Resources Network Workshop on the Complementarity of Feed Resources for Animal Production in Africa, Gaborone (Botswana), 4-8 March.

Leng, R.A. (1986). Constraints to ruminant production and concepts to increase productivity from low-digestibility forages. Proceedings of the 5th International Conference on Livestock Production and Diseases in the Tropics held in Kuala Lumpur, Malaysia, 18th - 22nd August, 1986. p. 145.

Madibela, O.R., Mosimanyana, B.M., Boitumelo, W. S. and Pelaelo, T.D. (2002). *S. Afr. J. Anim. Sci.*, 32:14-22

Marston, T.T., Lusby, D.S., Wettemann, R.P. and Purvis, H.T. (1995). *J. Anim. Sci.*, 73: 657-664.

McDowell, L.R. (1985). Minerals in Animal and Human Nutrition (Tony J. Chunha ed.) Academic Press, New York.

National Research Council. 1996. Nutrient Requirements of Beef Cattle, seventh revised edition. Washington, D.C.: National Academy Press.

Ndlovu, L.R. (1992). Reproductive performance of indigenous goats in traditionally managed flocks in North-East of Zimbabwe. In: Small Ruminant Research and Development in Africa. Eds. Lebbie, R.B. & Reynolds, S.H.B., Proc. First Biennial Conf. Africa Small Ruminant Network. ILRAD, Nairobi, Kenya, Dec. 1990. ILCA, Nairobi, Kenya. pp. 177-184.

Ocen,W.G. (1992). Performance of cattle given crop residues supplemented with high-quality forages and agro-industrial by-products. LRRD., 4(1).

Orskov, E. R. (1982). Protein Nutrition in Ruminants. pp 41-84. Academic Press, New York.

Orskov, E.R. (1986). *J. Anim. Sci.*, 63:1624-1633.

Poppi, D.P.and McLennan, S.R. (1995). *J. Anim. Sci.*, 73:278-290.

Prabowo, A., J. E. van Eys, I. W. Mathius, M. Rangkuti and W. L. Johnson. 1984. Studies on the mineral nutrition of sheep in West Java, Indonesia. Small Ruminant CRSP Working Paper No. 40, Res. Inst. for Anim. Prod., Bogor (indonesia) and North Carolina State Univ., Raleigh.

Prakash, P., Reddy, D.V., Reddy, R.R. and Krishna, N. (1996). *Anim. Feed Sci. Tech.*, 63: 229-243.

Rastogi, A., Dutta, N. and Sharma, K. (2006). Effect of strategically supplemented pregnancy allowance on nutrient utilization and reproductive performance of goats. LRRD., 18 (11).

Schauer, C.S.D., Bohnert, W., Ganskopp, D.C., Richards, C.J. and Falc, S.J. (2005). *J. Anim. Sci.*, 83:1715-1725.

Sharma, K., Dutta, Narayan and Pattanaik, A.K. (2004). Final Report ICAR Cess Fund Scheme on-farm studies on possible technological interventions for improving the feeding systems of dairy animal through supplementation and strategic feeding.

Sibanda, L.M., Ndlovu, L.R. and Bryant, M.J. (1997). *J. Agri. Sci.*, 128: 469-477.

Singh, B. and Makkar, H.P.S. (2000). The potential of mulberry tree foliage as an animal feed supplement in India. FAO Electronic Conference on Mulberry for Animal Production, April 2000, Rome, Italy.

Sutton J.D. (1989). *J. Dairy Sci., 72*: 2801–2814.

Van Niekerk, B.D.H. and Jacobs, G.A. (1985). *S. Afr. J. Anim. Sci.*, 15: 133 -136.

Wanapat, M., Pimpa, O., Petlum, A. and Boontao, U. (1997). Cassava hay: A new strategic feed for ruminants during the dry season. LRRD., 9 (2).

Wiltbank, J.N., Rowden, W.W., Ingalls, J.E., Gregory, K.E. and Koch, R.M. (1962). *J. Anim. Sci.*, 21:219-225.

Winter, K. A. and Pigden, W. J. (1971). *Can. J. Anim. Sci.*, 51: 777-781.

Woods, B. C. 1997. Effect of inclusion of urea and supplement frequency on intake, digestion, and performance of cattle consuming low-quality, tall grass prairie forage. M.S. Thesis. Kansas State University, Manhattan, Kansas.

□□□

Animal Nutrition, 2012
eds. Dr. (Mrs.) Usha R. Mehra et al., pp. 459-473
Satish Serial Publishing House e-mail : info@satishserial.com; website : www.satishserial.com

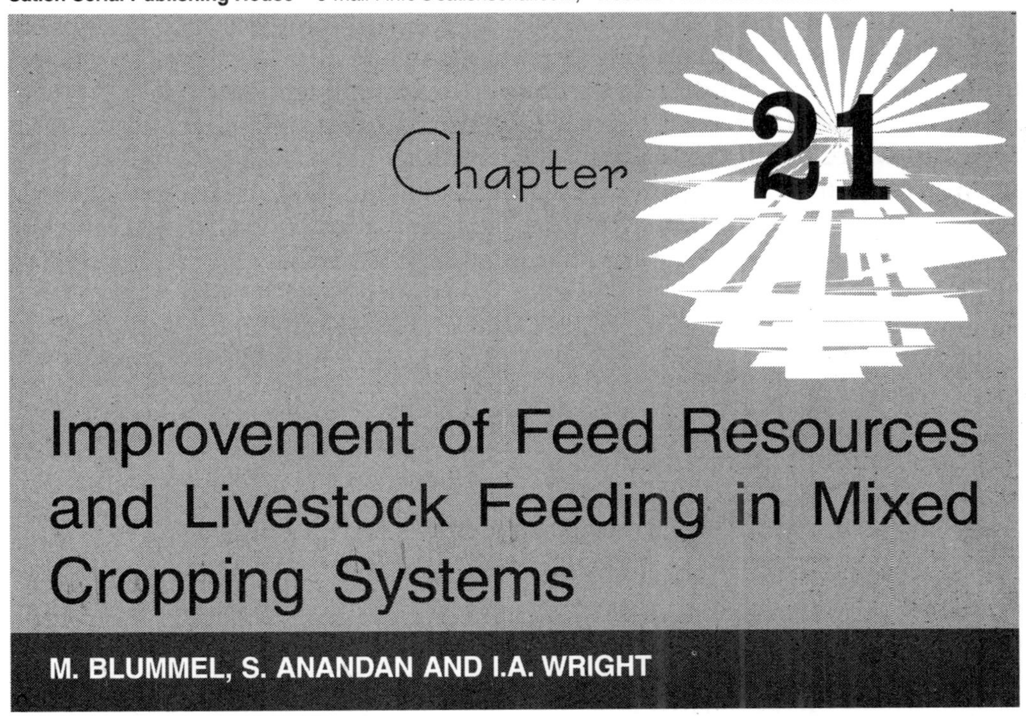

Chapter 21

Improvement of Feed Resources and Livestock Feeding in Mixed Cropping Systems

M. BLUMMEL, S. ANANDAN AND I.A. WRIGHT

The inability of producers in developing countries to feed animals adequately throughout the year remains the major technical constraint in most livestock systems (Ayantunde *et al.*, 2005). Meeting the predicted future demand for meat and milk (Delgado *et al.*, 1999) in a way that poor livestock keepers benefit more from their animal assets will require sustainable inputs of labor, land, water and nutrients to produce the feed required. While the increasing demand for livestock products offers market opportunities and income for small holder producers and even landless thereby providing pathways out of poverty (Kristjianson, 2009), livestock production globally faces increasing pressure because of negative environmental implications (Steinfeld *et al.*, 2006). Besides green house gases, high water requirement in livestock production is a major concern. Conventionally, water requirements for livestock have been thought of in terms of drinking water requirements and water in feed while in fact most of the water used by livestock is lost through evapo-transpiration in producing the feed. Water required to produce maintenance feed for one Tropical Livestock Unit is about 100 times more than the water required for drinking (Peden *et al.*, 2007). In regions with strong competition for land and water resources, land and water scarcity emerge as major constraints for increased feed production in small-holder systems. For instance in Northern India, water-use efficiency was found to be low in systems with high reliance on irrigated forages (Singh *et al.*, 2004). Singh and colleagues reported for Gujarat that on average 3 400 litres of water were required to produce one litre of milk - the world average is 900 liters. Clearly water requirement – and more generally sustainable natural resource use - needs to be a concern to those who work in feed resource development and livestock nutrition.

Strategic Investment into Feed Resources

Through coordinated central government and state efforts, India has systematically quantified fodder resources, building up a data base from district level (NIANP, 2003). Feed sources were classified into greens (subclasses: cultivated fodder, grass from grazing, grass from forests), crop residues (subclasses: coarse and fine cereal residues, leguminous residues) and concentrates (subclasses: grains, cakes, bran, chunnies). Subclasses from crop residues (CR) are further differentiated to list the contributions from specific crops (NIANP, 2003). This feed resource data base showed that crop residues were the most important single fodder resource. At the same time fodder from common property resources (CPR), forests, pastures and fallow lands constituted less than 18% of the available fodder and was declining. Also notable was that concentrates represented a very low proportion (< 4%) of the available feed resources, and there was no indication of any rapid increase in the use of concentrates. Recently Ramachandra *et al.* (2007) have pointed out that CR will provide more than 70% of the feed resources for Indian livestock by the year 2020. Worldwide total CR is estimated to be 3.8 billion metric tons with cereals contributing 74%, sugar crops 10%, legumes 8%, tubers 5% and oil crops 3% (Lal, 2005). Crop residues are generally considered to be of low nutritive quality, but this statement implicitly relates to cereal CR, since leguminous CR can have excellent fodder quality. The widespread availability of CR and extent of their use as livestock fodder marks them as a strategic feed resource of the highest order. Furthermore, it is important to realize that CR are some of the few feed resources that do not need allocation of water and land, because the crops are grown for the production of the primary products of grains and pods. The work presented here focuses on variations in food-feed traits of key crops and the relationships between CR traits and grain and pod yields. The chapter will also comment on the possible further improvement in the use of CR by targeted genetic enhancement and by supplementation and feed processing.

Entry Points for Increasing Fodder Value of Crop Residues (CR)

Entry points can be classified into pre and post harvest approaches (Fig. 1). In the past, livestock nutritionists tended to focus on post harvest interventions and considerable efforts were expended on technologies for improving the nutritive quality of CR by chemical, physical or biological treatments. Chemical treatments have received maximum attention of researchers and can be categorized into using hydrolytic and oxidative agents. Widely used hydrolytic agents were NaOH, $Ca(OH)_2$, NH_3 and urea. Common oxidants were ozone, SO_2 and various de-lignifying agents such as chlorite, paracetic acid, permanganate etc. Physical processing include as diverse techniques as chopping, grinding, pelleting, steaming, irradiation and mechanical separation of morphological fractions have been tried with varying degrees of success. Except for chopping, comparative little uptake of these technologies was observed till now, mainly because energy input-output ratios are unsatisfactory. Similar conclusions hold true for biological treatments. As an aside: these perspectives might change with the advent of 2nd generation biofuels, which have attracted huge investments. The development of cost-effective technologies for the conversion of ligno-cellulose to sugars could herald a livestock feeding revolution. In the case of bioethanol production, economically viable use of ligno-cellulose complexes will depend on: cheap and efficient processes for the hydrolysis of plant cell walls for the release and recovery of a high proportion of sugars; and the cheap and efficient

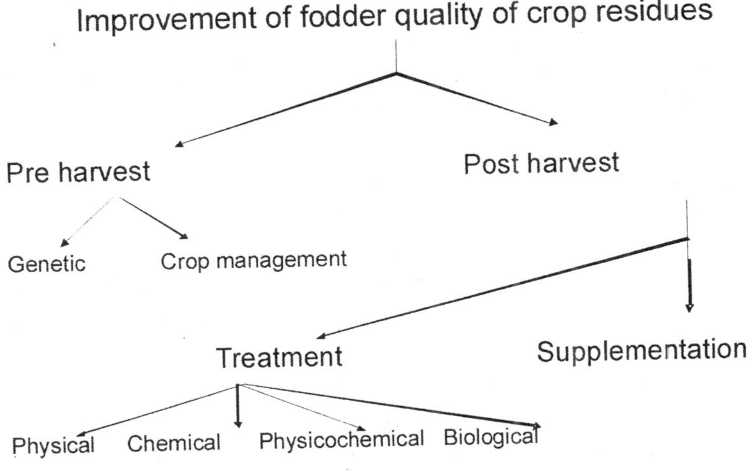

Fig. 1 : Entry points for improving fodder quality of crop residues

fermentation of sugars to ethanol. As the hydrolysis processes for bioethanol production become more efficient, straw, stover and woody material will become more valuable as livestock feed as the feeding value of roughages potentially match that of concentrates. Thus, it might become more attractive to use hydrolyzed ligno-cellulose for livestock rather than bioethanol production; and the effect on feed resources is uncertain (Dixon *et al.,* 2009).

Few of these interventions involving processing of roughages have been widely adopted (Singh and Schiere, 1993), giving way to a new research paradigm of targeted improvement of CR fodder value by plant breeding and selection (Reed *et al.,* 1988; Kristjianson and Zerbini, 1999). Until recently, the feed quality of CR was largely ignored in crop improvement, although farmers are aware of differences in the fodder quality of CR even within the same species (Kelley *et al.,* 1996). This neglect sometimes resulted in new cultivars that had been improved only for grain yields being rejected by farmers because of low CR quantity and quality (Kelley *et al.,* 1996). Interestingly, the Indo-Dutch Project on "Bio-conversion of Crop Residues for Animal Feed" had arrived at similar conclusions by the 1990s and shifted from a focus on straw treatment to breeding and management interventions. However, this occurred relatively late in the funding of the project and was not pursued with sufficient urgency after the project had ended. Increasing the feeding value of CR by multidimensional crop improvement depends upon: a) close collaboration between crop and livestock scientists, b) nutritionally significant cultivar-dependent variation in CR fodder quality; c) sufficient independence between CR fodder traits and primary traits such as grain and pod yield; and d) technologies for quick and inexpensive phenotyping of large set of samples for fodder quality traits. These conditions were found to be met in several key crops that were investigated in collaborative work between the International Livestock Research Institute (ILRI), the International Crops Research Institute for the Semi Arid Tropics (ICRISAT), the National Research Center for Sorghum (NRCS) and the International Rice Research Institute (IRRI).

Exploiting Variation in Crop Residue Fodder Quality in Available Cultivars

Farmers, fodder traders and dairy producers are well aware of differences in CR fodder quality within a species that are relevant for livestock nutrition. Blümmel and Rao (2006) surveyed six major sorghum stover traders in Hyderabad monthly from 2004 to 2005 and observed that a total of different six stover types were frequently traded. At any given time customers had usually the choice between two and sometimes three different sorghum stover types offered by the same trader. The poorest and best quality stover (perceived in terms of color, softness, sweetness etc) were sold on average for 3 and 4 IRs / kg dry matter, respectively. Blümmel and Rao (2006) investigated these traded stovers for laboratory fodder quality traits such as crude protein and *in vitro* digestibility and related these laboratory traits to stover prices (Fig. 2 and 3). While stover crude protein content was not related to stover prices, *in vitro* digestibility accounted for 75% of the variation therein. A difference of 5% in *in vitro* digestibility (47 versus 52%) was associated with a price premium for stover quality of more than 30%.

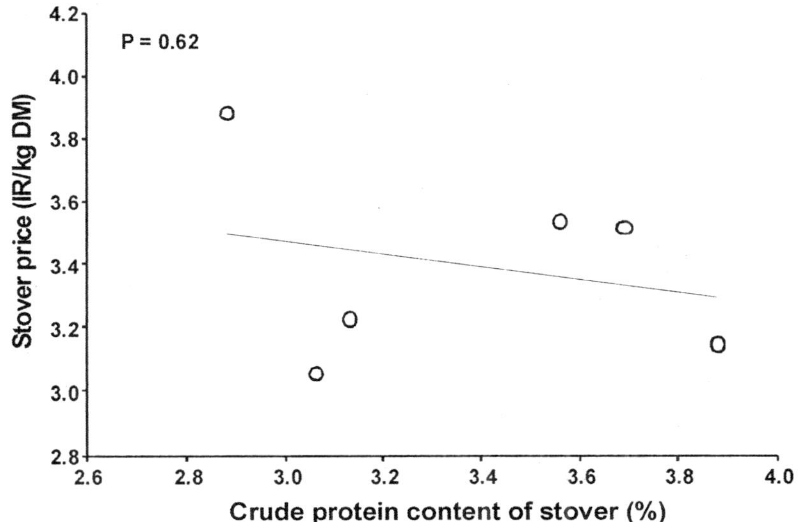

Fig. 2 : Relations between crude protein content of stover and price of stover

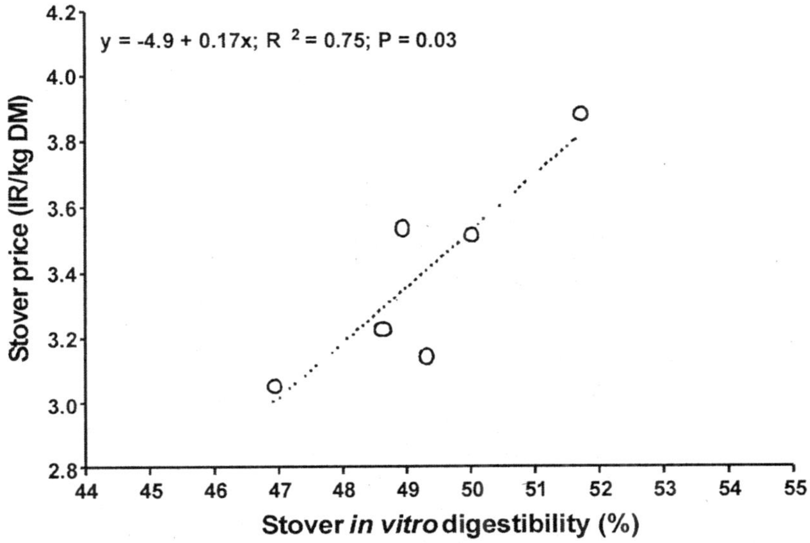

Fig. 3 : Relations between *in vitro* digestibility of stover and price of stover

These variations in stover fodder quality came about by chance, and the awareness of it and the development of differential pricing probably took considerable time. As shown by the collaboration of NRCS and ILRI in which new sorghum cultivars submitted for testing to NRCS for release have been phenotyped for fodder quality since 2002, such variations in stover quality can be targeted and exploited in a wide range of *Kharif* and *Rabi* sorghum with little or no trade-off between grain and stover traits (Fig. 4a-c). Sorghum stover digestibility in very high grain yielding *Kharif* cultivars varied by almost 10% (Fig. 4a) which is almost double the variation observed in samples collected in the studies of stover trading. Similarly stover digestibility was not negatively related to stover yield (Fig. 4b) and stover yield itself was quite independent of grain yield (Fig. 4c). There exists, therefore, a significant genetic variation for grain yield, stover yield and stover fodder quality and at the same time considerable independency between these traits. The strongest trade-off effects between stover quality and grain yield were observed for off-season (*Rabi*) sorghum, where stover digestibility accounted for 30% of the variations in grain yield (Fig. 1a). However, stover digestibility among the highest grain yielding cultivars still differed by more than 5% units and cultivars with superior stover quality could be chosen with out sacrificing grain.

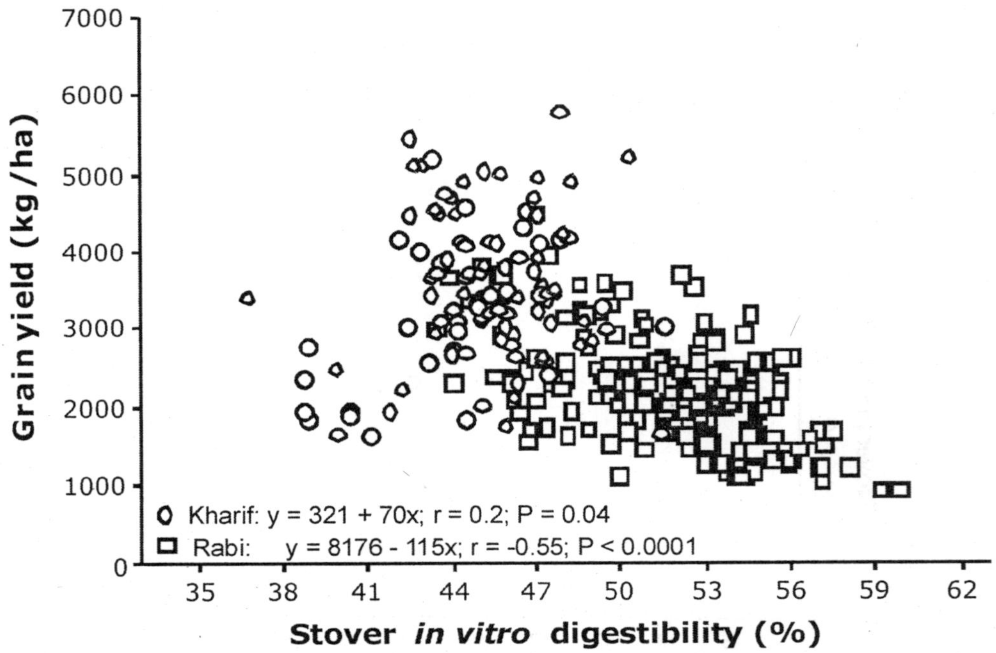

Fig. 4a : Relations between mean stover *in vitro* digestibility and grain yield in Kharif and Rabi sorghum cultivars submitted to NRCS 2002 to 2007.

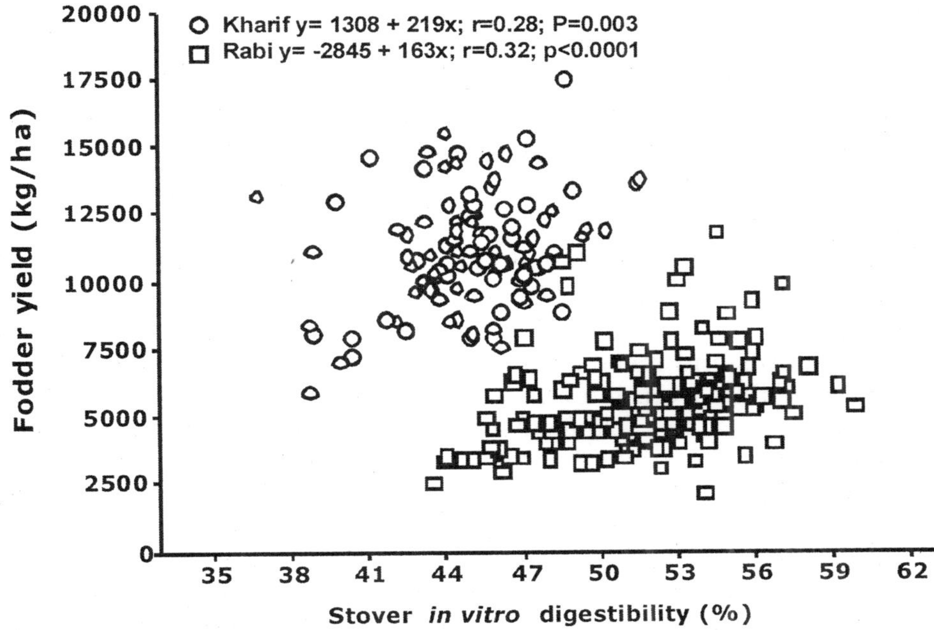

Fig. 4b : Relations between mean stover *in vitro* digestibility and stover yield in Kharif and Rabi sorghum cultivars submitted to NRCS 2002 to 2007.

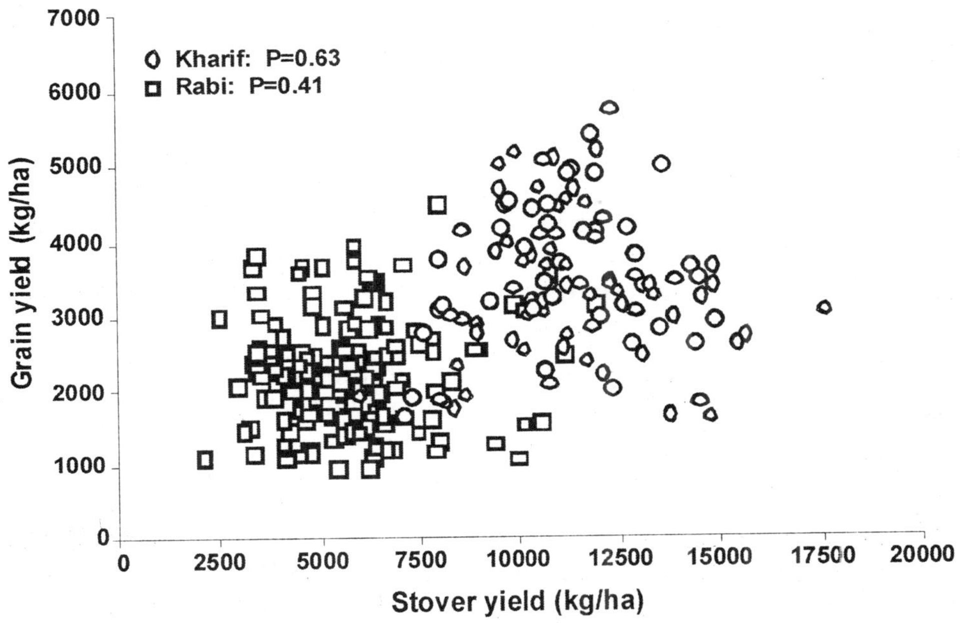

Fig. 4c : Relations between mean stover yield and grain yield in Kharif and Rabi sorghum cultivars submitted to NRCS 2002 to 2007.

Similar observations have been made for fine cereal CR (Table 1). Among most rice cultivar types variations for example in *in vitro* digestibility varied close to 10% with a minimum of 6.9% observed in New Planting Types (NPT). Interestingly, rice hybrids with on average the highest grain yields had also the highest mean straw *in vitro* digestibility (Table 1). As observed for sorghum, variations in rice straw digestibility came with little or no penalty to grain yields (Blümmel *et al.,* 2007).

Variations in CR fodder quality of importance to livestock nutrition were also observed in leguminous crops. Table 2 shows the example of groundnut. Haulm nitrogen content varied by almost twofold, *in vitro* digestibility varied by almost 10% units and metabolisable energy content varied by 3 MJ/kg. When feeding haulms from ten released groundnut cultivars *ad libitum* to growing male sheep as the sole feed sheep weight gains ranged from 63 to 151 grams per day. These were short term experiments and weight gain measurements might have been compounded by gut fill. However, nitrogen balances in the same experiments ranged from 6.6 to 11.4 g/day: almost a twofold difference between the low and high quality haulms. These nitrogen balances generally support the observed weight gains when allowing for some nitrogen sink (i.e. loss) into wool as is probable with the Deccani breed used in these experiments.

Crop productivity in smallholder crop–livestock systems is generally low relative to the genetic potential of the crops. In most national crop improvement programs new cultivars fulfill the releasing criteria if they outperform grain/ pod yields check cultivars by 10%. A mere 10% increase in grain/pod productivity may offer too little incentive for such cultivars to be widely promoted, multiplied and lastly to be adopted. As recently shown with a dual-purpose groundnut cultivar in India, a concomitant increase of about 10% in each of pod yield, haulm yield and haulm fodder quality (as reflected in higher milk yield) provided sufficient incentives for fast and large scale adoption of the new cultivar (Pande *et al.,* 2006). Release criteria for new cultivars intended for crop-livestock systems should therefore be revised and augmented to include CR fodder traits.

All laboratory analysis in the above studies was obtained using Near Infrared Spectroscopy (NIRS) after calibration with laboratory traits validated by extensive animal experimentation. NIRS instruments was also found to be capable of predicting quite sophisticated nutritional traits such as rate of fermentation (Prasad *et al.,* 2006) and extensively used, this technology for quick and inexpensive phenotyping of large set of samples for fodder quality traits. Based on extensive consultation between ILRI, ICRISAT and ICAR (crop and animal scientists) we estimate that 2 to 3 NIRS hubs could support multidimensional crop improvement in all India to exploit variation in crop residue fodder traits in existing cultivars.

Table 1 : Means and ranges in grain yield and nitrogen content, metabolizable energy content and in vitro digestibility of straw in different cultivars types of rice grown at the International Rice Research Institute

Cultivars Type	Grain yield (t/ha)			Straw N content (%)			Straw ME – content (MJ/kg)			Straw *in vitro* digestibility (%)		
	Mean	Range	SEM	Mean	Range	SEM	Mean	Range	SEM	Mean	Range	SEM
Aromatics (59)	6.2	4.9 – 7.5	0.09	0.61	0.49 – 0.78	0.009	5.56	4.41 - 6.17	0.04	41.4	34.8 – 45.2	0.03
Hybrids (53)	6.7	0.9 – 8.3	0.02	0.67	0.51 – 0.90	0.01	5.9	5.35 – 6.96	0.04	43.5	40.2 – 49.8	0.2
Indica (172)	6.7	4.5 – 8.1	0.05	0.60	0.47 – 0.75	0.005	5.6	4.72 – 6.27	0.02	41.3	36.6 – 45.8	0.11
NPT (92)	6.4	5.2 – 7.8	0.05	0.59	0.41 - 0.75	0.008	5.59	5.14 – 6.23	0.02	41.4	38.6 – 45.5	0.2
Varieties (61)	4.8	2.0 – 8.4	0.1	0.56	0.34 – 0.82	0.01	5.8	5.07 – 7.03	0.04	42.5	37.9 – 49.9	0.23

Table 2 : Means and ranges of nitrogen content, in vitro digestibility (OMD) and metabolizable energy (ME) content and their least significant difference (LSD) and probability values (P) for haulms of 860 groundnut genotypes

Haulm trait	Mean	Range	LSD	P	Correlation haulm trait (x) versus pod yields (y)
Nitrogen (%)	1.7	1.2 to 2.3	0.16	< 0.0001	y = 1427 + 1303x; r = 0.28; P < 0.0001
In vitro OMD (%)	56.3	51.7 to 61.1	1.9	< 0.0001	y = 2163 + 25.7x; r = 0.05; P = 0.13
In vitro ME (MJ/kg)	7.9	6.9 to 8.9	0.4	< 0.0001	y = 734 + 365x; r = 0.13; P < 0.0001

Table 3 : Response of dairy buffalo, sheep and bulls to densified total mixed ration (DTMR) feed blocks based on sorghum stover of different qualities

DTMR Feed Block	Animal	Intake	Production
DTMR Block Ex: Raichur (best stover Fig.3)	Dairy buffalo	3.6% of LW	8 liters of milk / day
DTMR Block Ex: Telangana (poorest stover Fig 3)	Dairy buffalo	3.3% of LW	7 liter of milk / day
DTMR Block Gold (commercial product)	Sheep	3.7% of LW	103 gram / day
DTMR Block Ex: Sweet Sorghum Stover	Sheep	3.4% of LW	113 gram / day
DTMR Block Ex: Telangana (poorest stover Fig 3)	Sheep	3.3% of LW	61 gram / day
DTMR Block Gold (commerci al product)	Bulls	2.5% of LW	742 gram / day
DTMR Block Ex: Sweet Sorghum Stover	Bulls	2.7% of LW	879 gram / day

Targeted Genetic Enhancement Towards Dual Purpose Traits

Till recently less effort was devoted to genetic enhancement of nutritive value towards food-feed cultivars than to directly exploiting existing variations in such traits as characterized by the work reflected (Fig. 4a-c, Table 1 and 2). We present here some recent proof-of-concept work assessing the gains in food-feed traits made by targeted genetic enhancement in pearl millet through recurrent selections and marker assisted breeding in pearl millet with the aim of producing a superior dual purpose variety. Within two recurrent selection cycles digestible organic matter intake measured in sheep increased from 12.9 to 15.1 g / kg live weight, an increase of 17%, and with the nitrogen balance changing from negative (-0.016 g/kg LW/d) to positive (0.05 g/kg LW/d). The improvement in stover fodder quality did not come at any penalty for grain or stover yield. Nepolean *et al.* (2009) used Quantitative Trait Locus (QTL) mapping to provide a better understanding of the genomic regions controlling stover quality and yield traits in pearl millet. Marker-assisted breeding would be an effective tool to exploit these genomic regions and to choose breeding lines having combinations of better stover quality and high grain yield without linkage drag between these traits. QTLs for stover *in vitro* organic matter digestibility (IVOMD) and metabolisable energy (ME) content were identified and introgressed into four parental lines of existing hybrids having good agronomic performance. Three generations of marker-assisted backcrossing and subsequent selfing of backcrossed progenies having target QTLs was carried out with the help of QTL-flanking microsatellite markers (SSRs). Single QTL introgression lines that were homozygous for target regions were identified. Improved hybrids were synthesized from these QTL homozygous lines and were evaluated in multi-location field trials. Results from the laboratory analysis of whole plant straw samples showed that one of the improved hybrids is at least 8.5% higher in ME and 6.3% higher in IVOMD compared to the control hybrid. The new hybrid also produced a 10% increase in grain yield and 4% increase in stover yield. These results suggest that new hybrids can be developed concomitantly improving grain and stover traits (Nepolean *et al.*, 2009).

Supplementation and Feed Processing for Optimizing Crop Residue Based Diets

As shown by Vogel and Sleper (1994), comparatively small differences of 3 to 5% units in forage digestibility can be important and were associated with 17 to 24% differences in animal performance. Similarly, Kristjanson and Zerbini (1999) calculated that a one-percentage unit increase in digestibility in sorghum and pearl millet stover would result in increases in milk, meat and draught power outputs ranging from 6 to 8%. These estimates appear very high, but they are broadly supported by the observed differences in prices of traded sorghum stover where a difference in digestibility of 5% was associated with price premiums of 30% and higher (Blümmel and Rao, 2006). As outlined in the present chapter, fodder quality differences in CR of this magnitude and more are available in a range of key crops (Fig. 4a-c; Table 1 and 2), generally without detriment to grain and pod yields. However, while improved (quantity and quality) CR will contribute to and support higher livestock productivity without overtaxing natural resource use. There is a limit to the level of production that can be achieved from feeding of CR alone.

Further increases in livestock productivity will only come through strategic supplementation. Principles of supplementation of crop residues are mostly well documented and understood (Van Soest, 1994). Still new, or perhaps less appreciated perspectives keep appearing, for example the potential of bypass protein even for lower producing livestock (Garg *et al.*, 2005; Krishna Mohan and Ramana Reddy, 2009). Also modern feed producers are aware that supplementation and feed processing and manufacturing are complementary; in addition to balancing nutrients by supplementation, physical processing of feeds like chopping, grinding, pelleting etc. increase intake (Naidu and Ramana Reddy, 2003). The final product has added value in the form of increased transportability, – important where some significant feed surplus areas exist as in India NIANP (2003) – storage ability and finally livestock productivity (Shah, 2007). Of the major physical forms, feed blocks, mash and pellets have attracted considerable attention from researchers (Sihag *et al.*, 1991; Singh *et al.*, 1998; Samanta *et al.*, 2003) and private industry (Shah, 2007). Miracle Fodder and Feeds PVT. LTD (Shah, 2007) designed so-called densified total mixed ration (DTMR) feed blocks that consist largely of by-products such as sorghum stover (about 50%), bran, oilcakes, husks (about 36%) with the rest contributed by molasses (8%), maize grain, urea, minerals, vitamins etc. Miracle Fodder and Feeds PVT. LTD offers DTMR feed blocks of three different qualities designed to produce daily (in dairy buffaloes) 11-16 liters (DTMR Diamond with 14.5 to 15% crude protein, 3.5% fat and 64-65% TDN), 7-11 liters (DTMR Gold with 13.0 to 13.5% crude protein, 3.0% fat and 62% TDN) and 5-7 liters (DTMR Silver with 11.5 to 12.0% crude protein, 2.5% fat and 60% TDN).

In a series of experiments with Miracle Fodder and Feeds PVT. LTD we tested these feed blocks with two objectives. First, to estimate probable maximum productivity levels on CR based diets. Second, to estimate the importance of the quality of the basic CR going into the blocks on overall livestock performance. In an experiment with a large private dairy two experimental feed blocks based on DTMR Diamond were produced from lower and premium quality sorghum varieties, Telangana and Raichur, respectively (Fig. 2). Daily milk yield on Raichur-based blocks was about 1 litre more than in the group that received Telangana based feed blocks. At the start of this trial the buffaloes were beyond peak lactation time (> 100 days into lactation) and their ME intakes relative to their ME requirements (ICAR, 1998) ended upto 151 and 130% in Raichur and Telangana groups, respectively. This ME intake above requirement (maintenance and actual level of milk production) would be sufficient for an additional milk yield of 8.7 and 4.8 litres daily the in Raichur and Telangana groups, respectively. The daily advantage in milk yield from premium stover based blocks would therefore be close to 5 litres. The overall potential production level would be 16.7 and 11.4 litres of milk daily, which agrees very well with the production level ascribed to DTMR Diamond. Similarly, live weight gains in sheep and buffalo responded significantly to improved sorghum stover quality in the feed blocks (Table 3).

Nutritionally significant cultivars are generally dependent on variations in crop residues and fodder quantity and quality exists in a range of important crops for the semi-arid tropics. Where crop improvement and livestock scientist collaborate closely these variations can be utilized for the benefit of farmers, livestock and natural resource management with little or no detriments to grain and pod yields. Improved crop residues strategically supplemented and properly physically processed can support very respectable levels of milk and meat production from almost completely by-product-based rations.

References

Ayantunde, A.A., Fernandez-Rivera, S. and McCrabb, G. (2005) (eds). Coping with feed scarcity in smallholder livestock systems in developing countries. Animal Sciences Group, Wageningen UR, Wageningen, The Netherlands, University of Reading, Reading, UK, ETH (Swiss Federal Institute of Technology), Zurich, Switzerland, and ILRI (International Livestock Research Institute), Nairobi, Kenya. 306 pp.

Blümmel, M., Seetharama, N., Prasad, K.V.S.V, Ravi, D., Ramakrishna, Ch., Khan, A.A., Anandan, S., Hash, C.T., Belum Reddy, Nigam, S. and Vadez, V. (2009). Food feed crop research and multidimensional crop improvement in India. Proceedings of Animal Nutrition Association World Conference, p. 17-19.New Delhi, India.

Blümmel, M., Virk, P. and Xianglin, L. (2007). Proceedings of the International Symposium on Production and Utilization of Paddy Rice as Feed, October 9-12, 2007, Japan, China, Korea, p 17-21.

Blümmel, M. and Parthasarathy, Rao, P. (2006). *International Sorghum and Millet Newsletter* 47: 97-100.

Delgado, C., Rosegrant, M., Steinfeld, H., Ehui, S. and Courbois, C. (1999). Livestock to 2020. *IFPRI Food, Agriculture and the Environment Discussion Paper 28, Washington, D.C., 72 p.*

Dixon, J., Xiaoyun, Li., Msangi, S., Amede, T., Bossio, D., Ceballos, H., Ospina, B., Howeler, R., Belum, V.S., Reddy, Abaidoo, R., Timsina, J., Crissman, C., Mares, V., Quiroz, R., Leon-Velarde, C., Herrero H., Blümmel M., Holmann F., Peters, M., White, W. Qadir, M. and Szonyi, J. (2009). *An Assessment Commissioned by the CGIAR System-wide Livestock Program* (In press).

Garg, M.R., Sheasia, P.L., Bhanderi, B.M., Gulati, S.K. and Scott, T.W. (2005). Effect of feeding rumen protected protein on milk production in low yielding crossbred cows. *Anim. Nutr. Feed Technol.* 5:1-8.

ICAR, (1998). Nutrient requirements of livestock. Indian Council of Agricultural Research, New Delhi.

Kelley, T.G., Parthasarathy Rao, P., Weltzien, R. and Purohit, M.L. (1996). *Exptl. Agric.*, 32:161-172.

Krishna Mohan, D.V.G. and Ramana, Reddy, Y. (2009). In: proc. Animal Nutrition Association World conference held during February 14-17, 2009, New Delhi, India. pp. 45-48 (Vol. 1).

Kristjanson. P. (2009). *Animal Nutrition, Association World Conference, 14-17 February 2009, New Delhi, India.* pp. 37-40.

Kristjanson, P.M. and Zerbini, E. (1999). Genetic enhancement of Sorghum and millet residues fed to ruminants. ILRI Impact Assessment Series 3, ILRI Nairobi.

Lal, R. (2005). *Environ. Inter.* 31: 575-584.

Naidu, M.M. and Ramana Reddy, Y. (2003). Improving nutritive value of poor quality roughages and agro-industrial by products. Feed Processing Technology. Ed Reddy, G.V.N., Krishna, N., Prasad, V.L.K., Reddy, J and Reddy, Y.R. Acharaya N.G.Ranga Agricultural University, Hyderabad, A.P.

National Institute for Animal Nutrition and Physiology (NIANP). 2003. FeedBase, Bangalore, 560-30.

Nepolean, T., Blümmel, M. and Hash, C.T. (2009). Improving straw quality traits through QTL mapping and marker-assisted selection in pearl millet. In (Eds Pahuja S.K., Jhorar B.S., Gupta P.P. Sheoran, R.S., Joshi, U.N. and Jindal Y.). Emerging Trends in Forage Research and Livestock Production, p.12, Forage Symposium-229, CAZRI, RRS Jaisalmer.

Pande S., Srinivasa Rao and Parthasarathy Rao, P. (eds.) (2006). Proceedings of the workshop on Farmers' Participatory Management of Diseases for Higher Yield and Nutritive Value of Crop Residues of Groundnut, Deccan Plateau India, 3-4 January 2005, ICRISAT, ILRI, DFID, ANGRAU, CPP, LPP. pp. 168.

Peden, D., Tadesse, D. and Misra, A.K. (2007). *In : D Molden (Ed) Water for Food, Water for Life: A Comprehensive Assessment of Water Management in Agriculture.* London: Earthscan, and Colombo: International Water Management Institute. pp. 485-515.

Prasad K.V.S.V., Reddy Ch. Ramakrishna and Blümmel, M. (2006). *IV Biennial Conference: Globalization – Challenges to Animal Nutrition.* November 20 to 22nd, Kolkata, India.

Ramachandra, K.S., Taneja, R.P., Sampath, K.T., Angadi, U. B. and Anandan, S. (2007). *Published by National Institute of Animal Nutrition and Physiology, Bangalore.*

Reed, J.D., Capper, B.S. and Neate, P.J.H. (eds). (1988). Proceedings of a workshop held at ILCA, Addis Ababa, Ethiopia, 7-10th December . ILCA Addis Ababa.

Samanta, A.K., Singh, K.K., Das, M.M., Maity, S.B. and Kundu, S.S. (2003). *Small Rumin. Res.*, 48, pp. 95–102.

Shah, L. (2007). Delivering Nutrition. Power Point Presentation delivered at the CIGAR System Wide Livestock Program Meeting 17th September 2007 at ICRISAT, Patancheru.

Singh, K. and Schiere, J.B. (eds) (1993). Feeding of Ruminants on Fibrous Crop Residues. Indian Council of Agricultural Research. Krishi Bhavan, New Delhi, India.

Sihag, Z.S., Rathee, C.S. and Lohan, O.P. (1991). *Indian J. Anim. Sci.*, 61: 1218–1221.

Singh, J., Lohan, O.P. and Rathee, C.S. (1998). *Indian J. Anim. Sci.*, 68: 480–483.

Singh, O.P., Sharma, A., Singh, R. and Shah, T. (2004). Virtual Water Trade in Dairy Economy. *Economic and Political Weekly*, 39: 3492–97.

Steinfeld, H., Gerber, P., Wassenaar, T., Castel, V., Rosales, M. and De Haan, C. (2006). Livestock's Long Shadow: environmental issues and options. FAO, Rome, Italy.

Van Soest, P.J. (1994). The Nutritional Ecology of the Ruminant. 2nd ed. Ithaca, N. Y: Cornell University Press.

Vogel, K.P. and Sleper, D.A. (1994). Alteration of plants via genetics and plant breeding. Pages 891-921 *in* Forage quality Evaluation, and Utilization (George. J. and Fahey, C., eds.) American Society of Agronomy. Madison, WI.

□□□

Animal Nutrition, 2012
eds. Dr. (Mrs.) Usha R. Mehra et al., pp. 475-498
Satish Serial Publishing House e-mail : info@satishserial.com; website : www.satishserial.com

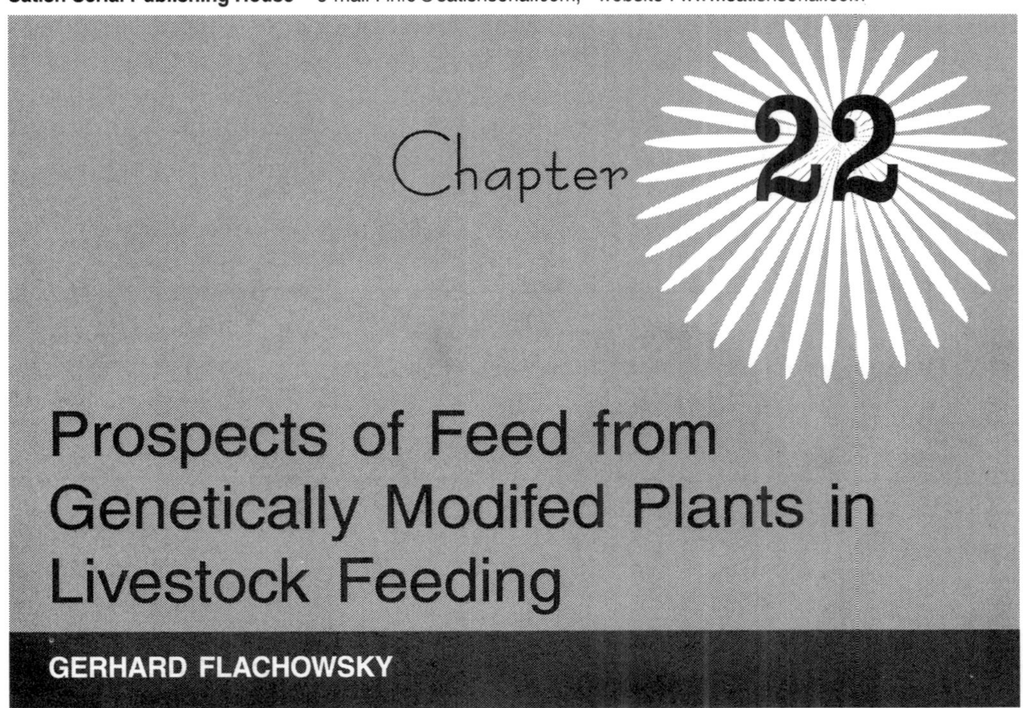

Prospects of Feed from Genetically Modifed Plants in Livestock Feeding

GERHARD FLACHOWSKY

In the future there will be a strong competition for arable land between feed/food, fuel, fibre areas for settlements and natural protected areas. According to the FAO statistics human population will increase from current about 6.5 to 9 billion people (about 40% more) on the earth in 2050 (Steinfeld *et al.*, 2006), but the estimated need for meat and milk will nearly double during this time (Table 1). The reason for such a development is a higher demand of food of animal origin with increased income in many countries (Keyzer *et al.*, 2005). The consumption of meat, fish, milk and eggs contributes to meet the human requirements in amino acids and many trace nutrients. Furthermore, foods of animal origin have a considerable enjoyment value and are considered as a parameter of living standard. The production of food of animal origin is consuming high amounts of resources (Flachowsky, 2002) and need much land for feed production but the arable land per person will decrease (Fig. 1).

Increasing feed/food demand requires very high natural resources and causes pollution of environment such as carbon dioxide (CO_2) from fossil fuel, methane (CH_4) from the anaerobic fermentation of carbohydrates or nitrogen-compounds (NH_3, N_2O) from the protein metabolism. Apart from the low input of limited resources a low output of greenhouse gases during feed/food production is a very important aim of sustainable agriculture (Flachowsky and Brade, 2007).

Table 1 : Challenges for animal production or "Livestock's long shadow" (Steinfeld *et al.*, 2006)

Year	Presently	2050	Percent increase
World population (Billion)	6.5	9.0	138
Meat production (MT)	229	465	203
Milk production (MT)	580	1043	180

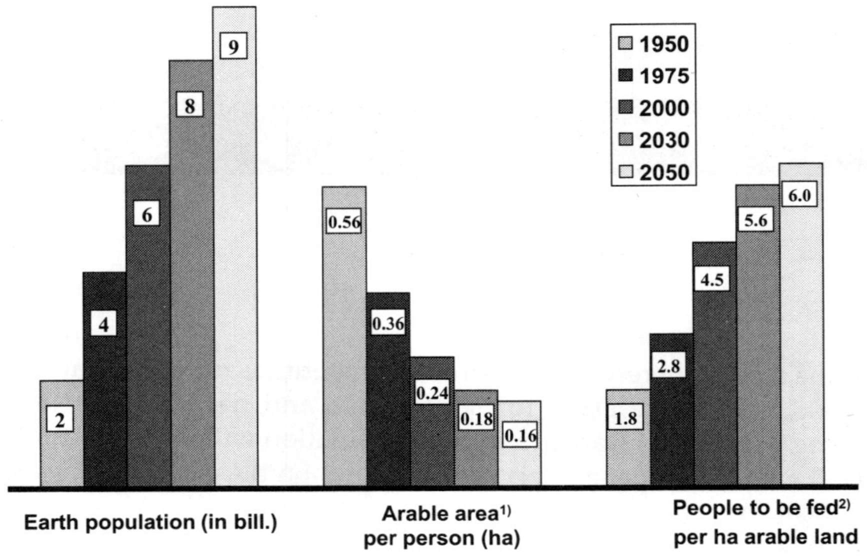

[1] » 1.5 bill. ha are available presently
[2] Number increases when area used to produce renewable resources increases

Fig. 1 : Development of the earth's population, the arable land area available and the number of people to be fed per hectare (FAO yearbooks)

In addition to the traditional competition of land use between production of vegetarian food for human consumption and feed production for animal production, land area is increasingly being used for bio-energy/fuel production in response to the challenge of global warming, as areas for settlements and as natural protected areas. Therefore, it is necessary to come from the shadows to the future (Miller, 2008). Possible strategies to overcome this situation include:

- Continued investments to increase plant yield and animal performances with traditional and innovative biotechnology.
- Improved efficiency of utilizing of limited resources (land, water, fertilizer, fuel etc.) and reduced pollution.
- Lower consumption of animal protein by people with current overconsumption.

Plant breeding and cultivation are the starting points for feed and food security during the next years. The perspectives mentioned above are real challenges for plant breeders all over the world. The most important objectives for plant breeders can be summarized as follows (Flachowsky, 2008).

- High yields with low external inputs (low input varieties) such as water, phosphorus, fuel, plant protection substances etc.
- Lower concentrations of toxic substances such as secondary substances, mycotoxins from toxin-developing fungi, toxins from anthropogenic activities or geogenic givens.
- Lower concentrations of substances that influence the use or bioavailability of nutrients such as lignin, phytate, enzyme inhibitors, tannin etc.
- Higher concentrations of the feed value determining components such as nutrient precursors, nutrients, enzymes, prebiotics, essential oils etc.

From the global view of feed and food security low input varieties have the highest priority. Furthermore, undesirable substances can not be removed from feedstuffs, or can only be removed with great effort. From the perspective of animal nutrition, this goal is of major significance for the improvement of feeds. An increase of essential nutrients (e.g. amino acids, vitamins, trace elements etc.) could be very favourable in some regions of the world, to meet the requirements of man and animal with trace nutrients, but it seems to be not so important, because of the availability of various feed additives in the market.

It is possible to fulfil the objectives mentioned above by conventional plant breeding. But in the future methods of biotechnology may be more flexible, more potent and faster. Presently, we are in the starting phase of this technology. Therefore, genetical engineering of plants seems to be a technology with a high potential to contribute to the solution of global problems. Of course, the technique needs further improvements and more public acceptance as presently. The current stage of nutritional assessment of feeds from Genetically Modified Plant (GMP) and future challenges will be analysed in the present contribution.

Current Status of Cultivation of GMP and Questions to Animal Nutritionists

The cultivation of GMP increased worldwide from about 1.7 (1996) to 114 million ha (James, 2007). Currently, soybeans (60), corn (24), cotton (11) and canola (5% of global GM area) are the most important GM-crops (Fig. 2).

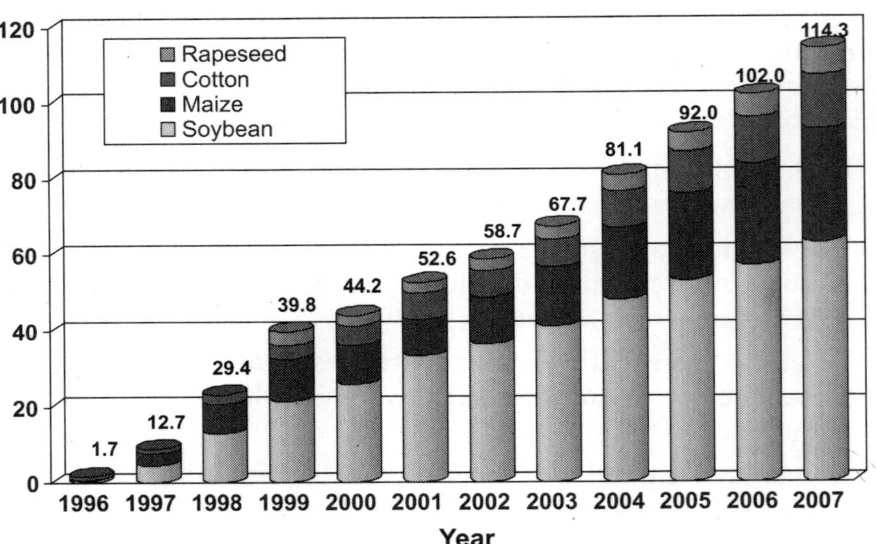

Fig. 2 : Global area of transgenic crops (GMP).

They are modified mainly for agronomic traits. Such plants are characterized by so-called input traits (GMP of the first generation) without substantial changes in composition or nutritive value. Animal nutritionists distinguish in GMP of the 1st and 2nd generation:

GMP of the 1st Generation

- Plants with agrotechnical traits (input traits)
- Without substantial changes in composition/nutritive value
- Substantial equivalent
- *Examples*:

  Bt-plants (corn, cotton), RR-plants (soybean), PAT-plants (corn, roots) etc.

GMP of the 2nd Generation

- Plants with output traits
- With substantial changes in composition/nutritive value
- Not substantial equivalent
- *Examples*:

  Golden rice, low phytate corn, changes in fatty acids or amino acids pattern etc.

GMP of the second generation (with output traits) should contain more nutrients (e.g. amino acids, fatty acids, vitamins, enzymes etc.) or less antinutritive substances (e.g. mycotoxins, inhibitors, allergens etc.). GMP of the 1st generation are considered as substantial equivalent to their isogenic counterparts. The definition of substantial equivalence (S.E.) some problems with the definition and future proposals are listed below:

The S.E. (OECD, 1993) embodies the concept that if a new food/feed is found to be substantially equivalent to an existing food/feed, it can be treated in the same manner with respect to safety as its traditional counterpart.

Problems

- Coarse frame work for evaluation; no safety and nutritional assessment
- What means traditional counterpart (isogenic plants or local average)?
- Irrational if changes in composition (e.g. lower content in mycotoxins or higher content of some nutrients, GMP of the 2nd generation).

Proposal

Various compartments should be considered as parts of S.E. as given below:

- Chemical/analytical equivalence.
- Nutritional equivalence.
- Safety equivalence.
- Exposure equivalence.

GMP can be used in a wide range to feed animals such as:

- Vegetative and generative plants or parts of plants (*e.g.* green forage, seeds, roots, tubers *etc.*).
- Conserved products from GMP (*e.g.* silage, hay).
- By-products of agriculture, fuel and food production, obtained from the processing of GMP e.g. straw, by products of milling, of the starch, oil, sugar and brewing industries or from production of bioenergy, such as dried distillers grain solubles, (DDGS).

Based on the present situation animal nutritionists are asked the following questions:

- Nutritional and safety assessment of feed and food of the 1st generation of GMP.
- Nutritional and safety assessment of feed and food of the 2nd generation of GMP.
- Influence of GM-feed on animal health and quality of food of animal origin.
- Studies on the degradation of novel protein, foreign DNA, unintended effects *etc.*

Studies with Feeds from GMP with Food Producing Animals

Feeds from GMP with Input Traits (1st generation)

Most of the area under GMP is cultivated with plants of the first generation. Numerous scientific associations and expert panels proposed guidelines for the nutritional and safety assessment of feeds from the first generation (EFSA, 2004). Based on the recommendations, nutritional studies with first generation GMP feeds have been undertaken worldwide. Since 1997, 16 studies were performed at the Institute of Animal Nutrition in Braunschweig to determine the effect of first generation GMP feeds on the nutrition of dairy cows, growing bulls, growing and finishing pigs, laying hens, chickens for finishing, as well as with growing and laying characteristics of quails. This research was recently summarized by Flachowsky *et al.*, (2007). The majority of feeds tested in the studies (Bt-maize, Pat-maize, Pat sugar beet) were grown under similar conditions to their isogenic counterparts in the experimental fields at the Institute. The composition of feeds was analysed, and animal studies were used to assess nutritional qualities, including parameters such as digestibility, feed intake, health and performance of target animal species, and effects on food quality derived from the animals. Reproduction was also considered in generation studies with quails (Fig. 3) and laying hens (4 generations).

Both chemical analyses and the animal studies reveal no significant differences between GMP feeds and their isogenic counterparts and hence strongly support their substantial equivalence. Our results agree with more than 100 studies published in the literature and reviewed recently (Flachowsky *et al.*, 2005a, 2007; Table 2).

Most experimental designs of previous studies were very simple. The authors compared only one feed (transgenic origin) with another one (isogenic counterpart) and neglected the normal biological range as impressively described in the OECD-consensus documents (OECD, 2001, 2002, 2003, 2004, 2005) or other feed value tables. Recent studies (Lucas *et al.*, 2007, McNaughton *et al.*, 2007) included three or more commercial isogenic plants to assess biological range of results. Such experimental designs are also recommended by ILSI (2007) and EFSA (2008) recently.

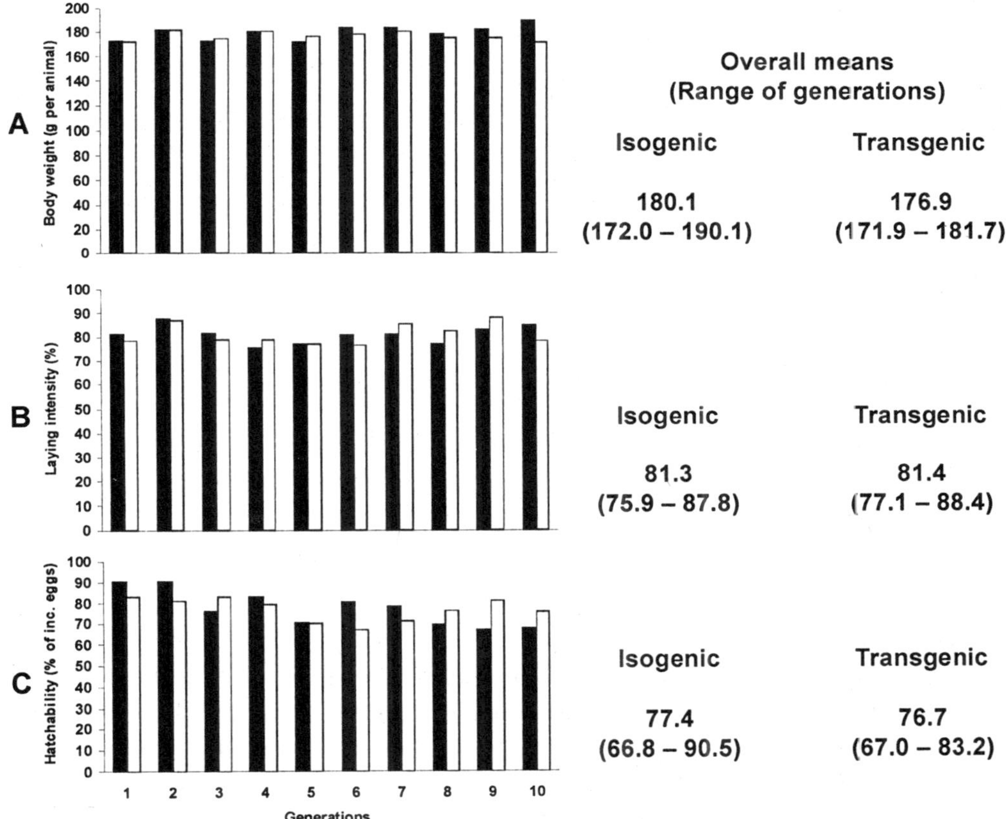

Fig. 3 : (A) Body weight of female quails (age: 6 weeks), (B) laying intensity and (C) hatchability of quails fed with isogenic and transgenic corn in a 10 generations experiment (Flachowsky *et al.*, 2005b).

Mycotoxin contamination of some GM crops is lower than that of non-GM which may be one exception to their substantial equivalence. For example, Bt maize is less severely attacked and weakened by the corn borer and might have a greater resistance to field infections, particularly *Fusarium* fungi, which produce mycotoxins. Evidence of reduced mycotoxin contaminated in GM crops has been demonstrated in some, but not all cases, as summarized by Flachowsky *et al.* (2005a).

Table 2 : Summary of published data to compare feeds from GM plants of the first generation (with input traits) with their isogenic counterparts.

Animal (Species/categories)	Number of experiments	Nutritional assessment
Ruminants		No unintended effects in composition (except lower mycotoxins concentration in Bt plants)
Dairy cows	23	
Beef cattle	14	
Others	10	
Pigs	21	No significant differences in digestibility and animal health as well as no unintended effects on performances of animals and composition of food of animal origin
Poultry		
Laying hens	3	
Broilers	28	
Others		
(Fish, rabbits etc.)	8	

In long-term studies, numerous researchers, investigated the influence of levels of corn borer infestation of isogenic and Bt hybrids on mycotoxin contaminated. Most researchers concluded that a lower level of mycotoxin contamination was observed in the transgenic hybrids, despite the considerable geographical and temporal variation observed (Figure 4). The lower input of herbicides and insecticides in GMP of the first generation may have some environmental gains as recently summarized by Brookes and Barfoot (2008).

During the last few years some reviews on nutritive and safety assessment of feeds from GM-plants were published (Clark and Ipharraguerre *et al.*, 2001, Flachowsky and Aulrich, 2001, Aumaitre *et al.*, 2002, Flachowsky *et al.*, 2005a, 2007, CAST, 2007, Alexander *et al.*, 2007). Furthermore, the documents by ILSI (2004, 2007) and EFSA (2004, 2008) summarize also the present stage of knowledge in feeding of GM-plants mostly of the 1st generation to target animals.

Feeds from GMP with Output Traits (2nd Generation)

Second generation GMP are characterized by either an increased content of desirable traits, such as:

- Nutrient precursors (β-carotene etc.)
- Nutrients (amino acids, fatty acids, vitamins, minerals etc.)
- Substances which may improve nutrient digestibility (enzymes)
- Substances with surplus effects (prebiotics)

- Improvement of sensoric properties/palatability (essential oils, aromas) or a decreased content of undesirable substances such as:
- Inhibiting substances (lignin, phytate etc.)
- Toxic substances (alkaloids, glucosinolates, mycotoxins etc.).

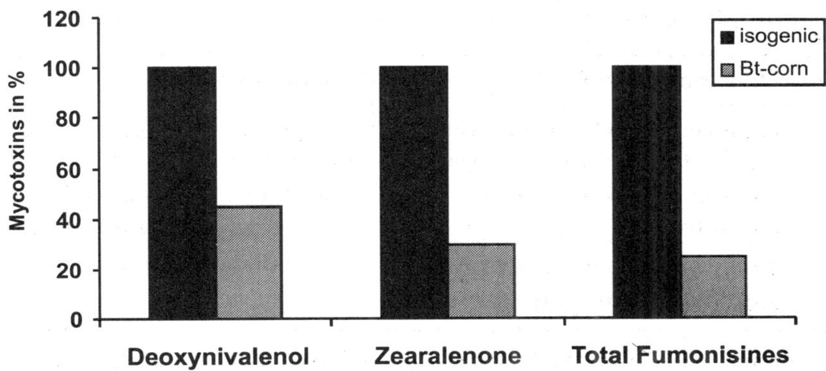

Fig. 4 : Mycotoxins in isogenic (100%) and Bt-corn (% of isogenic corn). Sources: Munkvold *et al.*, 1999; Cahagnier and Melcion 2000; Pietri and Piva, 2000; Valenta *et al.*, 2001; Bakan *et al.*, 2002, Reuter *et al.*, 2002a).

At present, test procedures are proposed to study the nutritive value of feeds from the second generation of GMP. Possible approaches for testing those feeds were reviewed by Flachowsky and Böhme (2005). Recommendations for nutritional and safety assessment of feeds from the second generation of GMP are developed by EFSA (2004, 2008) and ILSI (2007).

Tables 3 and 4 show examples to demonstrate the conversion of β-carotene as a vitamin A-precursor from maize into vitamin A. Howe and Tanumihardjo (2006) added to control maize poor in carotene b-carotene or vitamin A and compared the effects with carotene rich maize. Serum and liver were used as indicator organs (Table 4) to show the conversion of β-carotene into vitamin A. As well known, serum did not show any influence of β-carotene or vitamin A supply, but the liver showed significant effects. β-carotene from the maize was adequate to supplemented β-carotene, but less than half so active as supplemented vitamin A (Table 4).

Tables 5 and 6 show, a proposal to assess the lower phytate content in a GMP and results from a previous study. The authors compared control maize with a low phosphorus availability with a low phytate variety. The pigs fed with control maize needed a supplementation with inorganic P for adequate daily weight gain and strength of bones, but they excreted significantly more P. The results show that low phytate maize may contribute to a more efficient use of the limited resource phosphorus and may reduce the excretion of P. Further proposals for experimental designs to assess the nutritive value of GMP of the 2nd generation are given by EFSA (2008), Flachowsky and Böhme (2005) and ILSI (2007).

Table 3 : Proposal to assess the conversion of nutrient precursors from the second generation of GMP into nutrients (β-carotene)

Groups[3]	Diet composition	Measurements[2]
1[1]	Balanced diets including typical levels of isogenic counterpart + β-carotene (level/adequate to the transgenic crop)	Depends on the claim of genetic modification - Concentration of converted substances in target organs (vitamin A in liver)[2]
2[1]	Balanced diets with adequate amounts of transgenic crop	- Metabolic parameters

[1] equal feed for all animals, depletion of animals in preliminary period

[2] until a steady state is achieved in the target organs

[3] three or more groups with commercial isogenic plants to assess normal biological range (confidence interval) are recommended (ILSI 2007)

Table 4 : Experimental design to determine the conversion of β-carotene into vitamin A in maize (60 % of diet, Mongolian gerbils, n = 10, Depletion period: 4 weeks, Feeding: 8 weeks, Howe and Tanumihardjo, 2006).

	Unsupplemented control (Maize poor in carotene)	Carotene rich maize	Control + β-carotene supple mentation	Control + vitamin A supple mentation
β-Carotene/vitamin A (nmol/g)	0	8.8	8.8	4.4
Theoreticalretinolintake (nmol/d)	0	106	106	106
Retinol in serum mol/l)	1.23 ± 0.20	1.25 ± 0.22	1.23 ± 0.20	1.22 ± 0.16
Retinol in liver mol/g)	0.10[a] ± 0.04	0.25[b] ± 0.15	0.25[b] ± 0.08	0.56[c] ± 0.15

($p < 0.05$)

[a, b, c] Means with different letters differ.

Table 5 : Proposal to assess the effects of inhibitors of nutrient bioavailability (phytate)

Groups[1]	Diet composition	Measurements
1	Balanced diet including typical levels of isogenic counterpart, *ad lib.* feeding	Depends on the claim of genetic modification
2	Diets of Group 1 plus inhibited nutrient (P), *ad lib.* feeding	- Digestibility of inhibited nutrient
3	Balanced diet including transgenic counterpart in adequate levels to Group 1 (low phytatecrop)	- Growing experiment with target animals
4	Diets of Group 3 plus inhibited nutrient of Group 2	- Concentration of inhibited nutrient in indicator organs

Table 6 : Conventional and low-phytate maize (78.5% of the mixture) in the feed of fattening pigs (Spencer *et al.*, 2000).

	Control (0.3 g of available P per kg)		Low-phytate maize (1.7 g of available P per g)	
Inorganic P supplement	-	+	-	+
P content (g/kg)				
29 - 73 kg live weight	3.4	5.4 [1)]	3.4	5.4 [1)]
73 - 112 kg live weight	3.2	4.7 [2)]	3.2	4.7 [2)]
Feed intake (kg/d)	2.23 [a]	2.50 [b]	2.53 [b]	2.51 [b]
Live weight gain (g/d)	730 [a]	870 [b]	900 [b]	880 [b]
Feed per kg gain (kg)	3.05 [a]	2.87 [b]	2.81 [b]	2.85 [b]
P excreted (g/kg)	4.6 [a]	8.9 [c]	3.8 [b]	8.8 [c]
Strength (4th metacarpal bone, kg)	79.4 [a]	138.5 [bc]	132.2 [b]	153.9 [d]
Ash content (% in 4th metacarpal bone)	53.5 [a]	60.1 [bc]	59.3 [b]	61.2 [c]

a, b, c, d Different letters in one line indicate significant differences ($p < 0.05$)
[1)] +2.0 g P/kg [2)] +1.5 g P/kg

The Fate of Transgenic DNA and Transgenic Novel Protein in Food Producing Animals

The public is interested in the capability for transgenes or their products to be incorporated into animal tissues or products such as eggs and milk, concerning the fate of recombinant protein and DNA within the gastrointestinal tract of livestock. Therefore, many studies were done to contribute to answers to this question. The consumption of feeds from GMP resulted in the intake of transgenic DNA and proteins; therefore, studies were conducted on their fate during processing, within the gastrointestinal tract of animals, and the potential to which extent transgenes or their products may be incorporated into animal tissues (Flachowsky *et al.*, 2005a). Studies in this field were reviewed by Alexander *et al.* (2007) and Einspanier and Flachowsky (2008) recently.

The Fate of Transgenic DNA

The consumption of feeds from GMP resulted in the intake of DNA and proteins including transgenic DNA and proteins; therefore, studies were conducted on their fate during processing, within the gastrointestinal tract of animals, and the potential to which extent transgene or their products may be incorporated into animal tissues.

The amount of transgenic DNA ingested in the animal depends on the concentration of transgene in feed as well as feed intake. The quantity of DNA in most crops is less than 0.2 g/kg DM (Beever and Kemp, 2000), the transgene concentration is much lower (Beever and Phipps 2001, Van den Eede *et al.*, 2002). The actual total transgenic DNA intake may actually be lower, considering that ensiling GM plants quickly leads to degradation of large plant DNA fragments (Hupfer *et al.*, 1999, Aulrich *et al.*, 2004, Table 7).

Table 7 : Determined DNA-fragments in transgenic Corn Cob Mix (CCM) and Whole Plant Silage (WPS) as influenced by the ensiling period.

Duration of ensiling (days	Fragment 1016 bp		Fragment 680 bp		Fragment 194 bp	
	CCM	WPS	CCM	WPS	CCM	WPS
0	+	+	+	+	+	+
2	+	+	+	+	+	+
5	+	+	+	+	+	+
7	-	+	+	+	+	+
14	-	+	+	+	+	+
21	-	+	+	+	+	+
28	-	+	-	+	+	+
35	-	-	-	+	+	+
70	-	-	-	-	+	+
100	-	-	-	-	+	+
200	-	-	-	-	+	+

Longer DNA-fragments (> 1000bp) were already degraded after 28 days of ensiling (Table 7). While grinding has no and or heat application has little effect on DNA fragment size, it has been shown that processed feed samples may contain only short DNA fragments (Table 8).

Table 8 : Processing of rapeseed for oil production and determined DNA-fragments in final products of isogenic (i) and transgenic (t) rapeseed (Berger *et al.*, 2003)

Treatment		1	2	3	4
Processing		Crushing	Crushing	Crushing	Crushing
		-	-	Conditioning (96°C, 20 min)	Conditioning (103-111°C, 30 min)
		Pressing (69°C)	Pressing (95°C)	Pressing (95°C)	Pressing (95°C)
		-	Extraction	Extraction	Extraction
		-	Desolventizing Toasting (105°C)	Desolventizing Toasting (105°C)	Desolventizing Toasting (105°C)
Rape-final products					
Determined DNA-fragments (bp)					
21000 bp (intact DNA)	i	+	-	-	-
	t	+	-	-	-
248 bp	i	+	+	+	-
970 bp	i	+	-	-	-
194 bp	t	+	+	-	+
680 bp	t	+	-	-	-
1003 bp	t	+	-	-	-

There exist many studies in ruminants, pigs and poultry (more than 30 are published) where the authors analysed the fate of DNA in the digestive tract and in the animal body as summarized by Alexander *et al.* (2007) recently. Some of our studies were done over the whole growing/fattening period resp. the whole live spans (Table 9; Einspanier *et al.*, 2001, Reuter and Aulrich, 2003). Most authors did not detect fragments at tDNA in animal tissues (Alexander, *et al.*, 2007, Flachowsky *et al.*, 2005a). Also two transgenes (herbicide tolerance : mepsps and insect resistance : Cry 1Ab) in corn silage did not show tDNA in milk of cows (Calsamiglia *et al.*, 2007). But there are few studies where tDNA fragments in tissues were detected. Sharma *et al.* (2006) fed up to 15% Roundup Ready canola to lambs (n = 11) and pigs (n = 36) to slaughter. Some tDNA-fragments were detected in the intestine content samples and in the gastrointestinal tract tissues, but not in visceral tissues (liver, kidney) of lambs or in the spleen from pigs. However, one liver and one kidney sample from the pigs (different animals) were positive for a 278-bp fragment of the transgenic cp 4 epsps. Mazza *et al.* (2005) fed over 35 days eight piglets each with diets containing 50% isogenic or transgenic

(MON 810) maize. Blood, spleen, liver, kidney and muscle tissues from all animals were investigated for the presence of plant DNA. Fragments of specific maize genes (Zein, Sh-2) could be detected with different frequencies in all the examined tissues except muscle. A small fragment of the Cry 1A(b) transgene (519 bp) was detected in blood (30%), spleen (10%), liver (14%) and kidney (9% of investigated samples; Mazza *et al.*, 2005). The intact Cry 1A(b) gene (3500 bp) or its minimal functional unit (1800 bp) were never detected. All the authors (Alexander *et al.*, 2007, Mazza *et al.*, 2005, Sharma *et al.*, 2006) agree that recombinant DNA would be processed in the gut in the same manner as from endogenous feed ingested genetic material. The results indicate that the transfer of DNA-fragments may occur independently from the source and the type of the gene. The authors conclude that it would be unlikely that the occurrence of genetic transfer associated with GMP is higher than from conventional plants.

Table 9 : Studies from the Institute of Animal Nutrition on transfer of DNA fragments in food producing animals

DNA source	Animal species	Detection of transgenic DNA	Results Detection of "foreign" nontransgenic DNA	References
Bt-maize-grain and silage	Broilers Layers Growing bulls Dairy cows	No transgenic DNA in animal tissues	Plant DNA fragments in muscle, liver, spleen, kidneys of broilers and layers, not in blood, muscle, liver, spleen, kidneys of growing bulls, in eggs and feces of broilers and layers and in feces of dairy cows	Einspanier et al. (2001)
Bt-maize-grain	Pigs	Transgenic DNA fragments up to 48 hrs up to the rectum, not in blood, organs and tissues	Plant DNA fragments in the gastrointestinal tract, in blood, organs and tissues	Reuter and Aulrich (2003)
Bt-maize-grain	Broilers	Transgenic DNA in the gastrointestinal tract, no transgenic DNA in blood, organs and tissues	Plant DNA fragments in the gastrointestinal tract, in blood, organs and tissues	Tony et al. (2003)
Bt-maize-grain	Quails (10 generations)	Transgenic DNA fragments (211 bp) in the stomach and whole gastrointestinal tract, no transgenic DNA fragments in muscle, liver, stomach, spleen, kidney, heart and eggs	Plant DNA fragments in the gastrointestinal tract	Flachowsky et al. (2005b)
Bt-potato	Broilers	No transgenic DNA in muscle, liver, kidney and spleen	Plant DNA fragments in muscle, liver, kidney and spleen till 8 h after feeding	El Sanhoty (2004)
Gt-soybeans	Pigs	No transgenic DNA in muscle, liver, kidney and spleen	Plant DNA fragments in the gastrointestinal tract	Aulrich et al. (2002)
Inulin-potato-silage	Pigs	Transgenic DNA fragment (104 bp) in the stomach, no transgenic DNA fragments in animal tissues	Plant DNA fragments in the gastrointestinal tract, no plant DNA fragments in animal tissues	Broll et al. (2005)

The presence of antibiotic resistance marker genes e.g. against beta-lactam antibiotics in the first generation of GM crops raised concerns that these genes may be transferred to pathogenic bacteria making them resistant to specific antibiotics. This reasonable concern was acknowledged avoiding antibiotic resistance genes in the second generation of GM plants. The probability of transformation of intestinal microorganisms with feed derived from transgenic crops appears very low but still generates concern about health and safety of such constructs.

However, a recently published report (Demaneche *et al.*, 2008) clearly documents that a horizontal gene transfer of antibiotic-resistance genes present in some GM crops (Bt 176) is highly improbable.

Results on the fate of DNA can be summarized as follows:

- DNA is a permanent part of food/feed (daily intake: human: 0.1-1 g; pig: 0.5-4 g; cow: 40-60 g)
- DNA is mostly degraded during conservation (silage making) and industrial processing as well as in the digestive tract (pH, enzymes)
- Small fragments of DNA may pass through the mucosa and may be detected in some body tissues (especially leucocytes, liver, and spleen)
- Fragments of high-copy number genes from plants have been detected in animal tissues to a higher extent than from low-copy numbers
- Intact tDNA genes or their minimal functional units were never detected in animal tissues
- No data exists showing that tDNA is characterized by unique behaviour compared to native plant-DNA during feed treatment and in the animals
- From the present stage of knowledge, the fate of tDNA in the currently registered GM-plants need not to be included in feed safety assessment.

The Fate of Novel Proteins

Guidelines have been established by several organizations regarding assessment of the allergenic risk of each novel protein expressed in a GM plant, prior to market approval (FAO/WHO, 2000; Martens, 2000; Konig *et al.*,, 2004). These typically include comparison of amino acid sequence homology of the novel protein to known allergens and digestion of the protein in simulated gastric environments. While allergic reactions are primarily a concern for human consumption of GM foods, certain proteins in soybean have been shown to elicit allergenic reactions in calves and piglets (Van Dijk *et al.*,, 1988). It is common practice to apply heat to some feedstuffs to inhibit the actions of anti-nutritional proteins. Such is the rationale for toasting soybean, which contains trypsin inhibitors and haemagglutinins.

The fate of novel (transgenic) proteins in feed from GMP consumed by animals has also generated interest arising from consumers questions. Recently, an extensive review on the food safety of proteins from agricultural biotechnology was edited by Hammond (2008). Seale and English (2008) analysed the mode of action of bacterial protein toxins and concluded, that an interruption of the life cycle at any single step can render the protein nontoxic. For example, insecticidial toxins from Bacillus thuringiensis (Bt) have been shown to be rapidly degraded by simulated gastric fluid in *in vitro* studies (Astwood *et al.*, 1996). Transgenic proteins in feeds from Bt-plants are similar degraded as bacterial proteins (Federici and Siegel, 2008). This is in contrast to the stability of Bt toxins in insect guts where proteolytic activation of the protein occurs, leading to toxicity to insect cells.

Betz *et al.* (2000) tested the acute and subcronic oral toxicity of Bt-proteins. The "no-observed-adverse-effect-levels" (NOAELs) were in all cases the highest dosages that were tested (4000 mg Cry 1Ab-Protein per kg).

Hammond and Cockburn (2008) summarized the NOAELs in Acute High-Dose-Studies and in Subcronic Feeding Studies with different proteins introduced into crops developed through agricultural biotechnology. These studies confirm the absence of oral toxicity even the protein preparations were administered at very high dosage levels. The amount of transgenic protein ingested by livestock depends on the concentration of the protein in the feed and the amount of feed intake. Transgenic protein concentration varies with the transgenic event and the type of plant tissue in which it is expressed. The levels of introduced proteins in seeds of biotechnology, derived crops vary between 0.3 (Cry 1Ab in corn; Yieldgard Corn borer) and up to 580 mg/kg seed (cp 4 epsps in cotton; Roundup Ready Flex; Hammond and Cockburn, 2008).

Post-harvest feed processing can alter (likely decrease) transgenic protein concentrations (Alexander *et al.*, 2007). Anything affecting the concentration of transgenic protein in feedstuffs will also alter the total transgenic protein intake by livestock. Similarly, feed intake, which varies with animal and diet, will influence protein intake. Assuming intake of 10 kg of MON 810 grain per day, total daily Cry 1Ab intake by a dairy cow will be approximately 3.1 mg (10,000 g x 0.31 μg/g fwt = 3100 μg or 3.1 mg, Alexander *et al.*, 2007). Feed and protein digestion are also species-dependent. Thus, the presence of transgenic protein throughout animal digestive tracts and potentially in livestock products depends on multiple factors.

Alexander *et al.* (2007) summarized various studies where the authors analysed the fate of novel proteins in ruminants, pigs and poultry. Results from the studies can be summarized as follows:

- In ruminant feed, proteins are mostly degraded in the rumen, and microbial protein and bypass proteins are degraded by enzymes in the smaller intestine, similar to non-ruminants.
- The chemical and physiological properties (including microbial and enzymatic degradation) of novel proteins have been intensively tested.
- Intact novel proteins have not been detected outside of the digestive tract in target animals (also not in animal tissues and products).
- There is no evidence that novel proteins are characterized by unusual chemical/physical properties distinct from native protein.

Research Need

International studies have shown that in view of

(1) the increasing competition for agricultural area due to a higher demand for food/feed, for fuel, or raw material for industry, for settlements or for natural protection and in view of

(2) the increasing population with a higher income, the need for food from animal origin is increasing fast (Table 1).

Provision of enough animal feed is considered as a major challenge. Therefore, plant breeders invest in more efficient plants with higher yields and with lower inputs of limited resources (water, fossil fuel, phosphorus etc.). Also plants which are more resistant to biotic and abiotic stressors (heat, cold, drought) are considered of importance to increase high dry matter or energy yields of plants per area. Also for these new types of GM plants, basic research could provide insight into the possible unintended changes caused by these modifications as well as in the extend of background variability. Most of the biomass is used in animal nutrition. Therefore, plant breeders should consider the wishes of animal nutritionists and they should more collaborate in early stages of plant breeding (Flachowsky, 2008). Animal nutritionists developed various types of studies for nutritional and safety assessment of GM-products as shown in Table 10 and 11 shows some recommendations for feeding experiments to demonstrate the efficiency (and safety) of genetic modification.

Presently, most of the GMP don't meet the requirements mentioned above (Table 12). The more efficient use of limited resources should be one of the main aims of plant breeding to develop more low input varieties.

It can be expected that future GM plant generations will contain more complex traits, such as altered nutritional profiles and that a wider range of organisms will be used to introduce new traits via gene technology processes. Another possible scenario could be the production of multiple stacked (GM) varieties obtained by conventional breeding, carrying several GM traits within the same genome, and potentially having relevant nutritional implications. The new GM events or variety traits with specific nutritional and/or health claims would need additional basis and fundamental research to be conducted also by independent publicly funded research institutions/universities. Such basic research could provide insight into the possible unintended changes caused by these modifications as well as in the extend of background variability. Normally more side effects could be expected in GMP with more modifications as demonstrated by Cellini *et al.* (2004). In such cases studies according to the decision tree (Fig. 5) are recommended for the nutritional and safety assessment of GMP with target animals. The proposal can be modified in dependence on the questions asked (e.g. reproduction). It should be used on the base of case by case decisions. Presently the nutritional and safety evaluation of GM versus conventionally bred plants is not well balanced (Kok *et al.*, 2007). Therefore, it seems necessary to always adjust the screening frames on the basis of novel scientific criteria considering consumer and animal safety of different plant varieties liberated on the market.

Table 10 : Objectives of various types of studies with food producing animals (target species)

Type of study	Recommended to type of genetic modification	Objective/Measurements/ Endpoints
In vitro studies (outside of animals)	All types of genetic modifications	Properties of changed nutrients, in vitro digestibility/degradability of tDNA and novel proteins
Metabolism studies	Changes in concentration of valuable (e.g. nutrient precursor, nutrients) or antinutritive substances (e.g. phytate)	Bioavailability of nutrients in indicator organs: - e.g. vitamin A from β-carotene in the liver - Phosphorus from low phytate varieties in bones or faeces
Tolerance studies	GMP with many modifications	Studies concerning safety, including of very high level of GMP
Efficacy studies	Feeds from GMP, where effects on animal performance/ feed efficiency, could be expected (case by case studies)	See Table 11 for more detailed information
Long term studies	Studies with feeds from GMP, where long term effects could be expected (e.g. reproduction, case by case studies)	See Table 11 for more information

Table 11 : Some recommendations from the Best practices for the conduct of animal studies to evaluate crops genetically modified for input traits (GMP of the first generation); adapted from ILSI (2003)

Animals (species/categories)	No. of animals (Coefficient of variation 4 to 5%)	Duration of experiments	Compositition dies1	Measurements
Poultry for meat production	10 to 12 pens per treatment with 9 to 12 birds per pen	5 weeks or more	Balanced diets	Feed intake, gain, feed conversion
Poultry for egg production	12 to 15 replications per treatment with 3 to 5 layers per pen	18 to 40 weeks of age, at least three 28-day phases	Balanced diets	Feed intake, egg production, feed conversion, egg quality
Swine	6 to 9 replications per treatment with 4 or more pigs per replication	Piglets (7 - 12 kg), 4 - 6 weeks Growers (15 - 25 kg) 6 - 8 weeks	Balanced diets	Feed intake, gain, feed conversion, carcass quality
Growing and finishing ruminants	6 to 10 replications per treatment with 6 or more cattle per replication	90 - 120 days	Balanced diets	Feed intake, gain, feed conversion, carcass data
Lactating dairy cows	12 - 16 cows per treatment 28 cows per treatment	Latin square: 28 day periods Randomized block design	Balanced diets	Feed intake, milk performances and composition, body weight, Body Condition Score (BCS), cell counts in milk, animal health

1) Efficacy studies to evaluate feed from GMP with output traits (GMP of the second generation) should be done under consideration of recommendation by EFSA (2008) and ILSI (2007)

Table 12 : Assessment of present modifications of plants from the view of food safety and food security

Objectives	Present significance	Contributions to	
		Food safety	Global food security
More resistant against herbicides	⇑⇑⇑	⇑	⇑
More resistant against insects etc. (e.g. Europ. corn borer)	⇑⇑	⇑	⇑
More valuable ingredients	⇑	~	⇑
Less undesirable ingredients	⇑	⇑⇑	⇑
More efficient use of resources (water etc.)	⇑	⇑	⇑⇑⇑

⇑⇑⇑ extremely high ⇑⇑ very high high ~not important

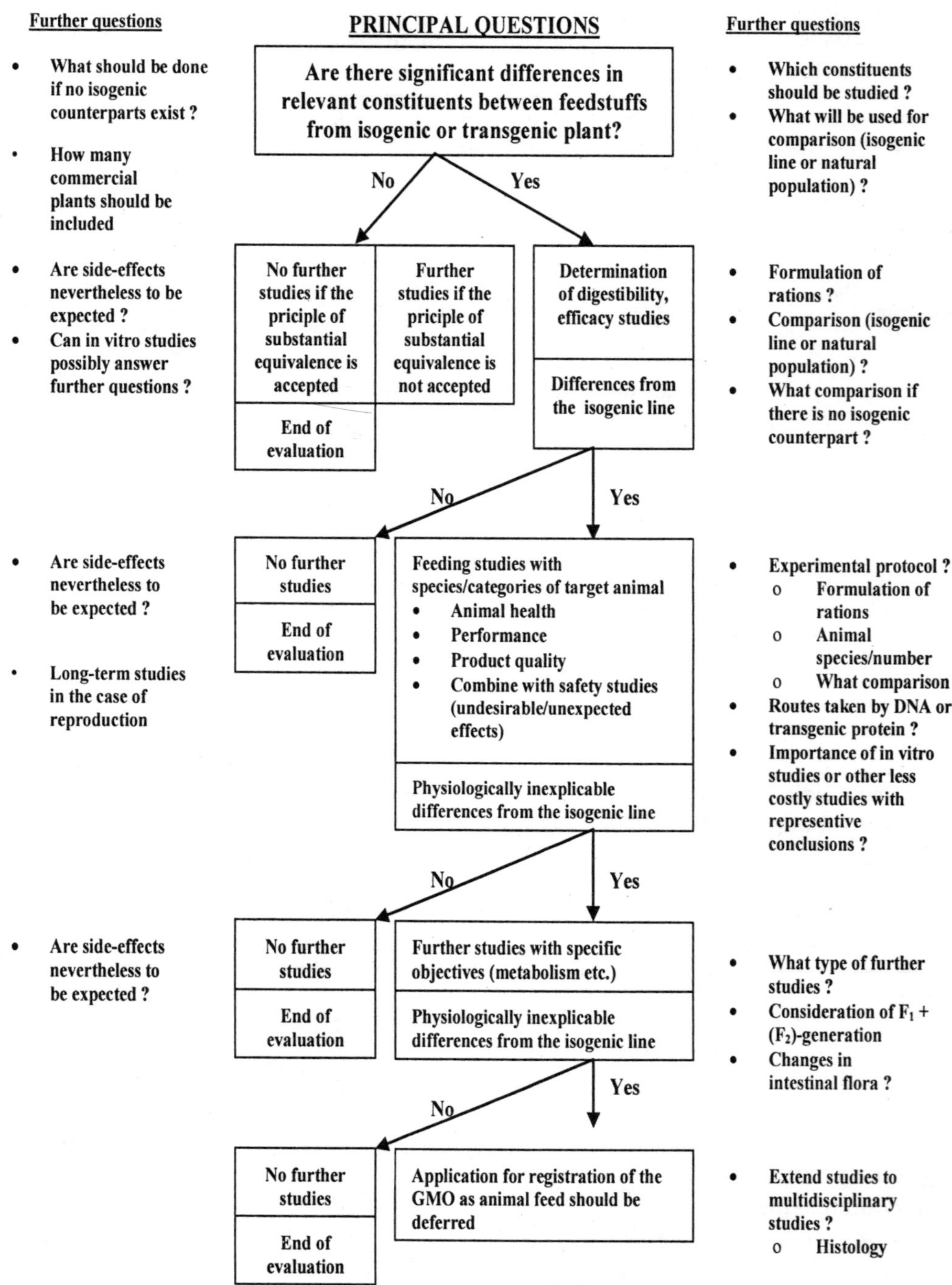

Fig. 5 : Proposal for a decision tree for nutritional assessment of feeds from GMP of the 1st and / or 2nd generation

There will be a strong competition for arable land between feed/food, fuel, fibre, areas for settlements and natural conservation in the future. Therefore, high yielding plants with low external inputs should be the main aim of plant breeding. Apart from traditional breeding plant biotechnology seems to have a certain potential to contribute to this objective. The cultivation of genetically modified plants (GMP) increased worldwide from 1.7 (1996) to about 114 million ha (2007). That means about 7% of arable land allover the world was cultivated by GMP in 2007. Nutritional and safety assessment of feed/food from GMP is urgently necessary. The contribution summarizes the present stage of knowledge. The results of the studies and the further research need can be summarized as follows:

- Up to now about 700 mio. ha of GM-crops have been cultivated allover the world
- Most animal studies were done with GM-crops of the 1st generation (with input traits)
- No unintended effects in composition (except lower mycotoxins) and nutritional assessment of feeds from GM-crops of the 1st generation were registered in more than 100 studies with food producing animals
- Other experimental designs are recommended for nutritional and safety assessment of feeds from GM-crops of the 2nd generation (with output traits)
- Transgenic DNA and novel protein did not show other properties as plant DNA or native proteins during feed treatment or in the animals
- Furthermore case by case studies seem to be necessary to answer open questions, more groups with isogenic counterparts should be included
- Feeding studies with food producing animals should be also used for safety assessment.

References

Alexander, T.W., Reuter, T., Aulrich, K., Sharma, R., Okine, E.K., Dixon, W.T. and McAllister, T.A. (2007). *Anim. Feed Sci. Technol.* 133: 31-62.

Astwood, J.D., Leach, L.N. and Fuchs, R.L. (1996). *Nat. Biotech.* 14: 1269.

Aulrich, K., Reuter, T. and Flachowsky, G. (2002). *Proc. Soc. Nutr. Physiol.*, 11: 187-188

Aulrich, K., Pahlow, G. and Flachowsky, G. (2004). *Proc. Soc. Nutr. Physiol.* 13: 112.

Bakan, B., Melcion, D., Richard-Molrad, D. and Cahagnier, B. (2002). *J. Agric. Food Chem.* 50: 728-731.

Beever, D.E. and Kemp, F. (2000). *Nutr. Abstr. Rev.* 70: 197-204

Beever, D.E. and Phipps, R.H. (2001). *J. Anim. Sci. 79 (E Suppl.)*, E290-E295.

Berger, B., Aulrich, K., Fleck, G. and Flachowsky, G. (2003). *Proc. Soc. Nutr. Physiol.*, 12: 108 (Abstract).

Betz, F., Hammond, B.G. and Fuchs, R.L. (2000). *Regul. Toxicol. Pharmacol.* 32: 156-165.

Broll, H., Zagon, J., Butschke, A., Leffke, A., Spiegelberg, A., Böhme, H. and Flachowsky, G. (2005). *J. Anim. Feed Sci. 14, Suppl.*, 1:337-340.

Brookes, G. and Barfoot, P. (2008). GMcrops: Global socio-economic and environmental impacts 1996-2006. PC Economics Ltd, Dorchester, UK, 118 p.

Cahagnier, B. and Melcion, D. (2000). *Feed Proc. Conference, 27-28 November, Piacenca*: 237-249.

Calsamiglia, S., Hernandez, B., Hartnell, G.F. and Phipps, R. (2007). *J. Dairy Sci.*, 90: 4718-4723.

Cellini, F., Chesson, A., Coquhonn, I., Constable, A., Davies H.V., Engel, K.-H., Gatehouse, A.M.R., Kärenlampi, S., Kok, E.J., Legnay, J.J., Lehesranta S., Noteborn, H.P.J.M., Pedersen, J. and Smith, M. (2004). *Food Chem.Toxicol.* 42: 1089-1123.

Clark, J.H. and Ipharraguerre, I.R., (2001). *J. Dairy Sci. 84: E. Suppl.*, E9-E18, 237-249.

Demanèche, S., Sanguin, H., Poté, J., Navarro, E., Bernillon, D., Mavingui, P., Wildi, W., Vogel, T.M. and Simonet, P. (2008). *Proc. Nat. Acad. Sci.*, 105: 3957-3962.

EFSA (European Food Safety Authority) (2004). Guidance document of the scientific panel on genetically modified organisms for the risk assessment of genetically modified plants and derived food and feed. *EFSA J.* 99: 1-93.

EFSA (2008). Safety and nutritional assessment of GM plant derived food and feed. The role of animal feeding trials. *Food and Chemical Tox.*, 46: 2-70.

Einspanier, R. and Flachowsky, G. (2008). Safety of meat, milk and eggs from animals fed genetically modified crops. Encyclopedia of Animal Science by W.G. Pond and A.W. Bell (Eds.). Health Sciences/Reference, Taylor & Francis Group, LLC, New York, USA (In Press).

Einspanier, R.; Klotz, A., Kraft, J., Aulrich, K., Poser, R., Schwägele, F., Jahreis, G. and Flachowsky, G. (2001). *Eur. Food Res. Technol.*, 212: 129-134.

El Sanhoty, R.M.E.S. (2004). Quality control for food produced by genetic engineering. *Diss., TU Berlin, 155 pp.*

FAO/WHO (2000). Safety Aspects of Genetically Modified Foods of Plant Origin. Report of a Joint FAO/WHO Expert Consultation on Foods Derived from Biotechnology. World Health Organization, Geneva.

Federici, B.A. and Siegel, J.P. (2008). Safety assessment of Bacillus thuringiensis and Bt crops used in insect control. In: Food Safety of proteins in Agricultural Biotechnology, by B.G. Hammond (Ed.) CRC Press, Taylor & Francis Group, 45-102.

Flachowsky, G. (2008). What do animal nutritionists expect from plant breeding? *Outlook on Agricult.* 37: 95-103.

Flachowsky, G.; Aulrich, K.; Böhme, H. and Halle, I. (2007). *Anim. Feed Sci. Technol.*, 133: 2-30.

Flachowsky, G. and Böhme, H. (2005). *J. Anim. Feed Sci.* 14: 49-70.

Flachowsky, G. and Brade, W. (2007). *Züchtungskunde* 79: 417-365.

Flachowsky, G., Chesson, A. and Aulrich, K. (2005a). *Arch. Anim. Nutr.* 59: 1-40.

Flachowsky, G., Halle, I. and Aulrich, K. (2005b). *Arch. Anim. Nutr.* 59: 449-451.

Halle, I., Aulrich, K. and Flachowsky, G., (2006). *Proc. Soc. Nutr. Physiol.* 15: 114, Abstract

Hammond, B.C. (Ed., 2008). Food safety of proteins in agricultural biotechnology, CRC Press, Taylor & Francis Group, Boca Raton, London, New York, 299 p.

Hammond, B. and Cockburn, A. (2008). In: Food safety of proteins in Agricultural Biotechnology, by B.G. Hammond (Ed.). CRC Press, Taylor & Francis Group, 259-288.

Howe, J.A. and Tanumihardjo, S.A. (2006). *J. Nutr.* 136: 2562-2567.

Hupfer, C., Mayer, J., Hotzel, H., Sachse, K. and Engel, K.H. (1999). *Eur. Food Res. Technol.* 209: 301-304.

ILSI (2007). Best practices for the conduct of animal studies to evaluate crops genetically modified for output traits. Int. Life Sci. Inst., Washington D.C.

James, C. (2007). Global status of commercialised transgenic crops: 2007. ISAA: Ithaca NY. http://www.isaaa.org.

Keyzer, M.A., Merbis, M.D., Pavel, L.F.P.W. and van Wesenbeck C.F.A. (2005). Diets shifts towards meat and the effect on cereal use: Can we feed the animals in 2030. *Ecological Economics* 55: 187-202.

Kok, E.J., Keijer, J., Kleter, G.A. and Kuiper, H.A. (2007). *Reg. Toxicol.Pharmacol.*, 50: 98-113.

Konig, A., Cockburn, A., Crevel, R.W.R., Debruyne, E., Grafstroem, R., Hammerling, U., Kimber, I., Knudsen, I., Kuiper, H.A., Peijnenburg, A.A.C.M., Penninks, A.H., Poulsen, M., Schauzu, M. and Wal, J.M. (2004). *Food Chem. Toxicol.*, 42: 1047-1088.

Luca, D.M., Taylor, M.L., Hartnell, G.F., Nemeth, M.A., Glenn, K.C. and Davis, S.W. (2007). *Poultry Sci.*, 86: 2152-2161.

Martens, M.A. (2000). *Int. Arch. Occup. Environ. Health.* 73 (Suppl.). S14-S18.

Mazza, R., Soave, M., Morlacchini, M., Piva, G. and Marocco, A. (2005). .*Transg. Res.* 14: 775-784.

McNaughton, I.L., Roberts, M., Rice, D., Smith, B., Hinds, M., Schmidt, J., Locke, M., Bryant, A., Rood, T., Layton, R., Lamb, I. and Pelaney, B. (2007). *Anim. Feed Sci. Technol.* 132: 227-239.

Miller, F.P. (2008). *Agronomy J.*, 100: 22-34.

Munkvold, G.P., Hellmich, R.L. and Rice, L.G. (1999). *Plant Disease,* 83: 130-138.

OECD (1993). Safety Evaluation of Foods Derived by Modern Biotechnology: Concepts and Principles, Paris, France.

OECD (2001). Series on the Safety of Novel Foods and Feeds No. 1. Consensus document on key nutrients and key toxicants in low erucic acid rapeseed (canola). Organization for Economic Co-operation and Development, Paris, France.

OECD (2002). Series on the Safety of Novel Foods and Feeds No. 3: Consensus document on compositional considerations for new varieties of sugar beet: Key food and feed nutrients and anti-nutrients. Organization for Economic Cooperation and Development, Paris, France.

OECD (2003). Series on the Safety of Novel Food and feed No. 7. Consensus Document on Compositional Considerations for New Varieties of Bread Wheat (Triticum aestivum): Key Food and Feed Nutrients, Anti-Nutrients and Toxicants. Organization for Economic Co-operation and Development, Paris, France.

OECD (2004). Series on the Safety of Novel Food and feed No. 10. Consensus Document on Compositional Considerations for New Varieties of Rice (Oryza sativa): Key Food and Feed Nutrients and Anti-Nutrients. Organization for Economic Co-operation and Development, Paris, France.

OECD (2005). Series on the Safety of Novel Food and feed No. 13. Consensus Document on Compositional Considerations for New Varieties of Alfalfa and other Temperate Forage Legumes: Key Feed Nutrients, Anti-nutrients and Secondary Plant Metabolites. Organization for Economic Co-operation and Development, Paris, France.

Pietri, A. and Piva, G. (2000). *Feed Produc. Confer.* 27.-28. November, Piacenca:226-236.

Reuter, T. and Aulrich, K. (2003). *Europ. Food. Res. Technol.* 216:185-192.

Reuter, T., Aulrich, K., Berk, A. and Flachowsky, G. (2002a). *Arch. Anim. Nutr.*, 56:23-31.

Seale, J.W. and English, L. (2008): The mode of action of bacterial protein toxis: The role of conformational changes in the life cycle of a protein toxin. In: Food Safety of Proteins in Agricultural Biotechnology, by B.G. Hammond (Ed.), CRC Press, Taylor & Francis Group, 31-44.

Sharma, R., Damgaard, D., Alexander, T.W., Dugan, M.E.R., Aalhus, J.L., Stanford, K. and McAllister, T.A. (2006). *J. Agric. Food Chem.* 54: 1699-1709.

Spencer, J.D., Allee, G.L. and Sauber, T.E. (2000). *J. Anim. Sci.* 78:675-681.

Steinfeld, H., Gerber, P., Wassenaar, T., Castel, V., Rosales, M. and de Haan, C. (2006). Livestock's long shadow: Environmental issues and options. Food and Agric. Organization of the United Nations (FAO), Rom.

Tony, M.A., Butschke, A. Broll, A., Zagon, J., Halle, I., Dänicke, S., Schauzu, M., Hafes, H.M. and Flachowsky, G. (2003). *Arch. Anim. Nutr.* 57: 235-252.

Van den Eede, G., Kay, S. and Anklam, E. (2002). *J. AOAC Int.* 85: 757-761.

Valenta, H., Dänicke, S., Flachowsky, G. and H. Böhme (2001). *Proc. of the Soc. of Nutr. Physiol.* 10: p. 182 (abstr.)

Van Dijk, J.E., Fledderus, A., Mouwen, J.M. and Holzhauer, C. (1988). *Vet. Res. Commun.* 12: 47-59.

□□□

Animal Nutrition, 2012
eds. Dr. (Mrs.) Usha R. Mehra et al., pp. 499-517
Satish Serial Publishing House e-mail : info@satishserial.com; website : www.satishserial.com

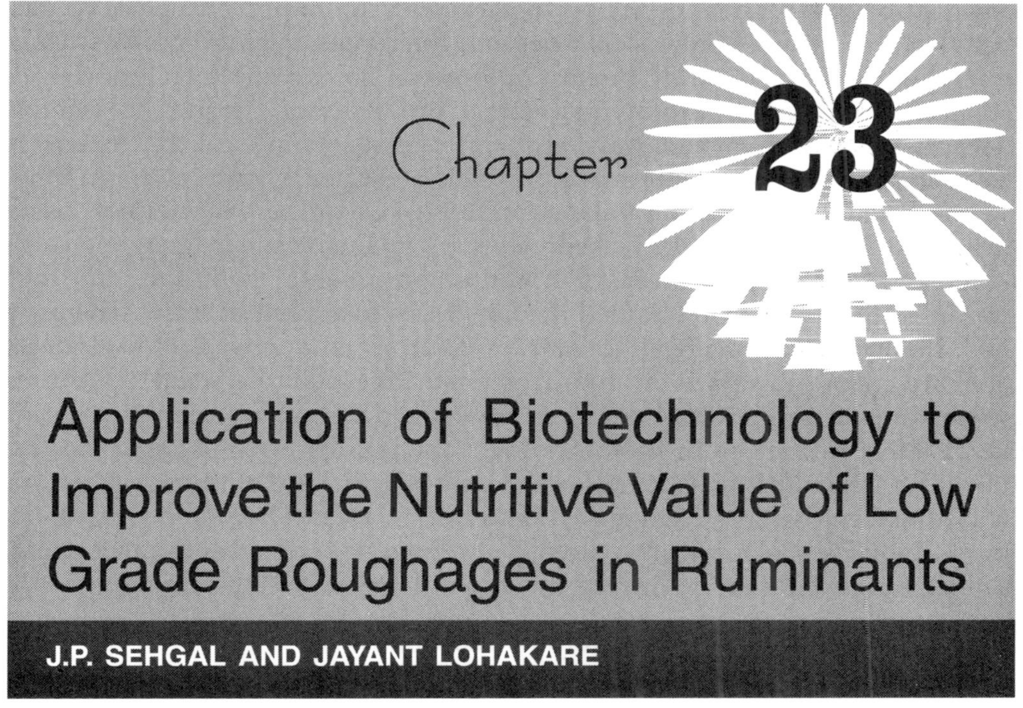

Chapter 23

Application of Biotechnology to Improve the Nutritive Value of Low Grade Roughages in Ruminants

J.P. SEHGAL AND JAYANT LOHAKARE

Ruminants have a unique ability to digest wide variety of fibrous feed in their digestive tract because of the presence of rumen microbes. In many tropical countries, the majority of the livestock subsist on poor quality crop residues those are bulky and poorly digested in rumen due to crystallite nature of cellulose and also due to the lignin-carbohydrates association. Thus, improvement of nutritive value of crop residue is a constant challenge for the researchers of ruminant nutrition for the last so many years. Its necessity could be felt from the fact that India being the highest milk producer in the world having a huge livestock population, faces an alarming deficit of quality concentrate feeds and fodder.

Utilization of Crop Residues

Wheat straw is one of the important crop residues and is fed in plenty to the animals in villages, but it is poor in nutritional quality because of low digestibility, low mineral and high lignin contents. However, it is a potential source of energy due to the presence of cell wall polysaccharides, such as cellulose and hemicellulose. High lignin contents of these straws reduce its digestible energy because lignin encrusts the cell wall and develops ester covalent bond with hemicellulose. In particular, lignin prevents close contact between the cell wall polysaccharides and the rumen microorganisms. Thus, upgrading the wheat straw quality in terms of its digestible energy (DE) is still a central issue for improving livestock productivity. During the past few decades research workers have shown interest in physical and chemical treatment of straws. Of the many physical treatments, only chopping and soaking were feasible under village conditions. Chemical treatment of straws using sodium hydroxide increased voluntary intake by sheep, goat and cattle However, excess requirement of water, environmental pollution, and high cost of sodium hydroxide limited the use of this treatment of straw. The urea-NH_3 treatment has received a major attention as an appropriate technology of treatment of straws, but the improvement in digestibility of urea-NH_3 treated wheat straw is temperature and moisture dependent and useful up to a certain level only. Advances in biotechnology opened up novel approaches for increasing the nutritive values of cereal straws by the use of fibrolytic bacteria and fungal cultivation to enhance their feeding values. Though the dry matter digestibility of the straws increased, but a huge loss of substrate dry matter during fungal cultivation limited the applicability of this technology.

Fibre Degrading Anaerobic Rumen Microbes

The *Butyrivibrio fibrisolvens, Ruminococcus albus,* R. *flavefaciens,* and *Fibrobacter succinogenes* are regarded as the primary fiber degrading bacteria in the rumen. The genetic diversity and phenotype of *Ruminococcus* have received little attention and very few investigations have been carried out in a systematic manner, but for other fibrolytic bacteria, a number of studies are available. The 16S rDNA analysis has confirmed the DNA–DNA hybridization results of B. *fibrisolvens* and showed that the bacterium is polyphyletic. A study to assess the genotype and extent of fiber digestion of a medium quality grass varied from 0-16%. The genotype was based on ribosomal DNA sequence analysis. It is believed that, if this phenotypic diversity is represented within an individual rumen, than increasing the number of highly fibrolytic *Ruminococci,* it could potentially improve the rates of cell wall digestion in the rumen. Krause *et al.,* (1999) also collected the highly fibrolytic *Ruminococcus* strain and evaluated them for their ability to colonize the rumen and to enhance fiber digestion. Tracking systems based on strain specific 16S rDNA sequences indicate that inoculated *Ruminococcus* strain did not persist for more than 3 weeks before reaching undetectable levels. Hence, the biggest problem is the ability to introduce bacterial strain and maintain the same in the mixed rumen population, and its survivability is not well understood.

Simultaneously, interest in the rumen anaerobic fungi developed after their discovery by Orpin in year 1975. These anaerobic fungi act on sclerenchyma tissue of the low grade roughages through secretion of their esterases, which breakdown the bonds between lignin and hemicelluloses. Thus, anaerobic fungi (those having higher hydrolytic activity) were isolated from the cattle, buffaloes, sheep, goat, and wild ruminant. Fungi isolated from domestic and wild ruminants were administered in domestic animals (cattle and buffaloes) fed on a ration consisted of straws and concentrates, showed higher growth rate and improved nutritive value of the straws, and increased milk yield. *Neocallimastix* GR1 isolated from browsing goat was found to be promising fungi to act as probiotics in the rumen of buffalo calves. But it is not practicable to administer anaerobic fungal cultures to the animal on day-to-day basis to improve the digestibility of low grade roughages. Thus, it was essential to develop the fungal zoospore from fungal culture by augmenting zoosporogenesis. An attempt was made to maximize the zoosporogenesis with normal and deficient media and it was found that the zoosporogenesis start in the normal media after 96 h and completed by 144 h of incubation. Incorporation of fungal zoospores of *Neocallimastix* GR1 at a concentration of 250 x 10^6 tfu per ml in straw based total mixed ration and complete feed blocks, showed an improvement in growth rate, digestibility of nutrients, rumen fermentation pattern and also reduction in methane in buffalo calves.

Further rumen microbes have the ability to synthesize S- amino acids viz. methionine, cysteine and cystine from degradable inorganic sulphur. Utilization of nitrogen, assimilation, and metabolism of number of microelements in body depends upon sulphur. The activity of superior anaerobic fungi, which play a significant role in the structural degradation of fiber in the rumen, requires and necessitates the dietary sulphur and contributes in the synthesis of S- amino acids. As urea is a constituent of the concentrate mixture in practical ration, the proliferation of rumen microbes, especially, growth of rumen anaerobic fungi necessitates the dietary sulphur in the ration. Addition of sulphur enhanced fermentative activities, with the increased number of rumen anaerobic fungi proliferated in the rumen through complete feed blocks incorporated with rumen fungal zoospores, and enhanced the digestibility of nutrients and nutritive value in terms of total digestible nutrients in buffalo calves.

In this essay, progress and problems related to manipulation of rumen ecosystem through inoculation of natural rumen micro-organisms will be discussed.

Rumen Anaerobic Fungi

Rumen, the anaerobic chamber of ruminant digestive system and place for microbial-based fermentation of feed, contains mainly four kinds of microbes- a) Bacteria, b) Protozoa, c) Fungi, d) Bacteriophages. The fungi found in rumen are mainly of two kinds: Aerobic and Non-Aerobic. Some yeast and aerobic fungi are also normal inhabitants of rumen and intestines. But they are transient, non-functional and entering rumen with the feed. Nine species of yeast of four genera (*Candida, Trichosporon, Rhodtorula* and *Saccharomyces*) each are found in rumen. Some species of yeast and aerobic fungi like *Aspergillus fumigatus, Mucor rouxii, Rhizopus* sp. *and Sporormia minima* are the causative agent of bovine ill thrift and could survive in the rumen. However, yeast might be concerned with sugar fermentation, suppressed growth of pathogens and helped in synthesis of B-complex vitamins.

Although in very small number (10^3/ml), some parasitic fungi could also be present in the rumen. Like chytrid fungi, a parasite on ciliate protozoa is known as *Sphaerita hoari.* This fungus is also a parasite on *Eremoplastron bovis.* In light infection ciliates continue to divide but heavily infected ciliates degenerate. *Spagittospora cameroni* was also found to be parasitic on *Diplodinium minor and Eudiplodinium magii* that killed the host cells. The difference between these parasitic fungi and rumen anaerobic fungi is that these fungi have non-flagellate spore and plasmodial thallus, which on maturity produce a sporangium. But these parasitic fungi don't play any important role in digestion and metabolism in rumen.

Distribution of Anaerobic Fungi in Different Species of Livestock

Anaerobic fungi were isolated from both ruminants and monogastric herbivores. So far, they are comprised of 6 genera and 18 species. They are isolated from: Ruminants / foregut fermenters - such as Cattle, Sheep, Goat, Buffalo, Red deer, Reindeer, Musk ox Yak, Blue bull and in pseudo-ruminants: Grey Kangaroo, Wallaroo, Swamp wallaby, Camel, Ilama. These rumen microbes were also isolated from monogastric herbivores such as ass; horse.

Factors Affecting Fungal Population

There are so many factors, such as composition of diet, feed pretreatment, feeding frequency, defaunation, inophores, fungistats, probiotics and dietary phenolic compound, and interaction with rumen microbes that affect fungal population.

Diet composition: It has been observed in general that if fibre content is more in feed, fungal population increases. Few anaerobic fungi were seen in the rumen of animals that were fed lush pasture (either legume or grass when green and leafy) compared with the same pasture when it was mature. Thus, fibre or lignocellulose content of the diet was a critical factor for the growth of fungal population. The influence of diet composition on rumen fungal population by offering successively to a rumen fistulated cow 11 different diets rich in fibre, starch or soluble carbohydrates, was studied. At the same time, the colonization of four different plant substrates introduced into the rumen in nylon bags was investigated. They found that the population of rumen anaerobic fungi particularly was abundant with lignocellulose rich diets, decreased with starch or soluble-carbohydrate and the fungi selectively colonized the plant tissue with thick or lignified cell wall. If free lipid content of feed increased, fungal population decreased. Feeding of free lipids to ruminants could have a detrimental effect on rumen fermentation, retarding fibre digestion. Perhaps coating effect of fats on fungal cells could explain this.

The addition of grass lipids (extracted from fresh alfalfa grass) to the medium has significantly decreased fungal growth and cellulase activity. However, low chain fatty acids (palmitic, stearic and oleic acids) did not have any significant inhibitory effects on fungal growth and enzyme activities. Unsaturated fatty acids (oleic, linoleic acids) addition increased fungal growth and activities perhaps due to utilization as alternative hydrogen sink. But, linolenic acid showed an inhibitory effect. The size of anaerobic fungal population in the rumen increased dramatically either after an application of S to the pasture used to make the hay, or due to an S- containing dietary supplement to the low S-hay. It has been reported that microbial growth enhanced with the supplementation of S in the diet of ruminants. Further, it is also reported that the addition of the sulfur supplementation resulted in increased feed intake and increased flow of microbial protein to the small intestines when the animals were fed a poor quality roughage low in S (0.1%) and N. Both supplements improved rumen function by stimulating the microbial population to incorporate more ammonia N for protein synthesis. The study also demonstrated that the animals would benefit from additional supplemental urea for complete utilization of the S based supplements.

Feed pre-treatment : Alkali treatment (ammonium hydroxide) increased the *in vitro* digestibility of wheat straw by an efficient fibre degrading anaerobic fungus. Earlier it was reported that ammoniation of wheat straw increased the dry matter digestibility of the feed by 8-10% and normally faunated sheep consuming it had higher fungal counts in the rumen (1.6-3.0 folds). The microscopic studies of structure and rumen fungal colonization in sheep fed different alkali treated wheat straw and showed the effects of chemically treated wheat straw with calcium oxide (CaO), sodium hydroxide (NaOH), and alkaline hydrogen peroxide (AHP) on its subsequent colonization and degradation *in-sacco* by rumen fungi in sheep. AHP caused the greatest fragility to straw particles followed respectively, by NaOH and CaO treatments. Untreated straw showed relatively less fungal colonization compared with treated straws being heavily colonized by rhizoids and thalli. The thalli of this study resembled mono- and poly-centric genera of anaerobic *Chytridiomycete* fungi.

The fibrolytic activities of rumen fungi in terms of dry matter loss, plant cell wall degradation, and enzyme (cellulase and xylanase) activities, when grown *in vitro,* on either untreated or sodium hydroxide treated stems of barley straw over a 12 day period. It has showed that *in vitro* degradation of cellulose and hemicellulose was higher in the treated than that of untreated cultures. Although, comparatively, xylanase activity was higher than that of cellulase, the cellulose fraction of the straw was degraded more than hemicellulose in both treated and untreated straws. *Piromyces spp.* WNG-12 from Nilgai had shown better digestibility of urea-NH_3 treated wheat straw than *Orpinomyces* C-14 from cattle *in vitro.*

Defaunation : Ionic detergents caused increased populations of rumen fungi and it was found that with the increase in rumen anaerobic fungal count there was a decrease in protozoal count, but the bacterial count was more in the rumen of buffalo calves fed wheat straw based ration incorporated with superior fungal culture.

Ionophores : Monensin, tetronasin, salinomysin, polyoxins were found to decrease fungal count. The effect of the antibiotic lasalocid on the rumen anaerobic fungus *Neocallimastix frontalis* RK 21 was examined as it was thought that lasalocid increased the efficiency of feed utilization by cattle by altering the rumen fermentation. The effect of steroidal saponins from *Yucca schidigera* extracted from rumen microbes concluded that steroidal saponins from *Y. schidigera* inhibited cellulolytic rumen bacteria and fungi, but their effects on amylolytic bacteria were species dependent and similar to the effects of ionophores.

Fungistats : Sodium propionate had no effect on the number of fungi in sheep at a rumen dose rate of 20-40 g/ day, only *Neocallimastix* become dominant over *Piromyces.*

Other fungal probiotics : Feeding of live *S. cerevisiae* to sheep had no effect on the numbers of fungal zoospores in the rumen. The effects of a live yeast strain of *Saccharomyces cerevisiae* on zoospore germination, metabolism, and cellulolytic activity of the anaerobic rumen fungus *Neocallimastix frontalis* was observed and results showed that yeasts could enhance plant cell wall colonization by *N. frontalis.* The yeasts could therefore also be a good tool to optimize the microbial degradation of lignocellulosic materials on certain diets. The effects of *Aspergillus oryzae* fermentation extract, Amaferm, on the rumen fungus *Neocallimastix frontalis* showed that the secretion of cellulase was increased by 67% and rhizoid development was increased by 3.8-fold in the presence of this extract. These results supported the idea that by accelerating fungal growth and metabolism, Amaferm increased the rate of fibre degradation caused by rumen fungi and that this, in turn, may contribute to enhanced animal performance.

Dietary phenolic compounds viz. lignin and phenolic acids : Lignin and lignocellulosic content in feed increased fungal count as fungi showed chemotactic response to phenolic acids such as p-coumaric acid, ferulic acid and syringic acids, often found in lignified tissue of plant. The effect of coumarin (1, 2 benzopyrone) on glucose utilization by the anaerobic rumen fungi *Neocallimastix frontalis* and *N. patriciarum* was compared with the effect of p-coumaric acid. Both compounds largely inhibited glucose utilization by *N. patriciarum* strain Cx, when present in the medium at a concentration of 2.5 mM, and had a similar effect on *N. frontalis* strain RE1 at 5 mM.

The effect of condensed tannins from birdsfoot trefoil on endo-glucanase activity and the digestion of cellulose filter paper by rumen fungi viz; *Neocallimastix frontalis, Neocallimastix patriciarum, Piromyces communis,* and *Orpinomyces joyonii* were studied. For all four fungi, inhibition of endo-glucanases was evident at 100 micrograms condensed tannins/ml with nearly complete inhibition at 300 micrograms condensed tannins/ml. Mycelia of fungi grown with condensed tannins were covered by filamentous material, which may have arisen from the formation of condensed tannin-protein complexes. But the minimum inhibitory concentration of tannins appeared to be much higher for fungi than for bacteria, and anaerobic rumen fungi might be more tolerant to tannins than the bacteria which compete with them.

Interaction with fibrolytic bacteria : Co-culture with *Ruminococcus albus* and *R. flavifaciens* resulted in less efficient degradation of a variety of fibrous substance, such as xylans, filter paper, or straw compared with fungal monocultures. Extracellular factors of *R. flavifaciens* inhibited the growth of anaerobic fungi on cellulosic substrates. The supernatants of fungal cultures inhibited xylan degradation by *R. flavifaciens.* In contrast to interactions with *Ruminococci,* co-cultures of other fibrolytic bacteria with fungi gave increase in fibrolytic activity over what occurs with fungi or bacteria alone. Thus the digestion of straw was greater with a mixture of *Neocallimastix* and *Fibrobacter succinogenes* and likewise the digestion of xylan was greater when fungi were grown with *Butyrivibrio fibrisolvens* or *Prevotella ruminicola* and hydrogen utilizing bacteria.

Interaction with methanogens : The anaerobic fungi resulted in interspecies hydrogen transfer, with the methanogen providing the low H_2 environment that encouraged the flow of carbon through hydrogenosomes and results in a shift in the end products towards acetate, H_2 and. Fumarate. The fungal co-cultures with methanogens increased the activity and yield of polysaccharide degrading enzymes and there was an increase in fungal biomass in co-cultures. The degradation of fresh ryegrass by methanogenic co-cultures of rumen fungi grown in the presence or absence of *Fibrobacter succinogenes* was observed. The *N. frontalis* and *Piromyces* isolates showed the greatest rates of stem degradation. When interactions between *Fibrobacter succinogenes* and methanogenic co-cultures of fungi growing on ryegrass stem were investigated *N. frontalis* inhibited *F. succinogenes*. In contrast, a *Caecomyces* spp interacted positively with *F. succinogenes* to increase stem degradation, suggesting that *F. succinogenes* and *Caecomyces* spp may have complementary fibrolytic activities. Thus showed the superiority of fungi in the degradation of intact stem in *in vitro* studies. A decrease in methane production by feeding complete feed blocks based on wheat straw and incorporated with fungal zoospores of *Neocallimastix* GR-1 has also been reported in latest studies. Co-cultures of anaerobic fungi with H_2 utilizing bacteria have yielded similar results to experiments with methanogens. Thus, the acetogenic species such as *Eupatorium limosum Acetitomaculum ruminis* and *Clostridium* spp and the sulphate reducing bacterium *Desulfovibrio sp* shifted the fermentation products towards acetate and H_2 from lactate to reduce methane production.

Interaction with other bacteria and protozoa: It has been demonstrated that the saccharolytic bacterium Succinovibrio dextrinosolvens stimulated hemicellulose degradation by anaerobic fungi possibly by fermenting arabinose with resultant minimization of feedback inhibition by this sugar. The lactate utilizing bacteria such as Megasphaera elsdenii and some strains of Selenomonas ruminantium stimulated fungal cellulolysis in co-culture, whereas other strains of S.ruminantium inhibited this process. The chitinolytic bacteria and their cell free culture medium inhibited both the growth and cellulose degradation by polycentric fungi. One of the observed consequences in most experiments where protozoa have been removed from rumen has seen an increase in the number of fungal zoospores. The interaction of rumen fungi with protozoa showed that the protozoa act as a predator on the anaerobic fungi and digest them. Generally the presence of protozoa inhibits the level of cellulolytic activity in the co-cultures. Some workers have reported that protozoa number in rumen decreases with the incorporation of fungal culture of Neocallimastix spp GR1.

Degradation of Different Nutrients

Role of fungi in feed intake: There is a definite relationship between fungal population in rumen and fibrous feed intake. There is also a positive relationship between presence of anaerobic fungi in rumen and voluntary intake of herbage diets of low digestibility. The intake of forage by early weaned calves was 35% higher in *Neocallimastix* spp dosed calves (from 1.35-1.85 kg DM/day) and dosing of fungus free sheep with *Neocallimastix* spp increased 40% intake of straw based diet. A 10% increase in DM and OM intake of straw based complete feed mixture in crossbred calves dosed with *Orpinomyces* spp C-14 has also been observed.

Fibre degradation : The crop residues are the most abundant renewable resources having potential as animal feed. These are characterized by low protein, low energy, low mineral and low vitamins, but contain a potential source of digestible energy due to the presence of cell wall carbohydrates such as cellulose and hemicellulose. These polysaccharides are not available to the ruminants because of the presence of high lignin. High lignin content has been implied to be a major hindrance to unlock energy from cellulose.Which is a linear polymer of D-anhydro-glucopyranose units linked by b-1, 4 glucosidic bonds with a degree of polymerization. Cellulose contents of wheat straw in 40.3 percent and that of barley and oat straw are 41.3 and 42%, respectively, although the percentage of cellulose depends upon the varieties and proportion of leaves in straws. Hemicelluloses are chemically the most complex plant polysaccharides and consist largely of heteropolymers of xylose and smaller quantities of arabinose, glucose, galactose, mannose, and rhamnose. The bulk of hemicelluloses are based on a linear chain of b-1, 4 linked D-xylopyranose units with varying amounts of side branches containing other sugars. Wheat straw contains 26.9 percent hemicelluloses, whereas barley and oat have 29.6 and 24.3%, respectively.

Lignin is a major component of straws, apart from the structural carbohydrates. It is a complex three-dimensional polymer arising from an enzyme-initiated dehydrogenative polymerization of three primary precursors: trans-p-coumaroyl alcohol, trans-coniferyl alcohol and trans-sinapyl alcohol. Wheat straw, maize, and alfalfa hay contain 12.3, 1.2 and 8.0% acid detergent lignin, respectively. It has been reported that the presence of 5.8 to 15.0 percent lignin limits the voluntary dry matter intake as well as digestibility of cereal straws. In particular, lignin prevents close contact between the cell walls and the rumen microorganisms. Rumen anaerobic fungi help in degrading the fibre portion of low grade cereal straws. Rumen fungi get attached to thick lignified tissues of cereal straws to degrade these by following ways:

- By breakdown of the cell wall structural protein (like extensin) covering fibre by metalloprotease enzyme, which decreases integrity as well as increases the extent of cell wall degradation.
- By physical disruption of feed particle with rhizoid penetrating deep into it and thereby favoring other rumen microorganisms to attack.
- By producing a vast range of degrading enzymes, especially feruloyl and p-coumaroyl esterase, which helps in breakdown of ester bond of lignocellulose and thereby freeing and increasing availability of hemicellulose and cellulose.

There exists a role of anaerobic fungi in *in vitro* forage degradation. Forages used as substrate for rumen microorganisms were coastal Bermuda grass and alfalfa. It was found that the NDF, ADF and cellulose digestion was 1.3, 2.4 and 7.9 percentage units higher, respectively, for Bermuda grass substrate than alfalfa. *In vitro* studies involving pure cultures showed that about 40-50% of dry weight of wheat straw fragments was lost and 50% of cellulose and hemicellulose was digested by causing a loss of 16% of plant lignin content. It was further observed that stems of Bermuda grass and Alfalfa incubated with rumen fungi got weakened by 57% and 55% whereas; in case of rumen bacteria only it got weakened by 29% and 42%. Fungi (*Neocallimastix spp and Piromyces spp*) solublize 30-40% fragments of barley straw whereas, *R. albus* solublize only 8%. Another significance of anaerobic fungi to ruminant nutrition is probably to weaken the structure of forage plants so that less effort is expended by the animal in rumination and digestion leading to conservation of energy.

Polysaccharide degradation : Cereal straws are characterized as a potential source of polysaccharides such as celluloses and hemicelluloses. And then digestion is through hydrolytic and fermentative activity of some of the fungal isolates in rumen. Their degradation is as as follows:

Amorphous cellulose: All rumen fungal Isolates can degrade it.

Crystalline cellulose: Some species of *Caecomyces, Piromyces,* and *Anaeromyces* cannot degrade it.

Starch and Glycogen: Some species of *Caecomyces, Piromyces,* and *Anaeromyces* don't ferment these.

Xylan: All isolates can degrade it although some relatively poor and slowly.

Carbohydrate fermentation : Fungi can use glucose, fructose, xylose, cellobiose and gentiobiose as substrate. Galactose and mannose utilization by anaerobic fungi were variable and L-arabinose was not used.Anaerobic fungi use only EMP pathway for catabolism of glucose to pyruvate and produce lactate, ethanol, succinate. In cytoplasm; and acetate, CO_2 and H_2 in hydrogenosome. Hydrogenosomes are unique structure of anaerobic fungi equivalent to eukaryotic mitochondria and said to be evolved from mitochondria.

Lignin degradation : Rumen fungi colonize on thick- walled sclerenchyma and vascular tissues and other lignified tissues. They solublize lignin but can not ferment it. They produce feruloyl and p-coumaroyl esterases and break ester linkages between lignin and hemicelluloses but, unable to break either the ether bonds between the phenolic moieties and polysaccharides or the inter-phenolic bonds found in the lignin complex. Selected strains of anaerobic fungi were found to solublize about 35% of the labeled $_{C}14$ (lignin) lignocellulose preparation and more than 34% of the lignin component of sorghum stem was removed by the anaerobic fungus *N. patriciarum* .

Zoospores of *N. frontalis, P. communis, O. joyonii,* and *Anaeromyces* spp also showed chemotactic response to phenolic acids such as p-coumaric acid, ferulic acid, syringic acids, often found in lignified tissues of plant. Fungal esterases such as p-coumaroyl esterase and p-feruloyl esterase are 20-fold more active than bacteria's esterases. Perhaps this is the answer why rumen fungi attack highly lignified tissue. The digestibility of lignin was higher with the incorporation of fungal zoospores in complete feed blocks based on wheat straw in buffalo calves.

Pectin degradation : Pectin is also disrupted by endopectin lyase and polygalacturonase enzymes produced by both monocentric and polycentric fungi but fermentation of pectin degradation products has not been reliably detected. Whole tract digestibility of wheat based ration was found to be higher with the incorporation of fungal culture or fungal zoospores in buffaloes.

Protein degradation : Rumen fungi also have protease activity and it may have role in plant cell wall degradation as it degrades plant structural proteins such as. The protease activity is due to a Zn metalloprotease with a trypsin like specificity working at neutral or slightly acidic pH.Majority of the strains did not degrade casein while producing several peptidase activities but a strain of *O. joyonii* was able to degrade casein.

Lipid degradation : Effective dietary lipid degradation potentiality not detected in anaerobic fungi and a lipid based diet or addition of more unsaturated fatty acids (UFA) in diet decrease anaerobic rumen fungal population but certainly an anaerobic ä-desaturase enzyme is operative in these organisms which could synthesize oleate from stearate.

Value of Anaerobic Fungi as a Nutrient

Rumen fungi flows from rumen to intestine like other microorganisms, and is also used as a protein source by host animals. Fungal biomass is about 8% of total microbial biomass in rumen. *N. patriciarum and P. communis* contained 24% and 30% protein by dry weight, respectively, and ammonia alone as nitrogen source supports growth of fungi. Digestibility factor for fungal protein is 0.91-0.98, for bacteria is 0.66-0.77, and for protozoa is 0.88. Rumen fungi have high level of some of the essential amino acids such as lysine, isoleucine, phenyl alanine, and S-amino acids. Fungal cells composed of proteins with a well-balanced combination of amino acids, are highly digestible and available to ruminant host. The amino acids profiles of fungi were compared favorably with casein and Lucerne fraction 1 protein. If an increase in the biomass of anaerobic fungi in the rumen is feasible, supply of high quality microbial protein to the host ruminant would be enhanced.

Influence of Rumen Anaerobic Fungi Culture on *in vitro* Digestibility of Cereal Straws

Incubation of wheat and paddy straws with different fungal isolates from cattle and buffalo showed an increase in IVDMD of wheat straw from 34.0 to 54.0% with addition of *Orpinomyces* spp $_C$14 from cow, and 31.4 to 35.5% with addition of *Orpinomyces* spp B-13 from buffalo @ 10^3 cfu/ml; and increase in IVDMD% of wheat straw from 37.9 to 55.3%, and paddy straw from 33.7 to 44.8%, decrease in NDF% from 79.9 to 64.1 in wheat straw, and 72.6 to 57.1 in paddy straw; decrease in ADF% from 41.1 to 27.1 in wheat straw, and 39.1 to 27.4 in paddy straw; decrease in ADL% from 12.3 to 6.25 in wheat straw, and 10.9 to 5.9 in paddy straw by addition of *Orpinomyces* spp $_C$14 from cow @10^6 cfu/ml and concluded that *Orpinomyces* spp $_C$14 from cow was most promising isolate than other isolated fungi studied from these two species of livestock. Thus, rumen fungi isolated from cattle was found to be better than rumen fungi isolated from buffaloes. Comparison of *Piromyces* spp (WNG-12) from Nilgai with *Orpinomyces* spp. $_C$14 isolated from dairy cattle for the *in vitro* biodegradation of urea -NH_3 treated wheat straw shown *Piromyces* spp (WNG-12) from Nilgai was most effective in enhancing digestibility of nutrients and TVFA production. Also, *in vitro* studies on *Piromyces* spp (WNG-12) showed higher growth rate, higher digestibility of nutrients than *Orpinomyces* spp isolated from cows.

Forty fungi were isolated from sheep and goat and their enzymatic activity was compared *Anaeromyces* spp SR4 isolated from sheep rumen and *Neocallimastix* spp GR1 isolated from grazing goat, were most efficient in enzymatic activity. The anaerobic fungi definitely increase fibre digestibility and thereby might increase nutritive value of crop residues. Also different strains of fungi isolated from different animal showed different extent of activities. So fungi, if administered *in vivo* the digestibility of nutrients and livestock productivity may increase. The effect of a daily administration of the rumen fungus *Neocallimastix* spp, strain R1 (a fungal based probiotic; FBP) into the rumen of calves on feed intake and calves performance was assessed and they concluded that the use of a fungal based probiotic stimulated forage intake in early weaned calves, and enhanced live weight gain without causing any obvious side effect. *Orpinomyces spp.* isolated from Korean native goat and dosed with 200 ml culture (7 days incubated) @ 10^6 cfu/ml to 4 sheep daily intraruminally, with other treatments containing 4 sheep each dosed with 200 ml broth (control) and 200 ml autoclaved culture (containing fungal enzymes only) per day. The sheep were fed with Orchard grass hay 560 gm/day and concentrate mixture 240 gm/day (roughage: conc ratio 80:20). Fungal culture administration showed an increased nutrient digestibility (DM digestibility from 71.5 to 75.2%, NDF digestibility from 65.1 to 68.9%; ADF digestibility from 57.3 to 62.9%), nitrogen retention, increased population of total bacteria (2-fold), cellulolytic bacteria (1.3-fold) and fungi (2-fold), increased rumen VFA concentration (TVFA concentration increased from 6.57 to 8.33 mM) and fibrolytic enzyme activities, but fungal enzyme administration could not show any effect as they being proteins rapidly degraded in rumen without any effect.

The rumen degradation of DM and fibrous components, besides gas production profile by anaerobic fungi which were compared in cattle and buffalo, were influenced by cell wall structural carbohydrate and varied between cattle and buffalo. The overall NDF disappearance among feedstuff differed but remained alike owing to source of rumen fungi. They observed that the fibrous moieties of hay were maximally degraded by both ruminant fungi, though, magnitude of ADF disappearance exceeded in buffalo than cattle for Berseem and Oat hay. *Orpinomyces spp.* C^{14} isolated from cow and dozed to 6 crossbred calves of 10 months of age @ 160 ml (10^6 cfu/ml)/animal/ week. The calves were fed wheat straw: conc. mix 50:50 on DM basis with 1 kg green oat/animal/day. Average daily gain was significantly higher (15.37%); FCR and feed efficiency also increased significantly. Nutrient digestibility was increased significantly for CF, NDF, and ADF after fungal administration. DE value also increased in terms of TDN. The pH and NH_3-N were lower, whereas TVFA, Total -N, TCA-N and number of zoospores were increased significantly in rumen of fungi fed group.

Piromyces spp isolated from blue bull and fed to 8 growing male buffalo calves of 16 months of age @ 200 ml culture having 10^6cfu/ml by daily mixing with concentrate mixture for a short period of 26 days. The calves were given a diet consisted of wheat straw: conc. mix: 50:50. Except CP and EE, digestibility of all other proximate and detergent fractions was increased significantly. *Neocallimastix* spp GR1 incorporated in ration on alternate days gave higher digestibility of nutrients of a total mixed ration based on wheat straw in female buffalo calves. An increase in milk production with the incorporation of fungal culture in straw based total mixed ration in buffaloes has also been reported at NDRI Karnal.

Microbial Requirements of Sulphur and its Utilization by Ruminants

Working with purified diets low in sulphur, indicated that supplemental sulphur is beneficial in increasing *in vitro* cellulose digestion and nitrogen retention by rumen microbes. Nitrogen retention and ADF digestion increased when organic or inorganic source of sulphur content in the diet was increased from 0.20% to 0.32%. Because the rumen microorganisms can reduce oxidized forms of sulphur to forms which can be incorporated into organic compounds, ruminants have the ability to obtain their sulphur supply from inorganic sources of sulphur. Inorganic sulfate can be substituted for organic sulphur sources such as methionine and vice versa. However, elemental sulphur used as sulphur source, has generally been shown not to be so readily available than sulfate or organic sources, probably owing to its lower solubility in the rumen fluid Sulphur from elemental sulphur and sodium sulfate was 30% and 50% as available as that of methionine. However, true retention data concluded that sulphur from elemental sulphur and sodium sulfate was 38 and 80% as available, as sulphur from methionine, respectively. Addition of sulphur to urea-based supplements for ruminants consuming mature forages increased N retention and forage digestibility. The reason for the increase in intake and digestibility of dry matter and organic matter when sodium sulfate is added to diets can be explained by the better utilization of the nitrogen present. However, the effect of sulphur supplementation is present only if the level of nitrogen is adequate in the diet Moreover, with the addition of sulphur to the diet of spear grass and urea, the concentration of rumen ammonia is reduced and more nitrogen is retained. In the N: S ratio of 11:1 each gram of added dietary sulphur yields 69 g of bacterial protein in the rumen. A mean value of 18.5:1 ratio (N: S) for mixed rumen bacteria, ranging between 8.6: 1 and 30.8: 1, and a mean value of 21.6:1 for protozoa, ranging between 14:1 and 38:1. From this, they concluded that a ratio of 20: I between available nitrogen and available sulphur should be adequate to meet the requirements of rumen microbes. Recent studies have indicated that the optimal dietary sulphur level for maximum daily gain of goat kids was approximately 0.22% of dietary dry matter with N: S ratio of 10: 1. Therefore, the optimal dietary sulphur level presumably improved performance by enhancing bacterial protein synthesis in the rumen and improving the amino acid balance. However, in vivo digestibility was highest with 0.11 % of sulphur as calcium sulfate in the diet. Apparent digestibility of dry matter, organic matter, ADF, and crude protein were increased linearly by adding 0.6, 0.28, and 0.36% sulphur as calcium sulphate in the diet.

There is an availability of several sources of sulphur and it was found that a N: S ratio of 10: 1 resulted in major microbial protein synthesis *in vitro* when sulphur was supplied through sulfate salts of sodium, potassium, calcium, iron, and ammonium, as well as through methionine. However, the best level with zinc sulfate or cysteine was 40: 1. Use of elemental sulphur at 15:1 ratio in dwarf goats and sheep showed better N retention and apparent digestibility of dry matter compared with 28: 1, 7: 1, and 6:1 ratio (N:S). No difference in apparent digestibility of dry matter, NDF, and ADF among lambs was observed. This sub-optimal level of minerals is indicated by enhanced fibre digestibility. In particular sulphur supplement has been reported to enhance the breakdown of cellulose and lignocellulose by rumen microorganisms. In recent years, the sulphur content of forage diets has been recognized as a significant factor governing the size of the rumen fungal population whereby, a deficiency of dietary sulphur could limit their growth in the rumen, and hence limit their contribution to plant tissue digestion. Anaerobic fungi were not detected in sheep fed *Digitaria pentzii* hay harvested from sulphur deficient plots, whereas the hay collected from the same plots after an application of sulphur fertilizer supported an active population of rumen fungi, the number of zoospores per ml were 4,000 to 6,000, and with methionine supplementation (4.5 g/day) the amount was only of 4,100 per ml. An increase in bacteria, protozoa, and sporangia of rumen anaerobic fungi in sheep supplemented with sulfate was reported however the sulphur content of wheat stubble affects the number of rumen fungi. Unlike low sulphur, *Digitaria pentzii* fungi were found in sheep receiving low sulphur wheat straw even though they were present only in low numbers. This difference between *Digitaria* and straw may be due to varying components of the feeds or, more probably, to the ability to detect small populations of rumen anaerobic fungi, ability which has been gained with wider experience.

Rumen anaerobic fungi have been found in the rumen of sheep fed tropical hay, and they appeared to contribute to digestion when there was adequate dietary sulphur. In a study of sulphur deficient wheat straw fed to sheep it was found showed that two types of anaerobic fungi were present in the rumen. In culture, one fungus produced an obvious mycelium, whereas the other produced a sporangium from spherical bodies. The straw diet did not support normal populations of these fungi. However, dietary methionine supplementation allowed the proliferation of the mycelial type (MT) but not the non-mycelial type (NMT). In addition to cellulose digestion, the fungi apparently degrade other structural elements of plant tissues, such as hemicellulose and pectin. It has been seen that rumen fungi are abundant with lignocellulose-rich diets, and selectively colonize plant tissues, especially those with thick or lignified cell walls. The development of fungi depends not only on the substrate on which they become attached, but also on the rumen medium. This fact can explain the results on the change of the sulphur status of the feed had no detectable effect upon numbers of viable bacteria. However, changing the feed from sulphur (+) to sulphur (-) grass increased the number of cellulolytic fungi. This effect probably was caused by the increase of fiber in grasses without sulphur fertilization.

Plant cell wall compounds stimulated zoospore production resulting in their higher population, zoosporogenesis was also induced by heme-type compounds. In Australia, sulphur fertilized grass and methionine supplemented diets resulted in increased fungal populations. And increased rumen fungi populations occurred with alfalfa versus Bermuda grass and mature versus immature wheat forage diets.

Sulphur can be utilized by *N. patriciarum* when supplied as L-cysteine, methionine or sodium sulfide. Sulfate, or reduced sulphur sources including dithiothreitol, 2-mercaptoethanol and thioglycollate were not utilized, but did not interfere with the utilization of cysteine S or sulfide S. The amino acid methionine acted as a source of sulphur only in the presence of compounds which generated a low redox potential in the medium, such as dithiothreitol or 2-mercaptoethanol. The low redox potential in the rumen would ensure the availability of L-cysteine and sulfide from the microbial hydrolysis of dietary proteins and sulphur containing amino acids. Sulphur containing amino acids and sulfide can be detected in rumen contents at any time and are unlikely to limit the growth of *Neocallimastix* spp *in vivo*.

The digestibility of sulphur amino acids in rumen bacterial protein was less than that of rumen fungi; this suggested that increasing fungal populations in the rumen at the expense of bacteria would be unlikely to cause deleterious effects on the quality of protein available for absorption at the small intestine. This may have important implications in sheep grazing low quality forages if procedures can be developed to increase the rumen fungal population thereby enhancing the voluntary feed intake and rate of fiber degradation. In many sulphur-deficient areas of the world sulphur fertilization has been used to promote forage production, and under these conditions the probability of a deficiency of this element occurring in animals fed forages and grains has become more remote. However, the total sulphur and others minerals content in forages may not always be a reliable indicator of availability to the rumen microorganisms. Thereby, with poor quality forages or with forages grown on sulphur deficient soil or with these forages fed non-protein nitrogen, sulphur supplementation will most likely be needed to meet the sulphur requirements of the animal. However, demonstrated that voluntary intake and dry matter digestibility of sulphur fertilized grass was lower than that of the control grass when the determinations were made with sheep supplemented with sulphur.

Supplementation with sodium sulfate or methionine with a semi-purified diet containing 4% urea and the S-content increasing from 0.05 to 0.15% through either sodium sulfate or methionine, both cellulose digestion and nitrogen retention were increased. The rumen population in animals feeding with low-quality roughage and supplemented with 0.21 % sulphur, contain 10% more bacteria, 22 % more protozoa, and 69% more fungal zoospores. The proportional increase in rumen fungi population was coupled with a

16% increase in fiber digestion. The ratio of nitrogen to sulphur retention is determined by the amounts of nitrogen and sulphur deposited in body tissue. Generally, diets supplying more sulphur tend to result in higher retention of both nitrogen and sulphur. It was suggested that an increased biomass of rumen fungi in sheep may result in increased quantities of essential and sulphur amino acids being absorbed from the small intestine. This would be expected to stimulate wool growth and may have important implications for wool production in sheep grazing low-quality roughages.

The utilization of inorganic sulfate by rumen microorganisms in the synthesis of the sulphur containing amino acids has been well substantiated long back and its role to synthesize rumen fungi has been studied in recent past. But numerous studies have indicated that methionine is one of the amino acids limiting rumen microbial growth and substrate fermentation rates in the rumen. For instance, sulphur has long been recognized as an essential element for rumen microorganisms. Sulphur and nitrogen metabolism are closely associated in ruminants. The action of the rumen microflora may completely alter the dietary form of both of these elements; for instance, the degradation of dietary protein to yield ammonia and sulfide or the synthesis of microbial protein from dietary urea and inorganic sulphate. When rumen microorganisms are incubated with radioactive sulfate, radioactive sulphur can be found in cysteine, cystine and methionine of the bacterial proteins. But, in order for sulphur amino acids to be synthesized in the rumen, sulphur must be present in the diet. In addition, the sulphur containing vitamins, such as thiamine and biotin are synthesized by the rumen microbes; moreover, sodium sulfate and methionine have been shown to stimulate the synthesis of riboflavin and vitamin B_{12} by rumen microorganisms to a greater degree than when the source of sulphur was cysteine or elemental sulphur.

As sources of sulphur, sodium sulfate, calcium sulfate, and methionine were equal at equal sulphur concentration in their ability to promote *in vitro* lignocellulose digestion with rumen bacteria; the optimum was 0.16 to 0.24% S as sodium sulfate or calcium sulfate and 0.32% S as methionine. The theory which best explains the results of this study, is the one in which the supplemental sulphur stimulates bacterial activity in the rumen. Although some pure strains of rumen microorganisms have a preference for certain forms of sulphur, due to the symbiotic relationship of a mixed culture of rumen microorganisms, the form of sulphur does not appear to have a significant influence on their activity. However, some strains isolated from the rumen were able to synthesize cysteine and methionine from inorganic sulfate. The structural components of forage have been considered to play a part in limiting forage digestibility. In addition to structural components, mineral levels in forage are often inadequate for efficient microbial activity and fiber degradation. Moreover, the total sulphur content in forages may not always be a reliable indicator of sulphur availability to the rumen microorganisms. Sulphur supplementation enhanced the breakdown of cellulose and hemicellulose by enhancing the proliferation of rumen anaerobic fungi in the rumen through zoospores of rumen fungi incorporated in the complete feed block diet of the ruminants for enhancing the nutritive value of low grade roughages

The above-discussed literature suggested that introduction of rumen anaerobic fungi into the rumen of animals having natural fungi can improve the nutrient utilization of straw based diets for enhancing productivity from low grade roughages. So, as and when the zoospores elite fungi are administered in the wheat straw based complete feed blocks for feeding ruminants; some sulphur sources must be added for the proliferation of the rumen anaerobic fungi for further enhancing the digestibility and nutritive value of wheat straw.

References

Akin, D.E. and Windham, W.R. (1989). Influence of diet on rumen fungi. Page 75, In: The roles of Protozoa and Fungi in Ruminant Digestion.

Borneman, W.S., Ljungdahl, L.Q., Hartley, R.D. and Akin, D.E. (1992). *Microbiol.* 58: 3762.

Bray, A.C. and Hemsley, J.A. (1969). *Aust. J. Agric. Res.* 20: 759.

Breton, A., Bernalier, A. Dusser, M. Fonty, G. Gaillard, B. and Guillot, J. (1990). *Microbiol. Lett.* 70: 177.-182.

Calderon-Cortes, J.F., Elliot, R. and Ford, C.W. (1989). Influence of rumen fungi on the nutrition of sheep fed forage diets. In: The Roles of Protozoa and Fungi in Ruminant Digestion (J.V. Nolan, R.A. Leng and D.I. Demeyer, eds.). Penumble Books, Armidale, Australia, pp.181-187.

Dayanand, T., Nagpal, R., Puniya, A.K., Sehgal, J.P., Singh, K. (2007). *J. Anim. Feed Sci.*, 16: 484-489.

Dey, A., Sehgal, J.P., Puniya, A.K and Singh, K. (2004a). *Asian-Aust. J. Anim. Sci.*, 17: 820-824

Dey, Avijit, Sehgal, J.P and Puniya, A.K. (2004b). *Indian Vet. Med. Jour.*, 28 (4): 325-327.

Givens, D.I., Everington, J.M. and Adamson, A.H. (1989). *Anim. Feed Sci. Tech.*, 26: 323-335.

Ho, Y.W., Barr, D.J.S., Abdulah, N., Jalaludin, S. and Kudo, H. (1993). *Mycotaxon*, 47:285-293.

Joblin, K.N. (1990). Bacterial and protozoal interactions with ruminal fungi. In: Microbial and Plant Opportunities to Improve Lignocellulose Utilization by Ruminants ed. Akin, D.E., Lungdahl, L.G., Wilson, J.R. and Harris, P.J. pp. 311-324. New York: Elsevier.

Kopecney, J., Hodrova, B. and Stewart, C.S. (1996). *Lett. Appl. Microbiol.*, 23: 1999-2002.

Kostiukovosky, V.A., Okunev, O.N. and Tarakanov, B.V. (1991). *J. Gen.Microbiol.*, 137: 1759-1764.

Krause, D.O., Dalrymple, B.P. Smith, W.J. Mackie, R.I. and McSweeney, C.S. (1999). *Microbiol.* 145: 1797-1807.

Orpin, C.G. (1977). *J. Gen. Microbiol.*, 101:181-189.

Paul, S.S., Kamra, D.N., Sastry, V.R.B., Sahu, N.P. and Agarwal, N. (2004). *Anim. Feed Sci. Technol.*, 115 (1-2): 143-157.

Prashant K., Shelke, S.K., Chabra,A. and Sehgal, J.P. (2008). *Ind. J. Anim. Nutr.*, 25:7-383.

Samanta, A.K., Walli, T.K., Batish, V.K., Grover, S., Rajpoot, Y.S. and Mohanty, A.K. (1999). *Ind. J. Anim. Nutr.*, 16: 275–278.

Sanjay (2009). Development of complete feed blocks based on low grade roughage fortified with potential anaerobic fungal zoospores and their evaluation in buffaloes. Ph.D. Thesis, NDRI, Karnal.

Sehgal, J.P., Neelkhantan, J., Puniya, A.K., Singh, Kishan and Prasad, K.S.N. (2002). Use of ruminal anaerobic fungi to improve the nutritive value of cereal straws. Annual Report of National Dairy Research Institute, (ICAR) Karnal.

Shelke, S.K., Chhabra, A, Puniya, A.K. and Sehgal, J.P. (2009). *Annals Microbiol.* 59(3) 415-418.

Thareja A., Puniya A.K., Goel G., Nagpal R., Sehgal J.P., Singh P., Singh, K. (2006). *Arch. Anim. Nutr.*, 60: 412-417.

Theodorou, M.K., Beever, D.E., Haines, M.J. and Brooks, A. (1990). *Anim. Prod.*, (Abstract) 50:577.

Tripathi, V.K., Sehgal, J.P., Puniya A.K., Singh, K. (2007a). *Anaerobe*. 13:36-39.

Tripathi, V.K, Sehgal, J.P, Puniya, A.K. and Singh, K. (2007b). *Arch. Anim. Nutr.*, 61: 416.

□□□

Animal Nutrition, 2012
eds. Dr. (Mrs.) Usha R. Mehra et al., pp. 519-528
Satish Serial Publishing House e-mail : info@satishserial.com; website : www.satishserial.com

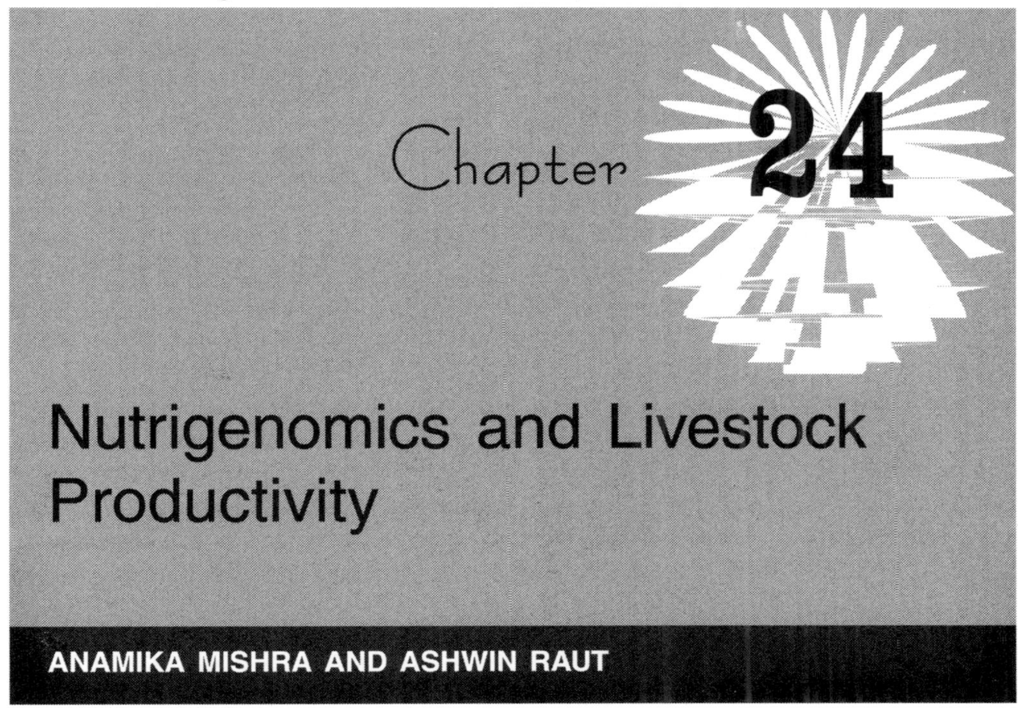

Chapter 24

Nutrigenomics and Livestock Productivity

ANAMIKA MISHRA AND ASHWIN RAUT

The relationship of nutrition with health and production is long known but how the components of diet exert their effects is being gradually unraveled. In the post genomic era it is becoming evident that the genome, which is the hereditary information of an individual, is in fact the blueprint of the life of an organism. The differences in the genetic make up or the DNA sequence between individuals result in the difference in their performance potential, response to external factors and also decide their very ability to survive under certain conditions. The genes present in the genome of an individual exert their impact biologically by coding for certain proteins this is called the expression of the gene. It is well established that all genes present in an individual's genome are not expressed always. Expression of genes varies between individuals, between the different cells of same individual and also the genes expressed by the same cell differ over a period of time and under different conditions. There is a constant switching on and off of the genes going on under the influence of genetic and environmental factors and all physiological processes and pathological events are the direct or indirect results of an intricately orchestrated expression of a particular set of genes. Studies in humans, animals and cell culture systems demonstrate that bioactive molecules originating from diet are one of the key environmental factors and can regulate gene expression in diverse ways (Mead, 2007).

Nutrient-gene interactions are known as widespread, ancient features across species. However, with the advent of high throughput molecular biological tools and analysis systems, information in the field of nutrient-gene interactions has rapidly accumulated in the past decade. We have thus started uncovering the mechanism by which mammals sense nutrient status and regulate their metabolism accordingly. With this, a new area of study called nutrigenomics has emerged (Roche, 2006). Nutrigenomics is a term coined to describe the use of cutting-edge molecular technologies in the understanding of diet-gene interactions and human or animal health. It is the study of molecular relationships between nutrition and the response of genes, with the aim of extrapolating how subtle changes in nutrition can affect health and productivity. It includes how diet affects the way genes are expressed, the effect of genes on how the body uses nutrients, and the effects of nutrients on molecular level processes in the body.

Another apparently similar term is nutrigenetics, which encompasses studies to understand how the genetic makeup of an individual coordinates their response to diet (Ordovas and Mooser, 2004) and thus considers underlying genetic polymorphisms Polymorphism is nothing but variations in the DNA sequences of a particular gene in different individuals in a given population. In the short, nutrigenomics is the measuring of nutrition responsive genome activity, whilst nutrigenetics is the science of population variation [Figure-1] (Mariman, 2006). Both these fields have distinct approaches to elucidate the interaction between diet and genes but with a common ultimate goal to optimize health and production through the personalization of diet. They provide powerful approaches to unravel the complex relationship between nutritional molecules, genetic polymorphisms and the biological system as a whole.

Fundamentals of Nutrigenomics

The primary goals of nutrigenomics research are: 1) to establish dietary recommendations that have a high predictive value with respect to disease prevention, and account for modifying the effects of genetic variation; and 2) to design effective dietary regimens for efficient productivity and management of complex disease (Stover, 2004). The identification of alleles that contribute to polygenetic production traits is expected to catalyze organism-based research that will support the rational design of targeted dietary regimens for the high performance phenotypes. Such expectations from nutrigenomic research are based on the facts that 1) Common dietary chemicals act on the genome, either directly or indirectly, to alter gene expression or structure (Clarke and Abraham, 1992). 2) Under certain circumstances and in some individuals, diet can be a serious risk factor for a number of diseases. 3) Some diet-regulated genes (and their normal, common variants) are likely to play a role in the onset, incidence, progression, and/or severity of chronic diseases and productivity. 4) The degree to which diet influences the production efficiency may depend on an individual's genetic makeup. 5) Dietary intervention based on knowledge of nutritional requirement, nutritional status, and genotype (i.e., "individualized nutrition") can be used to prevent chronic diseases as well as to enhance or economize livestock production (Kaput, 2005).

Pathways of Nutrient Action on Gene Expression

Until quite recently, most scientists thought that food had basically one job: it was metabolized to provide energy for the cell. Indeed, that is what happens to most dietary chemicals - but not all. Some don't get metabolized at all; instead, the moment they are ingested, they peel off and become ligands - molecules that bind to proteins involved in "turning on" certain genes to one degree or another. A diet that's particularly out of balance, thus causes gene expressions that nudge us towards chronic illness unless a precisely-tailored "intelligent diet" is employed to restore the equilibrium. Dietary chemicals can affect gene expression directly or indirectly. At the cellular level, nutrients may: 1) act as ligands for transcription factor receptors 2) be metabolized by primary or secondary metabolic pathways, thereby altering concentrations of substrates or intermediates; or 3) positively or negatively affect signal pathways (Kaput and Rodriguez, 2004). Here nutrients are seen as signals that target a specific cell in the body and elicit specific reactions. The nutrients are detected by a sensory system in the cell. Such a sensory system works like sensory ecology whereby the cell obtains information through the signal, the nutrient, about its environment, which is the diet. The sensory system that interprets information from nutrients about the dietary environment includes transcription factors together with many additional proteins. Once the nutrient interacts with such a sensory system, it changes gene, protein expression and metabolite production in accordance with the level of nutrient it senses. As a result, different diets elicit different patterns of gene and protein expression and metabolite production. Data indicate that nutritional factors, e.g., various vitamins regulated through dietary intake, can interact with other regulatory networks, such as tissue-specific, developmental, and hormonal factors, as well as dietary fat or carbohydrates - to regulate gene expression. It is worth mentioning here that the mechanism of regulation of gene expression is not a universal one. The stage at which nutritional intervention can occur differs with the gene as well as with the nutrient involved. While in most lipogenic enzymes the regulation is at the transcriptional level in response to nutrition, nutritional regulation of G6PD gene expression is posttranscriptional. Change in the rate of synthesis of the mature G6PD mRNA involves regulation of the efficiency of splicing of the nascent G6PD transcript (Salati *et al.*, 2004). Amino acid availability can modify the expression of target genes at the level of transcription, mRNA stability and translation (Averous *et al.*, 2003).

Bioactive Food Components and Targets

There are numerous examples to state and scientifically prove how micro and macronutrients control the expression of gene and thus influence the health and physiology of the organism. However, since the pathways branch and sub-branch into various conditional and alternative pathways the influence of certain of the dietary components are not easy to comprehend and analyze. Dietary fats, carbohydrates, proteins, vitamins and minerals all have their respective say in regulation of gene expression though they may differ in their mechanisms of action, target gene or tissue and magnitude of impact.

Specific fatty acid regulated transcription factors have been identified, these factors include peroxisome proliferator-activated receptors (PPARα, -β/δ and -γ), oestrogen receptors (ERs) and sterol regulatory element binding proteins (SREBPs) (Fekete and Brown, 2007). All these receptors are regulated either by direct binding of (oxidized) fatty acids, fatty acyl-coenzyme A or oxidized fatty acid (eicosanoid) regulation of cell surface receptors and that of intracellular calcium levels as well as activation of signaling cascades (Jump, 1999). At the cellular level, the physiological response to fatty acids depends on the quantity, chemistry and duration of the fat ingested. Dietary carbohydrates, both independently and through insulin effect, deeply influence the transcription of the fatty acid synthase gene in a number of species. In ruminants, the presence of glucose in the intestine increases sodium-dependent glucose transporter 1 (SGLT1) mRNA abundance by 2-fold, with a 60- to 90-fold increase in cotransporter number (Drackley *et al.*, 2006). Protein-rich diets cause a shortage of mRNA necessary for expression of the fatty acid synthase gene in the adipocytes, resulting in the moderation of total body fat. Amino acids by themselves can play, in concert with hormones, an important role in the control of gene expression (Averous *et al.*, 2003). Bivalent metals like zinc or cadmium enhance the transcription rate of the metallothionein (MT) gene in intestinal tissue (Ouellette *et al.*, 1982). Iron influences transferrin and ferritin concentrations by exerting an effect on mRNA stability and the translation rate (Bremner and Beattie, 1990). Vitamin D can both downregulate and upregulate mitochondrial transcription in a tissue specific manner. Vitamin D receptor directly binds to DNA at vitamin D responsive elements as a homodimer or heterodimer to activate gene transcription. Vitamin A in the form of retinoic acid upregulates the transcription of several mitochondrial as well as nuclear gene. Growth hormone, glycerolphosphate dehydrogenase and leptin genes are the vitamin A responsive genes and the target tissues are in the adrenal glands, testes, cerebellum, kidneys, prostate, cerebral cortex, skin and the viscera (Scribner *et al.*, 2005). Hyperammonaemia due to significant depression of ornithine transcarboxylase gene expression is seen in biotin deficient subjects (Yuichi *et al.*, 1996).

Livestock Performance

Practically speaking, animal nutritionists have always been using dietary manipulations to affect and control the phenotype/performance. However the exact genetic cascade that was being targeted by such manipulations were not known. Since the central dogma of molecular biology states that DNA makes RNA makes protein, the application of molecular biology to understand nutrient metabolism centers on identifying conditions that lead to the amplification of genetic information and synthesis of several copies of RNA and ultimately the initiation and progression of protein synthesis. The ultimate end point of these processes in livestock is a coordinated change in cellular and tissue metabolism to maintain homeostasis or to undergo homeorhesis to support a new physiological state (Dackley *et al.*, 2006). On these lines of action theoretically it is possible to control the performance of animals for all traits having a genetic component by nutrient management and manipulation.

Nutrigenomic studies in livestock are still rare, but they will become more important as we develop an understanding of the relationship between nutrition, genetics, animal performance, and product quality. Advances in the recent past are providing new evidences and biomarkers that have not been elucidated in the past. The recognition that fatty acids are regulators of metabolism and act in the cell nucleus to control expression of genes for fatty acid synthesis has been extended to investigations on the origins of milk fat depression in dairy cows. The reduction in milk fat when fish oil is fed is due to decreased mRNA abundance of lipogenic enzymes like acetyl CoA carboxylase, fatty acid synthase, and stearoyl-CoA desaturase (Ahnadi *et al.*, 2002). Also the reduced milk fat synthesis in lactating dairy cows caused by *trans*-10, *cis*-12 CLA involves a reduction in mRNA for acetyl CoA carboxylase, fatty acid synthase, stearoyl-CoA desaturase, lipoprotein lipase, fatty acid binding protein, and glycerol phosphate acyltransferase (Bauman *et al.*, 2008). These changes are directly linked to a substantial reduction in lipogenic activity in explant cultures in vitro. These data provide understanding of the molecular basis for milk fat depression, a practical milk production problem that has been recognized for several decades.

The importance of maternal nutrition during pregnancy on the gene expression and development of offspring was demonstrated in sheep (Han *et al.*, 2004). In pigs, nutrient excretion was shown to vary depending on breed, suggesting differences in metabolism due to genotype (Rivera-Ferre *et al.*, 2006). Flushing effects (sow, ewe) can partly be explained by the effect of excess portions (i.e. high-carbohydrates with the concentrate intake) that activate fat synthesis by strikingly enhancing the fatty acid synthase transcription rate (Fekete and Brown, 2007). This again is a management practice since long but the reason why the impact of flushing differs between populations can be explained better now with the nutrigenomic approach.

Possible Application in Animal Production and Health

As the understanding about how bioactive food components modify genetic events becomes clearer, the current conundrum surrounding appropriate dietary recommendations should evolve into rational and personalized intervention strategies to improve health, production and minimize the risk of disease. Nutrigenomical databanks may make possible the selection for metabolic disease resistance. Data will enable us to screen susceptible breeds or individuals and to give guidance for optimized or individualized diets to prevent the onset of polygenic, nutrition-related disorders in genetically predisposed individuals. Hopefully, in future, it may become possible to determine cell-physiologically appropriate nutrient allowances for production animals. Nutrigenomics and nutrigenetics respectively, are potentially of huge importance to the health care system and to the food industry, as well as to those seeking to understand the biology underlying normal homeostasis and disease.

Some of the areas where nutrigenomics can make is presence felt and enhance the rate of achievement in the field of animal productivity are lean meat production, designing of daily rations for transient high-yielding dairy cows, reduced milk fat production during the critical periods of dairy cows in a controlled manner, finding biomarkers of nutritional status and diseases etc.

Diet is a potent mechanism for altering the environment of cells in most organs, particularly the gastrointestinal tract which is inhabited by a great number of microbes. This microbiotic genome comprises approximately 100 times more genes than the body of monogastric animals. The modern terms gaining currency for such populations are microbiotome or microbiota rather than microflora. The role of the gut microbiotome in systemic responses to dietary nutrients, drugs and toxins is just as important as tissue metabolism (Nicholson *et al.*, 2005). Manipulation of the diet may be a way of changing microflora to treat intestinal disorders indirectly in addition to direct effects of changing the character of nutrient supply on gene function that controls intermediary metabolism.

Other genomic outcomes, including embryo rescue (Pennisi, 2002), are emerging as criteria for establishing tolerable upper limits during reproductive ages. Individual nutrients, when administered in supra-physiological levels during critical developmental windows, can rescue severe genetic lesions. This is the concept of nutritional rescue of genetic mutations, or "good diet hides genetic mutations". The prevalence of this rescue phenomenon is not established, but animal studies indicate that nutrients can modify the viability of genomes, including genomes that confer atypical nutrient requirements to the surviving fotus. Nutrition has a critical role in DNA metabolism and repair and this awareness is leading to the development of the new field of Genome Health Nutrigenomics. A deficiency in a micronutrient required as a cofactor or as an integral part of the structure of a DNA repair could mimic the effect of a genetic polymorphism that reduces the activity of that enzyme.

Because of the vast improvements made in veterinary medicine and companion animal nutrition in recent years, dogs and cats are living longer than ever before. Now, instead of being troubled by intestinal parasites or succumbing to viral infections (e.g., canine distemper), many companion animals are living long enough to suffer from obesity. Renal disease, arthritis and several diseases associated with abnormal immune function (e.g., ulcerative colitis, atopic disease) also are becoming more prominent in cats and dogs (Swanson *et al.*, 2003). Nutritional genomics and proteomics will definitely play a vital role in enhancing our understanding of metabolism and optimizing companion animal nutritional and health status and pet foods designing.

There are high expectations that nutrigenomics, when coupled successfully with more traditional methodologies, will provide previously unreachable information on the dynamics of metabolic control in response to nutrient supply, will serve to clarify the causal factors of metabolic disorders, and will shape future feeding strategies to enhance productive efficiency and animal well-being.

Limitations

As of yet, nutrigenomics with relevance to animal production is in its infancy. Although this area of research is promising, the evidence remains weak at this stage. The enthusiasm of designing individualized diets is tempered by an inability to identify low-penetrant contributing alleles in multigenic traits (Schork *et al.*, 2000), insufficient knowledge to accurately modify genome function and cell physiology through diet, and an inability to address and minimize the potential for unintended consequences resulting from the administration of nutrients at intake levels that cannot normally be achieved with a healthy and natural food-based diet (German *et al.*, 2003). The development of bovine-specific metabolic maps is necessary for greater understanding of the complex molecular basis of nutrient metabolism in support of traits like milk production, growth and reproduction.

The tools to study protein expression and metabolite production have not yet developed to the point as to enable efficient and reliable measurements. Transcript profiling using DNA microarrays or candidate gene analysis is a static measure of the pool size of individual mRNA in a cell or tissue and does not provide any information on the dynamics of mRNA synthesis (transcription) or RNA degradation (RNA stability). Determining the rate of mRNA synthesis typically involves use of nuclear run-on assays that measure the relative amount of new transcripts made from the previously initiated RNA polymerases and provides a measure of the *in vivo* rate of transcription of DNA to mRNA. Levels of some key proteins (e.g., the transferrin receptor) are regulated at the level of RNA stability; however, measures of RNA degradation rate are presently not easily attainable *in vivo* and therefore nutritional impacts on gene expression usually are only described for transcription rate and mRNA abundance. All these technologies are still in the process of development. There is a need to develop guidelines and standards, which incorporate the state-of-the-art techniques and enable and encourage researchers to apply the 'omics' technologies in ways that can be replicated, so that comparisons between laboratories can be made and facilitate pooling of samples and data. Also once such data has been created, it will need to be integrated together in order to produce results and dietary recommendations. Since the diet comprises of a multitude of nutritional and chemical molecules each capable of regulating disparate biological processes, and thus an approach similar to the pharmaceutical industry, i.e., the "one drug one target" paradigm cannot be used for nutrigenomics (Robert *et al.*, 2001). Also nutritional requirements are recognized to be complex traits that are subject to modification by both genetic background and by nutrient-nutrient interactions. A comprehensive understanding of the mechanisms that underlie the reciprocal interactions of dietary components with the genome is not attainable by genomic profiling approaches alone (Stover, 2004). Hence to enable the manipulation of genome expression and stability for benefit through diet with high predictive value extensive research and data interpretation with multidisciplinary expertise is imperative.

Nonetheless nutrigenomics holds great promise to revolutionize the way we think about measuring nutritional effects and evaluating the nutritional value of dietary components.

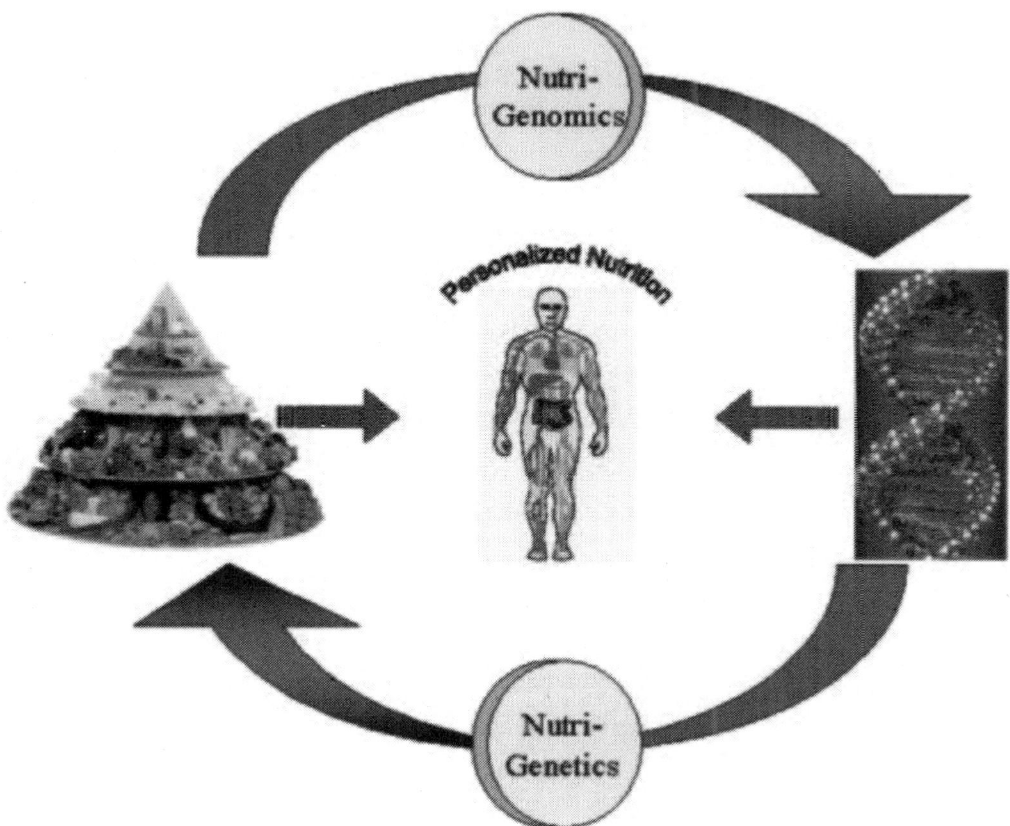

Fig. 1 : Nutrigenomics and nutrigenetics: two sides of a coin. For the target goal of personalized nutrition to be realized, the effects of diet on whole-body metabolism (i.e., genes, proteins, and metabolites) and the influence of genotype on nutritionally related disease must be considered. Food pyramid image obtained from: http://www.shb.ie/content454667358_1.cfm

References

Ahnadi, C.E., Beswick, N., Delbecchi, L., Kennelly, J.J. and Lacasse, P. (2002). *J Dairy Res.*, 69: 521-531.

Averous, J., Bruhat, A., Mordier, S. and Fafournoux, P. (2003). *J. Nutr.*, 133: 2040S–2045S.

Bauman, D.E., Perfield, J.W. 2nd, Harvatine, K.J. and Baumgard, L.H. (2008). *J. Nutr.*, 138: 403-409.

Bremner, I. and Beattie, J.H. (1990). *Annu. Rev. Nutr.*, 10: 63-83.

Clarke, S.D. and Abraham, S. (1992). *FASEB Journal*, 6: 3146-3152.

Drackley, J.K., Donkin, S.S. and Reynolds, C.K. (2006). *J. Dairy Sci.*, 89: 1324-1336.

Fekete, S.G. and Brown, D.L. (2007). *Acta Vet. Hungarica.* 55: 229–239.

German, J.B., Roberts, M.A. and Watkins, S.M. (2003). *J. Nutr.,* 133: 2078S-2083S.

Han, H.C., Austin, K.J., Nathanielsz, P.W., Ford, S.P., Nijland, M.J. and Hansen, T.R. (2004). *J. Physiol.,* 558:111-121.

Jump, D.B. (1999). *Annu. Rev. Nutr.,* 19: 63-69.

Kaput, J. and Rodriguez, R.L. (2004). *Phy. Genomics,* 16:166-177.

Kaput, J. (2005). *Annals New York Acad. Sci,* 1055: 64-79.

Mariman, E.C.M. (2006). *Biotech. Appl. Biochem,* 44:119-128.

Mead, M.N. (2007). *Environ. Health Perspect.,* 115, 584-589.

Nicholson, J.K., Holmes, E. and Wilson, I.D. (2005). *Nat. Rev. Microb.,* 3:431-438.

Ordovas, J.M. and Mooser, V. (2004). *Curr. Opin. lipidology,* 15:101-108.

Ouellette, A.J., Aviles, L., Burnweit, C.A., Frederick, D. and Malt, R.A. (1982). Am. J. Physiol., 243: G396.G403.

Pennisi, E. (2002). *Sci.,* 296:1010–1011.

Rivera-Ferre, M.G., Aguilera, J.F. and Nieto, R. (2006). *J. Anim. Sci.,* 84:3346-3355.

Roberts, M.A., Mutch, D.M. and German, J.B. (2001). *Curr. Opin. Biotech.,* 12: 516–522.

Roche, H.M. (2006). *J. Sci. Food Agric.,* 86:1156-1163.

Salati, L.M., Szeszel-Fedorowicz, W., Tao, H., Gibson, M.A., Amir-Ahmady, B., Stabile, L.P. and Hodge, D.L. (2004). *J. Nutri.,* 134: 2437S–2443S.

Schork, N.J., Fallin, D. and Lanchbury, J.S. (2000). *Clin. Genet.,* 58: 250–264.

Scribner, K.B., Odom, D.P. and McGrane, M.M. (2005). *J. Nutri.,* 135:2774-2779.

Stover, P.J. (2004). *Physiol Genomics.,* 16: 161–165.

Swanson, K.S., Schook, L.B. and Fahey, J.G.C. (2003). *J. Nutr.,* 133: 3033-3040.

Yuichi, M., Sumio, K., Yochiaki, I., Kazuto, F., Igura, T. and Matsuzawa, Y. (1996). *J. Nutr.* 126:61.66.

□□□

Animal Nutrition, 2012
eds. Dr. (Mrs.) Usha R. Mehra et al., pp. 529-548
Satish Serial Publishing House e-mail : info@satishserial.com; website : www.satishserial.com

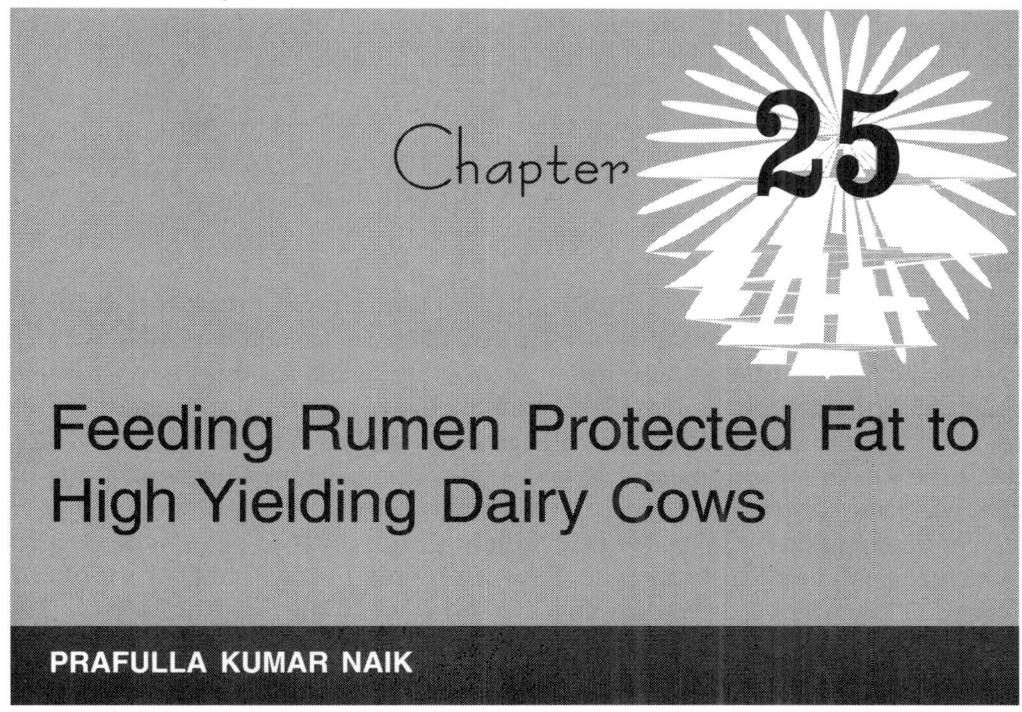

Feeding Rumen Protected Fat to High Yielding Dairy Cows

PRAFULLA KUMAR NAIK

In modern dairy farming system, there is an increasing trend of maintaining high yielding dairy cows by the progressive livestock farmers. In India, dairy cows having daily milk yield of more than 15 kg are generally treated as high yielders (Reddy, 2003). Immediately after parturition, there is decline in feed intake due to changes in rumen environment and various hormone profiles, which is resumed later than the peak milk yield. However, following peak, milk yield decreases with simultaneous increase in feed intake of the animal to normal level. Tremendous energy output associated with milk fat secretion and decline feed intake, puts high yielding dairy cows in negative energy balance, particularly during early lactation (first three months postpartum). Inability of high yielding dairy cows to maintain a positive energy balance during early lactation imposes considerable metabolic stress (Bell, 1995) leading to metabolic disorders and suboptimal milk production (Drackley, 1999), for which they need scientific and systematic feeding practices. With limited dry matter (DM) intake, energy intake of animal can be enhanced by making the diet energy dense, which can be achieved by incorporating either concentrates (cereal grains) or fat. Addition of concentrates at higher level decreases fibre intake and leads to acidosis (Palmquist and Jenkins, 1980). As fat is the most energy dense nutrient (contains 2.25 times more energy than carbohydrate and protein), its dietary supplementation is the best alternative for enhancement of energy density of ration without lowering fibre intake (Naik *et al.*, 2009[a]).

Basic Concepts on Fats

Lipids are group of substances of plant and animal origin, insoluble in water but soluble in common organic solvents, which are structurally categorized as simple, compound and derived lipids. Simple lipids contain only alcohol and fatty acids (FA), which include fats, oils and waxes. In fats and oils, alcohol is trihydric, known as glycerol or glyceride. Glycerol, in which all three alcohol groups are estrified with FA are known as neutral fat or triacylglycerol or triglyceride (TG), which may be either simple (same types of FA) or mixed (different types of FA). Although, fats and oils have same general structure and chemical properties, they differ only in physical characteristics. Generally, at room temperature fats are solid, while oils are liquid. In waxes alcohol is mostly a monohydroxy or rarely a dihydroxy of higher molecular weight and FA are long chain.

Compound lipids contain glycerol or sphingosine (amino alcohol) along with FA with or without phosphate and nitrogen base or inositol or hexose sugar. Based on type of alcohol or nitrogen base, compound lipids can be broadly grouped into phospholipids (phosphatides) and glycolipids. Phospholipids may be phosphoglycerides or phosphoinositides or phosphosphingosides (sphingolipids). Phosphoglycerides contain glycerol, FA, phosphate and a nitrogen base, which may be either choline or ethanolamine or serine. Thus, based on type of nitrogen base, three important phosphoglycerides are lecithin (phosphatidyl choline), cephalin (phosphatidyl ethanolamine) and phosphatidyl serine. Phosphoinositides contain glycerol, FA, phosphate but the nitrogen base is replaced by inositol. Phosphosphingosides (sphingolipids) may be sphingomyelins or cerebrosides. Sphingomyelins contain sphingosine, FA, phosphate and either choline or ethanolamine; while cerebrosides contain sphingosine, FA, phosphate and hexose sugar (galactose or glucose). Glycolipids contain glycerol, FA and hexose sugar, which are mostly galactose (galactolipids) and rarely glucose (glucolipids).

Derived lipids include steroids (sterols, cholesterol, ergosterol, bile acids and salts, glucocorticoids, mineralocorticoids and sex hormones), terpenes (carotenoids, xanthophyll, chlorophyll and essential oils), fatty aldehydes, ketones and hydrocarbons.

Thus, FA are important constituents of all types of lipids and the type and proportions of FA determine physical and chemical properties of fat. FA contain chain of carbon atoms with a methyl group at one end and a terminal carboxyl group at other end. Based on number of carbon atoms, FA are grouped into short chain (less than 6 carbons), medium chain (6-12 carbons) and long chain (more than 12 carbons). Chain length of FA is determined by saponification number, which is defined as number of milligrams of alkali (KOH) required to saponify 1.0g of fat. Larger the saponification number, smaller is average FA chain length. FA may be without (saturated) or with double bonds (unsaturated). When FA contain more than one double bond, it is known as polyunsaturated fatty acids (PUFA). Degree of unsaturation of FA can be determined by iodine number, which is defined as number of grams of iodine absorbed by 100g of fat. Higher the iodine number, more is unsaturation of FA. Physical characteristics of fats and oils depend upon chain length and presence of double bonds in FA. Melting point of FA increases as chain length increases, but addition of double bond lowers the melting point of FA for a particular chain length. Carboxyl carbon atom of FA is numbered as carbon atom 1, where as carbon atoms 2 and 3 are designated as alpha (α) and beta (β), respectively. Methyl carbon atom at distal end of chain is designated as omega (Ω) carbon. Position of double bond in unsaturated fatty acids (USFA) is indicated with reference to carbon atom 1. Based on position of double bond nearest to omega carbon atom, PUSFA are grouped into oleic (Ω-9), linoleic (Ω-6) and linolenic (Ω-3) FA. Configuration of double bond of USFA may be in *cis* (hydrogen atoms on same side of double bond) or *trans* (hydrogen atoms on opposite side of double bond), giving a range of isomers (McDonald *et al.*, 2002).

Fat Content of Dairy Ration

In proximate analysis, dietary fats are expressed as ether extract (EE), which includes both true fats (FA) and ether soluble non-FA substances. In dairy ration, EE is mostly contributed by green fodder and concentrates (oil seeds, oil seed cakes, cereals and their byproducts). There is almost no variation in EE content of commonly grown fodder for livestock feeding, which is around 3% on DM basis. However, due to advances in various feed processing technologies, there is a large variation in EE content of concentrates, available in market. As per specifications of Bureau of Indian Standards (BIS), EE content of concentrate mixture should be at least 2.5-3.0%. EE content of most commonly used feed ingredients for livestock feeding (Gupta *et al.*, 2004) has been given in Table 1.

Table 1 : Ether extract (EE) content of commonly used feed ingredients

Feed ingredients	EE (%)
Cereal grains	
Wheat	2.0
Rice kani	1.8
Maize	2.5
Bajra	3.8
Barley	2.4
Triticale	1.3
Oil seeds	
Cottonseed (whole)	20.0
Soybean (whole)	20.0
Cereal byproducts	
Rice bran	16.0
Rice bran (ext.)	0.8
Wheat bran	3.5
Vegetable cakes	
Mustard seed cake	9.8
Mustard seed cake *(papri)*	2.5-3.5
Deoiled mustard seed cake (ext.)	0.5-1.0
Canola	8.0
Soybean meal (ext.)	0.9
Sunflower cake (ext.)	1.2
Cottonseed cake	8.8
Maize gluten meal	2.5
Groundnut cake (ext.)	1.0
Guar meal	5.0

Green fodder mostly contains galactolipids with linolenic acid ($C_{18:3}$) as predominant FA. Fat of concentrate sources are mostly TG with linoleic acid ($C_{18:2}$) as predominant FA. Besides, dairy ration also contains palmitic acid and oleic acid as most common FA and mono-unsaturated fatty acid (MUFA), respectively. Most FA of naturally occurring fats and oils are of straight chain, even numbered carbon atoms and with *cis* configuration (McDonald *et al.*, 2002). Non-FA lipid components of plant leaves are cuticular waxes, pigments, carotene, chlorophyll and other unsaponifiable materials. Up to 50% of forages and 20% of grain ether extractable materials may be of non-FA nature (Palmquist and Jenkins, 1980).

Ruminal Metabolism of Dietary Fat

Dietary fats entering rumen consist of high proportion of estrified FA as TG, phospholipids and galactolipids containing oleic acid, linoleic acid and linolenic acid as predominant FA. These dietary fats are metabolized by rumen micro-organisms for synthesis of microbial lipids, which involves two important steps i.e. lipolysis and biohydrogenation (Jenkins, 1993). Lipolysis causes release of free fatty acids (FFA) from dietary fats; however, it also causes little accumulation of mono- or di-glycerides. Lipolysis is followed by biohydrogenation, in which USFA are converted to saturated fatty acids (SFA), via isomerization reaction to *trans* fatty acids (TFA) intermediates followed by hydrogenation (reduction) of double bonds to SFA, predominantly stearic acid. Thus, depending upon condition of rumen and type of FA, various proportions of stearic acid and TFA (conjugated isomers) are produced during ruminal metabolism of dietary fat.

Conjugated isomers of linoleic acid (conjugated linoleic acid) produced during ruminal biohydrogenation have very significant role in dairy nutrition. Conjugated linoleic acid (CLA) is a mixture of positional and geometric isomers of linoleic acid (18:2) containing conjugated double bonds, both in *cis* and *trans* configurations. Linoleic acid (*cis*-9, *cis*-12-18:2) has all *cis* double bonds. Isomerization reaction mediated by *cis*-12, *trans*-11-isomerase converts the *cis*-12 double bond of linoleic acid to a *trans*-11 isomer and forms conjugated *cis-trans* double bond. Thus, linoleic acid (*cis*-9, *cis*-12-18:2) is converted to *cis*-9, *trans*-11-18:2 (rumenic acid). Formation of *trans*-11 bond in isomerization reaction is followed by hydrogenation (reduction) of the *cis*- 9 double bond of rumenic acid by microbial reductase converting it to *trans*-11-18:1 (vaccenic acid), which is finally hydrogenated to stearic acid (18:0). Rumenic acid, the most biologically active isomer of linoleic acid is naturally formed by both biohydrogenation of linoleic acid in rumen and 9-desaturation of vaccenic acid in mammary tissue and has beneficial role in human health due to its anticarcinogenic properties (Jenkins and McGuire, 2006). In normal situation, rumenic acid and vaccenic acid are the most abundant isomers produced during rumen biohydrogenation. Besides, different CLA and TFA isomers ranging from *trans*-3 to *trans*-16 (Piperova *et al.*, 2000) are also produced in rumen having significant role related to milk fat depression (MFD).

Milk Fat Depression

MFD represents a diet induced temporary situation, where milk fat yield can be reduced up to 50-60% from normal levels (NRC, 2001) without alteration in yield of milk and milk protein (Bauman and Griinari, 2003) and therefore, can be used as a management tool to alleviate negative energy balance of high yielding dairy cows during early lactation (Giesy *et al.*, 2002).

Earlier, influences of diet on MFD have been related to changes in rumen volatile fatty acids (VFA) and its subsequent effect on metabolism, but recently it is associated to changes in rumen biohydrogenation process and not changes in rumen VFA patterns (NRC, 2001).

Dietary factors, which cause MFD includes high levels of concentrate, finely chopped forages and high level of PUFA. Rumen acetate: propionate molar ratio has been frequently used as an indicator of fermentative changes during MFD (Tyznick and Allen, 1951). In MFD caused by feeding high levels of concentrate or finely chopped forages, there is decrease in rumen acetate: propionate molar ratio due to decrease in rumen acetate concentrations, a precursor for *de novo* FA synthesis in mammary gland or increase in propionate production without decrease in acetate production (NRC, 2001). Specific positional isomer of TFA double bond produced during rumen biohydrogenation process is important as MFD occurs only when *trans*-10, *cis*-12-CLA (Baumgard *et al.*, 2000) or *trans*-10-18:1 isomer (Griinari *et al.*, 1998) is increased compared with normal situations, where *cis*-9, *trans*-11-CLA and *trans*-11-18:1 isomer is most abundant. Mechanism by which TFA causes MFD is by reduction in *de novo* FA synthesis (NRC, 2001).

MFD is mainly affected by two factors i.e. level of dietary PUFA and rumen pH. Dietary PUFA are potential sources of CLA and TFA production in rumen. MFD occurs when rumen pH falls below 6.0 (Erdman, 1988). As rumen pH is related to fibre content of diet, inadequate dietary fiber results in low rumen pH causing MFD. Supplemental PUFA causes MFD in low forage diets (low rumen pH) and even addition of high levels of PUFA in diets with normal forage level does not cause MFD (Griinari *et al.*, 1998). During MFD, mostly milk FA of less than 16 carbons ($<C_{16}$) are decreased due to reduction in *de novo* FA synthesis, but TFA in milk are increased (NRC, 2001). MFD can be corrected by either increasing rumen pH by maintaining normal dietary fibre or addition of dietary buffer (Erdman, 1988) or restricting amounts of dietary PUFA as potential sources of CLA and TFA (NRC, 2001). Addition of dietary buffers to high concentrate diets reduces duodenal flow of TFA, decreases milk TFA content, and increases milk fat percent (Kalscheur *et al.*, 1997).

Microbial lipid synthesis in rumen occurs from both exogenous uptake of dietary long chain fatty acids (LCFA) and endogenous sources (*de novo* synthesis). LCFA are directly taken up by rumen microbes for exogenous microbial lipid synthesis. FA synthesized *de novo* from various precursors mainly include LCFA ($C_{16:0}$ and $C_{18:0}$), straight chain even numbered carbon FA, straight chain odd numbered carbon FA, branched chain FA and MUFA. As fat content of diet is increased, uptake of exogenous lipid by microbial cells is increased and *de novo* synthesis is declined. Lipid content of rumen bacteria dry mass varies from 10-15% (Bauchart *et al.*, 1990) and microbial lipid synthesis is estimated as 15g/kg of lipid free organic matter (OM) digested in rumen (Jenkins, 1993). Approximately, 85-90% of FA leaving rumen are FFA and 10-15% are microbial phospholipids (NRC, 2001). Finally, dairy animals utilize FA of both dietary and microbial origins.

Use of Dietary Fat in Dairy Animals

In dairy animals, dietary fat is used to enhance metabolic efficiency of energy utilization for milk production by generating ATP more efficiently than VFA or protein; lowering heat production; incorporating preformed FA into milk fat, thus sparing energy for other productive functions in mammary gland; and substituting for rapidly fermentable carbohydrate to optimize forage fibre intake and rumen function, thereby promoting nutrient partition towards milk production (Palmquist, 1994). Although, energy obtained from oxidation of LCFA is relatively small, yield of ATP is 10% more efficient than oxidation of acetate (Schauff and Clark, 1992). Milk fat of dairy animals consists of a mixture of TG containing a wide range (short, medium and long chain) of SFA and USFA. Milk FA of less than 16 carbons ($<C_{16}$) are synthesized *de novo* in mammary gland, FA of more than 16 carbons ($>C_{16}$) are derived from diets (uptake of preformed FA), while FA with 16 carbons (C_{16}) are synthesized from both diet and *de novo* synthesis (Castaneda-Gutierrez *et al.*, 2005).

Limitations of Fat Supplementation in Dairy Ration

Although, dietary fat has a great potential to enhance metabolic efficiency of energy utilization in dairy animals, various factors limit its use in large amounts in ration. These include, inhibitory effects on ruminal fermentation leading to decrease in fiber digestibility, lower intestinal absorption at higher intake, low contribution to total oxidation of nutrients and sensitivity to nutrient imbalance causing reduced energy intake (Palmquist, 1994). Extent of hydrolysis of dietary free (rumen active) fat in rumen is very high (85-95%), which causes reduction in fiber digestibility. Devendra and Lewis (1974) explained four theories on reduction of fiber digestibility by dietary fat, which include (i) coating of fibrous portion of diet with lipids thereby preventing attack by rumen microorganisms (ii) modification in rumen population concerned with cellulose digestion (iii) inhibition of the activity of rumen microorganisms due to an effect on cell permeability brought about by absorption of FA on cell wall or due to an antimetabolite effect (iv) reduction in availability of minerals (Ca and Mg), essential for microbial activity due to formation of mineral complexes with FA.

Rumen Protected Fat

Dietary fat, which resists lipolysis and biohydrogenation in rumen by rumen microbes, but gets digested in lower alimentary tract, is known as rumen protected fat (PF). Frequently, this is also known as bypass fat or inert fat. Due to its inertness in rumen, it can be supplemented to dairy animals at higher levels than active fats. As FA are absorbed directly from lower alimentary tract, it is easier to modify the FA profile of milk by feeding specific fat (FA) in protected form. Besides, as it is dry at room temperature, it is easily transportable and can be mixed into diets without any specific equipment.

Natural Dietary Rumen Protected Fat

Oil seeds provide natural partial protection from lipolysis and biohydrogenation in rumen due to their hard outer seed coat (Ekeren *et al.*, 1992). However, ruminal protection is very inconsistent as processing (ground, extruded, pelleted) of oilseeds reduces their resistance to biohydrogenation. Cottonseed and full fat soya are good sources of both rumen protected protein and fat. Feed ingredients containing SFA are less toxic to ruminal microorganisms and minimize adverse effects of feeding fat, as they react more readily with metal ions, forming insoluble salts in rumen (Jenkins and Palmquist, 1982) and do not go for further ruminal biohydrogenation (Chalupa *et al.*, 1986).

Preparation of Rumen Protected Fat

Various physical and chemical treatments imparted to dietary fats (FA) to make protected from ruminal lipolysis and biohydrogenation have been discussed in brief.

Crystalline/ Prilled Fatty Acids

It is made up of SFA or from hydrogenated fat by liquifying and spraying under pressure into a cooled atmosphere. Due to high melting point, these FA do not melt at ruminal temperature, there by resisting ruminal hydrolysis and are less likely to associate with bacterial cells or feed particles (Chalupa *et al.*, 1986).

Fatty Acyl Amides

Fatty acyl amides are amides of USFA, which resist biohydrogenation in rumen. Protection of amides from ruminal biohydrogenation depends up on the specific FA and amide linkage. Generally, fatty acyl amide is supplemented in diet of lactating cows to increase the desired FA (especially USFA) content of milk fat. Butylsoyamide is a fatty acyl amide consisting of an amide bond between soy FA and a butylamine, which increases linoleic acid content of milk fat (Jenkins, 1998). Conversion of oleic acid to fatty acyl amide (oleamide) increases MUFA concentration in milk, when fed to dairy cows (Jenkins, 1999), while amide of soybean FA is effective in enhancing post-ruminal flow of oleic acid (Lundy *et al.*, 2004).

Formaldehyde Treatment of Oil Seeds

For formaldehyde treatment of oil seeds, crushed oil seeds are treated with formaldehyde (1.2 g per 100g protein) in plastic bags or silos and kept for about a week. During this process, internal FA content of oilseeds is protected from ruminal lipolysis and biohydrogenation by the formaldehyde treated protein coat. Major limitation of this technology is the inconsistency in the level of rumen protection due to physical break down of the treated oil seeds during mastication by animal. Casein-formaldehyde coated fat has been used as PF by earlier workers (Bines *et al.*, 1978).

Calcium Salts of Long Chain Fatty Acids

Calcium salts of long chain fatty acids (Ca-LCFA) are insoluble soaps, produced by reaction of carboxyl group of LCFA and calcium salts (Ca++). However, degree of insolubility (inertness) of Ca-LCFA depends upon rumen pH and type of FA of Ca soaps. In rumen, Ca-LCFA is inert, if pH remains more than 5.5. At normal rumen pH, dissociation of Ca salts of USFA is relatively higher than Ca salts of SFA (Sukhija and Palmquist, 1990). As dissociation constant (pKa) of Ca-LCFA is 4 to 5, dissociation is significant, when rumen pH decreases to 6.0 (Chalupa *et al.*, 1986). In acidic pH of abomasum, FA is dissociated from Ca-LCFA and then absorbed efficiently from small intestine. Ca-LCFA can be prepared by two methods.

Double Decomposition Method

In double decomposition method, Ca-LCFA is prepared in two steps (Jenkins and Palmquist, 1984; Sampelayo *et al.*, 2004). In first step, fat (FA) is heated and an alkali (aqueous solution of sodium hydroxide) is added to it with constant stirring till FA are dissolved (saponified) completely (soluble Na soap). In second step, heating is stopped and calcium chloride solution is added slowly to warm soluble Na soap with constant stirring, which causes formation of Ca soaps (Ca-LCFA). Excess water is removed by filtration and then Ca-LCFA (PF) is dried at low temperature and ground.

Fusion Method

In fusion method, Ca-LCFA is prepared in single step by treating fat (FA) with either calcium oxide or calcium hydroxide in presence of catalyst. (Naik *et al.*, 2007[a, b]) has developed a simple, indigenous technology for preparation of Ca-LCFA (PF) by treating vegetable FA oil with calcium hydroxide under specific conditions (Naik *et al.*, 2009[a]). For bulk preparation, 4 kg rice bran fatty acid oil (RBO), a byproduct of rice bran oil refinery industry is heated in an aluminum vessel and 120 ml concentrate sulphuric acid in 500 ml tap water is mixed in it (Fig. 1). After few minutes (when effervescence almost subsides), 1.6 kg technical grade calcium hydroxide dissolved in 10 liters of water, is added to it and boiled for 30 minutes without cover on medium heat (Fig. 2). When product (Ca-LCFA) becomes granular and non-sticky, it is filtered through cloth with repeated washings (Fig. 3&4) under running tap water and then sun dried (Fig. 5). After mixing with butylated hydroxy toluene (BHT) @ 0.05% as an antioxidant, Ca-LCFA (PF) is kept in air tight container in cool place. The product (PF) contains 70-75% fat, 7-8% Ca and is 80-85% rumen protected. This technology of preparation of Ca-LCFA (PF) is user-friendly and pro-small farmer.

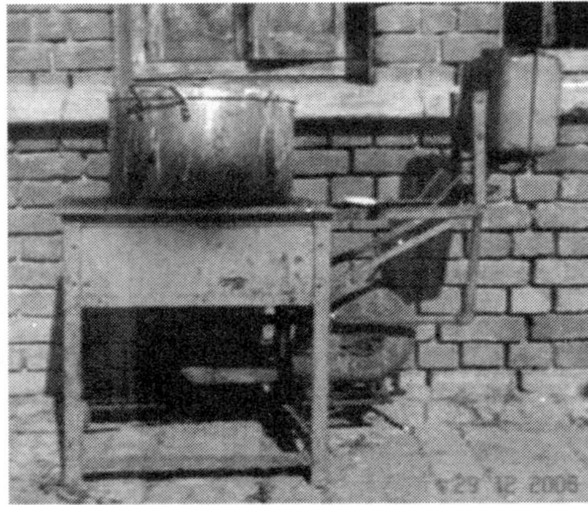

Fig. 1 : Equipment used for preparation of Ca-LCFA (PF)

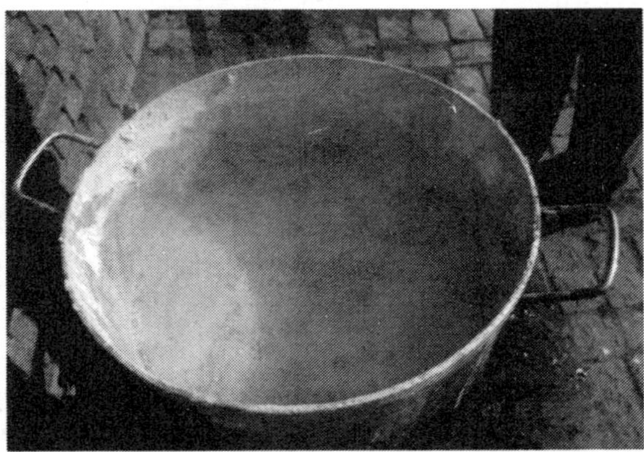

Fig. 2 : Boiling stage

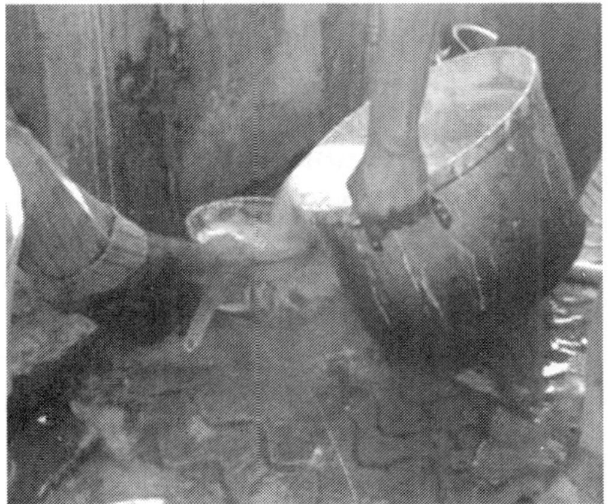

Fig. 3 : Washing and filtration of Ca-LCFA (PF)

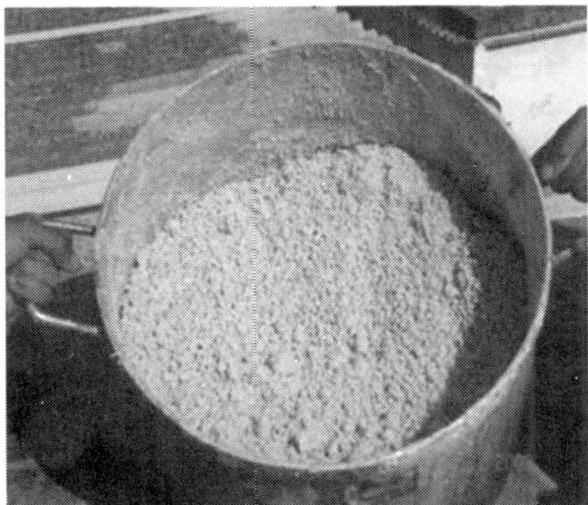

Fig. 4 : Washed and filtered Ca-LCFA (PF)

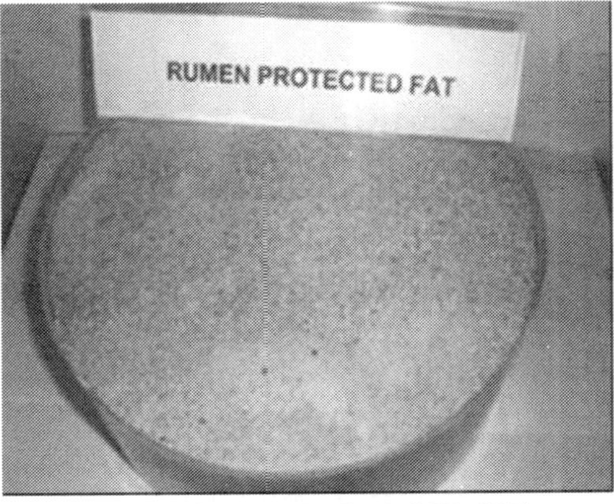

Fig. 5 : Sun dried Ca-LCFA (PF)

Level of Fat Supplementation in Dairy Ration

In developing countries, generally, concentrate mixture forms up to 50-60% of dairy ration and rest parts consist of green fodder and crop residues. Theoretically, efficiency of nutrient utilization for milk production is maximal, when supplemental dietary fat provides 15-20% of dietary metabolizable energy or 7-8% of dietary fat on DM basis (Scott *et al.*, 1995). As per NRC (2001), dairy ration (mixture of cereals and forages) contains about 3% fat, and total dietary fat in ration should not exceed 6-7% of DM. This means, only up to 3-4% of dietary DM can be provided through supplemental fat. Addition of 3-5% fat of total ration DM has beneficial effect on milk production (Palmquist and Jenkins, 1980); and decrease in production occurs, when fat level exceeds 6% of ration DM (Jenkins and Palmquist, 1984), which probably results from the effects of fats, especially unesterified FA on rumen cellulolytic microbial activity. However, fats that are insoluble or unavailable in rumen like PF can be included in diet in higher amount (West and Hill, 1990).

Although, PF can be incorporated up to 9% of dietary DM due to its inertness in rumen (Sharma, 2004), feeding Ca-LCFA at 9% of dietary DM is not beneficial in lactating dairy cows (Schauff and Clark, 1992). However, it is always better to supplement different types of fat in dairy ration. First 3% fat of DM intake of animal should be provided by oilseed sources and that in excess of 3% should be as PF (Palmquist, 1990) or rations of high yielders should have 4-6% fat, containing 1/3rd fat from each source of natural feed, oil seed and PF (Sharma, 2004).

Effect of Rumen Protected Fat on Various Parameters

Effect of supplementation of PF (Ca-LCFA) on rumen fermentation, DM intake, apparent nutrient digestibility, milk yield, milk composition, body weight (BW), body condition score (BCS) and reproductive performance of dairy cows has been discussed in brief.

Rumen Fermentation

Supplementation of Ca-LCFA has no adverse effect on rumen fermentation of dairy animals up to 6-8% of ration DM (Naik *et al.*, 2010); but, when Ca-LCFA, especially of highly USFA are fed, dietary buffers should be added to maintain ruminal pH and minimize dissociation of Ca salts in rumen (Chalupa *et al.*, 1986). Ruminal pH, ammonia nitrogen and VFA level are not affected adversely by supplementation of Ca soaps up to 5% of dietary DM in lactating cows containing 60% forages (Ohajuruka *et al.*, 1991). With increase in level of dietary Ca-LCFA, ruminal fluid pH and TVFA concentration is not changed, but molar percentage of acetate and acetate to propionate ratio are increased linearly (Schauff and Clark, 1992).

Dry Matter Intake

DM intake involves limitations of gut fill as well as energy satiety factors. Amount of Ca-LCFA required to limit DM intake is a function of amount of energy provided by basal ration and energy requirement of dairy cow (Chilliard *et al.*, 1993). DM intake decreases quadratically as EE content of diet increases (Hayirli *et al.*, 2002). However, decrease in DM intake is not observed, when lipids are provided instead of concentrates based on their energy value (Elmeddah *et al.*, 1994). DM intake of dairy animals either decreases linearly (Chouinard *et al.*, 1997) or is not altered (Chouinard *et al.*, 1998), as percentage of Ca-LCFA is increased in diets. Palatability may be a problem, when Ca-LCFA is fed to dairy cows and therefore, should be diluted with grains to overcome the problem (Grummer *et al.*, 1990). DM intake of animal is affected by type of FA of Ca salt and ADF digestibility of ration. DM intake is reduced quadratically, with increase in unsaturation of dominant FA in Ca salts and increase in ADF digestibility (Chouinard *et al.*, 1998). Addition of dietary buffers (Na or K bicarbonates) to diets containing Ca-LCFA has no effect on DM intake of animals (Erdman, 1988; Chouinard *et al.*, 1997).

Apparent Digestibility of Nutrients

Effect of supplemental Ca-LCFA on apparent digestibility of various nutrients depends upon level of supplementation. There is no effect of supplemental Ca-LCFA on apparent digestibilities of DM and OM (Garcia-Bojalil *et al.*, 1998), which may be due to its non-interference and relatively stable nature causing minimum dissociation in rumen. Digestibility of nitrogen or CP is either increased linearly (Schauff and Clark, 1992) or not altered (Garcia-Bojalil *et al.*, 1998), when Ca-LCFA is supplemented in diet. Generally, with increase in fat intake, apparent fat digestibility increases quadratically and true fat digestibility decreases (2.2%/100g fat consumed) linearly (Palmquist, 1991). Increase in digestibility of fat indicates that added fat is more digestible than fat of basal diet or fat supplementation dilutes endogenous lipid secretions, resulting in more accurate estimate of true lipid digestibility (Grummer, 1988). However, at higher level of fat supplementation, fat digestibility is decreased, which may be due to limited capacity of small intestine to absorb fat (Jenkins and Palmquist, 1984) or masking effect of endogenous faecal fat (Ngidi *et al.*, 1990). Ruminants digest SFA more efficiently than non-ruminants. Digestibility of SFA decreases with increase in chain length, while unsaturation of FA increases digestibility, thus palmitic acid is more digestible, and stearic acid is less digestible than average FA mixture in ruminants (Palmquist, 1994). Beside fat (FA), digestibility of soluble residues (SR) is also increased quadratically by addition of Ca-LCFA in ration of lactating dairy cows (Schauff and Clark, 1992). On increasing level of Ca-

LCFA in diet, NDF digestibility is either increased linearly (Ngidi *et al.*, 1990) or not affected (Garcia-Bojalil *et al.*, 1998). When PF is supplemented with replacement of some part of starch of ration, then apparent digestibilities of DM, CP, EE and NDF are increased (Chouinard *et al.*, 1998). Reduction in readily fermentable carbohydrates in rumen influences microbial protein synthesis resulting in loss of ammonia nitrogen (Palmquist *et al.*, 1993) and lower amount of starch available at large intestine causes lower excretion of CP in faeces (McCarthy *et al.*, 1989), which in turn is responsible for higher apparent digestibility of CP. Increase in total tract apparent digestibility of NDF in cows fed Ca-LCFA is due to increase in post-ruminal degradation (Chouinard *et al.*, 1998). However, at low level of supplementation of Ca-LCFA, digestibility of ADF is not affected (Schauff and Clark., 1989). Digestibility of ADF and cellulose varies with level of Ca-LCFA supplementation in diet. There is cubic effect of Ca-LCFA supplementation on digestibility of ADF and cellulose, as digestibilities increased up to 6% of supplementation and decreased at 9% supplemental level (Schauff and Clark., 1992). Type of FA of Ca salt also influences digestibility of ADF. Apparent digestibility of ADF is altered quadratically, when unsaturation of dominant FA in Ca salts is increased, as ADF digestibility was lowest for rations supplemented with Ca-LCFA from soybean oil ($C_{18:2}$) and highest from canola oil ($C_{18:1}$) and linseed oil ($C_{18:3}$); however, it was not observed for NDF (Chouinard *et al.*, 1998). Hemicellulose digestibility is either not altered (Schauff and Clark, 1992) or increased (Garcia-Bojalil *et al.*, 1998) with inclusion of Ca-LCFA in diet. With supplementation of Ca-LCFA, improved hemicellulose digestibility causes increase in NDF and decrease in ADF digestibility in cows during early lactation (Erickson *et al.*, 1992).

Milk Yield

Effect of supplemental Ca-LCFA on milk yield and fat corrected milk (FCM) yield is dependent upon breed, parity, stage of lactation of animal; level of supplementation and FA composition of Ca-LCFA. Although, there is no significant interaction with breed of cow, effect of supplemental Ca-LCFA on milk yield tends to be greater in Holstein cows than Jersey cows (West and Hill, 1990). Effect of supplementation of Ca-LCFA in dairy cows on milk yield and FCM yield is more in primiparous cows than multiparous cows (Sklan *et al.*, 1994). Supplemental effect of Ca-LCFA on milk yield and FCM yield is generally more in early and peak lactation (Schneider *et al*, 1988). Transfer efficiency of plasma FA to mammary tissue decreases as lactation progresses; therefore, increase in production is maximal during early and peak lactation than mid or late lactation (Grummer, 1988). Cows fed Ca soap produces more milk (60 days postpartum) and more FCM (90 days postpartum) in early lactation, which may be due to higher energy intake, more efficient use of fat by mammary gland and enhancement of tissue mobilization before peak production (Sklan *et al.*, 1991). During early lactation, milk yield increased 3.2 kg/d (19.6 %) and FCM yield increased 2.8 kg/d (22.3%) on supplementation of Ca-LCFA in crossbred lactating cows (Naik *et al.*, 2009[b]). Supplemental Ca-LCFA increases FCM yield of lactating cows up to 6% of dietary DM, but yield is decreased at 9% of dietary DM (Schauff and Clark, 1992). Yields of milk, solid corrected milk (SCM) and total solids (TS) alter in quadratic pattern to supplemental Ca-LCFA, being highest at 2% and lowest at 0 or 4% of DM; as at higher level of supplementation, Ca-LCFA interferes with digestion of other nutrients and impairs benefits of supplemental fat on energy utilization and thus, has a negative impact on lactation performance of dairy cows (Chouinard *et al.*, 1997). With increase in unsaturation of dominant FA in Ca salts, milk yield increases linearly in early lactation (Chouinard *et al.*, 1998). However, milk yield is not affected by dietary supplementation of Ca salts of CLA in lactating animals (Castaneda-Gutierrez *et al.*, 2005).

Milk Composition

Effect of supplemental Ca-LCFA on milk composition is dependent upon breed, parity, stage of lactation of animal; level of supplementation and FA composition of Ca-LCFA. Among milk components, fat content is the most sensitive to dietary changes. Milk protein is more responsive to diet than lactose, but is less responsive than fat (Jenkins and McGuire, 2006). Similar to milk yield, although there is no significant interaction with breed of cow, effect of supplementation of Ca-LCFA on milk composition tends to be greater in Holstein cows than Jersey cows (West and Hill, 1990). On supplementation of Ca-LCFA, milk fat percentage increased only in multiparous cows but not in primiparous cows; however, total fat yield increased both in primiparous and multiparous cows (Sklan *et al.*, 1994) which is due to increase in milk production. In general, on supplementation of Ca-LCFA to lactating animals, milk fat percentage is either increased (Sklan *et al.*, 1991) or decreased (Chouinard *et al.*, 1998) or not altered (Naik *et al.*, 2009[b]). Percentage and yield of milk fat decreases linearly with increase in level of dietary Ca soap; and Ca-LCFA from a saturated fat source have little influence on milk fat content (Chouinard *et al.*, 1997), while increase in unsaturation of dominant FA in Ca salts has positive linear effect on milk fat percentage of lactating cows (Chouinard *et al.*, 1998). Supplementation of Ca-LCFA in diet of lactating cows decreases proportions of short and medium chain SFA ($C_{6:0}$ to $C_{16:0}$) of milk fat due to reduction in *de novo* FA synthesis in mammary gland and increases proportions of LCFA ($C_{18:1}$, $C_{18:2}$, $C_{18:3}$) due to increase uptake of preformed LCFA from blood (Mishra *et al.*, 2004). Proportions of odd numbered FA ($C_{15:0}$, $C_{17:0}$) of milk fat decreases because ruminal bacteria, which are major source of odd chain FA of milk fat prefers to use preformed FA, and *de novo* FA synthesis is reduced (Chouinard *et al.*, 1997). Supplemental Ca salts of CLA (*cis*-9, *trans*-11-CLA and *trans*-10, *cis*-12-CLA) reduces milk fat content (Selberg *et al.*, 2004; Castaneda-Gutierrez *et al.*, 2005) and *de novo* synthesis of $C_{8:0}$, $C_{10:0}$ and $C_{12:0}$ FA, but increases CLA (*cis*-9, *trans*-11-CLA and *trans*-10, *cis*-12-CLA) content of milk fat in a dose dependent manner (Giesy *et al.*, 2002). Supplementation of rumen protected CLA to pregnant, lactating cows promotes MFD with no apparent adverse effects (Perfield *et al.*, 2002). Very often, CLA induces reduction in milk fat content but milk yield is simultaneously increased, so there is no overall improvement in energy balance (Bernal-Santos *et al.*, 2003). At higher dose, CLA induced MFD decreases milk energy output, but this is not reflected in a statistically significant improvement in net energy balance or reduction in use of body fat reserves as evaluated by changes in BW and BSC (Castaneda-Gutierrez *et al.*, 2005). Effect of supplemental Ca-LCFA on milk protein content is not influenced by the breed of animal (West and Hill, 1990), but influenced by parity and stage of lactation of animal. Decline in milk protein content is reported both in multiparous cows (West and Hill, 1990) and primiparous cows (Sklan *et al.*, 1992); but decline is apparent only in late lactation, not in early lactation (Sklan *et al.*, 1992). Supplementation of Ca-LCFA frequently has a negative effect on milk protein percentage; an overall effect of 0.12 percentage unit (Chouinard *et al.*, 1998). Decrease in milk protein is related to dilution of milk protein as higher milk volume synthesized is not synchronize with uptake of amino acids by mammary gland (DePeters and Cantt, 1992). Further, dietary fat impairs amino acids transport to mammary gland and decreases milk protein synthesis by inducing insulin resistance (Palmquist and Moser, 1981). If protein or amino acids are inadequate, lipoprotein synthesis may be decreased. Consequently, fat and protein transport to mammary gland is reduced leading to decrease in milk protein percentage, which usually occurs and decrease in milk fat percentage, which sometimes occurs. Dietary protein should be increased, when fat supplemented diets are fed to animals (Palmquist and Moser, 1981). However, always, supplemental Ca-LCFA has no negative effect on milk protein percentage or may not alter it; but total yield of milk protein is increased due to more milk production (Sklan *et al.*, 1994; Naik, *et al.*, 2009[b]). Supplemental effect of Ca-LCFA on milk total solid (TS) is influenced by parity of animal, which is greater for primiparous cows than multiparous cows (West and Hill, 1990). Concentration and yield of lactose is altered in quadratic pattern, when level of supplemental Ca-LCFA is increased in diet, being highest at 2% and lowest at 0 or 4% level of supplementation (Chouinard *et al.*, 1997).

Body Weight and Body Condition Score

Effect of supplemental Ca-LCFA on change of BW is influenced by parity of animal. Loss of BW is more and longer lasting in primiparous cows than multiparous cows (Sklan *et al.*, 1994). BCS is a useful management tool to assess body fat stores of dairy cows and has therefore, received considerable attention in nutritional studies (Waltner *et al.*, 1993). General pattern of change in BCS over lactation is an initial fall continuing for 2-3 months and then a lower recovery over mid lactation (Treacher *et al.*, 1986). Although, there is no significant effect of supplemental Ca-LCFA on changes of BW and BCS of dairy cows, recovery of BW and BCS losses are better in Ca-LCFA supplemented cows in early lactation (Naik *et al.*, 2009[b]).

Reproductive Performance

Dietary supplementation of Ca-LCFA has positive effect on reproductive performance of dairy cows, which is further dependent upon the specific FA profile of Ca salt. Feeding Ca-LCFA increases pregnancy rate and reduces open days (Sklan *et al.*, 1991). Several hypotheses are suggested regarding role of FA on improvement of reproductive performance of dairy animals (Sklan *et al.*, 1994). These include (i) improved energy balance, resulting in an earlier return to post-partum ovarian cycling; (ii) increase linoleic acid may provide increase PGF2α and stimulate return to ovarian cycling and improve follicular recruitment; and (iii) increase in progesterone secretion either from improvement energy balance or altered lipoprotein composition of dietary fat. Dietary supplementation of Ca-LCFA reduces number of artificial inseminations required per conception (Naik *et al.*, 2009[b]), which indicates better reproductive performance of dairy animals. However, changes in reproductive performance associated with fat supplementation are related to magnitude of milk response of fat supplementation (Scott *et al.*, 1995).

References

Bauchart, D., Legay-Carmier, F., Doreau, M. and Gaillard, B. (1990). *Br. J. Nutr.*, 63:563.

Bauman, D. E. and Griinari, J. M. (2003). *Ann. Rev. Nutr.*, 23: 203-227.

Baumgard, L. H., Corl, B.J. Dwyer, D. A., Saebo, A. and Bauman, D. E. (2000). *Am. J. Physiol. Regulatory Integrative Comp. Physiol.*, 278: R179-R184.

Bell, A.W. (1995). *J. Anim. Sci.*, 73: 2804-2819.

Bernal-Santos, G., Perfield, J.W., Barbano, D.M., Bauman, D.E. and Overton, T.R. (2003). *J. Dairy Sci.*, 86: 3218-3228.

Bines, J.A., Brumby, P.E., Storry, J.E., Fulford, Rosemary J. and Braithwaite, G.D. (1978). *J. Agric. Sci. Camb.*, 91: 135-150.

Castaneda-Gutierrez, E., Overton, T.R., Butler, W.R. and Bauman, D.E. (2005). *J.Dairy Sci.,* 88: 1078-1089.

Chalupa, William, Vecchiarelli, Bonnie, Elser, Andrew E., Kronfeld, D.S., Sklan, David and Palmquist, Donald L. (1986). *J. Dairy Sci.* 69: 1293-1301.

Chilliard, Y., Doreau, M., Gagliostro, G. and Elmeddah, Y. (1993). *Inst. Natl. Res. Agro. Prod. Anim.,* 6: 139-150.

Chouinard, P.Y., Girard, V. and Brisson, G.J. (1997). *J. Dairy Sci.,* 80: 1185-1193.

Chouinard, P.Y., Girard, V. and Brisson, G.J. (1998). *J. Dairy Sci.,* 81: 471-481.

DePeters, E. J. and Cant, J. P. (1992). *J. Dairy Sci.,* 75: 2043-2070.

Devendra, C. and Lewis, D. (1974). *Anim. Prod.,* 19:67-76.

Drackley, J.K. (1999). *J. Dairy Sci.,* 82: 2259-2273.

Ekeren, Peg A., Smith, Dana R., Lunt, David K. and Smith, Stephen B. (1992). *J. Anim. Sci.,* 70: 2574-2580.

Elmeddah, Y., Doreau, M., Rouel, J. and Chilliard, Y. (1994). *Ann. Zootech.* (Paris), 43: 341.

Erdman, R.E. (1988). *J. Dairy Sci.,* 71: 3246-3266.

Erickson, P.S., Murphy, M.R., and Clark, J.H. (1992). *J. Dairy Sci.,* 75: 1078-1089.

Garcia-BoJalil, C.M., Staples, C.R., Risco, C.A., Savio, J.D. and Thatcher, W.W. (1998). *J. Dairy Sci.,* 81: 1374-1384.

Giesy, J.G., McGuire, M.A., Shafil, B. and Hanson, T.W. (2002). *J. Dairy Sci.,* 85: 2023-2029.

Griinari, J. M., D. A. Dwyer, M. A. McGuire, D. E. Bauman, D. L. Palmquist, and K. V. V. Nurmela. (1998). *J. Dairy Sci.* 81: 1251- 1261.

Grummer, R.R. (1988). *J. Dairy Sci.,* 71: 117-123.

Grummer, R.R., Hatfield, M.L., and Dentine, M.R. (1990). *J. Dairy Sci.,* 73: 852-857.

Gupta, B.K., Bhardwaj, B.L. and Ahuja, A.K. (2004). Nutritive value of fodder crops of Punjab. Dept. Anim. Nutr., PAU, Ludhiana.

Hayirli, A., Grummer, R.R., Nordheim, E.V. and Crump, P.M. (2002). *J. Dairy Sci.,* 85: 3430-3443.

Jenkins, T.C. (1993). *J. Dairy Sci.,* 76: 3851-3863.

Jenkins, T.C. (1998). *J. Dairy Sci.,* 81: 794-800.

Jenkins, T.C. (1999). *J. Dairy Sci.,* 82: 1525-1531.

Jenkins, T.C. and McGuire, M.A. (2006). *J. Dairy Sci.,* 89:1302-1310.

Jenkins, T.C. and Palmquist, D.L. (1982). *J. Anim. Sci.,* 55:957-963.

Jenkins, T.C. and Palmquist, D.L. (1984). *J. Dairy Sci.,* 67: 978-986.

Kalscheur, K. F., B. B. Teter, L. S. Piperova, and R. A. Erdman. (1997). *J. Dairy Sci.*, 80: 2104–2114.

Lundy, F.P., Block, E., Bridges, W.C. Jr., Bertrand, J.A. and Jenkins, T.C. (2004). *J. Dairy Sci.*, 87: 1038-1046.

McCarthy, R.D., Klusmeyer, T.H. Jr., Vicini, J.L., Clark, J.H. and Nelson, D.R. (1989) *J. Dairy Sci.*, 72: 2002-2016.

McDonald. P., Edwards, R.A., Greenhalgh, J.F.D. and Morgan, C.A. (2002). Anim. Nutr., sixth eds., Pearson Education (Singapore) Pte.Ltd., Indian branch, 482 F.I.E., Patparganj, Delhi, India.

Mishra, Siddhartha, Thakur, S.S. and Raikwar, Rakesh (2004). *Indian J. Anim. Nutr.*, 21: 22-25.

Naik, P. K., Saijpaul, S. and Rani Neelam. (2007[b]). *Indian J. Anim. Nutr.*, 24: 212-215.

Naik, P.K., Saijpaul, S. and Rani, Neelam (2007[a]). *Anim. Nutr. Feed Technol.*, 7: 95-101.

Naik, P.K., Saijpaul, S. and Rani, Neelam (2009[a]). *Anim. Feed Sci. Technol.* 153: 68-76.

Naik, P.K., Saijpaul, S., Sirohi, A.S. and Raquib, M. (2009[b]). *Indian J. Anim. Sci.*, 79: 1045-1049.

Naik, P.K., Saijpaul, S. and Kaur, K. (2010). *Indian J. Anim Sci.*, 80: 902-905.

Ngidi, M.E., Loerch, S.C., Fluharty, F.L. and Palmquist, D.L. (1990). *J. Anim. Sci.*, 68: 2555-2565.

NRC (2001). Nutrient Requirements for Dairy Cattle. 7th rev. ed., Natl. Acad. Sci., Washington, DC.

Ohajuruka, O.A., W.U., Z. and Palmquist, D.L. (1991). *J. Dairy Sci.*, 74: 2601-2609.

Palmquist, D. L. (1990). In Proc. International Anim. Nutr. Symp., Natl. Renderer's Assoc., Brussels, Belgium, p. 35.

Palmquist, D. L. and Moser, E. A. (1981). *J. Dairy Sci.*, 64: 1664-1670.

Palmquist, D.L. (1991). *J. Dairy Sci.*, 74: 1354-1360.

Palmquist, D.L. and Jenkins, T.C. (1980). *J. Dairy Sci.*, 63: 1-14.

Palmquist, D.L., Weisbjerg, M.R., Hvelplund, T. (1993). *J. Dairy Sci.*, 76: 1353-1364.

Palmquist, Donald L. (1994). *J. Nutr.*, 124 : 1377S-1382S.

Perfield, J.W., Bernal-Santos, G., Overton, T.R. and Bauman, D.E. (2002). *J. Dairy Sci.*, 85: 2609-2617.

Piperova, L. S., B. B. Teter, I. Bruckental, J. Sampagna, S. E. Mills, M. P. Yurawecz, J. Fritsche, K. Ku, and R. A. Erdman. (2000). *J. Nutr.*, 130: 2568– 2574.

Reddy, D.V. (2003). Applied Nutrition (Livestock,Poultry,Human,Pet, Rabbit and Laboratory Animal Nutrition). Oxford & IBH Publishing Co. Pvt. Ltd., New Delhi. p. 60.

Sampelayo, M. R. Sanz, Alonso, J. J. Martin, Perez, L., Extremera, F. Gil and Boza, J. (2004). *J. Dairy Sci.*, 87: 1796-1802.

Schauff, D.J. and Clark, J.H. (1989). *J. Dairy Sci.*, 72: 917-927.

Schauff, D.J. and Clark, J.H. (1992). *J. Dairy Sci.*, 75: 2990-3002.

Schneider, P., Sklan, D., Chalupa, W. and Kronfeld, D.S. (1988). *J. Dairy Sci.*, 71:2143-2150.

Scott, T.A., Shaver, R.D., Zepeda, L., Yandell, B. and Smith, T.R. (1995). *J. Dairy Sci.*, 78: 2435-2451.

Selberg, K. T., Lowe, A. C., Staples, C. R., Luchini, N. D. and Badinga, L. (2004). *J. Dairy Sci.*, 87: 158-68.

Sharma, D.D. (2004). All India Dairy Husbandry Officers' Workshop. Dairy Extension Division, National Dairy Research Institute, Karnal, India, p.28-33.

Sklan, D., Ashkenazi, Ruth, Braun, A., Devorin, A. and Tabori, K. (1992). *J. Dairy Sci.*, 75: 2463-2472.

Sklan, D., Kaim, M., Moallam, U. and Folman, Y. (1994). *J. Dairy Sci.*, 77: 1652-1660.

Sklan, D., Moallem, U. and Folman, Y. (1991). *J. Dairy Sci.*, 74: 510-517.

Sukhija, P. S. and Palmquist, D. L. (1990). *J. Dairy Sci.*, 73: 1784-1787.

Treacher, R. J., Reid, I. M. and Roberts, C. J. (1986). *Anim. Prod.*, 43: 1-6.

Tyznick W. and N. N. Allen. (1951). *J. Dairy Sci.*, 34:493.

Waltner, S.S., McNamaara, J.P. and Hillers, J.K. (1993). *J. Dairy Sci.*, 76: 3410-3419.

West, J. W. and Hill, G. M. (1990). *J. Dairy Sci.*, 73: 3200-3207.

□□□

Animal Nutrition, 2012
eds. Dr. (Mrs.) Usha R. Mehra et al., pp. 549-559
Satish Serial Publishing House e-mail : info@satishserial.com; website : www.satishserial.com

Chapter 26

Feeding Behaviour of Domestic Animals

GYANENDRA SINGH AND B.C. DAS

Depending upon the food habits, the animals are classified as carnivorous, herbivorous and omnivorous. The carnivorous animals like dogs, which live on food like meat and meat products, have their simple stomach and digestion is mostly enzymatic and non-fermentive in nature and with a limited microbial digestion in the lower alimentary tract. The domestic herbivorous live on straw, grasses and some amount of concentrates. The omnivorous animals feed on both plant and animal products. The digestion in these species is mostly enzymatic or non-fermentive. The domestic pig falls in this category. Depending upon the food habits of animals, feeding behaviour also changes likewise and which is species specific.

Behaviour as Influenced by Structural and Functional Peculiarity

The oral cavity is externally guarded by lips. In cattle, the lips are thick and upper lip is comparatively immobile. The middle part of the upper lip and the surface in between the nostrils is known as muzzle (Hughes and Reid, 1951). In case of sheep, goat and horses the lips are shorter and flexible. It helps picking up fodder, however, in cattle lips do not serve any major function in feed intake. Cheeks help in placing the food between the teeth for proper mastication. For all domestic animals, tongue helps in prehension of food and in case of cattle it functions as main prehensile organ. The distribution of taste buds for different species is different in terms of shape and size.

Theories of Feed Intake

Glucostatic theory: it states that voluntary feed intake is under the control of circulating blood glucose level. A lower blood level stimulates feeding centre. It is also suggested that an acute release of insulin increases rate of utilization of glucose and as a result low blood level stimulates voluntary feed intake in farm animals.

Thermostatic theory: it states that in animals food intake is directly related with maintenance of internal homeothermy. During hot environmental temperature, the homeothermic animals reduce feed intake to limit the metabolic heat production as a part of maintenance of heat balance in the body. But during the period of low ambient temperature animals increase feed intake to accelerate metabolic heat production and keep the body temperature constant (Larkin, 1954).

Lipostatic theory: explains that the feed intake is governed by certain constituents of fat in the circulation. The theory of feed intake favours that some function of energy intake or storage is monitored by brain which then controls the feed intake to preserve the constancy of body conditions. Thus energostasis concept supports that energy supply to some tissues is monitored by brain and is then used to control the feed intake (Kennedy, 1966).

Factors Affecting Feeding Behaviour

- Voluntary feed intake of farm animals is under the control of hypothalamus in the brain. The centre located in the lateral hypothalamic area called feeding centre is responsible for stimulating urge for feeding in animals. In the medial hypothalamus area there is another centre called satiety centre, which controls the animal's reluctance to consume food any further (Wagon, 1963).
- In simple stomach animals, the feed intake is restricted by the gastric distension and is influenced by hunger contraction. In ruminant animals, the distension of stomach is restricted by rumen capacity, the digestibility of feed materials and rate of passage of food from the rumen. In ruminants feeding behaviour is not controlled according to nutrient requirement because of lack in correlation between meal size and pre and post meal interval. However, products of digestion may act as negative feedback signals.

- Physical filling of digestive tract and characteristic of feed constituents are considered very important. There are stretch receptors in the wall of stomach. The signals from the stretch receptors in the stomach wall depend on degree of stretch and number of stretch receptors involved. Stretch receptors in most or all parts of the gut relay information on the wall of the gut to the brain via the nervous system to inhibit feed intake. This act as a negative feedback pathway. There are evidences suggesting presence of chemoreceptors in the duodenum of the gut. But relative important of the stretch due to distension and chemical stimulus varies under different situation depending mainly on the type of feed. Rumen is sensitive to pH of its content and acetate in the rumen has been shown to depress the feed intake.
- Chemoreceptors in the wall of stomach and in liver are also considered to have a definite role in deciding feed intake.
- Gut peptides like Cholecy Stokinin (CCK), pantagastrin, endorphin all influence feed intake through their effect on chemoreceptors.
- Liver has been shown to be sensitive to glucose in monogastric animals as propionate in case of polygastric animals and the information is transmitted to the brain via autonomic nervous system. The local section of vagus and or splanchnic nerve blocks the transmission of such impulses to the brain.
- The level of many metaboilites and hormones in the blood has also been suggested to inform brain about the state of metabolism in the body. The changes in the ionic composition of Cerebrospinal Fluid (CSF) also influence the feed intake. The Ca^{++} and Mg^{++} ions stimulate feed intake but Na^{+} and K^{+} ions depress the feed intake in farm animals (Redick *et al.*, 1973).
- Grazing pattern of animals is different for different species and it is influenced by number of factors (Hancock, 1952) like animal factors (age, physiological status and nutritional need) and plant factors (herbage yield, palatability and plant height, etc.).
- Lactating dairy cows increase their energy intake in response to the demands for milk synthesis but this increase typically lags several weeks behind the increase in milk yield. There is usually a high correlation between milk production and nutrient intake. Lactating cows commonly lose body weight in early lactation, but the weight loss normally is recovered later as milk yield declines, but feed intake remains high. Thus, over the entire lactation, energy demands are generally matched by intake (Selman *et al.*, 1967).

Responses to Changes of Heat Exchange with Environment

Heat stress causes reduced feed intake and general performance. Continuous heat stress may reduce feed intake to such an extent that negative energy balance results and ruminants may not eat at all when a climatic temperature of 40°C is maintained. Although the critical temperatures or environmental conditions at which growth or lactation are reduced by heat stress vary with species and breeds within a species, animals have a relatively uniform productions rate and efficiency over a range of conditions. Under severe cold conditions, which cause increase heat loss, feed intake increases and efficiency of production is reduced (Hamilton, 1967).

The influence of heat balance on feeding is demonstrated also by direct heating or cooling of internal organs. Increasing the temperature of rumen contents in cattle, from the normal 38.0°C to 41.3°C with heating coils in the rumen, depressed intake by 15%. Decreasing the temperature of the rumen of cattle by adding cold water (0.5°C) resulted in a decrease in body temperature (0.5°C) and increased intake by 24%.

Control of Feeding Behaviour

The smallest units of feeding are individual bites, but a more frequently studied unit of feeding behaviour is the meal. Some sensory and metabolic stimuli affect feeding by changing meal frequency, while others affect feeding by changing meal size. Due to conditioning associated with feeding, factors affecting meal size in animals fed *ad libitum* may not be the same as those in animals adapted to feeding schedule (LaMagen, 1971). While meal size varies greatly, the amount taken in some extent of meals must be controlled to maintain energy balance. Signals of satiety controlling meal size must change during the course of a meal and, thus, must have short time constants compared with the signals that regulate long-term energy balance. Although many physiological functions change as a consequence of feeding and have been considered for possible satiety factors, only a few appear to have an influence in controlling meal size.

Sensory Cues

It appears that ruminants use the same sensory cues as other mammals for selection of feed. It is also likely that these cues play a role in initiating a meal. There is likely an interaction between sensitivity to sensory inputs and state of energy balance. Sheep, for example, may be most choosy when nearly satiated and eat almost all parts of plants when hungry (Tribe, 1955).

Although sensory aspects of feeding are important in feed selection and under some conditions may influence the quantity eaten, such as with dry feed acceptance in young calves, other oropharyngeal factors are probably not important. Cows in which the boli were removed from the rumen continued to eat for much longer times and consumed larger quantities of feed than during normal feeding. It is unlikely; therefore, that exhaustion of salivary glands or fatigue of jaw muscles limits or acts as a control for feed intake. Also, there is no evidence that a monitoring of volume of feed swallowed might influence feeding.

Gastrointestinal Factors

There is an increase in volume of ruminal contents during feeding despite prandial increase in rate of emptying of the rumen. It may be a possibility that the amount eaten at a meal might be limited by capacity of the rumen. When cattle were offered feed for about 6 h/day, the increase in total weight of digesta in the rumen during this period was 48% and the increase in weight of dry matter in the rumen was 96%. The consistency of these results, considering the range of feeds and types of cattle included, supports the concept that with roughages at least, cattle eat until a certain ruminal distention is achieved. This distention must be variable, however, and may be acting as a safety valve to prevent distress. In the ruminant stomach there is evidence for tension receptors with various neural adaptation times. These receptors have not yet been identified histologically. Sheep reduced their feed intake more in response to reticular distention. Thus, the actual stretch receptors for the feeding response to distention may be located in the reticulum.

Feeding can influence rumen fluid pH and the importance of pH on fermentation in the rumen is well studied. It is likely that feed intake is depressed when rumen fluid pH falls below 5.0-5.5 because of the resulting ruminal stasis. Receptors sensitive to changes in pH in rumen epithelium have already been described. This evidence may be against the likelihood of rumen pH as a physiological controller of intake, although under pathological conditions it may be a principal cause of an accompanying hypophagia.

As volatile fatty acids (VFA) have importance in ruminant energy metabolism, their effects on feed intake have been investigated in many experiments. During and after feeding, concentrations of VFA in rumen fluid and in blood increases. While this change is most apparent in cattle and sheep adapted to restricted access to feed. There is evidence that smaller increase occurs during and after spontaneous meals. Differences in VFA concentrations are large in different parts of the rumen for several hours after large meals because of the relatively slow mixing in the rumen.

Acetate is produced and absorbed in greatest quantities of all VFA, and it may play a major role in the control of meal size. Intra-ruminal injections of acetate solutions of various concentrations before or during a scheduled meal depressed intake in cattle, sheep, and goats. Several attempts have been made to identify receptor sites for the effect of acetate on feeding. Injections into the dorsal area of the rumen had greater effect on intake than injections into the ventral rumen, reticulum, or abomasum. Exposure of as little as 5% of the total rumen to high concentrations of acetate was sufficient to decrease feeding. Infusion of sodium acetate into the rumen causes depression in feed intake in goat, however, the depression in feed intake was lesser when the same amount is injected into the jugular vein. This suggests that on the lumen side of the rumen contain receptors sensitive to acetate that are not activated by acetate in blood.

A second major metabolite, propionate, also may have a role in controlling meal size. Intra-ruminally injected propionate depressed feed intake of cattle, sheep, and goats, and intravenous injections in cattle decreased intake. Despite similarities between effects of acetate and propionate on feeding, the receptors probably are different because similar depression in intake occurred whether propionate was injected into dorsal rumen, ventral rumen, reticulum, or abomasum. In addition, injections of propionate into the ruminal vein were more effective in depressing intake than were injections into the lumen of the rumen, mesentric or portal veins, or carotid artery. This suggests that propionate receptors may be in the ruminal vein walls and possibly also on the luminal side of the rumen but not in liver or in brain. Recent evidence showed that propionate receptors may be in the liver of sheep. Intra-ruminal injections of butyrate into goats resulted in little more than caloric compensation in feed intake in contrast to effects of injections of acetate and propionate.

While an animal is eating, it may be possible that because of increased rate of fermentation, stratification of digesta, and slow mixing in the rumen, the concentration of rumen fluid around the papilli may change substantially more than the average of the whole ingesta. Thus, VFA action on receptors, either at the surface or after absorption, would be enhanced. Apparently acetate and propionate are effective in ruminants' because of receptors in the ruminal area.

Metabolites

Glucose has long been regarded as a part of the controlling system for feeding in monogastric animals. Although severely reduced rates of utilization of glucose from insulin induced hypoglycemia or glucose analogues like 2-deoxyglucose do cause hunger and feeding, however, hyperglycemia and increased glucose utilization rates had little effect on feeding. In ruminants, blood glucose concentration, venous differences of glucose and, probably glucose utilization rates generally have decreased rather than increased with feeding even with ruminants adapted to a single daily meal of concentrate diet. Deoxyglucose causes feeding in ruminants when injected peripherally or intra-cerebroventricularly (Redick *et al.*, 1973).

There is little evidence that glucose concentration or utilization rate has a significant role in controlling feeding in ruminants; in fact, there is much evidence to the contrary. The hunger-satiety system of ruminants may be different from that of monogastric animals. It has been suggested that with starvation, the increased free fatty acids (FFA) concentration in plasma might act as a signal to induce feeding even though FFA increase with feeding in animals adapted to a daily feeding schedule. Intra-duodenal injections of long-chain fatty acids or fats in sheep depressed intake, but it was not clear whether this was due to depression in rumino-reticulum movements or to changes in blood fatty acid composition. Therefore, little information is available to show that FFAs are a cause rather than an effect of changes in feeding.

Amino acids in plasma have also been considered for roles in control of feeding. In sheep, the amino acids decline for a few hours after a single daily feeding and then increase to a maximum about 24 h after feeding. It is unlikely that meal size of ruminants is controlled by absorbed amino acids since amino acids are absorbed mainly from the small intestine several hours after ingestion. Diets containing even 40% protein were tolerated by cattle; although blood ammonia exceeds 100 mg/100 ml, feed intake was near normal. In regard to imbalances of amino acids or protein deficiencies the suckling pre-ruminant lamb decreased its intake about 50% in response to dietary deletion of either threonine or isoleucine and when a low total protein was fed (8% of gross energy as protein and amino acids). It is unlikely that the feed intake of ruminants fed balanced diets is affected directly by amino acid changes in plasma.

Hormones

Concentrations in plasma of some hormones, e.g., antidiuretic hormone, insulin, renin, change during feeding, but it is not known whether one or more of these changes affects feeding. When injected into sheep during spontaneous feeding, neither insulin nor growth hormone affected daily intake. Epinephrine and norepirephrine depressed intake only when injected at near lethal doses (Redick *et al.*, 1973).

Glucocorticoids caused increased feed intake in sheep when injected intramuscularly over several weeks. Hydrocortisone injected intravenously during spontaneous meals did not affect feed intake of sheep, although during the short injection periods the rate of hormone administration was 1000 times the rate at which 17-OH-corticosteriods normally are secreted in sheep. It is likely that corticosteroids act indirect1y on feed intake via their effect on energy metabolism (Tarttelin & Gorski, 1973).

Body Temperature

Ruminants have, relative to carnivores, a high specific dynamic action, and a substantial proportion is due to ruminal fermentation. Blood and skin temperatures rose during feeding in both cattle and sheep and fell when feed was removed. Hypothalamic temperature increased when goats and sheep became active at the time of day at which feed normally was offered, even when feed was withheld. Conversely, intra-ruminal force-feeding had no effect on hypothalamic temperature. It appears, therefore, that feeding is not related causally to increased hypothalamic or peripheral temperature in ruminants (Hamilton, 1967).

Changes of hypothalamic and surface temperatures during feeding are more related to nonspecific activity than to feeding. There seems to be little evidence that temperature changes per se act under most conditions as a signal for the hunger-satiety system. Hot or cold environmental conditions can influence feed intake but may involve only indirectly control of feeding through the energy balance regulatory system. Severe heat loads inhibit feeding, and this response often may be related to stress rather than to a normal signal for satiety.

Role of Central Nervous System in Feeding Behaviour

The hypothalamus has been identified as one of the important in control of feed intake among the various central nervous system (CNS) structures in behavioural control. Studies in rodents involving electrical or chemical stimulation or lesion of various hypothalamic areas have identified certain areas, which appear to be important components of the system involved in control of feeding and regulation of energy balance. The ventromedial hypothalamus (VMH) generally has an inhibitory effect on feeding, and lesions of this area can result in hyperphagia and obesity. The lateral hypothalamus (LH) appears to be responsible for initiation of feeding, and lesions in LH result in aphagia and weight loss (Kennedy, 1966).

Evidence of a similar system or regulating energy balance in ruminants is that lesions of the VMH but not other areas of the hypothalamus of goats caused hyperphagia. However, in sheep VMH lesions have not produced hyperphagia. Lesions in the LH of goats and sheep have caused sustained aphagia or adipsia. As in other animals, electrical stimulation of the LH caused feeding in satiated goats and sheep while stimulation of the VMH reduced feeding activity of goats (Rabin, 1972).

Further evidence for existence of an energy balance regulating system for ruminants has been obtained with injections of neural depressants into the cerebrospinal fluid (CSF) to suppress the inhibitory action of the medial hypothalamus on the feeding system. Satiated goats, sheep, and calves eat voraciously during perfusion of the CSF with pentobarbital. Neural depressants also cause feeding when injection directly into the medial hypothalamus of goats and sheep. It seems likely the VMH has an inhibitory action on feeding in ruminants similar to that in other mammals (Smith and Epstein, 1969).

Although these particular areas do appear to have important roles in the control of feed intake, the neuronal mechanisms involved in the information transfer have not yet been fully determined. However, inter-neuronal communication is probably via neurotransmitters, and many of the traditional neurotransmitter agents have been tested for a possible role in feeding behaviour.

A variety of agents injected into the brain can elicit feeding in cattle and sheep. To date it has not been possible to delineate any series of neurotransmitters that form a feeding circuit.

It is also likely that some agents act on combinations of several systems. Recently, role for certain brain peptides as neuro-hormones or neurotransmitters in both hunger and satiety has been indicated. The opiate peptides, the endorphins and enkephalins, have been implicated in several behavioural control systems including feeding behaviour. It has been suggested that in ruminants, an opiate peptide receptor system is involved in initiation of hunger. Some evidences showed CNS peptide involvement in satiety. Cholecystokinin octapeptide (CCK-OP) is in high concentrations in the CNS of ruminants and is localized primarily to cortical and hypothalamic areas. Results from experiments indicated that CCK-OP may have a physiological role in satiety. The CCK-OP probably acts specifically to decrease feed intake, since neither water intakes nor body temperatures are affected. In pigs, increase in osmoconcentration in the duodenum during a meal can inhibit feeding behaviour and inhibition is proportional to the hypertonicity of the duodenal content. This inhibition may be because of arrival of chime in the duodenum also trigger the release of CCK (Cholecystokinin) as exogenous CCK inhibits feeding and may acts as a satiety or inhibitory signal during meals (Houpt, 1984).

Under certain conditions, effect of CCK-OP on feed intake was longer. In sheep adapted to a 6-h feeding, injection of CCK-OP throughout that period resulted in decreased cumulative feed intake for up to 2 days. Thus, it appears that more chronic elevations of CCK-OP in the CNS could result in negative energy balance.

Bombesin, a nonapeptide structurally different from CCK, has been found in both, CNS and peripheral tissues. Peripherally bombesin has both cholecystokinetic and pancreozyminic effects but acts via its own receptors.

Bombesin was equally as potent as CCK-OP in suppressing feeding when injected into the LV of sheep. Thus, there may be two CNS peptide receptor systems involved with satiety. Moreover, it has been suggested that CCK-OP in the brain is released during feeding into the CSF, which then transports to CCK receptors responsible for initiating satiety and related physiological changes.

Recent reports indicated an important signal controlling feeding behaviour in a large number of species is NPY produced in the arcuate nucleus of the hypothalamus (Kalra *et al.,* 1999). Clark *et al.* (1984) and Miner et al (1989) have shown that intracerebroventricular injection of NPY stimulates, whereas that of an antibody or antisense oligodeoxynucleotide against NPY suppresses feeding behaviour (Akira *et al.,* 1994). The studies in goats suggests that NPY is released in the hypothalamus of goats episodically with an interval of approximately 2.5 h, which probably drives spontaneous feeding as a physiological signal in this ruminant species (Mogi *et al.,* 2003).

Factors Limiting Feeding Behaviour

Many factors limit feed intake and alter energy balance. These factors usually act independently of energy needs of the animal and, thus, can reduce production (La Magnen, 1971).

Feeding drive is suppressed by apparent restrictions related to the state of the rumino-reticulum, palatability, nutritional deficiencies, and metabolic disorders (Oatley & Toates, 1973). In ruminants the neutral detergent fraction of the feed has been proposed as the major limitation to feed intake of fibrous feedstuffs. Pregnancy places restrictions on the energy regulatory system as a result of a significant physiological stress including severe hormonal shifts and fetal displacement of the rumino-reticulum.

Feed intake is reduced quickly during most metabolic diseases such as pregnancy toxemia acetonemia, lactic acidosis, ketosis, or bloat (Fibiger et al., 1973). Most gastrointestinal disorders of either infectious or parasitic origin as well as many systemic diseases result in decreased feed intake. Mechanisms for the feeding response these diseases probably are varied and not related to signals normally controlling feed intake. Some feeds such as tall fescue contain intake-depressing components under certain conditions.

Many forms of stress decrease feed intake, probably for a number of reasons. Heat stress, and its effect on feed intake, is probably one of the most easily studied and documented forms. Stress caused by dehydration decreases feeding in ruminants.

References

Akira, A., Claes, W., Jesline, T.A., Leibowitz, S.F. (1994). *Mol. Brain Res.*, 21:55–61.

Clark, J.T., Kalra, P.S., Crowley, W.R., Kalra, S.P. (1984). *Endocrinology*, 115:427–9.

Fibiger, H.C., Zis, A.P. and McGeer, E.G.(1973). *Brain Res.*, 55:135-48

Hamilton, C.L.(1967). Food and temperature. In Handbook of Physiology, ed. Code, C.F., vol.-I, Washington, D C.: American Physiological Society.

Hancock J. (1952). *Proc 6th Intl Grassld Congr.*, 1999-1407.

Hughes G P and Reid D. (1951). *J Agric Sci., Camb.*, 41, 350-66

Houpt, T R. (1984). *J. Anim. Science*, 59(5):1345-1353.

Kalra, S.P., Dube, M.G., Pu S, Xu, B., Horvath, T.L., Kalra, P.S. (1999). *Endocr. Rev.*, 20:68–100.

Kennedy, G.C. (1966). *Br. Med. Bull.*, 22, 216-20

LaMagen, J.(1971). In Progress in Physiological Psycology,ed. Stellar, E. & Sprague, J M., pp.203-61. New York: Academic Press

Larkin R M. (1954). *Qd. J. Agric. Sci.*, II, 115-41

Miner J L, Della-Fera, M,A,, Paterson, J.A., Baile, C.A. (1989). *Am. J. Physiol.*, 257:R383–7.

Mogi, K., Yonezawa, T., Chen, D.S., Li, J.Y., Sawasaki, T. and Nishihara, M. (2003). *Domestic Anim. Endocrin.*, 25:175–182.

Oatley, K. and Toates, F.M. (1973). *J. Comp. Physiol. Psychol.*, 82, 415-27

Rabin, B.M. (1972). *Brain Res.*, 43, 317-42

Redick, J.H., Nassbaum, A.I. and Mook, D.G. (1973). *Physiol. Behav.*, 10, 543-7

Selman, I.E., Fisher, E.W. and McEwan, A.D. (1967). *Proc. Soc. Ethology*, 1, 7-8

Smith, G.P. and Epstein, A.N. (1969). *Am. J. Physiol.*, 217, 1083-

Tarttelin, M.F. and Gorski, R.A. (1973). *Acta. Endocrine.*, 72, 551-68

Tribe, D.E. (1955). *J. vol. II*, p. 285. London: Butterworths.

Wagon, K.A. (1963). *Calif. Agric. Expt. Sta. Bull.*, No.799

□□□

Animal Nutrition, 2012
eds. Dr. (Mrs.) Usha R. Mehra et al., pp. 561-569
Satish Serial Publishing House e-mail : info@satishserial.com; website : www.satishserial.com

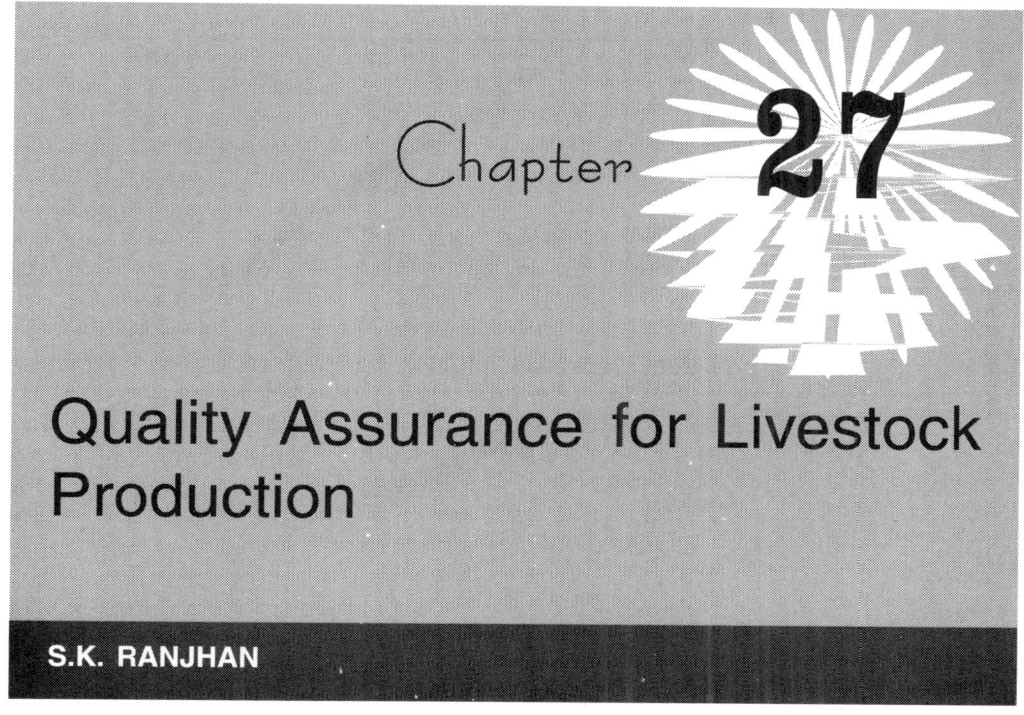

Quality Assurance for Livestock Production

S.K. RANJHAN

India has the largest livestock population in the world comprising of 185 million cattle, 97 million buffaloes, 63 million sheep, 120 million goats, 423 million poultry and 96 million broilers (DAHD, GOI, 2004), (Table 1). The animal food production through these sources is projected at about 96 million tonnes of milk (first position), 6.1 million tonnes meat (fifth position), 44 billion eggs (Fourth Position) and 1.6 million tonnes of poultry meat (4th position) in the world (Table 2).

The contribution of livestock sector to the food security in India has been very significant - increasing steadily at 4-5 per cent annually, despite the decreasing pasture land and availability of green fodder from only 4% of cultivable aerable land. This shows that the crop livestock integrated farming system being practiced by the Indian farmer is ideal where the crop residues from the main cereal/oil/commercial crops are routed through the animal system with adequate supplement with feeds to produce high biological value added products in the form of milk, meat and fibre.

Table 1 : Present Status of Livestock Population (2004) Millions

Species	World	India	% Share
Cattle	1339.3	185.5	13.9
Buffaloes	172.3	97.7	56.7
Pigs	947.8	14.3	1.5
Goat	782.9	120.0	15.3
Sheep	1058.6	62.5	5.9
Poultry	16352	425.3	2.6

Source: FAO, 2006

Table 2 : Present Status of Meat Production (2004) Millions Tonnes.

Species	World	India	% Share
Cattle	59.2	1.48	2.5
Buffaloes	3.11	1.48	47.5
Pigs	100.8	0.49	0.5
Goat	4.37	0.48	11.3
Sheep	8.21	0.24	2.9
Poultry	78.61	1.71	2.2
Others	5.0	0.14	27
TOTAL	**259.4**	**6.03**	**2.3**

Source: FAO, 2006

Linkage of Quality of Feed with Livestock Production

The quality and safety of animal food products (milk, meat, pork and poultry) has a direct bearing on the quality and safety of feed on which the animals are raised. The animals are to be fed as per the nutrient requirements for growth (meat), milk, egg and broiler production. There are various standards of feeding being practiced in India, namely, National Research Council of USA (2003) and Indian Council of Agricultural Research (1997). If the animals are underfed or overfed, the quality and safety of animal products are also affected.

The technologies of urea treatment of straws, feeding of bypass proteins, protected fats, probiotics etc., improve the animal performance thereby improving the production of animal products. Some of them have been discussed briefly below:

Urea Treatment of Poor Quality Roughages

Most of the research work has shown urea as a partial replacer for crude protein requirement in ruminants along with some high energy ingredients like maize, starch, molasses etc., for growth. (Ranjhan, 2001). The most practical method of feeding urea is, its ensiling with straws.

The urea treated straws improve the palatability of the straw and increase the nitrogen content. About 4% (W/W) urea solution in water is sprinkled on the straw which is uniformly mixed and the treated straw is ensiled for four weeks before using it. This method has been accepted on a large scale in Indonesia, China and some of the South-East Asian countries.

Feeding of bypass proteins

The microbial intervention in the reticulo-rumen may be beneficial or disadvantageous to the host animals depending upon the type of nitrogen source in the diet. With the intake of NPN compounds and proteins of low quality, the microbial protein synthesis improves the quality of the protein, but with the good quality protein, the fermentation in the rumen lowers its biological value.

The bypass protein technology is mainly used in high producing dairy animals (cows, crossbred cow/buffaloes). The content of rumen un-degradable protein are passed through the rumen which are then enzymatically digested in the intestines. The good quality proteins (having about 65% and above rumen un-degradable proteins) are then available for milk synthesis. The good sources of bypass proteins are cottonseed cake, soyabean cake, guar meal and maize gluten etc.

Various methods have been used to decrease the ruminal degradation of proteins to increase its Biological value, namely, physical (heat), and chemical methods, (formaldehydes). The protection of amino acids has also been tried. The NRC nutrient requirements now recommend the protein requirement for cattle in terms of rumen undegradable protein (UDP) so that more proteins are available for enzymatic degradation in the small intestines rather than fermented by the microbial enzymes in the rumen.

Feeding of Protected Fats

The protected fats increase the energy density of ration of high producing animals. The concept of protected fats feeding is the same as the protected proteins. The protected fats pass through the rumen undegraded and then digested in the intestines. They have effect on the quality of the fat deposited in the body and fats secreted in the milk. For milk production, poly unsaturated fats are protected and fed to lactating animals to secrete unsaturated fats in the milk to prevent cardio-vascular disease in human beings.

Feeding of Probiotics

Although the use of probiotics feeding in India is not prevalent at present, but when used in the diets of high producing animals, their performance is improved.

Climate Change and its Effect on Green Animal Production

Ruminants are blamed to produce methane which is one of the important green house gas affecting the climate. Ruminants (cattle, buffalo, sheep, goats) contribute 15-25 per cent of global gas annually (Leng: 1990, Melbourne). Methane is also produced by biomass burning, landfills, oil and gas production, coal- mining, rice cultivation and other natural resources.

Methane emission from ruminants in developing countries is difficult to quantify. However, Food and Agriculture Organization (FAO) of the United Nations indicates that these countries contribute significantly since more than half of the ruminant population inhabits in these areas. India alone accounts for one quarter of the cattle population which is fed on agricultural byproducts such as wheat straw, rice straw etc., low in digestible protein and energy. These poor quality roughages produce higher levels of methane which could be as high as 15% of digestible energy of the feed (Leng 1990). It has been established that ammonia levels, the most critical nutrient for stimulating efficient microbial growth and fermentation in the rumen, is inadequate in such diets. Supplementation of these diets in cattle and buffaloes suitably with NPN compounds and protein could increase rumen fermentation efficiently and reduce methane production and provide better nutrition essential for growth, pregnancy, lactation and work.

A few technologies have been developed to reduce the production of methane in the ruminants for efficient utilization of feeds like supplementation, defaunation etc.

Food Safety Requirements

Consumer priorities have changed tremendously during the last one decade both in India and abroad. Hence, there has been a conscious outlook for safety, welfare, ethics, reliability and zero risk factors for the consumer of animal products. India has accordingly taken many steps to improve the Sanitary and Phytosanitary (SPS) measures to follow strict surveillance on animal diseases conforming to World Trade Organization (WTO) norms on International Trade. However, domestic consumers are not very much aware about the quality and safety aspects of animal products. The animal food safety measures for domestic consumers are not properly monitored as is being done for the international market / consumers. Besides infective agents, residues of drugs, antibiotics, hormones, pesticides and heavy metals, are monitored as quality measures.

The International Organizations concerned with Food Safety are: Food and Agriculture Organization of the United Nations (FAO), World Health Organization (WHO), International Animal Health Organization (OIE), International Plant Protection Commission (IPPC) and Codex. Food Safety is ensured through quality control programmes which are in-built in the plant as well as regulated by the approved agencies. Some of these are: Hazard Analysis Critical Control Point (HACCP), Good Manufacturing Practices (GMP), Good Agricultural Practices (GAP), International Standards Organization (ISO) etc. Livestock Management has a major role to play in food safety, particularly with regard to pesticides and veterinary drug residues and introduction of pathogens and food spoilage organisms.

Risk Analysis

Hazard Analysis Critical Control Point (HACCP) is a risk management tool which provides a scientific approach to the control of manufacturing and processing products rather by traditional inspection and quality control of the end products. The codex Alimentarius Commission has promulgated the concept of HACCP by adopting guidelines for application of the system during its 20th session. The Critical Control Points in processing safe and hygienic meat followed at meat processing plants are a model code, have been given in **Annexure 1.**

Individual Identification and Traceability

In the identification of risk in food trade, traceability has become very important. Indian livestock production is by "masses rather than mass production" observed in some developed countries. Thus, the production of animal products and their safety problems are unique. The Codex standards state that the ***"farm to fork"*** concept of food safety has to be adopted which starts at the primary production level with the farmers where the animals are to be raised under disease free conditions with an individual record of all the drugs and feed resources utilized for feeding the animals so as to prevent the residual effect of drugs, pesticides etc., in the feed which may affect the animal products and thereby the health of the consumers.

Status of Organization International Des Epizooties (OIE) - List 'a' and List 'b' Diseases in India

Prevention, control and eradication of diseases are important in safe animal food production and trade.

Among the trade related diseases of cattle and buffaloes, except for Foot and Mouth Disease, India is free from all other diseases namely, Rinderpest, Vesicular Stomatitis, Contagious Bovine Pleuropneumonia, Lumpy Skin Disease and Rift Valley Fever.

In the case of FMD, effective control measures are in place actively supported by Central and State Governments. The entire State of Uttar Pradesh has not reported any FMD outbreak since January 2001 (OIE Reports 2002-2007). For control of FMD, 54 districts were identified during the 10th Five

Year Plan where 100% vaccination programme was undertaken from August 2003. The animals were vaccinated every six months under the programme. During the 11th Five Year Plan (2007-2012), 200 districts have been selected in the programme (including 54 districts of 10th Plan).

In addition, for meat exports, the practices followed in India are as per OIE guidelines given in Chapter 2 on FMD of Animal Health Code for Terrestrial Animals which completely eliminates the FMD risk from Indian buffalo meat, namely, de-boned and de-glanded frozen buffalo meat is first chilled at 2-4°C for 24 hours to bring the pH below 6. In a study sponsored by Agricultural and Processed Food Products Export Development Authority (APEDA) to assess the risk free status of Indian buffalo meat in respect of FMD, it was reported that acidic pH below 6 in the meat significantly eliminates FMD Virus in the meat. Data of more than 3,000 samples of buffalo meat showed an average of pH less than 6, suggesting that Indian deboned and deglanded lean buffalo meat is risk free which was confirmed by absence of FMD virus using ELISA and cell culture isolation tests (Kondaiah *et al.*, 2005).

India is free from BSE (Bovine spongiform Encephalapathy), Anjeszky's Disease, Heart Water, Trichanellosis and Enzootic Bovine Leukosis.

Vaccination and other control measures, including ante mortem and post mortem inspection, are followed in modern meat processing plants to ensure safety of meat.

Regulation of Animal Food Safety

The Indian animal products exports are regulated as per Export (Quality Control and Inspection) Act, 1963 and the Export (Quality Control and Inspection) Rules, 1964. Under the Act, Export of Raw Meat (Chilled/Frozen) Quality Control and Inspection Rules 1992 (Amended Rules 1993) and Processed Meat (Quality Control and Inspection) Rules, 1995 have been made for regulation of fresh, frozen and processed meats. Similarly, dairy and poultry products are also regulated for the quality control.

Registration of abattoirs and meat processing plants with APEDA, a Government of India Organization, is mandatory for export of meat from India. APEDA is assisted by Meat Plant Inspection Committee with members drawn from the Ministry of Agriculture, Ministry of Food Processing Industries, Export Inspection Council, Veterinary Experts from Central and State Veterinary Departments etc. The Committee inspects the infrastructural facilities, operation and sanitary aspects as per the meat export rules. A Plant Registration Certificate is issued by APEDA which is renewed every year. Thus, the quality aspects of meat for export are monitored and assured effectively at every step.

Similarly, dairy and poultry processing plants are also registered with Agricultural and Processed Food Products Export Development Authority (APEDA) for export of dairy and poultry processing products.

Animal Welfare and Meat Quality

Animal welfare issues are important in the production of quality meat and international trade. India follows the Act on the Prevention of Cruelty to Animals SPCA, 1960.

Food Safety Regulations in India

- The Food Safety and Standards Act, 2007
- Milk and Milk Product Order, 1992,
- Meat and Meat Product Order, 1973
- Water (Prevention and Control of Pollution) Act 1974
- Air (Prevention and Control of Pollution) Act, 1981
- Prevention of Food Adulteration Act, 1954
- The Prevention of Cruelty to Animal Act, 1960
- Export (Quality) Control and Inspection) Act, 1963
- Export (Quality Control and Inspection) Rules 1964
- Export of Raw Meat (Chilled/Frozen) Rules 1992
- Export of Processed Meat (Quality Control and Inspection) Rules 1995

Food Regulatory Authority in India

The National Food Regulatory Authority (FRA) has been created under the Ministry of Health and Family Welfare. It is a statutory body established by an Act of the Parliament under the Food Safety and Regulatory Act. The FRA will bring under one roof all the standards for inspection, quality, safety etc., for food including animal products. These standards will also harmonize with the International Standards. The animal food standards will jibe with the Codex Standards for dairy, meat and poultry.

The National Food Regulatory Authority has been established recently. The Indian Standards on milk and milk products, meat and meat products and eggs will be revised and upgraded to the international standards, taking into consideration the technological development in dairy, meat and poultry production under the OIE / WTO regulations. The up-gradation of national standards would provide quality safe animal products for the domestic market and further promote the export of Indian meat, dairy and poultry products.

Annexure 1 : Process Flow Chart of Safe and Hygeinic Meat Products in Meat Plants

Receiving & holding

Ante mortem

Lairage

CCP-1

Animal Race + Washing

Halal

Tieing of oesophagus

Skinning & Hide removal

Evisceration

Post mortem examination

CCP-2

Washing

Weighing

Chilling

CCP-3

Deboning

Processing

Packing material

QC Inspection

Packing, Cartoning & Shrink Wrapping

Metal Detector

Weighing of packed Cartons

Freezing

Cold Storage

Despatch

CCP - Critical Control Points of HACCP

References

Codex Alimantarius, (2006). Guidelines for Hygienic Meat Production, Production Joint FAO / WHO Committee Report.

DAHD, GOI (2004). Basic Animal Husbandry Statistics, Government of India, Min. of Agriculture, Krishi Bhawan, New Delhi-110001

FAO of the United Nations 2006. Animal Production Year Book.

Kondaiah, N.K. (2005). Safe Animal Food Production. Asian Buffalo Magazine - Page 30.

Leng R.A. (1990). Improving Ruminant Production and Reducing Methane Emission from ruminants by Strategic Supplementation. Report submitted to Environment Protection Agency (EPA), Washington, USA.

Ranjhan, S.K. (1997). Chemical Composition of Indian Feeds and Feeding of Farm Animals, ICAR, New Delhi.

Ranjhan, S. K. (2001). Animal Nutrition in the Tropics, Vikas Publishing House, New Delhi.

SPCA (1960). Society for Prevention of Cruelty to Animals Act, GOI.

□□□

Animal Nutrition, 2012
eds. Dr. (Mrs.) Usha R. Mehra et al., pp. 571-600
Satish Serial Publishing House e-mail : info@satishserial.com; website : www.satishserial.com

Chapter 28

Assessing Quality and Safety of Animal Feeds

D. NAGALAKSHMI AND S.V. RAMA RAO

Animal feed is a critical component of human food chain that has a direct impact on animal health, welfare and food safety. The most important previous objective of animal feeding was to meet the nutrient requirements of animals so as to achieve its maximum production with higher efficiency. But, in recent times food safety has become an emotive issue, having a high degree of public awareness. The situation has arisen from a series of food safety scares commencing with the *Salmonella* species contamination problems in poultry of the 1970s, shortly followed by the appearance of BSE (Bovine spongiform encephalopathy) or 'mad cow disease' in cattle in the 1980s, its resurgence in continental Europe in 2000 and appearance in Asia in 2001. Also, there have been increasing concerns expressed about the development of bacteria resistant to antibiotics. The issue of dioxin contamination of feed fats in 1999 and the introduction of genetically modified crops (GMOs) further increased public concern over various aspects of food safety. These events have underlined its impact on public health, feed and food trade, and food security. These food scares have generated demands for new legislative controls on animal feeds and animal production. The safety of food from animal origin starts with safe animal feed. Therefore feed manufacturers, farmers and food operators have primary responsibility for food safety. Quality assurance and feed-food safety are therefore are of paramount importance to all stake holders involved in the production chain.

Animal feed quality comprises of two distinct components-wholesomeness and safety. Total quality management deals with managing both the components to an acceptable level. Quality assurance (QA) is everything that goes into producing a product from the initial concept, to the ingredient specifications, to the formulation of the feed, to the manufacturing and distribution, to the feed trials to ensure performance, to customer service, to employee commitment and dedication to producing quality products. While, feed/food safety means a minimum or the lowest practical relevant content of undesirable/anti-nutritive substances so that it does not pose health hazard to the consuming animal or to humans consuming these animal products. Feed/food safety should be considered along the food chain. For animal nutritionists, maximizing of animal production remains an important criterion, but now there is also a need to achieve a satisfactory balance between maximizing production volumes, minimizing costs and ensuring food safety and customer satisfaction. An effective solution to these demands requires new strategies for animal nutrition that involve the aspects of health maintenance, disease avoidance and general nutrition, all considered as requirements of feeds.

This chapter deals with quality control in feed manufacturing, methods for evaluating nutritional quality and feed safety assessments.

Quality Control in Feed Manufacturing

Quality assurance is a comprehensive program which ensures the production of products that consistently meet their predetermined quality standards. The American Feed Industry Association (AFIA) has defined feed quality-control programs as: 'All actions directed toward ensuring the product meets the specifications established by the manufacturer'. Any good feed quality-control programme contains four components i.e., ingredient quality, process control, finished feed quality and control of undesirable substances.

Ingredient Quality

Ingredients account for 70-90% of the cost of feed production (Jones, 1989) and could be still higher in larger feed mills. About 40-70% of variation in finished feeds could be associated with quality of raw ingredients. Thus the incoming ingredient quality is important for economic reasons besides minimizing the variability of finished feeds.

Ingredient specifications are essential in a feed quality assurance programme and is the first step in establishing QA for incoming raw materials. Specifications serve as the basis for purchasing agreements, feed/ration formulation and for ingredient inspection. Ingredient specifications for feeds and feed ingredients in India are given by Bureau of Indian Standards (BIS). The ingredients should be evaluated for its specifications and any adulterants or incriminating substances by physical examination or chemical analysis or both. The physical and chemical analysis is discussed in later section of the chapter.

In-Process Quality Control

The process of using high quality ingredients into high quality feeds involves three components within the feed mill: personnel, machinery and procedures. If quality is lacking in any of the above mentioned components consistently high quality feed production is unlikely (Jones, 1992). The feed should be produced following current good manufacturing practices. Clean out of equipment between batches to prevent cross contamination (to avoid contamination of another feed) is very important. Magnets must be placed at strategic locations, regularly inspected and cleaned. Scalping and cleaning equipment must be in place and functioning properly to remove superfluous materials. All the materials handling equipments, viz. conveyors, elevators, valves, turn heads and spouts must be regularly inspected, maintained in good working order, properly cleaned and free from misalignments and leaks to prevent cross contamination and/or housekeeping problems (McEllhiney, 1979). The feed bins must be inspected for proper functioning of bin level indicators and cleaned on regular basis. The frequency of cleanouts vary with type of material, season of the year, region, to ensure that ingredients or feeds do not build up (Jones, 1992) for molds and other toxic substances. The particle size reduction equipment in feed mill (grinders, roller mills, etc) should be periodically examined for screens as these affect the final texture and appearance of the products. Batching system validation should be conducted at least on a half yearly basis. All batching scales should be cleaned, inspected and calibrated on monthly basis. Volumetric and gravimetric feeders need more frequent checking i.e., once each shift or in some cases with every product change (McEllhiney, 1979). Batch mixers should be inspected and cleaned weekly and, should contain no buildup. Mixing time tests should be conducted at least twice a year. All the packing scales, lines and packing area should be cleaned and scales should be checked verified with standard weights. Usually the first 10 bags should be weighed when the packer is operating in its normal rhythm with no stops and starts.

Finished Products Quality Control

Finished product should meet the specifications as per the formulation and as per customer's satisfaction. The pellets should be of high durability with minimum number of fines. The packaging station, along with bulk loadout, is the last line of defence for quality control in a feed manufacturing plant. Here the samples of the finished feeds are collected for physical or chemical analysis. The bulk weights and package should be accurate for which it is coded.

Quality Evaluation of Feed Ingredients/Finished Feeds

The quality of ingredients/feeds could be evaluated by physical, chemical or biological methods. For any type of evaluation, appropriate sampling technique should be adopted for analysis of incoming ingredients and finished feeds. Gehrt and Poundstone (1976) stated that 'No analysis can be better than the sample from which it was made'. Good analytical data require that samples be representative of the whole and that their integrity has been ensured during transport to the laboratory and during their preparation (drying and grinding). Standard sampling procedures depending on the type of sample and nutrient to be analysed is available (AOAC, 1995). Appropriate sampling equipment should be selected for dry or liquid ingredients, those in bags or bulk, etc. The most common sampler used for dry materials is trier or probe. For bag samples, a trier of 1" diameter double tube without compartment is recommended. Take > 500g sample, 1kg preferred as follows: Lay bag horizontally and remove core diagonally from end to end. Determine number of cores as follows: From lots of 1-10 bags, sample all bags; from lot of > 11, sample from10 bags. Take 1 core from each bag sampled, except that for lots of 1-4 bags take enough diagonal cores from each bag to total > 5 cores. For bulk truck loads, rail or ship loads a trier of 1-3/8" diameter is recommended. For most bulk ingredients, the cross cutter or diverter type samples is recommended that cuts the entire stream being conveyed and sampler should be held in horizontal position in the stream established, approximately 30cm below the end-gate of the truck. Samples should not be taken from the first or last portions of a load. About 3 samples of approximately 2kg each should be taken in the middle of each third of the load. For open truck shipments, where automated sampling systems are not available- the trier should be inserted at an angle of 10°C to vertical and at least 5 locations would be probed, with at least one at centre of the load. Use slotted single or double tube, all with pointed ends. For bulk feeds draw > 10 cores from different regions; in sampling small containers (<10lb) 1 package is enough. After sampling, further sub sampling should be done to the desired amount, preferably by riffling, or by mixing thoroughly on clean oil-cloth or paper and quartering. Place samples in air-tight container. Further sample preparation for chemical analysis

(950.02; AOAC, 1995) grind sample to pass sieve with circular openings 1mm in diameter and mix thoroughly. If sample cannot be ground, reduce to as fine condition as possible. Do not grind molasses feeds. For liquid samples continuous flow method is preferred, also known as drip or petcock method. For drums of liquid, an oil thief should be used. Number of drums to be sampled depends on packages in shipment with at least 10% of the packages. Roll the drum to mix the contents thoroughly and insert the oil thief slowly through the bung.

Physical Evaluation

Physical evaluation is easy but rough in nature. One must be highly trained to identify the changes in the nature of the raw material/feeds. The physical evaluation includes examining the colour, taste, smell, sound and touch.

Colour: Change in the normal colour of the feed ingredients indicates the maturity state of the grain, storage conditions, presence of toxins, and contamination due to sand, possible use of insecticides/fungicides which gives dull and dusty appearance. Black coloured fish meal indicates the rancidity of fish oil. Dark brown colour of meat meal indicates over cooking.

Size: Size of the grains governs its energy and protein due to proportional decrease/increase in seed and its coat. Smaller the grain lower will be the nutrient contents due to more proportion of seed/grain coat. To evaluate the weight of cereals about 100grains or fixed volume is taken. Higher weight indicates a higher ME value. This technique is called Test Weight.

Homogeneity: Presence of contaminants like other grains, broken grains, husks, weed seeds, infested seeds is viewed. In the oil seed cakes, closer observation will reveal the presence of fibrous material like hulls in de-oiled groundnut cake, rice polish contaminated with husk. Presence of clumps in oilseed meals indicates inadequate cooling of the cake before packing. Clumps may contain fungal growth. Clumps in mineral ingredients are not suitable for premixing.

Smell: Standing near the stock immediately indicate any difference from the normal smell. Musty odour indicates the beginning of fungal contamination or boring insects. To detect rancidity in oil rich feed ingredients this is the best method. Odour of petroleum products is suggestive of excessive pesticide or fungicides. Leather smell of meat meal indicates adulteration with leather meal.

Taste: Each ingredient has a different taste; any change in the taste like bitterness in grains and oilseed cakes indicates the presence of mycotoxins.

The level of salt can be detected by tasting. Bitter taste of rice polish indicates rancidity of fatty acids.

Touch: Feeling the raw material indicates dryness. Clumps can be found out by inserting the hand inside the bag. The clumps may be due to high moisture content, improper storage, packing of fresh warm solvent extracted meal that crumble on application of light pressure. Clumps formed due to excess moisture will be very hard.

Sound: Dry grains on pouring down or biting will produce sound of spilling coins, indicative of optimum moisture in grains.

Common adulterants in feeds and fodders: The feed ingredients should be checked for possible adulterants (Table 1). Adulteration is defined as the admixture of a pure substance with some cheaper and low quality substance, done intentionally usually to make money. The common contaminant or adulterant is husk or sand. Winnowing is the best method to detect husk in the feedstuff. Sieving can be done to differentiate contaminants based on particle size. To detect for the presence of sand a weighed quantity of grain is soaked in water and then by sieving with hand, the grains can be separated. The remaining water is decanted and the settled sand is weighed to assess the level of contamination. Low CP and high CF in oil seed meals is indicative of adulteration with fibrous material. The high CF alone is indicative of adulteration with urea and or some inferior quality oil seed meals like mahua, castor or karanja cake. The amount of acid insoluble ash is a good guide to the amount of sand or other dirt which may be present. Determination of peroxide content and free fatty acid in oily materials is indicative of rancidity and duration of storage, respectively.

Table 1 : Common adulterants of different feed ingredients

Feed ingredient	Adulterant
Groundnut cake	Groundnut husk, urea, non-edible oil cakes
Mustard cake	*Argimona maxicana* seeds, urea
Soybean meal	Urea, hulls, saw dust
Deoiled rice bran, wheat bran	Ground rice husk, saw dust
Fish meal	Common salt, urea, crustaceans, feather meal
Mineral mixture	Common salt, marble powder, sand, lime stone
Meat and bone meal	Sand, leather meal, blood meal, rock phosphate
Shell grit	Sand, dust
Molasses	Water
Maize	Cobs, cob dust, sand
Rice broken	Marble, grit
Dicalcium phosphate	Calcite powder, rock phosphate

Certain spot tests (quick check by chemical tests on spot) can be done to identify the presence of undesirable and incriminating factors and quality of feedstuffs (Table 2). Application of spot tests in feed ingredients and mixed feeds is rapid compared to elaborate chemical tests.

Table 2 : Most commonly used spot tests

Constituent	Test	Remark
Thiram (Pesticide in maize)	100g sample+ 50ml $CHCl_3$ & shake (5min). Filter the contents with Whatman filter paper 1. Add few crystals of cuprous iodide to filtrate and shake	Filtered chloroform extract turns amber to brown colour with in 1-2 min- indicative of thiram
HCN in feeds	Dip filter paper into 1% picric acid solution & dry. Then dip in 10% sodium carbonate solution & dry and preserve in stoppered bottles. Take test material in test tube and add few drops of $CHCl_3$ & stopper tube tightly.	The sodium picrate paper turns orange and brick red if positive for HCN.
Argimona seeds	Prepare water extract of test feed and add concentrated nitric acid	Appearance of brown-reddish colour indicates presence of Argimona seeds
Mahua cake	To water extract of test feed add conc. H_2SO_4	Violet or pink colour - presence of Mahua cake
Linseed meal	Test feed is treated with 1-2 drops or more of dilute H_2SO_4 in microtest tube. The mouth of test tube is covered with a disk of filter paper moistened with a drop of reagent	Depending upon the amount of HCN produced a more or less intense blue colour appears
Common salt	To 1g sample, add 100ml distill water, stir & filter. Add 8ml HNO_3 to filtrate	White turbidity indicates presence of salts
Leather meal	Pick up brown to black particles from sample and place on petridish, add 3-5 drops of ammonium molybdate, stand for 5-10min	No colour change-Leather meal; Greenish yellow colour-Meat & Bone meal
Fish meal quality (presence of NPN)	Put 2-3g of test sample in a 100ml beaker and add 10-15ml distill water & stir. After 2-3 min, add 3-5 drops of test extract on white porcelain plate and add 2-3 drops of mercuric-potassium iodide alkaline solution	Heavy orange colour indicates presence of NPN. Intensity of orange colour of precipitate depends on amount of NPN

Contd...

Decomposition test (animal & marine products)	5g test sample in 250ml flask. Prepare cork, to fit 2.25" of filter paper strip pinned to bottom & moistened with saturated lead acetate. Add 50ml dilute H_2SO_4 (5ml acid + 45ml distill water) & insert cork. Stand for 16h.	Test paper darkens quickly, if sample is badly decomposed
Hoof or horn	Place 2-3 particles of amber colour test sample into a evaporating dish, add 5ml glacial acetic acid, stand for 60 min	Test particles if hard & tough- hoof & horn; soft & swollen- gelatin
Urease activity in soybean meal	Spread the sample uniformly on petridish, glazed paper with white background. Spray cresol red (0.1% solution) and thymol blue (0.1% alcoholic solution) reagent mixture (80ml cresol red, 20ml glycerol/sorbitol, 2g urea and few drops of thymol blue) and examine for colour.	Inadequate heat treatment- particles turn red within a minute. Adequate heat treatment- Few particles (<10%) slowly develop red coloration. Excessive heat treatment- No particles show red coloration.
Urea	Mix 10ml of indicator solution (rub 0.15g Bromothymol blue powder with 0.1N NaOH solution, make to 50ml with distill water) with 10ml urease solution (0.2g urease in 10ml water) in a watch glass. Using clean tweezers, dip pieces of filter paper (No. 5) in solution (to avoid uneven distribution of indicator and enzyme, wet entire paper at one time by laying in surface of solution). Allow paper to dry in place free from ammonia, strong air currents, heat. Paper should be orange when dry.	Moisten urea test paper with few drops of distill water. Sprinkle feed evenly over the paper. A dark blue colour will develop if urea is present.

Feed Microscopy

Apart from physical evaluation and spot tests for quick evaluation of feed quality, feed microscopy is a basic and major tool to identify feed ingredients, adultrants and contaminants of raw materials and finished feeds. It uses microscopic techniques in the hands of trained personnel. Feed microcscopy offers an especially high return-on-investment when applied to incoming feed raw materials. It can provide 'quality analysis' as quick confirmation of ingredient identity and quality relative to stored samples. The technique also can be used for 'quantitative analysis' of adulterants and contaminants for example, percentage of foreign matter in feedstuffs. Feed quality can be either qualitative or quantitative. Qualitative feed microscopy identifies and evaluates ingredients and foreign materials, either alone or in mixtures, via surface features (stereomicroscopy) or via cellular or internal particle characteristics (compound microscopy). Quantitative microscopy is proportioned measurement of each ingredient in finished feeds or of contaminants and adulterants in ingredients. Acceptance and rejections decisions of incoming ingredients can be done based on microscopy. The basic equipment for feed microscopy is not expensive and its components are: 1. Sample sets of known ingredients and ingredient mixtures, which can be built-up as a 'reference library' over time given good storage conditions. 2. Stereomicroscope with widefield eyepieces (magnification range 7-45X) and zoom objective. 3. Compound binocular microscope (10X flat field, high eyepoint oculars coupled with 4X, 10X, 40X and 100X planachromatic objectives) with graduated mechanical stage, adjustable condenser (with filter carrier and field diaphragm). 4. Illuminator (dual-light fibre types preferred for cool light) with both top stage and bottom lighting (often built into compound microscopes). 5. Sieves (for sorting meal particles by size). 6. Laboratory balance or micro scale (0.1-0.01g accuracy). 7. Assorted hand equipment, 'spot plates' (white porcelain and black painted glass), various containers, filter paper, sample fraction surface. The feed microscopy involves sampling, reduction, grinding and microscopic examination.

Chemical Analysis

Chemical analysis could be done for proximate constituents (AOAC, 1995), fibre fractions (Van Soest et al., 1991), non starch polysaccharides, minerals, vitamins and incriminating/toxic constituents, etc. Proximate analysis includes moisture, crude fat, crude fibre, crude protein, total ash and nitrogen free extract. The moisture content can be determined by oven drying (at 105°C for 16h/125°C for 4h or 135°C for 3h), vaccum oven drying 95-100°C (AOAC, 1995) or at <70°C, Karl Fischer or toluene distillation for silages and high fat feeds (Crosby, 1995). Crude ash ((942.05) is determined either by ashing at 600°C for 2h or between 500-550°C for 12-16h. For crude protein, Kjeldahl method of nitrogen estimation is used and then multiplied by factor 6.25 (954.01). Under this method to reduce variability in results certain points like choice of catalysts, temperature and digestion times should be taken care of. The Dumas technique represents an alternative method for total nitrogen (968.08) based on combustion of the sample taking only 2-5 minutes per sample, but problem is with the small sample size (20 to 500mg) (Patterson et al., 1999). A quick analysis can also be made by Biuret method based on colorimetry (550nm) for wide variety of grains but requires initial calibration against protein values obtained by other techniques. Crude fat is based on solvent extractions with or without hydrolysis with fat solvents (preferably petroleum ether, 40-60°C) (945.16 and 920.39). The Rose-Gottlieb method is required for feeds containing milk products, as the alkaline pre-treatment frees occluded lipids from protein capsules (ISO 1211:1984). Similarly, canned dog foods require extraction with a series of solvents after hydrolysis (954.02). The crude fibre (978.10) is estimated by digestion with dilute acid and alkali and the residue is designated as fibre, but under this method the separation of digestible fraction (nitrogen free extract) and non-digestible fraction (fibre) was not proper. The Van Soest system was developed with proper fractionation of structural carbohydrates (neutral detergent fibre (NDF); acid detergent fibre (ADF); cellulose, hemicellulose and lignin) and cell contents (Goering and Van Soest, 1970) and adopted by AOAC (973.18). The Fibretec and Fibre bag systems are the automated instruments available for crude fibre, NDF and ADF estimations. The starch should be removed in concentrate samples for efficient filtration and requires pre-treatment with alpha-amylase either overnight (McQueen and Nicholson, 1979) or by using heat-stable alpha-amylase (Sigma product A3306) during the last 30 minutes of NDF extraction and filtration (Cherney *et al.*, 1989) or pretreatment with 8M urea (Van Soest *et al.*, 1991).

One of the innovations in modern feed evaluation is Near infrared reflectance spectroscopy (NIRS): NIR represents one of the truly rapid forms of analysis for nutritional components and requires limited sample preparation. It is a long-established and now a mature technology. The analysis depends on detecting the presence and intensities of spectral bands from overlapping overtones corresponding to various chemical bonds, particularly C-H, O-H and N-H. The advantages of NIRS are: rapid, minimal or no sample preparation, on-the spot analysis of whole sample, a non-destructive technique, allows simultaneous measurement of several parameters, environmental friendly, requires no chemicals, high precision, high throughput and thus makes NIR a cheap technique on a sample basis. Limitations of NIRS are high instrumental cost, accurate prediction depends on the volume of inputs and suitable for major feed components, complexity in choice of data treatment, calibration procedures that are matrix specific and time consuming. NIRS has been accepted as an official AOAC method for moisture (AOAC 991.01), crude protein and ADF (AOAC 989.03). Also determines starch, and non-starch polysaccharides, metabolizable energy, insect or weed seed contamination in feed grains (Wrigley, 1999), can be used to identify feeds and perform authenticity checks (De Boever et al., 1994) and can detect heat damaged protein, fungal contamination and adulteration with modern pattern recognition software (Givens and Deaville, 1999). NIR now-a-days is also used to predict animal responses to foods such as feed intake, nutrient digestibility, live weight gain, milk fat and protein or meat composition (Stuth and Tolleson, 2000).

Apart from analysis of chemical constituents in feed stuffs, the biological methods, i.e., *in vitro* rumen fermentation techniques are present for evaluation of nutritional quality of feed resources. The digestion or metabolism trials conducted in animals to arrive at the nutritive value of the feeds are used. These animal based studies are accurate but time consuming, tedious, costly, requires large number of animals and feeds. Therefore, needs for laboratory procedures based on *in vitro* techniques arises. These methods include two stage in vitro digestibility method (Tilley and Terry, 1963), modified Tilley and Terry technique (Goering and Van Soest, 1970), enzyme solubility (De Boever *et al.*, 1986), nylon bag (in situ) (Mehrez and Orskov, 1977), gas production (Menke *et al.*, 1979) and Rusitec (Czerkawski and Breckenridge, 1977), etc. Also, regression equations have been developed to predict digestibility from forage chemical composition. These *in vitro* methods are popular as they can accommodate large number of samples, furnish quick results, and require small quantity of sample, less laborious, simple and economical. These biological methods are more meaningful since microorganisms and enzymes are more sensitive to factors influencing the rate and extent of digestion than are chemical methods (Van Soest, 1994).

Animal Feed Safety and Risk Assessments

For feed safety assessments, it is important to establish guidelines that are generic enough to encompass the requirements of all ingredients and are flexible enough to allow for differences in ingredient types. Evaluations are often conducted on a case by case basis due to the specific characteristics and use of the ingredients which make up a complete feed. Safety assessments are often multifaceted. They usually consider both the safety of animals as the primary consumers of the feed, and safety of humans as the indirect consumers. In some cases, risk to people working with and mixing feed, and risk to the environment are assessed.

Understanding the risk posed by various food contaminants and residues forms the basis of controlling them. Risk basically a mathematical concept and can be defined as a product of hazard and exposure. Hazard is an intrinsic property of a substance to cause adverse effects, while exposure depends on environmental conditions and presence of contaminants. Exposure itself has two variables: quantity and time. Determination of all these factors is required for risk assessment associated with a particular hazardous substance and ensuring safety of food chain from it. On the basis of no observable adverse effect level (NOAEL) or lowest observable adverse effect level (LOAEL), the allowed daily intake (ADI) for residues and tolerable daily intake (TDI) for food contaminants are calculated (Renwick *et al.*, 2003). These values form the basis of maximum residue level (MRL) calculations and in absence of reference MRL for a particular food or feedstuff these calculations can be used for fixing MRL at Institute level. The assessment of feed and feed ingredients should be based on the Codex Principles for Risk Analysis (FAO, 2006). The risk assessment of microbiological and chemical hazards in feed and feed ingredients should be developed considering relevant Codex texts such as for pesticide residues, veterinary drugs, food additives, contaminants in foods (FAO, 2007) and microbiological risk assessment (FAO, 2001).

The steps for risk assessments are:

1. Hazard identification - for chemicals, the hazards are identified, including components, impurities, undesirable substances, and the toxicological profile or any other relevant assessment end points. In the case of micro-organisms the relevant pathogens and the microbiological profile of the feed are identified.
2. Hazard characterization - for chemicals the relevant reference values, especially for an oral route exposure are identified (e.g. LD_{50}, ADI) for all species of concern, including non-target species. For microbiological hazards, the nature and the severity of the adverse health effects are characterized and where possible a dose-response relationship established.
3. Exposure assessment - the potential exposure of animals and humans to undesirable substances or micro-organisms is determined based on the prevalence and concentrations of these hazards in the daily ration of the feed or feed ingredient, feed and food consumption data and consideration of any processing effects.
4. Risk characterization - the risk is characterized by combining information on the nature of the adverse health effect of the hazard and the potential for exposure to the hazard, with the inclusion of uncertainty factors. Toxico-kinetic or other models that can predict the transfer of potential residues or pathogens from feed to foods may be used.

A wide range of substances threatens the integrity of safe feed production chain that can be biological, chemical, physical or miscellaneous origin.

1. Biological hazards: All food pathogens like *Salmonella, Clostridium, Botulism, Prions* and many others.
2. Chemical hazards: Residues (pesticides, veterinary drugs), contaminants (environmental contaminants like heavy metals, dioxins, PCBs and mycotoxins; and process contaminants), plant endogenous toxins, feed additives, etc.
3. Physical hazards: Glass, wood, stone, plastic, metallic objects, radionuclide's, etc
4. Miscellaneous hazards: GM crops, novel and functional foods, etc.

Biological hazards: Animal feed or forage may be a source of a limited number of infections for farm animals that could lead to human illness. Probable organisms transmitted by animal feed are presented in Table 3.

Table 3 : Principal biological agents transmitted through animal feed (Hinton, 2000; D'Mello, 2004)

Category	Feed or feed ingredients	Dried/fermented forages	Pasture or grazing land	Waste food/ garbage
Infectious agents transmissible to humans from farm animals i.e., zoonoses	*Bacillus anthracis spiralis, BSE, Salmonella, E.coli, ND virus*	Toxoplasma	*Bacillus anthracis spiralis* spores; *Mycobacterium* spp. from wild life sources; E.coli including E.coli 0157; eggs of *Cysticercus bovis*	Trichinilla
Infectious agents or their products which cause disease in both farm animals & humans- Non-zoonotic	--	*Clostrodium bolulinum* toxin *Listeria monocytogens*	--	–
Infectious agents causing epidemic diseases in farm animals which may result in human hardship	Viruses of African swine fever, foot and mouth disease and swine fever			Viruses of African swine fever, foot and mouth disease and swine fever
Non-infectious agents which cause disease from farm animals & humans	Fungal hyphae and spores causing allergic disease	Fungal hyphae and spores causing allergic disease		
Products of non-infectious agents which cause disease in farm animals & humans	Mycotoxins	Mycotoxins	Mycotoxins	

Salmonella species: Many serotypes of *Salmonella* have been implicated in diseases of farm animals. The two most important serotypes associated with human disease are *enteriditis* and *typhimurium*. *S. typhimurium* is universally distributed while *S. enteriditis* has emerged as a regular pathogen of poultry and contaminant of eggs and chicken meat. Feed ingredients like meat cum bone meal, meat meal, fish meal and dried poultry manure used in ruminant diets, if not sterilized properly could be the sources of infection. Intensive pasture utilization and practice of spreading cattle slurry on to pastures are other potentially significant sources of infection. *S. enterica* commonly occurs in cattle feeds in US, Europe and South Africa with contamination rates ranging from 5 to 19 % (Krytenburg et al., 1998). The most effective means of eliminating Salmonella from feed is pasteurization (eg., 85°C with a residency time of 4 minutes).

Escherichia coli: There is particular concern over the occurrence of *E. coli* O157, as it is linked with human illness. Cattle feeds contain *E. coli* usually through faecal contamination with faeces. The application of slurry on to pastures has potential for transfer of faecal *E.coli* to grazing animals. Lynn et al (1998) reported 30% of cattle feed samples collected in USA were contaminated with *E. coli* (non-O157) and 25% from dried poultry litter fed to dairy animals (Jeffery et al., 1998).

Listeria monocytogenes: Occurs in big-bale and poor-quality silages with higher DM. Silage contamination with *Listeria* is important as it causes abortion, meningitis, encephalitis and septicaemia in animals and humans. Ensiling grasses under anaerobic conditions, at low pH regime excludes *Listeria*. However, in big-bale silages a degree of aerobic fermentation may occur, favoring growth of *Listeria*.

Clostridia: Two anaerobic *Clostridia* species i.e., *Cl. perfringens* and *Cl. botulinum* are of major concern in feed. Both could be a contaminant in inadequately ensiled feed materials. *Cl. perfringens* has been linked to bloat (gastric dilatation) in primates and necrotic enteritis in poultry (Annett et al., 2002). *Cl. botulinum* type B and/or C have been isolated from damp alfalfa hay, hay cubes, brewer's grains and mixed poultry feed (Wichtel and Whitlock, 1991). *Cl. perfringens* is resistant to heat in spore state and hence found in pellet feeds too (Greenham et al., 1987).

Brucella: *Brucella* infection could spread in animals via. plants contaminated with infected material from aborted animals in grazing fields or from which pasture is harvested and used for animal feed. If contaminated forage is fed to milking animals, the micro-organisms may be excreted in their milk. If this milk is not pasteurized prior to consumption by humans, it is a risk to food safety.

Bacillus anthracis: This organism causes Anthrax, sporulates on exposure to air and the resulting spores can survive for long periods in the environment and in contaminated feed particularly meat and bone meals prepared from animals which have died from anthrax. Cases have also been observed in people after consuming meat of infected animals.

Mycobacterium spp: Wildlife species e.g. the badger (*Meles meles*) in the UK and brush-tailed possum (*Trichosurus valpecula*) in New Zealand are both reservoirs of infection with *Mycobacterium bovis* and can pollute pasture land with faeces and urine. In these areas, screening is done on regular basis and reactors are slaughtered at an early stage in the infection and before they develop tuberculosis, pneumonia or mastitis. Tuberculosis remains a problem in cattle in many developing countries. There is a need to eradicate the infection from the cattle and hence reduce the risk of infection spreading to the human population.

Monitoring pathogens either in feed mixtures or feed ingredients requires direct detection of the pathogen. The feed and feed ingredients since comprises of large variety of products that differ in their composition, and could consist of complex matrices that can negatively affect microbiological analysis. Therefore for each microorganism the technical procedure should be adjusted, optimized and validated for different types of feeds in order to get reliable results. ISO has given Horizontal method for detection of *E. coli* 0157 (ISO 16654: 2001), *Coliforms* (ISO 4831: 2006), *Salmonella* (ISO 6579: 2002). The OIE Manual of Diagnostic Tests and Vaccines for Terrestrial Animals (OIE, 2004) have given analytical methods for Bovine *Brucellosis* (Chapter 2.3.1), *Salmonella* (Chapter 2.10.3) and Verocytotoxigenic *E.Coli* (Chapter 2.10.13), mostly in clinical samples, with some relevance to foods/feeds. Maciorowski *et al* (2002a) reported the use of low nutrient medium for microbial enumerations of fresh and stored animal feeds being comparable to traditional bacterial plating media. Molecular analysis could be applied as a surveillance method to detect microbial contamination in animal feed samples (Maciorowski et al 2005). These techniques are rapid and hence advantageous over accepted methods (involving the isolation of bacteria by enrichment, selective culturing and biochemical or serological identification). Traditional culturing methods can take up to 5-7 days to produce results versus 24-36h for molecular analysis. Based on molecular analysis numerous commercial PCR kits are available for *Salmonella* spp with more than 95% accuracy. Part of the difficulty with molecular assays lies with the problem of extracting and recovering representative samples from feeds for molecular analysis. A detergent-based initial detachment of micro-organisms from feeds followed by the modified procedure of Widmer et al (1996) was found to be the most robust extraction technique for removing inhibitory compounds (Maciorowski *et al.*, 2002b).

Transmissible spongiform encephalopathy (TSE): TSE's are non-febrile neurological disease of man and many animal species including ruminants. TSE's are associated with incompletely defined agents, currently termed prions which are resistant to normal heat treatment of feed and food. Prion proteins are normal animal tissue components with the capacity to transform into agents causing fatal neurological syndromes in a wide range of species. Sheep scrapie has been recognized for over 250 years, while Bovine Spongiform Encephalopathy (BSE) was 1st recognized in UK in 1986. The onset of BSE was attributed to the feeding of cattle with meat and bone meal prepared from carcasses of scrapie-infected sheep. The reported occurrence of a new variant of the human TSE, Creutzfeldt-Jakob disease (vCJD) has raised the possibility of an association with BSE in cattle with CJD in humans through consumption of BSE-contaminated beef. This led to extensive and stringent legislation in the European Union regarding the use of mammalian processed animal proteins (PAPs) (meat meal, meat cum bone meal, etc) in livestock feeding (Regulation 2001/999/EC, EU, 2001). Milk and milk products such as whey and egg and egg products are allowed for feeding to farmed animals. Feeding of by-products to the same species and the source is prohibited (species-to-species ban) by Animal By-product Regulation 2002/1774/EC (EU, 2002). Generally a zero tolerance for PAP in feed is applied.

Microscopic evaluation is currently the only accepted method for the detection and characterization of meat cum bone meal and other processed animal proteins (Directive 2003/126/EC, EU, 2003) and can detect processed animal proteins at the levels even below 1g/kg with great accuracy. But classical microscopy cannot discriminate between vertebrate classes (mammal versus avian; ruminant vs. non-ruminants) of animal proteins. Detection of DNA and specific proteins by polymerase chain reaction (PCR) are additional methods for identification of PAP's below 1g/kg and could detect the source in terms of animal species and breeds, could be a future method of detection, since it combines both requirements of a species specificity and high forensic value of the result, but full validation of this method is required (Van Raamsdonk et al., 2007). Other methods such as near-infrared spectroscopy (NIRS), near-infrared microscopy (NIRM), near infrared imaging, liquid chromatography and olfactometry techniques can be applied. NIRS is a non-destructive method and could be applied on-line in feed production plants. But the detection limit is too high to be applied in official control laboratories and method still requires validation. Lateral flow immunoassays (dip sticks) for detection of MBM in feeds are used at field level.

Endoparasites: Some endoparasites of animals, such as *Echinococcus, Toxoplasma gondii, Cisticercus* and *Trichinella,* present a risk to human health, and ingestive stages can contaminate animal feeds. These pathogens can colonize/infect farm animals, and may pose a threat to human health if infected or contaminated products are ingested. The protozoan *Toxoplasma gondii* causes abortion in pregnant ewes and neonatal deaths in lambs and potential source of infection in ewes is preserved forage or bedding contaminated with faeces of cats and rodents (hosts of parasite). Human may become infected by accidental ingestion of oocysts from cat faeces due to poor hygiene practices. In addition, the cysts of the parasite may be present in the muscles of meat animals, particularly sheep and pose a threat to human health, if the infested meat is eater raw or partially cooked. *Trichinella spiralis* is principally a parasite of pigs and viable cysts in the muscles act as source of infections consuming raw or partially cooked meat. The OIE (2004) Manual of Diagnostic Tests and Vaccines for Terrestrial Animals have given analytical methods for Cysticercosis (Chapter 2.10.1).

Non Biological Hazards

Chemical Contaminants

A variety of inorganic and organic chemicals present in the feedstuffs can either elicit allergic reactions (food sensitivities) or intoxications causing tissue damage or other negative impacts on the health of the animals or may pose public health. These chemicals can be broadly classified as contaminants, residues, feed additives or endogenous substances

Contaminants : Industrial processes emit several thousands of inorganic (heavy metals and nitrate) and organic chemicals (dioxins and aromatic hydrocarbons) in to environment.

Heavy metals: Pollution of pasture and other farm land with heavy metals may occur due to aerial spread of smelting plants and other types of industrial wastes or the spreading of human and animal waste onto land (Strauch, 1987). Heavy metals may be ingested by animals grazing the pasture and these metals subsequently pass on to the human population via meat or other products of animal origin (Miller *et al.*, 1995). Heavy metals cannot be degraded or destroyed, hence persistent every where. Heavy elements or metals (elements with at least 5 times higher specific gravity than that of water) of greatest public concern are cadmium, lead, mercury as well as arsenic. Heavy metals become toxic when they are not metabolized by the body, accumulate in the soft tissues and also irreversibly bind to body tissues eg: lead to bone or cadmium to kidneys. Dietary exposure of the heavy metals showed a dose response related increase in heavy metal concentration in liver and kidney, but less in muscle and milk (Kreuzer et al., 1981). Care should be taken with regard to use of toxic elements in animal diets (Table 4).

Table 4 : Recommended maximum levels of heavy metals and halogens in animal feed (Association of American Feed Control Officials, 1996)

Category	Maximum concentration (ppm)	Metal
Highly toxic	10	Cd, Hg, Se
Toxic	40	Ba, Co, Cu, Pb, Mo, Tu, Va
Moderately toxic	100	Sb, As, I, Ni
Slightly toxic	1000	Al, B, Br, Bi, Cr, Mn, Zn

Cadmium is present in many feed and feed ingredients, particularly in mineral salts, and forages grown near smelting and mining areas. The mineral carry-over to milk, meat and eggs from feed is very low or (>0.05%) (Bluthgen, 2000). Arsenic and mercury are heavy metals present in feeds of marine origin. Lead is also a ubiquitous contaminant. Major share of dietary mercury intoxications originate from the Hg-organic fungicides (dimethyl mercury; chloride and phosphate of methyl mercury; chloride and acetate of phenyl mercury). All these are extremely toxic, lipid soluble and bioaccummable (Table 5) Methyl mercury was used for seed toxin treatment and thus found its way in animal feed and caused death of livestock. Bluthgen (2000) reported a carry-over percentage from feed to milk of 0.1-1% for lead, less than 0.1% for mercury. The recycled trace mineral sources have a high chance of contamination with heavy metals, dioxins/PCBs (Mc Cartney, 2009). The risk management of these heavy metals should be based on HACCP approach, i.e., avoid the use of the contaminated feedstuffs.

Table 5 : Minerals, their sources and bioaccumulation in animal tissues (NRC, 2005)

Mineral	Sources	Bioaccumulation in animal tissue
Arsenic (inorganic)	Sea plants, fish products and supplemental minerals	Fish
Cadmium	Mineral supplements (eg., phosphates, zinc sources). Forage/grains (depending on geographical area) Manure, sewage, sludge or phosphate fertilizers	Kidney and liver Highest concentration in Shellfish, oysters, salmon and fungi, Low concentrations in dairy products, legumes, meats and eggs
Lead	Contaminated soil, lead paints, water from plumbing systems that contain lead, batteries. Mineral supplements ($CuSO_4$, $ZnSO_4$, ZnO)	Bone, brain and kidney
Mercury/ methyl Hg	Anthropogenic contamination, fish meal	Liver, kidney, skeletal muscles, brain Fish, marine animals

CEN has published a graphite-furnace (GF)-AAS method for lead and cadmium (EN 15550:2007), hydride generation (HG)-AAS method for arsenic and cold vapour (CV)-AAS for mercury. A CEN-method (EN 155510:2007) based on inductively coupled plasma atomic emission spectrometry (ICP-AES) could be applied for lead and cadmium.

Mycotoxins: Mycotoxins are ubiquitous and wide spread at all levels of food chain. Feedstuffs could simultaneously contain various mycotoxins from different sources of molds (Table 6).

Table 6 : Mycotoxins commonly identified in feed ingredients and their effect on animals

Major class of Mycotoxin	Mold	Nature of toxin & effects
Aflatoxin (B1, B2, G1, G2, M1, M2)	*Aspergillus flavus; Aspergillus parasiticus*	Hepatotoxin, Immunosuppresion, carcinogenic, teratogenic; Reduced feed intake, Reduced production
Trichothecenes (3-or 15-acety-deoxynivalenol, Deoxynivalenol, nivalenol, fusarenon X (type-B trichothecenes), T-2 toxin, HT-2 toxin	*Fusarium sp.*	Dermatoxins, immunologic effects, haematological changes & digestive disorders (Vomition, feed refusal, diarrhea), weight loss, reduced milk production,
Zearalenone (ZEA)	*Fusarium graminearum*	Estrogenic (vulvovaginitis, enlargement of uterus) & reproductive disorders (low birth weights, reduced litter size, abortion, swollen vents, reduced egg production
Ocharatoxin (OTA)	*A. ochraceus Penicillium* spp	Nephrotoxins (nephropathy, kidney dysfunction, gout) , immuno-suppression; Retarded growth, feed refusal, mortality
Fumonisin (B1, B2, B3)	*Fusarium moniloforme F. proliferatum*	Neurological disorders leukoencephalomalacia: blindness, head butting, and pressing, incordination), liver damage, pulmonary edema, pancreatic lesions
Ergot alkaloids (Ergometrine, ergosine, ergotamine, clavines)	*Claviceps purpurea, Cla. paspaspali, Cla. fusiformis*	Nervous or gangrenous syndrome

Mycotoxins transferred from feed to food are - aflatoxin B1 to liver, aflatoxin B1 to milk as M1, aflatoxin B1 to eggs as aflatoxicol; ochratoxin A to meat; deoxynivalenol to meat as DOM1; zearalenone to meat as zearalenol. The action limit set by the US FDA for aflatoxins is 100-300 ppb for maize, 0.5ppb for milk and for other food items limit has been set to 20ppb. While the limits set by European Union for aflatoxin B1 for all feed ingredients, complete feeds for adult cattle, sheep, goat, pigs and poultry is 20ppb and for calves, lambs is 10ppb and in milk and milk products (M1) is 0.05ppb.

FAO (2001) has suggested an HACCP concept for mycotoxin control. Various managemental practices was suggested by Edwards (2004). Emphasis should be to prevent during the growing phase of plants, as removal or inactivation of toxins often proved to be quite difficult or not economical. Mycotoxin control in field is however quite hard to be executed. Factors such as water activity of stored products, temperature, grain condition, gas composition of the intergranular air, microbial interactions and presence of chemical or biological preservatives influence toxin production (Shapira and Paster, 2004). Washing procedures using water or sodium carbonate solution reduced the mycotoxins in maize and other grains. The use of mould inhibitors or preservation by organic acids can reduce the amount of mould but not the content of toxins generated prior to treatment. Certain mycotoxin binding agents (bentonites), adsorbents (aluminosilicates, zeolitic minerals, clay etc) and glucomannans are used in livestock diets for reducing the toxic effects of mycotoxins.

The chemical diversity of mycotoxins and the equally diverse substrates in which they occur pose challenges for analytical chemistry. Mycotoxins are often produced in trace concentrations, so the sensitivity of the detection systems is also essential. Testing for mycotoxins involves in general, sampling, sample preparation and the analytical procedure. As the toxins are present in low concentrations (ppb) and often concentrated to a small fraction of the particles in the commodity sampling, sub-sampling and sample preparation become major sources of error (Whitaker, 2006). The variation associated with a mycotoxin test procedure is the sum of sampling, sample preparation and analytical variances, with sampling being usually the largest source of error (82% of variability). Aflatoxin contamination is not homogeneous; it is therefore very important to apply an appropriate sampling method. The AOAC (2000) has given methods for sampling, sample preparation and analytical methods for aflatoxin in various feed ingredients/feeds. Traditional methods have relied on solvents for clean-up steps and various chromatographic techniques for quantification; more recently, immunogenic assays that can be applied to samples with little or no clean-up have been developed. Mycotoxins are nonimmunogenic and can be conjugated to a protein carrier, and antibodies against almost all the major mycotoxins are now available. A variety of methods have been standardized, viz. a semi-quantitative ISO method based on thin-layer chromatography (ISO 6651:2001) and methods applying HPLC with fluorimetric detection after immuno-affinity clean-up. The latter method is commonly regarded as the reference method and has been adopted by AOAC (2000.02) and ISO/ CEN (ISO/EN 17375). For quality control of raw materials in feed mills, dipstick-like immunochemical screening methods are also applied. The rapid platform tests includes the immunological methods developed for testing aflatoxins, ocharatoxin, fumonisins, zearalenone and DON by fluorometer and ELISA methods. Some of the methods under investigation are minicolumn with adsorbent material, immuno affinity columns for selective adsorption for mixture of mycotoxins, mini column procedure for DON and a combination of chromatographic and mass spectrophotometer methods (based on minimal clean up of the sample).

Dioxins: Dioxins are stable, toxic and persistent organic pollutants. Chemically it is 2,3,7,8-tetrachlorodibenzo para dioxin (TCDD). Dioxins refer to a family of structurally and chemically related polychlorinated dibenzo para dioxins (PCDDs) and polychlorinated dibenzofurans (PCDFs). These are a group of polychlorinated aromatic compounds occurring naturally or as by-products of industrial activities. e.g. metal smelting, molding, or burning of chlorine containing organic chemicals such as plastics. Certain dioxin-like polychlorinated biphenyls (PCBs) with similar toxic properties are included under the term 'dioxins'. Sedimentation of dioxins from the atmosphere and into dietary plants leads to a unavoidable exposure of both animals and humans. Dioxin concentrates in fatty tissues of beef and dairy cattle, poultry, pork or seafood. Bovines accumulate dioxins from feed to their fat, with a transmission coefficient of 0-40%. The most important route for human exposure to dioxins is food consumption, contributing for more than 90% of total exposure of which products of fish and other animal origin account for approximately 80% of overall exposure. The Scientific Committee on Animal Nutrition (SCAN) reported that European fish oil and fish meals are the most heavily dioxin contaminated feed materials. PCBs are classified as probable human carcinogens and produce a wide spectrum of adverse effects in animals, including reproductive toxicity, immunotoxicity and carcinogenicity.

Since the Belgian dioxin crisis in 1999, dioxins have become important considerations for feed safety. Since then, numerous cases of contamination involving dioxin from unexpected sources have been reported. e.g. dioxins may be inherent to a product (e.g. clay minerals), can be formed during heat processing (e.g. lime in citrus pulp, dried bakery waste), or may arise through the use of treated wood in animal production, the grass meal or grass meal pellets produced from grass dried directly (e.g. coal-fired heating plants) and pasture placed near polluting plants. Dioxins may arise in animal feed via their presence in mineral sources (clays, recuperated copper sulphate, zinc oxide); food by-products; and fish by-products such as fish meal and fish oils.

The official method for estimation of dioxins comprises of extracting, concentrating and purifying dioxins using various chromatographic techniques and subsequent analysis using high resolution gas chromatography/mass spectrometer. High-resolution gas chromatography coupled with high resolution mass spectrometry (HRGC/HRMS) is currently the reference methods used in determination of very low concentrations of PCDDs and PCDFs. For rapid screening bioanalytical assays viz., enzyme immunoassay (EIA) and Dr. calux assay based on chemical activated luciferase gene expression (uses a dioxin sensitive cell, into which the gene that is responsible for making a firefly glow has been inserted) are followed.

Process contaminants: Now-a-days animal feed ingredients are exposed to variety of chemical and physical processes before reaching the animal, which may exhibit toxicity when ingested by animals. Polyaromatic hydrocarbons, heterocyclic amines, nitrosoamines, oxidized sterols, oxidizedtriacylglycerols, lysinsoalanine and acrylamide are some of the compounds that have been identified as process contaminants.

Residues

The presence of residues in feed may result from the application of a particular chemical during agricultural production or during treatment of animals.

Pesticides: Pesticides are widely used throughout the world in agriculture to protect crops and in public health to control diseases. e.g. insecticides, rodenticides, herbicides and fungicides. The pesticides can be divided into three major classes 1) compounds rapidly metabolized and excreted. e.g. Chlorpyrifos, 2,4-Dichlorophenoxyacetic acid, deltamethrin, diazinon, endosulfan, methoxychlor These compounds can be found during or shortly after exposure of animals. The risks for residues in animal products are considered to be quite limited. 2) Compounds with detectable accumulation in the animal. e.g. Chlordane, alpha hexachlorocyclohexane, lindane. These compounds can be found for some weeks after exposure of the animals. The risk management can consist of regular checking of feed ingredients from those areas in the world where the compounds are still in use. 3) Compounds with high accumulation. e.g. DDT, dieldrin/aldrin, endrin, Hexachlorobenzene, beta hexachlorocyclohexane, heptachlor. These compounds can be found in animal products for weeks or months after exposure of the animals. The risk management for these compounds should consist of regular checking of feed ingredients from those areas in the world where these compounds are still in use.

The methods of analysis for pesticides are very slow and expensive. High performance liquid chromatography, high resolution gas chromatography coupled with high resolution mass spectrometry is used for determination of pesticide residues. The ELISA can be used when large number of samples has to be screened that are rapid and easy. CEN has prepared two methods for persistent organochlorine pesticides like DDT, hexachlorobenzene and aldrin.

Veterinary Drugs/ Feed additives: Due to increasing intensification of animal production, the prophylactic use of drugs as a precaution against disease, hormonal drugs to control reproduction, tranquillizers to reduce stress and growth promoters are used. Typically, three kinds of risks are associated with the use of antibiotics or similar compounds viz., toxicological risks for human being, allergenicity to particular drug and risk of development of resistant strains of bacteria. Residues of veterinary drugs can be present in feed when ingredients of animal origin (terrestrial and aquatic) are used, but this is not a very significant route of exposure. Veterinary drug residues may be found in food products as a result of the carryover of veterinary drugs in feed during feed production. It is also important to take into account the illegal use of drugs in animal feed which may result in unsafe residues in meat, milk or eggs (e.g. chloramphenicol/nitrofurans in shrimps and chloramphenicol in milk powder). Volume 3 of the Codex Alimentarius contains, inter alia, MRLs for 15 veterinary drugs, guidelines for the establishment of a regulatory programme for the control of veterinary drug residues in foods, and a comprehensive set of definitions including acceptable daily intake, bio-available residue, bound residue, marker residue, maximum residue limit for veterinary drugs, non-extractable residue, veterinary drug and withdrawal and withholding time.

Many feed additives are being used in intensive animal production to improve the characteristics of feed, health and performance of animals. According to European Commission regulation (EC, 2003), feed additives are classified as Technological additives (antioxidants, preservatives, emulsifiers, preservatives, etc), sensory additives (flavours, colorants), nutritional additives (vitamins, trace elements), zootechnical additives (gut flora improvers, non microbial growth promoters) and coccidiostats. The excessive dosages and inappropriate use of these additives can pose a serious risk to public health through the development of resistances to certain antibiotics and intrinsic toxicity of certain products. Adequate administration and prescribed withdrawal times and due attention, when producing and using medicated feeds are important for reducing the risk from feed additives.

To check for carryover of antibiotic veterinary drugs and coccidiostats, at industry level, HPLC methods are frequently applied. For a number of these analytes immunochemical methods such as ELISA are also available. Microbiological inhibition assays are frequently used for multiscreening for antibiotics. Suspect samples can be confirmed with LC-MS/MS or liquid chromatography with diode array detector (LC-DAD) methods. For ionophoric coccidiostats (monensin, narasin and salinomycin) a multimethod based on HPLC has been published by ISO (ISO 14183:2005) and would become an official AOAC method. AOAC is working on HPLC methods for oxytetracycline (OMA-2004-Oct-017) and lasalocid (OMA-2005-Jan-002). For other analytes there is a need for method validation and standardization. For control of illegal use of chloramphenicol, immunochemical (dipstick-like and ELISA) screening methods are available. For other drugs, such as nitrofurans, HPLC can be used for screening. LC-MS methods are available for confirmation.

Endogenous plant toxicants: Many plant components have the potential to precipitate adverse effects on the productivity of farm livestock (D'Mello, 2000). These compounds are present in foliage and/or seeds of virtually every plant that is used for practical feeding. Typical concentrations for selected toxins are present in Table 7. Plant toxins may be divided into heat-labile group (lectins, protease inhibitors and cyanogens, which are sensitive to standard processing temperatures) and a heat stable group (antigenic proteins, condensed tannins, quinolizidine alkaloids, glucosinolates, gossypol, saponins, S-methyl cysteine sulphoxide, mimosine and phyto-estrogens). The toxic effects and potential presence of some toxic compounds in milk and meat are well documented.

Table 7 : Plant toxins: sources and concentrations (D'Mello, 1995)

Toxin	Principal sources	Typical concentrations
Lectins	Jackbean	73 units/mg protein
	Winged bean	40-320 units/mg protein
	Lima beans	59 units/mg protein
Trypsin inhibitors	soybean	88 units/mg
Antigenic proteins	soybean	--
Cyanogens	Cassava root	186 mg HCN/kg
Condensed tannins	*Acacia* spp.	65g/kg
	Lotus spp.	30-40g/kg
Quinolizidine alkaloids	Lupin	10-20g/kg
Glucosinolates	Rapeseed	100 mmol/kg
Gossypol	Cottonseed	0.6-12g/kg (free)
Saponins (steroidal)	*Bracharia decumbens*; *Panicum* spp.	--
S-methyl cysteine sulphoxide	Kale	40-60g/kg
Mimosine	*Leucaena leucocephala*	145g/kg(seed); 25g/kg (leaf)
Phyto-oestrogens	Clover, lucerne, soybean	--

However, there is lack of information about metabolic fates, residues and average daily intake for different toxicants. The risk pathway can be controlled by following Good Agricultural Practices (James *et al.*, 1994).

Physical Hazards

Radionuclides: The accidental emission of radioactive materials from nuclear power stations is a well-recognized problem having serious implications for the human and animal population, eg, Chernobyl disaster. The ingestion of contaminated feed and fodders with these radionuclides possess serious health hazard in the animal system and also in humans after it enters into the food chain via meat and milk. So, proper care should be taken while handling radionuclides in order to prevent its entry into food chain. The use of chemicals which either dilute the radionuclides with stable isotopes or analogous stable elements, or act as natural or artificial binding agents could be a possibility to reduce the risk of radionuclides.

Miscellaneous Hazards

Genetically modified organisms: Genetic engineering is the youngest branch of biotechnology. Its main products are genetically modified organisms (GMOs) mainly transgenic feed, food and fibre crop plants. The world wide cultivation of genetically modified plants (GMP) increased from 1.7 to 90 million ha/year from 1996 to 2005 with soybean, maize, rapeseed and cotton as predominant crops (James, 2005). The first generation GMP are characterized by input traits such as tolerance against pesticides or herbicides or against insects, while so-called second generation GMP are characterized by output traits as an increased content of valuable components (amino acids, fatty acids, vitamins, etc), an improved availability of nutrients or lower concentration of undesirable substances (eg. phytate, lignin, allergenic substances, etc) (ILSI, 2004). Animal studies conducted so far on 1st generation GMPs showed no significant differences in the nutritional value in comparison with non-GMP varieties (Flachowsky *et al.*, 2007). In certain experiments feeding of 2nd generation GMPs caused unfavourable side effects, which are of safety concern (Cellini et al., 2004). Though most DNA was degraded in the gastrointestinal tract (Wiedemann et al., 2006), some fragments have been found in animal tissue. Transgenic protein has not been detected in any animal tissues or products, but fragments of DNA from endogenous, high copy number chloroplast genes from plants have been detected in poultry, pig and ruminant tissues. Low copy endogenous and transgenic DNA in animal tissues have been detected but to a lesser extent than high copy genes (Alexander *et al.*, 2007). To ensure the safety of GM plants as animal feed, regulatory bodies have adopted the policy of substantial equivalence. Rigorous testing procedures for novel crops should be done, especially for 2nd generation GM crops and nutritional equivalence should be determined by performing trials on animals, in addition to substantial equivalence tests.

GMO tests detect either the novel DNA or the novel protein. Basically, there are 4 types of detection methods: Screening methods - have the broadest application because they can detect multiple GMO traits, 'Trait-specific methods'- detect a specific novel protein, 'Construct-specific' methods- detect a specific DNA construct used to introduce the novel trait and 'Event-specific' methods that provide unambiguous identification of a specific transformation event. Most screening, trait-specific or protein detection methods are immunoassays like ELISAs as they are easy to use, robust and relatively in expensive. The lateral flow strip formats requiring only minimal sample preparation are suited for on-site testing (in the fields or at the feed plant). Protein detection methods are best suited for raw or partially processed samples. Protein detection relies on the amount of protein produced or 'expressed' by the novel DNA construct and also on whether that protein is expressed in the part of the plant being tested. DNA detection methods are PCR based and very sensitive than other methods. This method can provide event specific results for plants expressing the same recombinant protein, but very expensive and sensitive.

International Standard-Setting Organizations

The international organizations engaged in food safety are World Trade Organisation, International Standards Organization (ISO), Codex Alimentarius Commission Office International des Epizooties (OIE of World Animal Health Organization), International Plant Protection Convention (IPPC) and Global Environment Monitoring System/Food Contamination Monitoring and Assessment Programme (GEMS/Food, 2003). The FAO, WHO, Codex and OIE are involved in many activities related to animal feeding, including risk assessment, development of international standards, capacity-building and technical assistance to their Members to promote feed safety. These organizations collaborate closely to ensure a coordinated approach along the food chain. The activities of FAO and WHO to ensure feed safety is development, compilation and dissemination of information; promotion of wide alliances and partnership with private sector; technical assistance and capacity- and institutional building and awareness raising and policy advice. The FAO and WHO provide the scientific basis to Codex through independent scientific expert meetings and consultations and through the Joint FAO/WHO Expert Committee on Food Additives (JECFA); the Joint FAO/WHO Meetings on Pesticide Residues (JMPR), the Joint Expert Meetings on Microbiological Risk Assessment (JEMRA) and the Joint FAO/WHO ad hoc Expert Meetings on Safety Assessment of Food Derived from Biotechnology.

The Codex Alimentarius Commission established the ad hoc Codex Intergovernmental Task Force on Animal Feeding in July, 1999 to address all issues relating to animal feeding. It developed guidelines or standards, as appropriate, on *Good Animal Feeding Practices* with the aim of ensuring the safety and quality of foods of animal origin. The objective of code is to help ensure the safety of food for human consumption through adherence to good animal feeding practice at farm level and *Good Manufacturing Practices* (GMPs) during the procurement, handling, storage, processing and distribution of animal feed and feed ingredients for food-producing animals. The Code applies to the production and use of all materials destined for animal feed and feed ingredients at all levels. The Codex Alimentarius Commission dissolved the Task Force in 2004. The standards relevant to animal feeding have been developed by other Codex Committees such as those on Food Additives and Contaminants (now split into the Codex Committees on Food Additives and on Contaminants in Foods), Meat Hygiene, Residues of Veterinary Drugs in Foods, Pesticide Residues and Food Labelling. The OIE guideline (OIE, 2007) is to provide guidance on animal feeding in relation to animal health and to complement the guidance provided by the Codex Code of Practice on Good Animal Feeding (CAC/RCP 54-2004) which deals primarily with food safety. This guideline aims at ensuring the control of animal and public health hazards through adherence to recommended practices during the production (procurement, handling, storage, processing and distribution) and use of both commercial and on-farm produced animal feed and feed ingredients for food producing animals (TAHSC, 2007).

Several international organizations world wide are involved in the preparation and publication of standardized methods for analysis of chemical substances in feed. International bodies are International Standardization Organization (ISO) (For feeds- Committee TC 34/SC 10 "Animal feeding stuffs" for chemical, biochemical, physical and microscopic methods; and Committee TC34/SC9 "Microbiology" for microbiological methods) and AOAC International. The Regional bodies like CEN (European Committee for Standardization) in Europe looks after the analytical methods and under this Committee TC 327 looks after the methods of sampling and analysis of 'Animal feeding stuffs'. The Quality Control of India (QCI) and Bureau of Indian Standards (BIS) lay the standards for foods and feeds in India. Various good practices codes like *Good Manufacturing Practices* (GMP), *Good Hygiene Practices* (GHP) and *Good Agricultural Practices* (GAP) have been drafted and adopted. These codes can function as proper basis for the application of other specific quality systems such as Hazard Analysis Critical Control Point (HACCP) system and ISO 9001:2000 family standards.

References

AAFCO. (1996). The AAFCO Official Publication, Association of American Feed Control Officials, pp. 108-110.

Alexander, T.W., Reuter, T., Aulrich, K., Sharma, R., Okine, E.K., Dixon, W.T., Mc Allister, T.A. (2007). *Anim. Feed Sci. and Technol.*, 133 (1-2): 31-62.

Annett, C.B., Viste, J.R., Chirino-Trejo, M., Classen, H.L., Middleton, D.M., Simko, E., (2002). *Avian Pathol.*, 31: 599-602.

AOAC, (2000). *Official Methods of Analysis*, Seventeenth Edition, Gaithersburg, MD, USA, AOAC International.

AOAC. 1995. Animal Feed. Chapter 4. In: *Official methods of analysis* 16th edition. (AOAC) International, Arlington, VI, USA. 30pp.

Bluthgen, A.H. (2000). *Bull. Int. Dairy Feder.* 356: 43-47.

Cellini, F., Chesson, A., Coquhonn, I., Constable, A., Davies, H.V., Engel, K.H., Gatehouse, A.M.R., Karenlampi, S., Kok, E.J., Legnay, J.J., Lehesranta, S., Noteborn, H.P.J.M., Pedersen, J., Smith, M. 2004. *Food Chem. Toxicol.* 42: 1089-1123.

Cherney, D.J.R., Patterson, J.A. and Cherney, J.H. (1989). *J. Dairy Sci.* 72: 3079-3084.

Crosby, N. (1995). *Encyclopedia of Analy. Sci.*, Vol. 1, pp. 120-136. Academic Press, London.

Czerkwaski, J.W. and Breckenridge, G. (1977). *Br. J. Nutr.*, 38: 371-384.

D'Mello, J.P.F. (1995). *Tropical Legumes in Animal Nutrition*, pp. 135-172. Wallingford, UK, CAB International.

D'Mello, J.P.F. (2000). *Farm Animal Metabolism and Nutrition.* pp. 383-403. CABI Publishing, Wallingford.

D'Mello, J.P.F. (2004). *Anim. Prod. and Health Paper No.* 160. Rome.

De Boever, J.L., Cottyn, B.G., Buysse, F.X., Wainman, F.W. and Vanacker, J.M. (1986). *Anim. Feed Sci. Technol.*, 14: 203-214.

De Boever, J.L., Cottyn, B.G., Vanacker, J.M. and Boucque, C.V. (1994). *Anim. Feed Sci. Technol.*, 47: 1-18.

EC, (2003). European Union. *Official Journal of the European Union* L 268/29, 18/10/2003.

Edwards, S.G. (2004). *Toxicol. Lett.* 153, 29-35.

European Union, (2001). *Off. J. Eur. Comm.* L147: 1-40.

European Union, (2002). *Off. J. Eur. Comm.* L273: 1-95.

European Union, (2003). *Off. J. Eur. Comm.* L339: 78-84.

FAO, (2001). *FAO Food and Nutrition* Paper 73. ISSN 0254-4725.

FAO/WHO. (2001). *Food and Nutrition/Codex Alimentarius* - Joint FAO/WHO Food Standards Programme, Rome. (http://www. codexalimentarius.net/download/standards/357/CXG_030e.pdf).

FAO/WHO. (2006). Rome. ftp://ftp.fao.org/codex/Publications/ProcManuals/Manual_16e.pdf)

FAO/WHO. (2007). *Joint FAO/WHO Food Standards Programme*. Rome.

Flachowsky, G., Aulrich, K., Bohme, H. and Halle, I. (2007). *Anim. Feed Sci. and Technol.* 133(1-2): 2-30.

Gerht, A.J. and B. Poundstone, (1976). *Feed Manufacturing Technol.*, 10: 253-256.

Givens, D.I. and Deaville, E.R. (1999). *Austral. Jour. of Agric. Res.*, 50: 1131-1145.

Goering, H.K. and Van Soest, P.J. (1970). *Agricul. Handbook 379*, ARS, USDA, Washington, DC. 20pp.

Greenham, L.W., Harber, C., Lewis, E., Scullion, F.T. (1987). *Vet. Rec.* 120: 557.

Hinton, M.H. (2000). *The Vety. Jour.*, 159: 121-138.

ILSI, (2004). *Compr. Rev. Food Sci. Food Safety*, 3: 36-104.

James L.F., Panter K.E., Molyneux R.J., Stegelmeier B.L. and Wagstaff D.J. (1994). *Plant Associated Toxins*, pp.83-88. Wallingford, UK, CAB International.

James, C. (2005). Global status of Commercialised Transgenic Crops, 2005. ISAA, Ithaca, NY. http://www. Isaaa.org.

Jeffrey, J.S., Kirk, J.H., Atwill, E.R. and Cullor, J.S. (1998). *Poul. Sci.*, 77: 808-811.

Jones, F.T. (1989). *Korean J. Anim.* 13(1): 25-39.

Jones, F.T. (1992). *Feedstuffs Reference Issue*, 64 (29): 136-139.

Kreuzer, W., Bunzl, K., Kracke, W., (1981). *Fleischwirtschaft*, 61(12): 1886-1894.

Krytenburg, D.S., Hancock, D.D., Rice, D.H., Besser, T.E., Gay, C.C. and Gay, J.M. (1998). *Anim. Feed Sci. and Technol.*, 75: 75-79.

Lynn, T.V., Hancock, D.D., Besser, T.E., Harrison, J.H., Rice, D.H., Stewart, N.T. and Rowan, L.L. (1998). *J. Dairy Sci.*, 81: 1102-1108.

Mc Cartney, D. (2009). *Feed Tech.* 13(1): 9-11.

Mc Ellhiney, R.R. (1979). *Feed Management*, 30(10): 28-30.

Mc Queen, R.E. and Nicholson, R. (1979). *Jour. of the Associa. of Official Analy. Chemists*, 62: 676-680.

Maciorowski, K.G., Jones, F.T., Pillai, S.D., Ricke, S.C., (2002a). *J. Rapid Meth. Automation Microbiol.* 10: 59-68.

Maciorowski, K.G., Pillai, S.D., Ricke, S.C., (2002b). *J. Environ. Sci. Health* B 37: 255-264.

Maciorowski, K.G., Jones, F.T., Pillai, S.D., Ricke, S.C., (2005). *Crit. Rev. Microbiol.* 31:45-53.

Mehrez, A.Z. and Orskov, E.R. (1977). *J. Agric Sci. (Camb.)*, 88: 645-650.

Menke, K.H., Raab, L., Salewski, A., Steingass, H., Fritz, D. and Schneider, W. (1979). *J. Agric. Sci.* (Camb.), 92: 217-222.

Miller, R.W., Azzare, A.S. and Gardiner, D.T. 1995. *Communication in Soil Science and Plant analysis* 26:5-6.

NRC 2005. Mineral tolerance of animals. National Research Council, Washington DC..

OIE, 2007. Draft guidelines for the control of hazards of animal health and public health importance in animal feed. Paris, World Organization for Animal Health.

OIE. 2004. Manual of diagnostic tests and vaccines for terrestrial animals, Fifth Edition. Paris. (available at http://www.oie.int/eng/normes/mmanual/A_summry.htm). (Chapter 2.3.1 for Bovine *Brucellosis* ; Chapter 2.10.1 for *Cysticerocosis* ; Chapter 2.10.3 for *Salmonellosis* ; Chapter 2.10.13 for Verocytotoxigenic *E. coli*).

Petterson, D.S., Harris, D.J., Rayner, C.J., Blakeney, A.B. and Choct, M. 1999. *Austr. J. Agric. Res.*, 50: 775-787.

Renwick, A.G., Barlow, S.M., Hertz-Picciotto, I., Boobis, A.R., Dybing, E., Edler, L., Eisenbrand, G., Greig, J.B., Kleiner, J., Lambe, J., Muller, D.J.G., Smith, M.R., Tritscher, A., Tuijtelaars, S., Van den Brandt, P.A., Walker, R., Kroes, R. 2003. *Food Chem. Toxicol.* 41: 1211-1271.

Shapira, R. and Paster, N. 2004. In: Magan, N., Olsen, M. (Eds.), *Mycotoxins in Food, Detection and Control*. CRC Press, Woodhead Publishing Limited, England, ISBN 1 855737337, pp. 190-223.

Strauch, D. 1987. *Animal Production and Environmental Health*. Elsevier Science Publishers.

Stuth, J., Jama, J. and Tolleson, D. 2003. Field Crops Research, 84: 45-56.

TAHSC, 2007. *Terrestrial Animal Health Standards Commission Report*, September 2007.

Tilley, J.M. and Terry, R.A. 1963. *J. Brit. Grassl. Soc.* 18: 104-111.

Van Raamsdonk, von Holst, C., Baeten, V., Berben, G., Boix, A and de Jong, J. 2007. *Anim. Feed Sci. and Technol.*, 133(1-2): 63-83.

Van Soest, P.J. 1994. Nutritional ecology of ruminants. 2nd Edition. Cornell University Press.

Van Soest, P.J., Robertson, J.B. and Lewis, B.A. 1991. *J. Dairy Sci.*, 74: 3583-3597.

Whitaker, T.B., 2006. Sampling foods for mycotoxins. *Food Addit. Contam.* 23(1): 50-61.

Wichtel, J.J. and Whitlock, R.H. 1991. *J. Am. Vet. Med. Assoc.* 1999: 471-472.

Widmer, F., Seidler, R.J., Watrud, L.S. 1996. Mol. Ecol. 5: 603-613.

Wiedemann, S., Lutz, B., Kurtz, H., Schwarz, F.J., Albrecht, C. 2006. *J. Anim. Sci.* 84: 135-144.

Wrigley, C.W. 1999. *Austr. J. Agric. Res.*, 50: 789-805.

□□□

Animal Nutrition, 2012
eds. Dr. (Mrs.) Usha R. Mehra et al., pp. 601-611
Satish Serial Publishing House e-mail : info@satishserial.com; website : www.satishserial.com

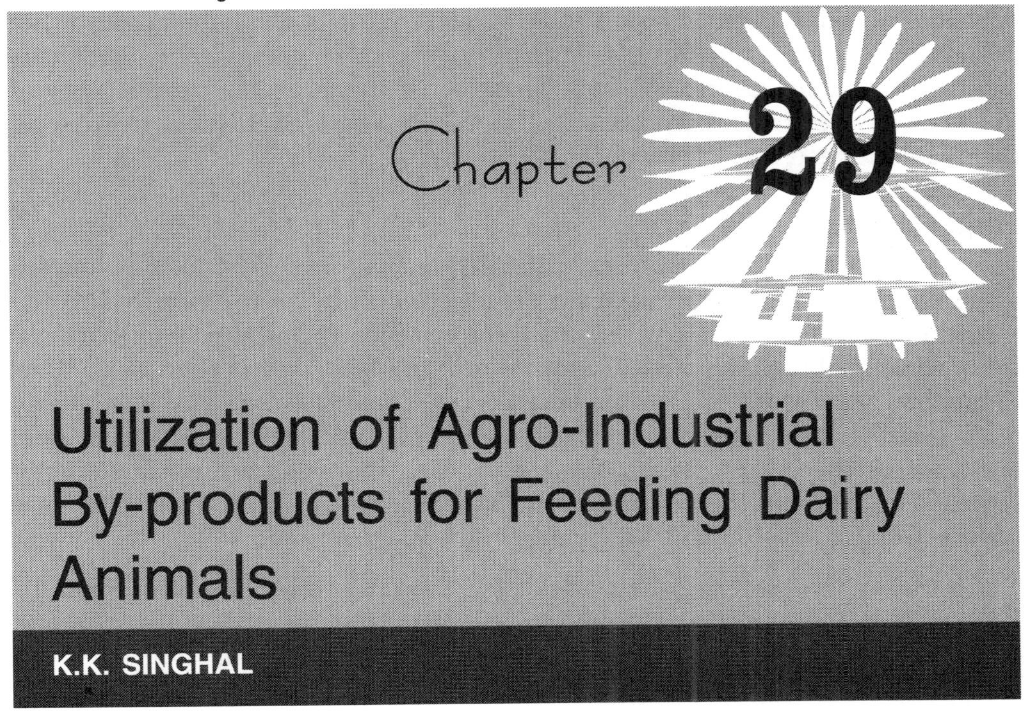

Chapter 29

Utilization of Agro-Industrial By-products for Feeding Dairy Animals

K.K. SINGHAL

Inspite of making big strides in annual milk production, the productivity per animal is still much lower in India than that in many developed countries. It is mainly attributed to the shortage of nutrients besides large prevalence of parasitic infestation, infectious diseases and mastitis. Since feed is the major input for milk production, efficient management of limited feed resources is of paramount importance for optimizing milk production in the country. As per the latest livestock census in 2003, India had 187.4 million cattle, 96.6 million buffaloes, 61.8 million sheep, 120.1 million goats and 16.8 million other animals, which are important for nutritional and economic security of masses as animal husbandry is being practiced along with agriculture in the country in a most integrated and sustainable manner. Crop residues and agro-industrial byproducts, which don't have any other utility for mankind, are being recycled through animals to get the food, draft power and fuel in rural India.

Farmers understand the value of good feeds and fodders for improving the productivity of their animals but in view of the limited area for fodder cultivation, they are forced to continue the feeding of agricultural wastes and our livestock has been adjusted to such feeding. It is clear that neither the area under fodder can be increased nor grains and other good quality feedstuffs can be utilized for animal feeding. Therefore, enhancing the productivity of livestock it is desirable to improve the nutritional status of animals by utilizing the available feed resources efficiently.

Feed Resources

Lack of information about availability and shortage of feed resources severely hampers the formulation of effective policies for improving the nutritional status of livestock. Efforts have been made in the past to work out the feed availability, feed requirements and the feed deficit (Jain *et al*, 1996; Ramachandra *et al.*, 2001). A data based on feed requirements and availability for livestock has been prepared by the scientists of National Institute of Animal Nutrition & Physiology, Bangalore in 2005. A gap between protein and energy required for the bovine population in the country and their availability has been estimated at 46.2 and 44.2%, respectively (Jain *et al.*, 1996).

Recently, an exercise was made at the National Dairy Research Institute, Karnal to project the total availability and requirements of DM, protein and energy for Indian livestock in view the latest productivity of different crops and the ratio of agricultural products and their crop residues, current population of different categories of livestock, cattle feed production and the availability of industrial products in the country (Table 1). DM availability appeared to be adequate but their wastage in handling, storage and transportation have not been taken into account. Availability of protein and energy appeared to be deficient due to the poor nutritional value of feedstuffs. It appears that deficiency of energy and protein will persist but magnitude will be reduced in view of declining trend of livestock population with increasing agricultural production. In a broader perspective it may appear good but concern have been expressed about the regional imbalances. Therefore, emphasis has to be given to increase the local feed resources besides making arrangements for the transportation and storage of feeds in the deficient areas as the trading and distribution of feed resources is totally under unorganized sector and needs to be streamlined for enhancing the livestock productivity.

Approximately, crop residues (637 million tones), green fodder (125 million tones) and conventional and non-conventional concentrate ingredients (82 million tones) worth Rs.2,34,800 crores at current prices are expected to be available in the country by the year 2020. Major part of available concentrate ingredients are either utilized for the poultry or exported, leaving ruminants to thrive only on unconventional feed ingredients along with crop residues. A report of Solvent Extractors Association of India indicated that

4.62 million tons of oil cakes worth Rs 69970 crores were exported from April 2008 to Jan. 2009. This is not only causing price escalation but also reducing the availability of nutritious material for our animals, thereby affecting their productivity. Potential and the methods for the utilization of agro-industrial products have been discussed by Mudgal and Singhal (1993) in a great length. However, for convenience, the major agro-industrial byproducts, which can be utilized for animal feeding, can be classified as follow, depending upon their source:

- Crop residues
- Food processing wastes
- Forest wastes
- Animal wastes
- Aquatic plants

Table 1 : Current status and projections of availability and requirement of nutrients (DM, CP and TDN) in India (x 10^6 MT)

Feed Resources	2005	2010	2015	2020
Green fodder & grasses	104.78	111.72	118.66	125.59
Crop residues	467.50	517.65	574.06	637.52
Oil cakes	19.29	21.65	24.32	27.31
Brans	7.32	8.24	9.27	10.43
Cereal grains	5.15	5.67	6.26	6.92
Top feeds	5.00	5.64	6.34	7.13
Vegetable & Fruits waste	5.24	5.49	5.77	6.06
Other agro byproducts	31.26	32.83	34.46	36.19
Total DM Availability	645.57	708.90	779.15	857.16
Total DM Requirements	622.37	626.74	642.57	670.92
Surplus/ Deficiency (%)	+ 3.73	+13.11	+21.25	+27.76
Total CP availability	34.946	38.083	41.563	45.435
Total CP Requirement	59.606	60.671	62.832	66.211
Surplus/ Deficiency (%)	- 41.37	- 37.23	- 33.85	- 31.38
Total TDN availability	268.36	298.56	332.59	370.96
Total TDN Requirement	354.58	358.86	369.61	387.50
Surplus/ Deficiency (%)	- 24.32	- 16.80	- 10.02	- 4.32

Jain and Singhal (unpublished data)

Crop Residues

These are usually low in protein, energy and mineral contents and methods for the utilization as well as nutritional improvement have been discussed in other chapter of this book.

Food Processing Waste

In the current era of economic liberalization, our country is experiencing a fast development of food processing industry with an estimated investment of Rs 38409 crores. Food processing wastes include the residual materials available after processing of foods for human consumption such conventional oil cakes, brans and fruits and vegetables, which are unfit for human consumption. Wastes from fruits and vegetables usually have high moisture content and sizable sugar levels, which cause their quick putrefaction; however, they contain low protein and moderate energy contents. Some food processing wastes such as animal processing wastes are usually high in protein. Wastes from the following food processing industries have a potential for animal feeding: Fruit and vegetable processing industry.

1. Starch industry
2. Egg, fish, meat and meat processing industry
3. Breweries

India is the second largest country for the production of fruits and vegetables and share over 13 % of the produce globally. It has been estimated that the annual total production of fruits and vegetables is about 64.8 and 86.0 million tones, respectively. About 33% of the produce is wasted during harvesting, marketing and processing. As per a recent estimate on the basis of production data published by GOI, the total availability of such wastes in India is about 5.24 million tons on DM basis, which can be utilized as a feed resource. However, small portion of such wastes is utilized as kitchen waste for animal feeding. Common vegetable wastes have reasonable nutrients (Table 2) and good palatability.

Ensiling of such wastes alone or in combination with dry roughages is a good technique for their preservation and utilization for animal feeding. Ration containing silage of carrot waste consisting crown and tail portion with small, split and woody carrots (treated with 0.25% urea and 0.5% common salt) and pea pods consisting empty shells and vines can replace berseem hay in a total mixed ration of growing and lactating animals without sacrificing their productive efficiency.

Apple is processed for manufacturing the juice, jam and other products. Apple pomace (25 to 35% of fresh apple) is the residual material after extracting the juice and contains 5.5% CP and 16.4% high quality fibre besides sizable level of minerals including calcium and phosphorus. Due to its high palatability it can be fed as fresh or after drying. Its nutritive value in terms of DCP and TDN is 1.62, and 64.84%. Urea treatment of fresh apple pomace under air tight condition for 2 days following its drying increases its nitrogen content. On replacing the maize grain with urea treated apple pomace in the concentrate mixture, the growth and milk production performance of dairy animals remained uninfluenced but cost of feeding reduced significantly (Table 3).

Table 2 : Chemical composition and nutrient digestibility of wastes of different vegetable (% DM basis).

Parameter	Cabbage	Cauliflower	Carrots	Pea pods	Pumpkin	Okra
DM	7.10	7.10	10.41	13.34	8.20	11.30
OM	90.95	85.35	91.9	95.40	96.10	92.40
CP	21.66	22.40	6.78	15.40	14.20	20.02
NDF	35.00	37.00	24.50	45.50	47.00	38.00
Calcium	0.68	0.74	0.38	1.35	0.66	0.98
Phosphorous	0.34	0.41	0.35	0.28	0.16	0.39
IVDMD%	54.55	50.60	58.52	50.98	51.22	51.98

Khan (2003)

Table 3 : Performance of growing and lactating cows on feeding urea treated apple pomace (AP) in place of maize grain in concentrate mixture.

Parameter	Control	Urea treated AP
Growth		
DM intake (kg)	483.6	483.4
Live wt gain (kg)	53.0	51.9
Daily wt gain (g)	541.6	529.8
Cost/kg gain (Rs)	13.8	10.75
Lactation		
DM Intake (kg)	6154	6268
Milk production (k g)	5137	5248
Total fat production (kg)	233.7	232.0
DM intake/kg milk yield (Kg)	1.2	1.2
Feed cost/ kg milk (Rs.)	1.25	1.04

Sharma *et al.*, (1989)

Treating the mixture of apple pomace and wheat straw (1:1) along with 4% urea (on DM basis) for 30 days under air tight conditions not only preserves the apple pomace but also improves the nutritive value of wheat straw. Similar approach can be employed for the utilization of other food processing wastes such as maize bran (from starch industry), spent grain (from breweries). In addition to the high moisture content, their seasonal availability is a constraint for their utilization for animal feeding.

Whey, a waste from milk processing industry, contains 0.7 to 0.9% CP, and 0.5 to 0.6% fat. It can also be used for feeding ruminants and swine as such or after drying, however, cost of drying is the major constraint in its utilization. Dried whey can be fed to young calves successfully; however, its use in poultry feed is restricted due to their lower lactose tolerance.

Aquatic Plants

Aquatic plants such as algae, water hyacinth, etc. are usually considered as a problem rather than an asset. Algae are higher in protein and minerals while low in fibre, but water hyacinth is high in fibre and low in protein. Aquatic plants have sizable nutritional value but their harvesting and processing are the major constraints in their utilization. India, having about 5700 km long coastal line, have a vast potential for such feed resources. Red, black and brown algae are available to the tune of 10, 30 and 60 million tones in west coast of Gujrat alone. It was also shown that dried brown algae (*Sargassum sp.*) contains 7-11% CP with good amino acid make up besides major and trace minerals. Incorporation of dried *Sargassum sp.* at 10 % level in the ration of lactating Sahiwal cows proved economical as the milk production of such cows was found to be similar to those supplemented with mineral mixture. Water hyacinth can yield 88 kg DM/ ha/day. If such a growth takes place even for 6 months in a year about 146 tons DM/ ha can be achieved against the yield of 11.3 tons DM/ ha from algae. Therefore, concerted efforts may be made for the harvesting and processing of aquatic plants for their utilization even as a source of minerals, whose deficiency has been reported in many parts of the country.

Forest Residues

Forests are the source of large number of unconventional feed ingredients such as tree leaves, oilseeds (neem, mahua, karanj, kosum, sal, etc.) and other biomass such as grasses. These ingredients have moderate protein content, but remain under utilized because of the presence of one or other incriminating factor. Collection and processing of these feed resources are other constraints as their availability is seasonal and unorganized.

In view of low availability of concentrate ingredients, research work on the use of unconventional feed resources was initiated at the Indian Veterinary Research Institute, during 1940's, which was further continued under All India Coordinated Research Project entitled 'Improvement of feed resources and nutrient utilization in raising animal production' by Indian Council of Agricultural Research from 1967 onwards. As a result, a number of byproducts, which were not utilized earlier, are now being used mainly by the compounded feed industry and these include rice bran, rubber seed cake, tapioca waste, tea waste, salseed meal, babool seed and pods, ambadi cake, mango kernels, cassia tora seeds and many others. However, several findings are yet to be adopted as these are based on replacement of a conventional ingredient with an unconventional (processed or unprocessed) one. However, feed industry utilizes a group of unconventional feed ingredients mainly in their unprocessed form. Presence of incriminating factors in these ingredients restrict their palatability and nutrient utilization thereby their use in animal ration (Table 4). For example, tannins, present in babool pods, salseed meal etc, not only affect the protein utilization adversely (tannins bind with the available protein in the GI tract) but also limit the feed intake. Technologies have been developed for the detoxification of some unconventional oil cakes. For example, treatment of mahua cake with 1% ammonium hydroxide for 2 days in closed conditions followed by sun drying removed its toxic mowrin to large extent. Detoxified mahua cake was found to be acceptable when incorporated at 25% level in the ration of growing animals without any adverse affect. Similarly, water washing of neem cake was found to be good for removing its incriminating factors. Such technologies, developed painstakingly, are not being utilized at the commercial level due to the economic constraints. However, certain methods such as toasting of guar meal and solvent extraction of karanj seeds are being adopted to remove their toxic factors.

During the processing of guar meal for gum extraction, its anti-nutritional factor i.e. anti-trypsin activity is taken care of and the cost of processing of guar meal is recovered from the sale of guar gum, which is in great demand for its utilization in many industries. If the same analogy is applied to other abundantly available oil cakes of neem, mahua, salseed etc, their use in animal feeding will be safer and economical and it will generate employment in rural/ tribal areas. The incriminating factors present in unconventional oil cakes may prove a potential as insecticide/ nematodicide/ anti-helmentic, etc. It will be a good idea to incorporate neem cake or its active principle in urea-molasses-mineral block lick as presence of molasses will mask its bitter taste. Alternatively, dietary incorporation of neem cake at lower level may control the parasitic infection in animals.

Table 4 : Agro-industrial by products, their availability (x 1000 MT), nutritional value (%) and incriminating factors.

Byproducts	Availability	DCP	TDN	Incriminating factors
Algae	NA	54.0	62.2	Moisture
Ambadi cake*	0.02			Cycloprene acid
Babul pods	NA	5.82	62.63	Tannins
Castor cake*	737			Ricin (protein) and Ricinine (alkaloid)
Cassia tora seeds	0.40	16.6	59.4	Crysophanic acid and tannins
Faba bean/ horse bean	NA			Vicine, Convicine (cyano gens)
Guar meal				Protease inhibitor
Karanj seed cake*	8.24	26.0	71.4	Karanjin, Gallabrin (proteins)
Kosum seed cake*	0.32	10.0	50.0	Prussic acid
Linseed cake*	2268			Linamarin (cyanogens), Linatine (amino acid)
Mango kernal*	7.6	6.1	50.0	Tannins
Mahua cake*	45.7	8.64	46.6	Mowrin (saponins), tannins
Mustard cake*	3864			Glucosinolates, Erucic acid
Neem cake*	52.9	8.8	57.8	Nimbin
Prosopis juliflora pods				Tripsin inhibitor, haemaglutinine
Rubber seed cake*	0.17	18.6	54.0	Prussic acid
Subabul le aves/ seeds				Mimosine (amino acid)
Salseed meal*	50.5			Tannins
Sugar beet pulp	NA	3.46	59.1	unidentified
Tapioca waste	65.0	-	71.1	Prussic acid
Tamarind seed*	22.0	5.34	60.1	Tannins
Thumba seed cake*	79.0			unidentified

*Mehta *et al.* (2000)

Recent reports suggest that tannins at the level of 3% of the total diet did not affect the intake and utilization of nutrients adversely on one hand and on the other hand cows fed on such diet excreted tannins metabolites in their milk, which have health benefits for human beings. In other words, dietary incorporation of tannins enhanced the nutraceutical value of milk and thus results in to value addition of the milk. Reports are appearing to show that plant extracts of various herbs have a potential to reduce the methane emission from ruminants, for which India is being blamed for global warming in view of its large animal population. Plants extracts contain some plant secondary metabolite(s), which control the protozoa population having a symbiotic relationship with methanogens in the rumen. If we could pinpoint the natural compound to reduce the methane emission from ruminants, it will be a great achievement.

Collection and processing of byproducts of forests origin, especially the non-conventional oil seeds have to be organized with an emphasis on their quality. During the process of their detoxification, pharmaceutical(s) should be isolated to recover the cost of processing.

Animal Waste

Animal wastes are low to fair in their energy, protein and mineral contents In spite of their potential for livestock feeding, the utilization is limited due to the presence of pathogens in animals waste. Moreover, it appears to be unethical to recycle the animals waste through ruminants, which are the source of human food. Large quantities of animal wastes are available in the country as excreta, waste from slaughter houses and other sources, such as poultry feathers, sea food processing, which can be converted into animal feeds. Poultry excreta generally have sizable nitrogen content besides energy and minerals and technologies have been developed to control the presence of pathogens by ensiling or drying the poultry waste prior to its mixing with feed. Ample evidences are available to show that properly processed poultry excreta can be incorporated in the ration of ruminants without affecting their productivity and quality of milk or meat. Utilization of poultry excreta as a feed resource for animals is not being adopted in India, in spite of shortage of nutrients, just because of ethical reasons.

Animal byproducts such as bone, meat, blood etc, are converted into meals for animal feeding, but as per Govt. of India circular in 2002 the byproducts of animal origin are banned in the ration of ruminants to control the 'Mad cow disease'. Therefore, these are not being used in cattle feeding. In view of high protein content in blood and meat meals and high calcium and phosphorous content in bone meal, these are being used in the ration of poultry, pigs and pet animals, but these should be decontaminated and processed thoroughly to make them free from pathogens, parasites and other harmful substances.

Level of Agro Industrial Byproduct in the Feed

Most of the unconventional byproducts contain some toxins and/or incriminating factors; therefore, their incorporation in animal feed results in poor palatability thereby poor productivity. Such byproducts may be included up to the level of 35-40% of the concentrate for low producing animals. To overcome the palatability problem, flavouring agents and sweeteners such as molasses may be added. To achieve the optimum performance of animals, it is recommended that dietary nitrogen level must be maintained at 30 g/ kg digestible organic matter by the supplementation of additional nutrients so that N requirements of ruminal bacteria can be fulfilled. To raise the N status to the desirable level, haulms of potato and groundnut, tops of sugarcane and cassava as well as tree leaves (such as subabool) may be incorporated after their processing such as chopping. Alternatively, commercially available urea-molasses-mineral block lick may be used for this purpose. Whatever may be the approach, the acceptability of the ration should not be compromised.

Strategies for Utilizing the Agro-Industrial Byproducts

Agro-industrial byproducts usually have problems of either low palatability or the low shelf life and a common farmer can not use them to their potential. Though cattle feed industry is utilizing such feed ingredients by their blending with the conventional feeds but large number of ingredients remains underutilized because of the low, scattered and seasonal availability. Scientific data has been generated during last several decades about the nutritional value of available agro-industrial byproducts. Therefore, it is desirable to use the information for the benefits of animals and the overall economy of the dairy farmer. National Dairy Development Board, has recently launched a country wide programme for the ration balancing. In this programme, field workers will be educated to use the computer for balancing the ration based on locally available feed resources. It is assumed that this strategy, appeared to gigantic, will succeed to improve the productivity of animals as majority of animals are fed on unbalanced ration. This approach will also ensure the better utilization of agro-industrial byproducts, wherever and whenever, they are available. Another approach for enhancing the utilization of agro-industrial byproducts is to utilize them in complete feed blocks. Of course, it needs the cooperation of feed industry as such ingredients may be blended in a duly processed complete feed as processing of the feeds is the only way to enhance their utilization in ruminants. This approach will not only reduce the cost of transportation and handling of feeds but will also be helpful in tackling the calamities such as drought and flood, which strike annually one place or other in the country.

Precise information about the availability of feed resources in different regions is required for strengthening the feed resources management and their processing as nutrient utilization of feeds improve following their processing, therefore, due emphasis must be given on processing aspects to remove the deficiency of nutrients in the ruminants ration. The feeding strategies have to be formulated for various agro-climatic zones keeping in view the type of animal and the availability of feed resources. Research work has to be taken up to exploit the potential of wastes from food industry whose availability is likely to show a quantum jump. Efforts have to be made to recover pharmaceuticals from non-conventional feeds by devising appropriate technologies to obtain the raw material free from incriminating factors, and pharmaceuticals may be utilized for industrial and agricultural application as insecticide/pesticide/anti-helmentics and/or mitigation of methane from ruminants. Critical analysis and review of policy for export of protein supplements such as oil cakes and fish meal needs to be done in view of local demands.

References

Jain, D.K., Sharma, K.N.S., Walli, T.K. and Rai, S.N. (1996). NDRI Publication No 281, National Dairy Research Institute, Karnal

Khan, Imran (2003). Ph.D. thesis, National Dairy Research Institute, Karnal, India.

Mehta, B.V. (2000). The Solvent Extractors Association of India, Mumbai.

Mudgal, V.D. and Singhal, K.K. (1993). Pashu poshan main krishi avam udyogon ke upodpad, Rajasthan Hindi Granth Academy, Jaipur.

Ramachandra, K.S., Anandan, S. and Raju, S.S. (2001). Proc. X Animal Nutrition Conference, National Dairy Research Institute, Karnal pp 134 -144.

Sharma, D.D, Bakalkar, R.K. and Singhal, K.K. (1989). Publ No. 149, National Dairy Research Institute, Karnal, India.

□□□

Animal Nutrition, 2012
eds. Dr. (Mrs.) Usha R. Mehra et al., pp. 613-640
Satish Serial Publishing House e-mail : info@satishserial.com; website : www.satishserial.com

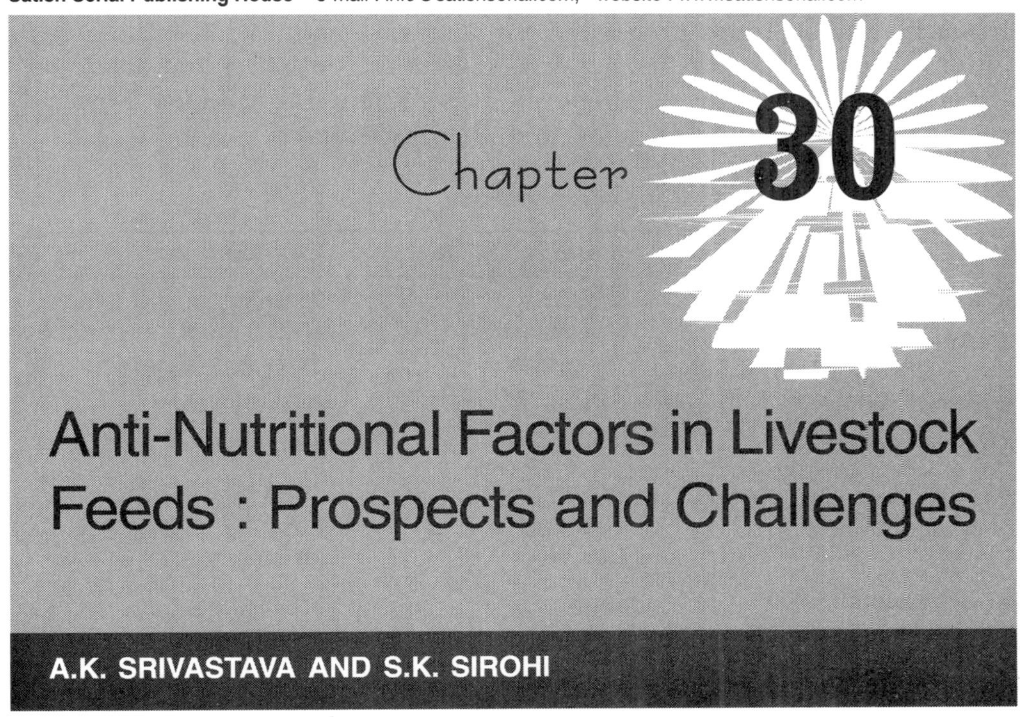

Anti-Nutritional Factors in Livestock Feeds : Prospects and Challenges

A.K. SRIVASTAVA AND S.K. SIROHI

Antinutritional Factors

The anti-nutritive factors may be defined as those substances generated in natural feed stuffs by the normal metabolism of species and by different mechanisms e.g inactivation of some nutrients, interference with the digestive process or metabolic utilization of feed which exert effects contrary to optimum nutrition. An anti-nutritional factor is a substance which under practical condition can impair/affect some aspect of metabolism and produce adverse biological or economic effects in animal production. The presence of endogenous anti-nutritional factors within plant feedstuffs is believed to be the largest single factor which limit their use within compounded animal feeds at high dietary levels. Although these factors vary in their individual toxicity to animals, a large proportion of these can be destroyed or inactivated by different treatment processes. Their presence at high dietary concentrations in untreated feedstuffs normally results in anorexia, reduced growth and poor food conversion efficiency. Typical concentrations for selected toxins are presented in Table 1. Plant antinutritional factors mainly divided into a heat-labile group, comprising lectins, proteinase inhibitors and cyanogens, which are sensitive to standard processing temperatures, and a heat-stable group including, antigenic proteins, condensed tannins, quinolizidine alkaloids, glucosinolates, gossypol, saponins, the non-protein amino acids S-methyl cysteine sulphoxide and mimosine, and phyto-oestrogens.

Table 1 : Plant toxins: Sources and concentrations

Toxin	Source	Concentration
Lectins	Jackbean Winged bean Lima beans	73 units / mg protein 40-320 units/ mg protein 59 units/ mg protein
Trypsin inhibitors	Soybean	88 units/ mg
Antigenic proteins	Soybean	-
Cyanogens	Cassava root	186 mg HCN/ kg
Condensed tannins	*Acacia* spp. Lotus spp.	65 g/ kg 30-40 g/ kg
Quinolizidine alkaloids	Lupin	10-20 g/ kg
Glusosinolates	Rapeseed	100 mmol/ kg
Gossypol	Cottonseed	0.6-12 g/ kg (free)
Saponins (steroidal)	*Brachiaria decumbens; Panicum* spp.	-
S-methyl cysteine sulphoxide	Kale	40-60 g/ kg
Mimosine 25 g/ kg (leaf)	*Leucaena leucocephala*	145 g/ kg (seed)
Phyto-estrogens	Clover; lucerne; soybean	-

Source: Compiled from D'Mello, 1995.

These anti-nutritional factors have major effects on monogastrics but have less effect on ruminants as microbial fermentation in the rumen can breakdown some toxic compounds such as the proteinase inhibitors. Natural toxicants can be classified on the basis of their chemical structure. With some exceptions, most are distributed among the following broad categories: alkaloids, glycosides, proteins, amino acids and derivatives, carbohydrates, lipids, glycoproteins, glycolipids, metal binding substances, resins, phenolics and sesquiterpene lactones. In addition to these, it is convenient to consider mycotoxins as a specific category. The chemical structure of different groups of anti-nutritional factors and their influence on animals are given as follows:

Alkaloids

Alkaloids are basic substances that contain nitrogen in a heterocyclic ring and it has been estimated that 15-20% of all vascular plants contain alkaloids. Most alkaloids are derived from amino acids. They have been regarded either as metabolic byproducts or substances that serve to repel insects and herbivorous predators. There is no doubt that in many cases their bitter taste does repel grazing animals also. Alkaloids are usually classified by their common molecular precursors, based on the metabolic pathway used to construct the molecule. Different alkaloid groups are-

Pyrrolizidine Alkaloids

The nucleus consists of two membered rings. These are responsible for toxicity of various *sececio* spp., crotalaria, *E. plantagenieum* and *Heliotropium europaeum*. Jacobine is one of the major pyrrolizidine alkaloids found in ragwort. The related pyrrolizidine alkaloid, monocrotaline was used in the experimental procedures. Monocrotaline was chemically oxidised to its pyrrolic derivative, dehydromonocrotaline (DHM) and exposed to equine plasma proteins.

Piperidine Alkaloids

The most important piperidine alkaloids in animal production are coiine and related alkaloids found in *Conium maculatum*. These alkaloids affect the central nervous system and are teratogens.

Pyridine Alkaloids

The most important pyridine alkaloid is nicotine, in *Nicotiana* spp.

Indole Alkaloids

Indole is derivatives of the amino acid tryptophan. The common indole alkaloids are the ergot alkaloids, perloline in tall fescue and bovine pulmonary emphysema causing alkaloid, 3-methylindole. Ergot, a fungal disease of cereal grasses, is caused by the fungus *Claviceps purpurea,* which produces active chemicals containing heterocyclic compounds known as indole alkaloids.

Quinolizidine alkaloids

The ergot alkaloids come from a fungus, *Claviceps purpurea,* which is a parasite on rye and wheat. The ergot alkaloids are responsible for ergotism (St. Anthony's fire), which manifests itself as gangrenous ergotism, resulting in loss of limbs, or convulsive ergotism, resulting in hallucinations. Some of the ergot alkaloids have been used to treat migraine headaches and sexual disorders in clinical applications. The most famous of these alkaloids is lysergic acid diethylamide (LSD), a powerful hallucinogen that is a synthetic derivative of the natural products.

The quinolizidine alkaloids occur in lupins and include lupinine, sparteine and lupanine. Bitter cultivars contain relatively high levels of total alkaloids and are not suitable as animal feedstuffs because of their negative effects on intake. In addition, cattle consuming certain lupin species during pregnancy may produce calves with multiple congenital deformities.

The quinolizidine nucleus consists of two six membered rings. Lupines contain these alkaloids, which cause acute poisoning in sheep and teratogenic effects in calves i.e. crooked calf disease.

Steroid Alkaloids

Solanum type (i.e. solanidine) - Found in green potatoes and tomatoes, they are central nervous system poisons and cholinesterase inhibitors.

Veratrum type- (i.e. veratramine) *Veratrum californicum* contain veratrum alkaloid that produce teratogenic effects in lambs and prolonged gestation in ewes.

Polycyclic Diterpene Alkaloids

This complex alkaloid found in *Delphinium* spp. and affects central nervous system acutely. The structure is given in Fig. 1 as shown below.

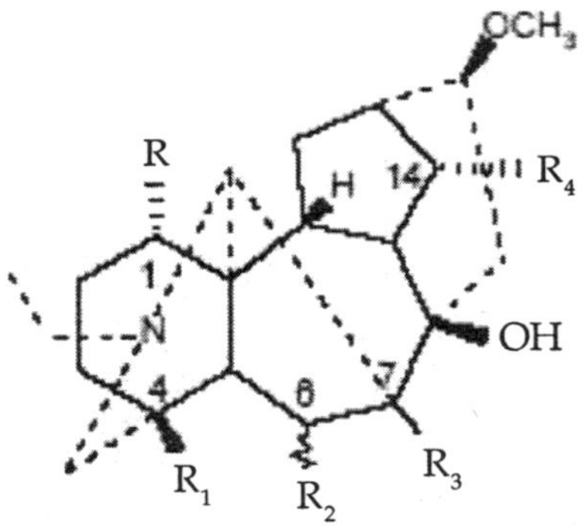

Compound	R	R_1	R_2	R_3	R_4
Neoline	OH	CH_2OCH_3	αOCH_3	H	OH
Isotalatisidine	OH	CH_2OCH_3	H	H	OH
Karakoline	OH	CH_3	H	H	OH
Delsoline	OH	CH_2OCH_3	βOCH_3	OH	OCH_3
Kondelfine	OH	CH_2OCH_3	H	H	$OCOCH_3$
14-Acerylvirescenine	OH	CH_2OCH_3	H	OH	$OCOCH_3$
Gigactonine	OH	CH_2OH	βOCH_3	OH	OCH_3
Lycoctonine	OCH_3	CH_2OH	βOCH_3	OH	OCH_3
Delectinine	OCH_3	CH_2OH	βOCH_3	OH	OH

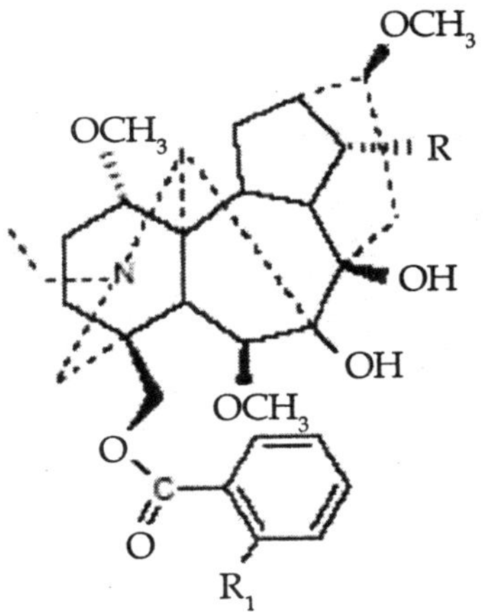

Fig. 1 : Structure of diference alkaloids found in delphinium spp.

Indolizidine alkaloids (Locoweed, Swainsona, Slaframine and Castanospermine Alkaloids types) – Indolizidine Alkaloids, such as swainsonine, the toxic component of *Swainsona* spp. and *Astragalus* spp. (locoweed). Slaframine is produced on red clover by a fungus.

Tryptamine Alkaloids

Tryptamine Alkaloids are found in *Phalaris tuberosa* and responsible for acute neurological signs and chronic muscular in coordination.

Tropane Alkaloids

Atropine found in *Datura* spp., is an example of alkaloid. It has a pronounced effect on central nervous system.

Fescue Alkaloids

Tall fescue (*Festuca arundinacea*) contains several alkaloids, with perloline and perlolidine being the major one. Perloline found in perennial ryegrass. Major problems associated with the use of tall fescue pasture are summer fescue toxicosis and fescue foot. An additional problem, fat necrosis, has also been linked to the grazing of fescue pastures.

Among the most famous of the alkaloids are the *Solanaceae or tropane alkaloids.* Plants containing these alkaloids have been used throughout recorded history as poisons, but many of the alkaloids do have valuable pharmaceutical properties. Atropine, the racemic form of hyoscyamine, comes from *Atropa belladonna* (deadly nightshade) and is used to dilate the pupils of the eye. Atropine is also a CNS stimulant and is used as a treatment for nerve gas poisoning. Scopolamine, another member of this class is used as a treatment for motion sickness. Cocaine is also a CNS stimulant. Caffeine was considered to be the major problem with the soft drink.

The morphine alkaloids, derived from the opium poppy, *Papaver somniferum* (dried latex of the seed heads), are powerful pain relievers and narcotics. Some derivatives of morphine have been developed and found use as opiate antagonists or as animal tranquilizers.

Vincristine, one of the most potent and widely used antileukemic drugs, was isolated in a search for diabetes treatment from *Vinca rosea* (now *Catharanthus roseus*) in the 1950's along with vinblastine, a homologue in which the N-methyl group is oxidized to an aldehyde moiety. Some important alkaloids occurring in plants are as follows:

Name of alkaloid	Plant
Atropine	Deadly nightshade
Cocaine	Leaves of coca plant
Coniine	Hemlock
Jacobine	Ragwort
Morphine	Dried latex opium poppy
Nicotine	Tobacco
Quinine	Cinchona bark
Ricinine	Castor plant seeds
Strychnine	Seeds of *Nux vomica*
Solanine	Unripe potatoes and potato sprouts

Tannins and Polyphenolic Compounds

Tannins

The term 'tannin' is difficult to define precisely, however the essential property of tannins is that they are naturally-occurring plant polyphenols which combine with proteins and other polymers such as cellulose, hemicellulose and pectin, to form stable complexes. Tannins are polyphenolic compounds which precipitate proteins from aqueous solution The term "tannin" is derived from the use of plant extracts (e.g., oak leaves) to tan the leather. Hydrogen bonds are formed between the phenolic hydroxyls and the peptide groups of collagen fibrils to form cross-links between adjacent protein chains. Oxidation of phenolic groups in the tannins to quinones may give rise to covalent bonds with the epsilon amino groups of lysine and arginine, further increasing the durability of the leather.

Tannins have the ability to precipitate proteins because they contain a number of functional groups which form strong complexes with protein molecules, producing a large cross- linked protein tannin complex. For this, the presence of o-dihydroxyphenols is required, forming hydrogen bonds with the protein, with hydrophobic binding also contribution to the stability of the protein tannin complex.

This property of tannins to form bonds with soluble proteins accounts for their adverse effects on animals. They can bind protein digestive enzymes to inhibit their activities, and can also bind with dietary proteins to prevent their digestion. They may bind with proteins in the intestinal mucosa and affect nutrients absorption. The interaction of tannins with the salivary proteins and glycol-proteins in the mouth causes the sensation of astringency. Astringency is the mouth puckering sensation experienced when one eats a green persimmon or a walnut, which, like most unripe fruits, contains tannins. The loss of astringency upon ripening is due to polymerization of the tannins, reducing their ability to react with proteins. Thus, tannins have pronounced effects on feed intake and palatability. Swain (1979) considers that tannins are the most significant plant components controlling the acceptability of plants to herbivores. Tannins are believed to have a major role in protection of plants from vertebrate herbivore, insect, bacterial, and viral attack by deterring herbivores with their astringent effects and by inactivating protein enzymes of insects and bacteria. The natural durability of many wood species may be due to the toxicity to microorganisms of phenolics deposited in the process of heartwood formation (Jung and Fahey, 1983).

Tannins and other similar compounds in plants are synthesized by rather by shikimic acid pathway or acetate-malonate pathway (Jung and Fehey, 1983). Tannins are generally classified as the hydrolysable (a) and the condensed (b) tannins. The ***hydrolysable tannins*** consist a carbohydrate moiety in which the hydroxyl groups are esterified to gallic acid (1) or m-digallic acid (2) gallotannins or hexahydroxydiphenic acid (3) ellagitannins. These tannins are easily hydrolysed either chemically or by enzymes, e.g. penicillium tannase. The ***condensed tannins*** consist, oligomers of the flavan-3-01s (the catechins) and related flavanol residues ,which typically produce anthocyanidins (e.g. cyanidin and pelargonidin) on acid degradation (Mangan, 1988). The condensed tannins do not have a carbohydrate core like the hydrolysable tannins, but occur as a range of polymers, an example being procyanidin. The tannins in sorghum grain and fava beans are of the condensed type. Salseed (Shroea robusta) meal, babul (Acacia nilotica) seeds, mango kernel and some other agro-industrial byproducts have sizable tannins content.

Hydrolyzable tannins (gallotannins, ellagitannins) consist of esters of glucose with gallic acid or related compounds. They can be readily hydrolyzed by hot mineral acids or esterases to yield the sugar core and the constituent acids. An example of the group of hydrolysable tannins with detrimental effects on livestock is the tannins in oak. There are other tannins which do not fit into either the condensed or hydrolysable groups such as chlorogenic acid, which is found in sunflower meal and alfalfa.

Oak Poisoning

Consumption of oak buds, leaves, twigs, and acorns causes poisoning in cattle. Tannins, such as tannic acid and its phenolic acid constituent (gallic acid) are the causative agents. The tannin content of leaves and acorns tends to be highest in the immature stages. The initial signs of oak poisoning include anorexia, depression, clear watery nasal discharge, rumen stasis, excessive thirst, and frequent urination. Initial constipation is followed by excretion of dark, thin, mucoid and often bloody faeces.

The principal lesions are gastritis and nephritis. The abomasum and small intestine are often inflamed and hemorrhagic. The major lesion of oak poisoning is necrosis of the renal tubules. Affected kidneys are pale and swollen. There is impaired kidney function, with elevated blood urea nitrogen. Supplemental feeding with a mixture containing calcium hydrogen has been recommended as a preventative measure. Treatments of tannins containing feeds such as supplementation of PEG (polyethylene glycol) and NaOH treatment showed variable reduction of tannins, however, these could not be adopted at commercial scale due to economic reasons.

Gossypol

Gossypol, a phenolic compound found in pigment glands of cottonseed (*Gossypium* spp.), was isolated and the name is derived from *Gossypium* phenol. While gossypol is the major phenolic in cottonseed, there are at least 15 other closely related compounds. The phenolic groups on the molecule are chemically reactive, so it reacts readily with various substances, including minerals and amino acids.

The cell wall of pigment glands is composed of cellulose, pectin, hemicellulose, and uronic acid, which is resistant to rupture. During the extraction of cottonseed oil, gossypol remains in the meal. Heat treatment of the seed causes gossypol to bind with the lysine of protein present in the seed.

Free gossypol is important for the feeding of animals as bound gossypol is physiologically inactive, and lowers the biological value of protein because of its binding with lysine of the protein. Besides reducing the hatchability of eggs, free gossypol causes olive green yolks in hen's eggs due to the reaction between gossypol and yolk iron, and taken as a most sensitive indicator of physiological activity. The cyclopropenoid fatty acids in cottonseed meal, cause pink albumins. They enhance the yolk discoloration by accelerating the increase in yolk pH during cold storage of eggs. In most of non-ruminant animals, gossypol causes a depressed appetite, loss of weight, liver and lung lesions, including edema and congestion of the lungs, and congestion and hemorrhages of the liver. The most common effect is cardiac irregularity; death is generally ascribed to cardiac failure. Labored breathing occurs in swine, with pulmonary edema a common feature in most animals. Anemia may occur, with reduced erythrocytes, hemoglobin, and packed cell volume, due to a complexing with iron.

At low levels, gossypol blocks spermatogenesis and reduces sperm motility. In the diets of non-ruminants, the free gossypol level should not exceed 0.01% or about 9% cotton seed meal. The addition of iron salts, such as ferrous sulfate, inactivates the gossypol and can be used in a 1:1 ratio of iron to free gossypol. High dietary protein levels have a protective effect by reacting with free gossypol. Gossypol does not normally affect ruminant animals, presumably because of inactivation in the rumen where binding of gossypol to protein occurs. However, if high levels of whole cottonseed are fed for a prolonged period, cardiac damage can occur. Indian farmers cook the cottonseed prior to the feeding of dairy animals.

Glycosides

Cyanogens

Cyanogens are glycosides of sugars (usually glucose) and a cyanide-containing aglycone. They can be hydrolyzed by enzymatic action with the release of hydrogen cyanide (prussic acid), which is a potent toxin, inhibiting the terminal respiratory enzyme cytochrome oxidase. The major cyanogenic glucosides, important for the animal nutrition point of view are:

Amygdalin (laetrile)

This glycoside is found in Rosaceae, such as chokecherries, wild cherries, mountain mahofany, Saskatoon and the kernels of almonds, apricots peaches and apples. Prunasin is also found in these plants; it has the same structure as amygdalin except it has one glucose rather than two attached to the aglycone.

Dhurrin

This occurs in sorghum species such as grain sorghums, forage sorghums (Sudan grass, hay grazer) and Johnson grass.

Linamarin

This compound is found in white clover, flax (linseed), cassava, and lima beans. The glycosides occur in vacuoles in plant tissue, while the enzymes are found in the cytosol. Damage to the plant from wilting, trampling, mastication, frost, drought, bruising (cassava), brings the enzymes and glycosides together, causing HCN to be released as a result of enzymatic action. These enzymes are also produced by rumen microorganisms. The optimal pH for the enzymes is near neutrality, so, release of HCN is more rapid in the highly acid stomach of the non-ruminant animals. For this reason ruminants are more sensitive to cyanogens than non-ruminants.

Glucosinolates

The glucosinolates are a class of organic compounds that contain sulfur, nitrogen and a group derived from glucose. They occur as secondary metabolites of many plants of the order Brassicales (especially in the family Brassicaceae). Plants use substances derived from glucosinolates as natural pesticides and as defense against herbivores; these substances are also responsible for the bitter or sharp taste of many common foods such as mustard, horseradish, cabbage and brussels sprouts.

Glucosinolates are water-soluble anions and belong to the glucosides. Every glucosinolate contains a central carbon atom, which is bound via a sulfur atom to the glycone group, and via a nitrogen atom to a sulfonated oxime group (Fig. 2). In addition, the central carbon is bound to a side group. Different glucosinolates have different side groups.

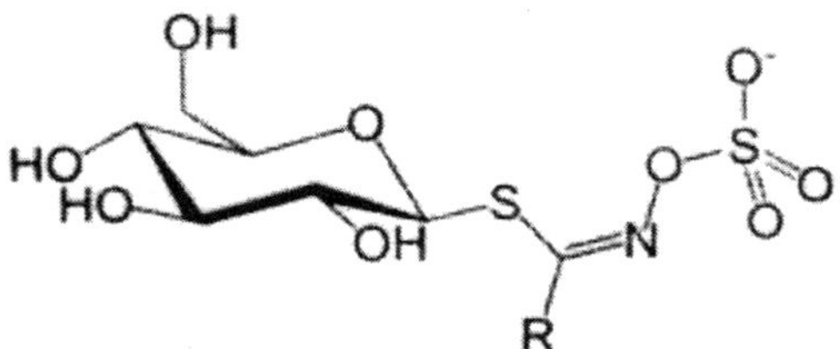

Fig. 2 : Glucosinolate structure; side group *R* varies

About 120 different glucosinolates are known to occur naturally in plants. They are synthesized from certain amino acids: methionine, phenylalanine, tyrosine or tryptophan. The plants contain the enzyme myrosinase which, in the presence of water, cleaves off the glucose group from a glucosinolate. The remaining molecule then quickly converts to a thiocyanate, an isothiocyanate or a nitrile; which are the active substances that serve as defense for the plant. To prevent damage to the plant itself, the myrosinase and glucosinolates are stored in separate compartments of the cell and come together only under conditions of stress or injury.

Because of the pungent and hot taste of the isothiocyantes and thiocyanates, the glucosinolate-containing plant materials have low palatability, therefore, plant breeders have developed low glucosinolates variety of some crops such as canola. On the other hand, plants producing large amounts of glucosinolates are also desirable, because substances derived from these can serve as natural pesticides and are under investigation in the prevention of cancer (with sulforaphane in broccoli being the best known example). Other examples of glucosinolate containing plants are as follows:

Glucosinolates	Plant
Amoracia lapathifolia	Horseradish
Brassica oleracea	Cabbage, Brussels sprouts, Cauliflower, kohlrabi, broccoli, kale
Brassica chinensis	Pak -choi (Chinese white cabbage)
Brassica campestris	Turnips
Brassica napus	Rutabaga, rape
Brassica nigra	Black mustard
Crambe abyssinica	Crambe
Limnanthes alba	Meadowfoam
Nasturtium officinalis	Water cress
Raphanus sativus	Radish
Thlaspi arvense	Stinkweed
Eruca sativa	Taramira

Metabolic Effects of Products from Glucosinolates

A major effect of the hydrolysis products of glucosinolates is inhibition of the function of the thyroid gland. The thyroid produces hormones that are important in regulating the rate of cellular metabolism (metabolic rate). Antithyroid agents have four general effects. They may interfere with iodine uptake by the thyroid, interfere with iodination of tyrosine, suppress thyroxine secretion, or act as metabolic antagonists to thyroxine in the tissues. The effects of some of the hydrolysis products of glucosinolates, such as goitrin, thiocyanates, isothiocyanates and nitriles are discussed briefly.

Goitrin

Goitrin from rapeseed meal inhibits thyroid function. It causes reduced growth rate, hyperplasia and hypertrophy of the thyroid. The oxazolidine-2-thiones act by inhibiting the incorporation of iodine into precursors of thyroxine and by interfering with thyroxine secretion. The anti-thyroid effect is not overcome by adding increased iodine to the diet.

Thiocyanates and Isothiocyanates

Thiocyanate inhibits iodine uptake by the thyroid. The effect is most pronounced when dietary iodine is low and can be overcome by increasing the iodine level of the diet. Since isothiocyanates are irritating to mucous membranes, they are probably not consumed as such in toxic amounts. However, if they are consumed as the glucosinolates precursor, with the isothiocyanates released in the gut, they may act as antithyroid agents.

Nitriles

Nitriles are formed from glucosinolates in crambe meal (*Crambe abyssinica*) and rapeseed meal. Nitriles are toxic, causing poor growth, liver and kidney lesions, including bile duct hyperplasia, liver necrosis, and megalocytosis of the kidney tubular epithelium. The biochemical cause of this effect is not clear. Paik *et al.* (1980) suggested that since nitriles may be metabolized by mixed function oxidases, they may cause enzyme induction and a consequent increase in liver size. Rapeseed meal nitriles may be partially converted to thiocyanate. Dietary thiosulfate overcomes part of the growth depressing effects of high-nitrile rapeseed meals (Paik *et al*,. 1980).

Poultry and swine, fed raw rapeseed meal, exhibit enlarged thyroids and growth depression. Additional problems noted in poultry include perosis, lowered egg production, off-flavors in eggs, and liver damage. Liver hemorrhage in poultry fed rapeseed meal may be caused by nitriles. Swine may have enlarged livers when fed rapeseed meal. Levels of 5-10% rapeseed meal have been acceptable for non-ruminants. Indian cattle and buffaloes can tolerate high levels of dietary rapeseed meal with no ill effect in long term feeding trials. They are less sensitive to glucosinolate and their derivatives than non-ruminants, presumably because of rumen metabolism of these compounds. Supplementation of copper sulphate to the mustard/rapeseed meal reduced their adverse effect not only in young calves but also in swine.

Saponins

Saponins, the naturally occurring surface-active glycosides, are mainly produced by plants and derive their name from their ability to form stable, soap-like foams in aqueous solutions. Saponins consist of a sugar moiety usually containing glucose, galactose, glucuronic acid, xylose, rhamnose or methylpentose, glycosidically linked to a hydrophobic aglycone (sapogenin) which may be triterpenoid or steroid in nature. The aglycone may contain one or more unsaturated C–C bonds. The oligosaccharide chain is normally attached at the C_3 position (monodesmosidic), but many saponins have an additional sugar moiety at the C_{26} or C_{28} position of the aglycone structure.

Saponins occur constitutively in a great many plant species, in both wild plants and cultivated crops. In cultivated crops the triterpenoid saponins are generally predominant, while steroid saponins are common in plants/herbs. Triterpenoid saponins have been detected in many legumes such as soybeans,

beans, peas, lucerne, etc. and also in tea, spinach, sugar beet, quinoa, liquorice, sunflower, horse chestnut, and ginseng. Steroid saponins are found in oats, capsicum peppers, aubergine, tomato seed, alliums, asparagus, yam, fenugreek, yucca and ginseng. India is having large number of plant sources, which are rich in saponins and these are Mahua, Reetha, Shikakai, and many others such as Albizia leaves. *Yucca schidigera* is the most common commercial source of steroid saponins. Many forage legumes grown in temperate and tropical areas contain saponins and a number of factors, such as physiology, age, environmental and agronomic factors, have been shown to affect their saponins content. Generally, immature plants of a species have been found to have higher saponins contents than more mature plants of the same species. The saponins content of some plants have been presented in Table 2.

Table 2 : Saponin content of some plant materials (% DM basis)

Botanical Name (part)	English name	Hindi name	Saponins (% DM)
Achillea millefolium (Aerial)	Yarrow	Gandana	
Acorus calamus Linn. (Rhizome)	Sweet flag	Bach	12.13
Anethum sowa Kurtz (fruit)	Dill	Sowa	6.54
Asparagus adscendens Roxb. (root)*	-	Satavar	13.79
Berberis aristata Dc (Root)	Indian Berberry	Chitra basant	19.18
Emblica officinalis Gaertu (Fruit)*	Indian gooseberry	Amla	1.92
Equisetum arvense Linn.(Aerial)*	Field horse tail	-	12.9
Euycalyptus globules Labil (leaf)*	Blue gum eucalyptus	-	
Fagopyrum esculentum Moenck (Leaf)*	Common buckwheat	Phaphra	4.52
Feronia limolea Linn. (Leaf)*	Elephant(wood)apple	Balin, Kait	2.16
Medicago sativa**	Alfalfa	Rijka	
Trifolium alexondrinum**	Berseem	Berseem	
Acacia concinnd**	Shikakoi	Shikakai	
Sapindu strifoliatus**	Soapnut	Retha	
Rumex acetosa Linn. (Leaf)*	Garden sorrel	Khatti Palak	2.58
Terminalia bellerica Roxb. (Fruit)*	Bellerin myrobolan	Beheda	
Terminalia chebula Retz (Fruit)*	Chebulin myrolan	Harad	2.29
Tinospora cardifolia Mierr (Stem)*	Gulancha tinospora	Giloe Amint	5.31
Bassia latifolia (seed cake)#	-	Mahua	7.34

* Alexander (2005), ** Malik (2007), # Anamika (2007)

Saponins have a wide variety of biological effects, with both positive in reducing serum cholesterol level and risk of atherosclerosis in humans. On the negative side, they inhibit the productive performance of swine and poultry fed diets containing alfalfa.

The saponins in alfalfa are probably of the most important in animal production. The principal saponins in common alfalfa cultivars are medicagenic acid, soyasapogenol A and B, and lucernic acid. They differ in the hydroxyl and carboxyl groups attached to the sapogenin (aglycone). Medicagenic acid appears to be the major saponin in alfalfa with antinutritional effects. Low levels of dietary alfalfa meal reduce the growth rate of poultry and swine, primarily due to bitter taste and irritation of mucus membrane of mouth and digestive tract thereby affecting the palatability and feed intake adversely. Since saponins form insoluble complexes with cholesterol, therefore, alfalfa saponins may cause a reduction in tissue and serum cholesterol, reduced cholesterol absorption, however, Nakaue *et al.* (1980) found no difference in egg cholesterol from hens fed diets containing high/low saponin alfalfa meal. Sarsaponins also control ammonia levels in poultry houses (Johnston *et al.*, 1981).

Saponins are surface active agents producing stable foams. These are found in legumes that cause bloat. Steroid saponins such as sarsaponin occur in yucca (*Yucca schidigera*). Some saponins in *Yucca schidigera, Acacia auriculoformis* and *Quillaja saponaria* (Makkar *et al.*, 1998) have shown some beneficial effects on animals and suggested their use as feed additive as saponins partition the nutrients in such a manner that a higher proportion of digested substrate goes to the formation of microbial mass and a lower proportion to VFA and gases (Makkar *et al.*, 1998).

Feeding of the saponins rich fodder reduced protozoal population by 50-60 per cent (Moss *et al.*, 2000), which is responsible for the inter species hydrogen transfer to the methanogenic bacteria attached to them thereby reducing the hydrogen availability to the methanogens, resulting a decrease in methane production. This possibility was investigated for mitigating the methane emission from ruminants. Hess *et al.* (2003) reported that the daily inclusion of *Sapindus saponaria* (a saponin rich fruit) to the roughage based diet at 14 per cent level, decreased protozoal population by 54 per cent and methane emission by 20 per cent, which was attributed to the inhibition of hydrogen producing bacteria or pyruvate ferridoxin oxidoreductase producing bacteria, which metabolize pyruvate to acetyl Co-A (Wang *et al.*, 2000).

Lila *et al.* (2003) while studying the effect of sarsaponin on ruminal fermentation with particular emphasis to methane production *in vitro*, observed the significant reduction in methane emission following the supplementation of substrate with sarsaponin. They further reported that dietary supplementation of saponin (0.5 and 1% on DM basis) decreased ($P<0.01$) methane emission in Holstein heifers (Lila *et al.*, 2005). Hu *et al.* (2006) reported that methane emission was decreased with the increasing levels of dietary saponins. Recently, Malik and Singhal (2008, 2009) reported that incorporation of lucerne to the wheat straw based total mixed ration decreased the methane emission from crossbred and buffalo calves significantly. These results have opened a new vista for utilizing the traditional source of nutrients for mitigating the methane emission.

Beside some beneficial effects on ruminants, some saponins containing plants are toxic such as seeds of *Bassia latifolia*, leaf of *Panicum dichotomiflorum*, *Panicum virgetum* (switch grass) etc. Saponins toxicity leads to photosensitization followed by liver and kidney degeneration in ruminants and gut problems such as gastroenteritis and diarrhoea.

Coumarin

Sweet clover poisoning

Sweet clover (*Melilotus alba* and *Melilotus officinalis*) contains a glycoside called melilotoside, an ether of glucose and coumarin .Coumarin is metabolized by various molds, such as *Pencillium nigricans* and *Pencillium jensi*, producing dicoumarol. Dicoumarol is an inhibitor of vitamin K and induces a vitamin K deficiency. Vitamin K functions in blood clotting, so a deficiency is characterized by susceptibility to hemorrhaging. Sweet clover poisoning occurs almost exclusively in cattle. The predominant sign is hemorrhaging, either external or internal. Internal hemorrhaging results in obvious subcutaneous swellings caused by pooling of blood. The mucous membranes are pale and the animal becomes progressively weaker and dies without a struggle. Before internal hemorrhaging occurs, cattle fed moldy sweet clover hay have a prolonged blood clotting time. Minor surgery such as dehorning or castration may lead to profuse hemorrhaging and death (Kingsbury, 1964).

Vitamin K is involved in the activation of prothrombin. Dicoumarol inhibits this effect, so there is a deficiency of prothrombin in the blood of affected animals. Thrombin acts as an enzyme to split one or more peptides from fibrinogen altering its solubility and causing it to precipitate as a clot. Levels of above 10 ppm dicoumarol in sweet clover hay are suggestive for possible toxicity problems. Dicoumaral levels tend to be the highest in small and in round bales, where opportunity for mold growth is greater than in stacks. Crimping or conditioning of sweet clover hay should speed up drying and might reduce the amount of mold growth, although Benson *et al.* (1981) found no difference in dicoumarol lives of crimped vs non-crimped hay.

Sweet clover poisoning can be treated with injections of vitamin K and also by whole blood transfusion (Radostits *et al.*, 1980). Low coumarin varieties of sweet clover such as Polara have been developed (Goplen, 1971). Dicoumarol problems in livestock are not exclusively caused by moldy sweet clover. Hemorrhagic syndrome in cattle was caused by dicoumarol in sweet vernal grass (*Anthoxanthum odoratum*) hay. Sweet vernal grass contains coumrol by *Aspergillus* spp. fungi. Both sweet clover and sweet vernal grass have a pleasant or sweet odour caused by the presence of coumarins.

Metal Binding Substances

Phytic acid

Plant seeds contain phytic acid, an organic compound containing six phosphates. This phosphate is largely unavailable to non-ruminant animals. In ruminants bacterial phytases release the bound phosphate. The nutritional significance is that phytic acid can chelate with various minerals, producing phytates. This is of particular significance with respect to Zn. When soyabean meal was first used in large quantities as protein supplement for swine, a high incidence of parakeratosis (a classical Zn deficiency symptoms) was observed in swine. The tie up of Zn can be overcome by supplementing the diet with sufficient Zn to exceed the chelating capacity of soybean meal. Other elements such as Cu, Mn, Fe, Ca and Mg can also bound in phytate form and render their availability. The decreasing order of stability of phytate mineral complexes is Zn, Cu, Co, Mg and Ca. In mature cereal grain, 60-80% of total phosphorus is bound as phytic acid, while 50-60% of the phosphorus in soybeans is as phytic acid. Phytate is not destroyed readily by heat and soaking, but fermentation does liberate phosphates from phytic acid.

Oxalic acid

Oxalate is found in plants in two major forms. Some plants, have cell sap pH of about 2, and the oxalate exist as salt of acid oxalate (H_2CO_4), such as acid potassium oxalate. Other plants, such as halogeton, have a cell sap pH of about 6, and the oxalate exist as soluble sodium and insoluble Ca and Mg oxalates. The paddy straw contains about 1.6 per cent oxalic acid and major part is soluble in nature. The mode of action of oxalate in causing toxicity is not totally clear. Acute toxicity may be due to hypocalcaemia, while uremia from kidney damage may contribute to chronic toxicity. Oxalate also inhibits several respiratory enzymes, including succinic dehydrogenase. Enzymes activated by calcium and magnesium may be inhibited by oxalate. Dietary oxalate can be degraded by rumen microorganisms and ruminants adapted to diets with high oxalate content can tolerate oxalate levels that are lethal to non adapted animals. To reduce the adverse effect of oxalates of paddy straw, its water soaking or ensiling is recommended. Feeding of lime water or other source of calcium neutralizes the adverse effect of oxalates.

Nitrate/ Nitrite Toxicity

Common crops, pasture plants and weeds may accumulate toxic levels of nitrates (Table 3). In ruminants, nitrate is readily reduced to nitrite, which is absorbed and causes toxicosis. Nitrite ions oxidize ferrous iron in hemoglobin to produce methemoglobin. Methemoglobin can not react with oxygen, so anoxia occurs. Clinical signs of toxicity may be seen when methemoglobin levels reach 30-40% of total hemoglobin, while death occurs at levels of 80-90% methemoglobin. Abnormal accumulation of nitrate in plants is provoked by high levels of nitrogen fertilization, drought conditions, and herbicide treatment with phenoxyacetic herbicides such as 2, 4-D. Nitrate accumulates in the vegetative tissues, particularly in stalks with less in the leaves. Sudan grass, oats, rape, wheat, barley and corn accumulate nitrate. Heavy fertilization of grass pastures, especially with cool, cloudy weather, may result in toxic nitrate levels. Forage levels of 0.5% nitrate and above are potentially dangerous, with acute poisoning likely to occur if the nitrate level exceeds 1%. Levels of 200 ppm nitrate in water are potentially hazardous, with 1500 ppm causing acute toxicity. When silage is made from high nitrate forage, toxic silo gas may be produced. Anaerobic silage fermentation results in reduction of nitrate to oxide of nitrogen (NO_2 and N_2O_4). These gases are yellowish brown and may collect in barns in sufficient concentration to kill animals. Affected animals can be treated by intravenous injections of methylene blue, a powdered dye material. Methylene blue converts the methaemoglobin back to oxygen-carrying haemoglobin.

Table 3 : Common crops/ pastures and weeds containing nitrate/ nitrite

Crops/Pastures	Weeds
Oats	Capeweed
Sorghum	Variegated thistle
Maize	Mintweed
Rape	Crown beard
Lucerne	Pigweed
Kikuyu	Redroot
Turnip tops	Caltrop (cat's head)
Sugar beet tops	Marshmallow
Rye	Blackberry
Sudan grass	Fat hen
Soybean	
Wheat	
Barley	

Proteins and Amino Acids

Protease inhibitors

The protease inhibitors are typical examples of heat-labile factors with antinutritional activity. They constitute a unique class of proteins with the ability to react in a highly specific manner with a number of proteolytic enzymes in the digestive secretions of animals. The trypsin inhibitors of soybean are now well characterized (D'Mello, 1995) and is an important determinant of nutritive value. Protease inhibitors are also present in other leguminous seeds such as field beans, winged beans, pigeon pea and cowpea. In soybeans, the protease inhibitors are two types i.e. Kunitz inhibitor and Bowman- Birk inhibitor. Kunitz inhibitor has a molecular weight of 20,000-25,000 with few disulfide bonds. It contains 181 amino acids and one mole inhibitor inactivates one mole of trypsin. Bowman- Birk inhbitor have a molecular weight of 6000-10,000 with a high proportion of disulfide bonds. It has two active sites, one that binds trypsin and one that bind chymotrypsin. Some of the effects of feeding raw soybeans, particularly in nonruminants, include poor growth, reduced feed intake, and a reduction in protein digestibility, pancreatic hypertrophy and a deficiency of sulphur amino acids. Activity of trypsin inhibitors is destroyed over 95% by heat treatment at 100^{0}C for 15 min.

Hemagglutinins (lectins)

Hemagglutinins (phytohemagglutinins, lectins) cause the clumping or agglutination of red blood cells *in vitro*. They were first isolated from castor beans, which contain potent lectins called ricin. Lectins are proteins that have a high affinity for certain sugar molecules. Many contain covalently bound sugars and so classed as glycoproteins. Their biological effects are probably due to their affinity for sugars. There are carbohydrate moieties in animal's cell membranes which may bind to lectins and be altered in functional properties.

Lectins are found in soybeans and other field beans (*Phaseolus*) such as kidney, pinto and navy beans. The lectins in raw soybeans are relatively nontoxic but feeding high levels of raw kidney beans to rats will kill them due to lectin activity. Hemagglutinins cause various adverse effects, including reduced growth, diarrhea, decreased nutrient absorption, and increased incidence of bacterial infection. The major effects seem to be on the intestinal mucosa. The hemagglutinins bind to cells in the intestinal wall and cause a non-specific interference with nutrient absorption. In addition, there is evidence that lectins impair the immune system, leading to greater sensitivity to bacterial infection. Changes in gut permeability may lead to invasion by normally harmless intestinal micro flora. Pusztai *et al.* (1979) have reported that field bean lectins disrupt the brush borders of the cells lining the duodenum and jejunum and that an abnormally high rate of tissue protein catabolism occurs in rats administered lectins. A dramatic proliferation of *Escherichia coli* occurs in the small intestine (Wilson *et al.*, 1980). Lectins are destroyed by moist heat but resistant to dry heat, therefore, kidney and other beans should be soaked prior to cooking.

Antigenic proteins

Certain storage proteins of legume seeds are capable of crossing the epithelial barrier of the intestinal mucosa to elicit adverse effects on immune function in farm animals. In the case of the soybean, the antigenic proteins have been identified as glycinin and conglycinin. The antigenic proteins are characterized by their resistance to denaturation by conventional thermal processing procedures and to enzyme attack in the digestive tract of mammals. The most striking effects of antigenic proteins are embodied within the "immune hypersensitivity" syndrome. This condition occurs after feeding heated soybean to sensitized calves and piglets (D'Mello, 1991). The component antigens provoke extensive local and systemic immunological reactions together with severe intestinal damage. The resulting effects include abnormalities in movement of digesta, impaired nutrient absorption and a predisposition to diarrhoea.

Amino acids

A wide range of non-protein amino acids occur in the foliage and seeds of plants. Forage and roots of brassica crops contain S-methyl cysteine sulphoxide, while the aromatic amino acid mimosine occurs in the foliage and seeds of the tropical legume *Leucaena leucocephala* (D'Mello, 2000). Mimosine, the toxic, non-protein amino acid, contributes as much as 14.8% to the total nitrogen content of *L. leucocephala* seeds. Arora and Joshi (1986) found that mimosine content varied with temperature, being higher in winter than in summer. Uncontrolled feeding of brassica forage to ruminants causes organ damage with haemolytic anaemia, which is attributed to the intake of S-methyl cysteine sulphoxide. Abrupt feeding of *Leucaena* to sheep causes shedding of fleece, reduced intake, organ damage and death. In cattle, loss of hair, excessive salivation, lethargy, weight loss and enlarged thyroids are common features of *Leucaena* toxicity.

Seleno-amino acids

In some northern states of India viz. Haryana, Punjab and UP incidences of a disease have been reported in which animals, particularly buffaloes, suffer from the necrosis of body extremities such as mouth, ear tips, tail end and the hooves, when they are fed on paddy straw based diets during the month of November onwards due to the non availability of green fodders. These symptoms are similar to those reported for selenium toxicity and locally this disease is known as 'Degnala disease'. It was found that the soil in these areas is rich in selenium and taken up by paddy plants. Feeding of paddy straw, rich in selenium, enter into the digestive system and during the course of microbial protein synthesis formation of selenocystine and selenomethionine take place instead of cystine and methionine as selenium replace sulphur in these amino acids. Deficiency of essential amino acids and entry of 'strange' amino acids in the tissues cause imbalanced protein metabolism and animal start showing the symptoms of 'Degnala' disease.

It has been reported that in a herd of buffaloes fed on same paddy straw under similar feeding management, only few are affected by 'Degnala'. To avoid the selenium toxicity, animals should be fed on balanced feeding and in case of feeding paddy straw, it should be stopped immediately after visible symptoms of Degnala. To treat the animals, 'Decure mixture' developed by National Dairy Research Institute, Karnal may be offered @30g/day till the animal is cured.

Lathyrogens

Lathyrogens, found in legumes such as chick peas and vetch, are derivatives of amino acids that act as metabolic antagonists of glutamic acid, a neurotransmitter in the brain. When lathyrogens are ingested in large amounts by humans or animals, they cause a crippling paralysis of the lower limbs and may result in death. Lathyrism only occurs on an impoverished diet of vetch, sweet pea, or grass pea and is characterized by bone thinning and leg paralysis. Lathyrogens decrease collagen and elastin cross-linking by inhibiting lysine oxidase. The lathyrogens isoniazid and semicarbazide decrease liver pyridoxal phosphate and are teratogenic. All their effects are reversed by pyridoxal. Another lathyrogen, â-Aminopropionitrile does not affect liver pyridoxal phosphate, and its lathyrogenic and teratogenic effects are not reversed by pyridoxal.

Bacterial Contamination

Occurrence of *Escherichia coli* in animal feeds is a serious problem. In a study (Lynn *et al.*, 1998), 30 percent of cattle feed samples in USA, obtained from commercial sources and farms contained *E. coli*, although none of the tests for *E. coli* O157 were positive. Replication of faecal *E. coli*, including the O157 type, was confirmed in a variety of feeds in summer is likely to occur on cattle farms. Faecal contamination of feeds is an important route for exposure of cattle to *E. coli* and other organisms. The potential for exposure to bacteria also exists when poultry litters are fed to cattle. Heat-processing of feed minimize or even eliminate the risks of contamination with *E. coli*, *Salmonella* spp. and *Campylobacter* spp. (Jeffrey *et al.*, 1998). *Listeria monocytogenes* tends to occur in poor-quality silage and big-bale silage. When grass is ensiled under anaerobic conditions, the low pH regime ensures that *Listeria* is excluded from the resulting silage. However, in big-bale silage a degree of aerobic fermentation may occur, raising pH levels and allowing the growth of *Listeria*. These bacteria also survive at low temperatures and in silages with high levels of dry matter. Contamination of silage with *Listeria* is important as it causes abortion, meningitis, encephalitis and septicaemia in animals and humans.

Mycotoxins

Mycotoxins are those secondary metabolites produced by toxigenic fungi (molds). These natural toxins have had a great impact on the livestock industry worldwide for many centuries, particularly in certain geographical regions. In the tropics, *Aspergillus* is the predominant genus in dairy and other feeds (Dhand *et al.*, 1998). Other species include *Penicillium, Fusarium* and *Alternaria,* which are also important contaminants of cereal grains. Spores from moldy hay, silage, brewers' grain and sugar-beet pulp may be inhaled or consumed by animals with deleterious effects termed "mycosis". Feed contamination has resulted in livestock losses due to death and subtle effects. In addition, translocation of residues into meat, poultry and dairy products represents a serious public health concern. Mycotoxin contamination of forages and cereals frequently occurs in the field following infection of plants with particular pathogenic fungi or with symbiotic endophytes. Moisture content and ambient temperature are key determinants of fungal colonization and mycotoxin production. It is conventional to subdivide toxigenic fungi into "field" (or plant-pathogenic) and "storage" (or saprophytic/spoilage) organisms. *Claviceps, Neotyphodium, Fusarium* and *Alternaria* are classical representatives of field fungi while *Aspergillus* and *Penicillium* exemplify storage organism. Mycotoxigenic species may be further distinguished on the basis of geographical prevalence, reflecting specific environmental requirements for growth and secondary metabolism. Thus, *Aspergillus flavus, A. parasiticus* and *A. ochraceus* readily proliferate under warm, humid conditions, while *Penicillium expansum* and *P. verrucosum* are essentially temperate fungi. Consequently, the *Aspergillus* mycotoxins predominate in plant products emanating from the tropics and other warm regions, while the *Penicillium* mycotoxins occur widely in temperate foods, particularly cereal grains. *Fusarium* fungi are more ubiquitous, but even this genus contains toxigenic species that are almost exclusively associated with cereals from warm countries. Mycotoxins, based on biological effects may be classified as follows:

Hepatotoxins	Aflatoxin, spordesmin, rubratoxin B, sterigmatocystin, trichothecenes, ochratoxin A, phomopsin A
Nephrotoxins	Ochratoxin A, citrinin, aflatoxin,
Neurotoxins	Trichothecenes (e.g., vomitoxin, satratoxin), slaframine, penitrem A (and other tremorgens), ochratoxin A (poultry only), ergot alkaloids, lupinosis (ammonia accumulation)
Genitoxins	Zearalenone, ergot alkaloids
Pulmonary Toxins	4-ipomeanol
Dermitoxins	12, 13 epoxytrich othecenes (e.g., T-2 toxin, nivalenol)
Photosensitizing Agents	Sporidesmin (facial eczema)
Carcinogens	Aflatoxin, sterigmatoeystin, luteoskyrin, patulin, penicillic acid, T-2 toxin (possibly)
Teratogens	Aflatoxin, ochratoxin A
Immunosuppressant	Aflatoxin, trichothecenes (T-2 toxin), ochratoxin
Hematologic Agents	Dicoumarol, aflatoxin, trichothecenes

Aflatoxins

The importance of aflatoxins in animal health emerged in 1960, following an incident in the United Kingdom in which one million turkey poults died from acute necrosis of the liver and hyperplasia of the bile duct (Turkey X disease), attributed to the consumption of groundnuts infected with *Aspergillus flavus*. Studies showed that aflatoxins are acutely toxic to ducklings, but ruminants are more resistant.

Aflatoxins are potent toxic, carcinogenic, mutagenic, immunosuppressive agents, produced as secondary metabolites by the fungus *Aspergillus flavus* and *A. parasiticus* on variety of food products. Among 18 different types of aflatoxins identified, major members are aflatoxin B_1, B_2, G_1 and G_2. Aflatoxin B_1 (AFB_1) is normally predominant in food products. *A. flavus* typically produces AFB_1 and AFB_2, whereas *A. parasiticus* produce AFG_1 and AFG_2 as well as AFB_1 and AFB_2. Four other aflatoxins M_1, M_2, B_{2A}, and G_{2A} which may be produced in minor amounts were subsequently isolated from cultures of *A. flavus* and *A. parasiticus*. Aflatoxin M_1 and M_2 are major metabolites of aflatoxin B_1 and B_2, respectively, found in milk of animals that have consumed feed contaminated with aflatoxins. Aflatoxins normally refer to the group of difuranocoumarins and classified in two broad groups according to their chemical structure; the difurocoumarocyclopentenone series (AFB_1, AFB_2, AFB_{2A}, AFM_1, AFM_2, AFM_{2A} and aflatoxicol) and the difurocoumarolactone series (AFG_1, AFG_2, AFG_{2A}, $AFGM_1$, $AFGM_2$, $AFGM_{2A}$ and AFB_3). The aflatoxins display potency of toxicity, carcinogenicity, mutagenicity in the order of AFB_1 > AFG_1 > AFB_2 > AFG_2 as illustrated by their LD_{50} values for day-old ducklings. Structurally the dihydrofuran moiety, containing double bond, and the constituents liked to the coumarin moiety are of importance in producing biological effects. The aflatoxins fluoresce strongly in ultraviolet light (ca. 365 nm); B_1 and B_2 produce a blue fluorescence where as G_1 and G_2 produce green fluorescence.

Ochratoxins

Aspergillus ochraceus produces ochratoxins and ochratoxin A and ochratoxin B are two forms that occur naturally as contaminants, with ochratoxin A being more ubiquitous, occurring predominantly in cereal grains and in the tissues of animals reared on contaminated feed. Another mycotoxin, citrinin, often co-occurs with ochratoxin. The ochratoxins and citrinin are nephrotoxic to a wide range of animal species.

Fusarium Mycotoxins

Three types of *Fusarium* mycotoxins contamination of cereal grains and animal feed is found i.e. trichothecenes, zearalenone (ZEN) and the fumonisins (D'Mello and MacDonald, 1998). The trichothecenes are subdivided into four basic groups, with types A and B being the most important. Type A trichothecenes include T-2 toxin, HT-2 toxin, neosolaniol and diacetoxyscirpenol (DAS) whereas Type B includes deoxynivalenol (DON, also known as vomitoxin), nivalenol and fusarenon-X. The production of the two types of trichothecenes is characteristic for a particular *Fusarium* species. However, a common feature of the secondary metabolism of these fungi is their ability to synthesize ZEN which, consequently, occurs as a co-contaminant with certain trichothecenes. The fumonisins are synthesized by another distinct group of *Fusarium* species. Three members of this group (fumonisins B_1, B_2 and B_3) often occur together in maize. The *Fusarium* mycotoxins induce a wide range of effects in farm livestock (D'Mello, 2000). DON is a potent feed intake inhibitor in pigs and ZEN is associated with reproductive abnormalities in pigs and ruminants. Fumonisins have been linked with specific syndromes, namely porcine pulmonary oedema and equine leukoencephalomalacia. Fumonisin contamination of maize in South Africa has been correlated with the occurrence of oesophageal cancer in humans.

Control of Mould and Mycotoxins

Controlling mould growth and mycotoxin production is very important for producing the good quality feeds. Control of mould growth in feeds can be generally done by keeping moisture low, feed fresh, equipment clean and using mould binders and inhibitors during feed production. Grains and other dry feeds must be stored at a moisture level of less than 14 percent to prevent mould growth. Aeration of grain bins is important to reduce moisture migration and keep the feedstuff dry (Jones *et al.,* 1994). The use of chemical mould inhibitors is a well established and practice in the feed industry. However, mould inhibitors are only one of several tools useful in the complex process of controlling the growth of moulds, and they should not be relied upon exclusively. The main types of mould inhibitors are individual or combinations of organic acids like propionic, sorbic, benzoic and acetic acids, and salts of organic acids for example, calcium propionate and potassium sorbate. Further, copper sulphate (solid or liquid forms) work equally well if the inhibitor is evenly dispersed through the feed. Generally, the acid form of a mould inhibitor is more active than its corresponding salt (Jones *et al.,* 1994). Binding agents such as bentonite, aluminosilicates, spent canola oil, bleaching clays and alfalfa fibre have also been used in feeds containing mycotoxins to prevent intestinal absorption of the toxins (Smith and Seddon, 1998). Mineral clay products such as bentonites, zeolites and aluminosilicates have been found to be effective in binding/adsorbing mycotoxins. Among these, aluminosilicates have been found to be more effective. The molecular surfaces of these additives, when saturated with water, attract the polar functional atomic structure of the mycotoxin and trap it against its surface. This isolates the mycotoxin from the digestive process and thereby prevents it from entering into circulation. Hydrated sodium calcium aluminosilicate (HSCAS) at 1.0% of the feed (10kg/tonne) can significantly diminish the adverse effects of aflatoxin in chickens, pigs and cows (Scheildler, 1993). Now it is very important that mycotoxins will be of increasing importance for all those who involved in feed manufacturing, farming and food production. Quality of raw materials, prevention of the occurrence of mycotoxins, control and testing systems are all essential to reduce the exposure of humans and animals to mycotoxins.

Animal Originated Toxins

The prion proteins of mammalian meat and bone-meal have recently emerged as important feed contaminants. Prion proteins are harmless animal tissue components with the capacity to transform themselves into agents causing fatal neurological lesions in a wide range of species. The significance of prions has been highlighted following the emergence of bovine spongiform encephalopathy (BSE) as a major disease of cattle in the United Kingdom. The onset of this disease was attributed to the feeding of cattle with meat- and bone-meal prepared from the carcasses of scrapie-infected sheep. The latter disease is also caused by prion proteins, as is the human equivalent - new variant Creutzfeldt-Jakob disease (v CJD). The incidence of v CJD in humans has been linked to the consumption of BSE-infected beef. Specific regulations apply to the control of BSE in cattle. In the United Kingdom, it has been illegal to feed ruminants with any form of mammalian protein since November 1994. The feeding of mammalian meat and bone-meal to farmed livestock has been prohibited since April 1996. However, pigs and poultry may still be fed diets containing mammalian protein in forms other than mammalian meat- and bone-meal, e.g. processed catering waste.

All the animal feed and fodder may be contaminated with organic, inorganic compounds and particulates. Organic chemicals comprise the largest group and include plant toxins, mycotoxins, antibiotics, prion proteins and pesticides. Inorganic compounds include heavy metals etc. Particulates such as weed seeds and certain bacterial pathogens are common contaminants of animal feed. The effects of feed contaminants and toxins range from reduced intake to reproductive dysfunction and increased incidence of bacterial diseases. Comprehensive legislation is in place for the control of several of these chemical compounds and pathogens in feed. The scope for decontamination of feeds is limited and generally uneconomic, and prevention is the most effective practical strategy.

Prospects and Challenges of Anti-nutritional Factors of Feed Origin

India possesses large quantities of feed resources, which are either not being utilized or being under-utilized as animal feeds, in spite of the shortage nutrients in the ration of livestock. Such feeds include various natural plants and trees, which yield green matter (leaves), fruits and seeds. The main reason for not utilizing their potential is the presence of one or other anti-nutritional factor, which either restricts their palatability or causes the toxicity as discussed earlier. However, few of these feed resources, particularly the oilseeds are collected and processed for oil extraction, which have wide applications ranging from soap making, and manufacturing of varnishes and some pharmaceuticals etc and residual material such as neem cake, mahua cake, karanj cake, dhupa cake, jatropha cake, salseed meal, rubber cake etc are generally utilized as manure. In view of their nutrients composition including amino acids and minerals, these resources were evaluated as a constituent of animal ration under All India Coordinated Research Project by ICAR involving research institutions and State Agricultural Universities. Several technologies were developed for the utilization of these unconventional feed resources and recommendations were given accordingly. However, these technologies for the removal of anti-nutritional factors are being used because of high cost of processing.

Several unconventional feeds having anti-nutritional factors have shown other uses besides their potential for animal feeding. For example, insecticidal property of neem has been demonstrated. Neem seed cake (containing azaderone, azaderadione, vilasinin, nimbidin, azadirachtin, salanin nimbin, nimbolinin), mahua cake (containing saponins) and karanj cake (containing karangin and pongamol) etc have bitter taste and the acetone extract of neem (Bains *et al.*, 1971) and mahua cake or hot alcohol extract of neem seed cake (Mishra *et al.*, 1975) can play a role as nitrification inhibitors as rapid nitrification of urea following its application to the fields is a direct loss of N. The exact chemical constituent of neem/mahua cake or their extracts that causes regulation of urea mineralization has not been identified so far. Besides the neem based soap, tooth paste and mosquito repellents, neem oil have also shown the spermicidal activity as well as its use to control skin diseases such as furuculosis, arsenical dermatitis, scabies. Nimbin and nimbidin produce anti-inflammatory effect similar to a pharmaceutical known as cortisone acetate. For the insect control, neem based products have been developed such as Margosine-O in USA and Neem rich in India and sizable quantity of neem seed cake is being exported for its utilization as a source of pharmaceuticals.

Besides the use of saponins in fishery management, these may be used in soft drinks, fire extinguishers, wetting agent of photo films and the synthesis of steroidal hormone, which may have an application in birth control. Presence of saponins, terpenoids, phenylpropanoids, tannins etc, in plants also known as secondary metabolites have demonstrated their potential in modification of rumen microbial fermentation. Extract of saponins containing plants have also shown the possibilities for the mitigation of methane from ruminants, which is an important issue in view of peoples concern for global warming. This brief description indicates that the potential of anti-nutritional factors, present in under utilized feed resources may be exploited for the benefits of man kind; it will not only solve the problems of deficiency of nutrients but will add a new chapter in the services of society.

References

Alexander, P. (2005). Effect of Plant Extracts on Rumen Fermentation and nutrient utilization in sheep. Ph. D. thesis submitted to Indian Veterinary Research Institute, Izatnagar, UP.

Anamika (2007). Effect of plant extracts on rumen fermentation and methane emission. M.V.Sc. Thesis submitted to National Dairy Research Institute, Karnal.

Arora, S. K. and Joshi V. N. (1986). *Leucaena Res. Rep.*, 7:34-35.

Bains, S.S., Prashad, R. and Bhatia, P.C. (1971). *Fertil. News*. 16(3): 30.

Benson, M.E., Casper, H.H. and Johnson, L.J. (1981). *Am. J. Vet. Res.*, 42: 2014-2015.

Dhand, N.K., Joshi, D.V. and Jand, S.K. (1998). *Indian J. Anim. Sci.*, 68: 1095-1096.

D'Mello, J.P.F. (1991). Antigenic Proteins. *In:* Toxic substances in crop plants. (Eds) J.P.F. D'Mello, C.M. Duffus and J.H. Duffus. Cambridge, UK, Royal Society of Chemistry. p. 107-125.

D'Mello, J.P.F. (1995). Antinutritional substances in legume seeds. *In:* Tropical Legumes in Animal Nutrition. (Eds.) J.P.F. D'Mello and C. Devendra, CAB International, Wallingford, UK, pp. 135-172.

D'Mello, J.P.F. (2000). Antinutritional factors and mycotoxins. *In*: Farm Animal Metabolism and Nutrition. (Ed) J.P.F. D'Mello, CAB International, Wallingford, UK. pp. 383-403.

D'Mello, J.P.F. and Mac Donald, A.M.C. (1998). Fungal Toxins as Disease Elicitors. *In:* Environmental toxicology: Current developments. (Ed.) J. Rose, Gordon and Breach Science Publishers. Amsterdam, The Netherlands, pp 253-289.

Goplen B.P. (1971). *Can. J. Plant Sci.*, 51: 249-251.

Hess, H.D., Kreuzer, M., Diaz, T.E., Lascano, T.E., Carculla, J.E., Soliva, C.R. and Machmuller, A. (2003). *Anim. Feed Sci Tech.*, 109: 79-94.

Hu, W.L., Liu, J.X., Yan-Qiu, Wu. and Yue-Min. (2006). Proc. 12th AAAP Congress, Bushan, South Korea pp. 121.

Jeffrey, J.S., Kirk, J.H., Atwill, E.R. and Cullor, J.S. (1998). *Poult. Sci.*, 77: 808-811.

Johanston, N.L., Quarles, C.L., Fagerberg, D.J., and Caveny, D.D. (1981). *Poult. Sci.*, 60: 2289-2292.

Jones, F.T., Genter, M.B., Hagler, W.M, Hansen, J.A, Mowrey, B.A, Poore, M.H. and Whitlow, L.W. (1994). Understanding and coping with effects of mycotoxins in livestock feed and forage. North Carolina Cooperative Extension Service, pp: 1-14.

Jung, H.G. and Fahey, G.C. Jr, (1983). *J. Anim. Sci.*, 57: 206 – 219.

Kingsbury, J.M. (1964). Poisonous plants of the USA and Canada. Prentice-Hall, Englewood Cliffs. NJ.

Lila, Z.A., Mohammed, N., Kanda, S., Kawada, T and Itabashi, H. (2003). *J. Dairy Sci.*, 86: 3330-3336.

Lila, Z.A., Nazimuddin, M., Kanda, S., Kurihara, M. and Itabashi, H. (2005). *Asian-Aust. J. Anim. Sci.*, 18: 1746-1751.

Lynn, T.V., Hancock, D.D., Besser, T.E., Harrison, J.H., Rice, D.H., Stewart, N.T. and Rowan, L.L. (1998). *J. Dairy Sci.*, 81: 1102-1108.

Makkar, H.P.S., Sen, S., Blummel, M. and Becker, K. (1998). *J. Agric. Food Chem.*, 46: 4324-4328.

Mangan J.L. (1988). *Nutr. Res. Rev.*, 1, 209-231

Malik, P.K. (2007). Effect of different leguminous fodder on methane and nitrous oxide emission from ruminants. Ph.D. thesis submitted to National Dairy Research Institute, Karnal.

Malik P.K. and Singhal K.K. (2008). *Indian J. Anim. Sci.*, 78(3): 293-297.

Malik P.K. and Singhal K.K. (2009). *Indian J. Anim. Sci.*, 79: 422-425.

Mishra, M.M., Neelkanthan, S., Khandelwal, K.C., Bhardwaj, S.K. and Vyas, S.P. (1975). *Soil Biol. Biochem.* 7: 183.

Moss, A.R., Jouany, J.P. and Newbold, C.J. (2000). *Ann. Zootech.*, 49: 231-253.

Nakaue, H.S., Lowry, R.R., Cheeke, P.R. and Arscott, G.H. (1980). *Poult. Sci.*, 59: 2744-2748.

Paik, I.K., Robblee, A.R. and Clandinin, D.R. (1980). *Can. J. Anim. Sci.*, 60: 481-493.

Pusztai, A., Clarke, E.M.W. and King, T.P. (1979). *Proc. Nutr. Soc.*, 38: 115-120.

Radostits, O.M., Searcy, G.P. and Mitchell, K. (1980). *Can. Vet. J.*, 21: 155-158.

Scheildler, S.E. (1993). *Poult. Sci.*,72: 282-288.

Smith, T.K. and Seddon, I.R. (1998). (Eds.) Lyons, T.P. and Jacques, K.A., Nottingham University Press, Loughborough, U.K. 257-269.

Swain, T. (1979). *Tannins and Lignins. In : G.A. Rosenthal and D.H. Janzen, Academic Press, NY,* pp. 657-682.

Wang, Y., Mc Allister, T.A. Yanke, L.S. and Cheeke, P.R. (2000). *J. Appl. Microb.*, 88: 887-896.

Wilson, A.B., King, T.P., Clarke, E.M.W. and Pusztai, A. (1980). *J. Comp. Pathol.*, 90: 597-602.

□□□

Animal Nutrition, 2012
eds. Dr. (Mrs.) Usha R. Mehra et al., pp. 641-650
Satish Serial Publishing House e-mail : info@satishserial.com; website : www.satishserial.com

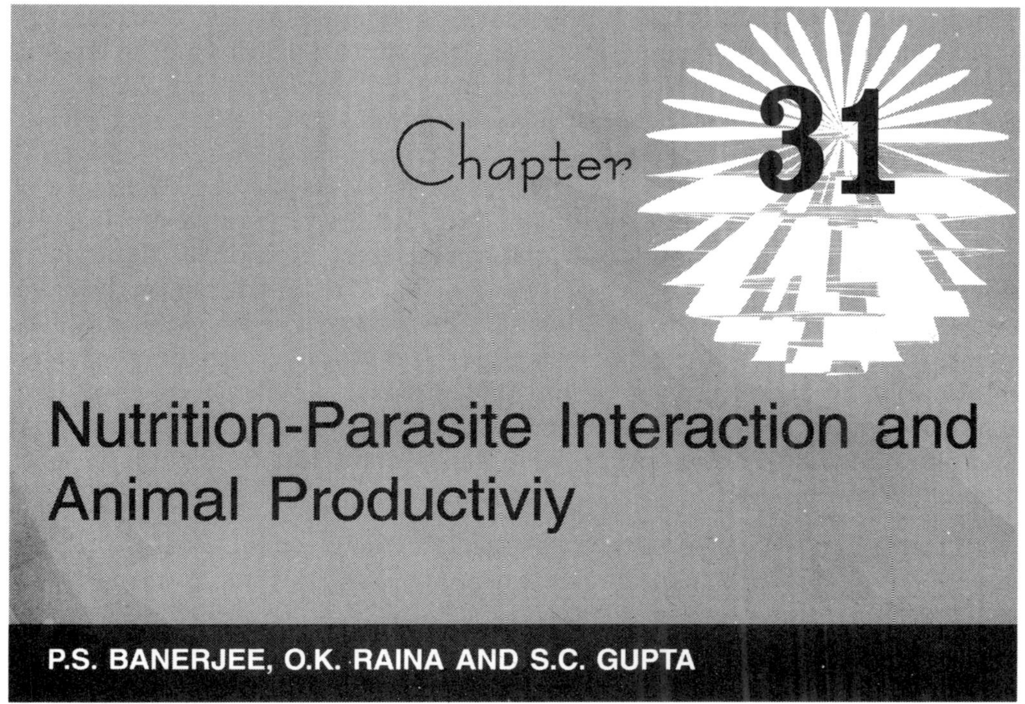

Chapter 31

Nutrition-Parasite Interaction and Animal Productiviy

P.S. BANERJEE, O.K. RAINA AND S.C. GUPTA

Parasitic infection of animals is one of the major causes of incessant and unnoticeable losses to the animal production industry. The infections can be encountered in most organs of the animals with their respective consequences. All parasites rob of the animals' nutrition by way of consuming either the digested food material or feeding upon various forms of hosts' tissues consequently resulting in metabolic disorders and pathophysiological conditions that are not possible to overcome with any sort of nutritional supplements until the parasites are expelled from the host's body. However, nutritional status of the host may greatly influence the establishment, fecundity and rejection of the incoming parasite population but it can not replace conventional parasite control strategy like chemotherapy. Animal nutrition of course is an important and essential component along with manipulation of management practices of an integrated approach in animal production for the control of parasitic infections. The effect of nutrition can be seen on the metabolic disturbances, reproduction and pathophysiology induced by the parasitism (Mehra *et al.*, 1999) on one hand and on the other the availability of nutrients may result on the ability of the host to mount an effective response against parasite establishment and/or induce parasite rejection. The level of nutrition can thus influence the 'resistance' and 'resilience' of the host to parasitic infection. The concept of "resistance" and "resilience" emerged to describe the ability of the host to withstand parasitic challenge. Resistance is the ability of the host by which it prevents or limits the establishment or development of a parasite. Breed, plane of nutrition, previous exposure and innate immunity determine the degree of resistance in animals. On the flip side, resilience is defined as the ability of the host to maintain reasonable level of production in the face of a parasitic infection (van Houtert and Sykes, 1996). Resilience to gastrointestinal (GI) nematodosis can be enhanced reasonably by increasing metabolisable protein supply. Increasing host resistance and/or resilience to parasitic infection through nutritional management can be one practicable component in integrated parasite management approach.

From a historical perspective, an interaction between parasitism and host nutrition long has been suspected. Scrimshaw *et al.*, (1968) set out a conceptual framework for the interaction between infection and host nutritional status, based on the assumption that interactions are more than the additive contribution or coexistence of nutritional factors and infection. These investigators classified the majority of interactions of malnutrition and infection as synergistic. That is, infection aggravated nutritional deficiencies and malnutrition aggravated infections. In contrast, these researchers also identified antagonistic interactions, that is, increasing degrees of malnutrition led to reduced levels or severity of infection. Imagine also a second form of antagonistic interaction, in which increasing levels of infection may lead to reduced degrees of malnutrition. This situation might occur when parasites synthesize nutrients that are required by the host, such as foliate, biotin, or vitamin K.

Over the past several decades, we have learned a great deal about how parasitic infection affects host nutritional status. In contrast, we understand much less about how host under nutrition influences parasitic infections. Host malnutrition leads to impaired immunity, and a functional immune system is required to control infections. Therefore, host nutritional status must be important for the parasite. This premise has formed the basis for the design and interpretation of most of the limited research in this area. Hypothetically, host nutritional status affects the parasite in many other ways as well. Under this chapter, we will explore a spectrum of ideas, many of which have not been tested but are logical extensions of current knowledge, based on independent observations made, distributed spatially and temporally by researchers globally.

One of the most challenging aspects of research in nutrition-infection interactions concerns methodologies. In the field and in the laboratory, investigations rely on qualitative or quantitative measures of infection and nutritional status, but the reliability with which chosen indicators actually measure infection or nutritional status is often low. Many of the indicators most valuable for assessing nutritional status are invasive, so their use is not warranted in the majority of studies. In this chapter, we discuss a few of the issues related to parasitism, choosing appropriate indicators of infection and nutritional status, and to interpreting the resulting data.

Parasitic diseases, especially parasitic gastroenteritis, caused by a number of gut-dwelling nematodes, blood sucking *Haemonchus contortus* being the most important, is a major constraint to economic small ruminant production around the globe. The situation is graver in tropical and sub-tropical countries including India. Environmental conditions in tropical countries are conducive for rapid development and survival of the free-living infective stages of gastrointestinal parasites round the year and the animals are continually exposed to heavy infection from the pasture. Classically, the problem is tackled by chemical intervention. However, due to tremendous biotic potential and short regeneration time of the parasites, the animals, within no time become reinfected. Thus, repeated medication is required to keep up the livestock production economically viable. Moreover, increased demand for animal protein food to cater the ever increasing world population resulted in adoption of intensive livestock management system by the producers. All the above factors led to over reliance on anthelmintics, which paved the way for rapid emergence of anthelmintic resistance in parasites. It is aptly said that "The present era is characterised by drugs more effective than ever before and by treatment failures more menacing than ever before". To add to the worry of the farmers, there is now increasing awareness amongst consumers about chemical residues in foods of animal origin. Consequently, producers are forced to minimise the use of chemicals for parasite control. The attention thus diverted towards integrating all available potential classical and alternate control strategies, which must be sustainable, i.e. "which meets the need of the present without compromising the ability of future generations to meet their own need."

Nutrition in Parasites

Cestodes or the tapeworms inhabit the intestinal tract of the animals. The important feature is that the tapeworms lack digestive system. The function of fulfilling their nutritional requirement is thus taken over by their body wall called the "tegument" which is metabolically a highly active interface between the host and the parasite. Tapeworms absorb all nutrients in the form of carbohydrate, proteins, minerals and vitamins essential for their survival and reproduction, in the digested form, from the host intestinal contents. Subsequently, this leads to severe deficiency of these essential food nutrients in the host despite of good nutritional diet under normal conditions (Smyth, 1994).

Trematodes or flukes may infect digestive tract, liver, lungs and vascular system of animals. Accordingly, they are called as intestinal or stomach flukes, liver flukes, lung flukes and blood flukes. Unlike tapeworms, flukes possess well-developed digestive system. Besides, their body wall is also metabolically active and provides an important interface for molecular and immunological interactions. Therefore, the flukes draw nutrition from the host through their digestive system as undigested material and through their tegument as digested nutrients.

Nematodes are ubiquitous parasites of the animals and have spared no organ of the animal in which they can not be found. Nematodes possess a well-developed digestive system and their cuticular body covering is least permeable to molecules. With their adaptive oral structures, they may feed on ingested food, browse on tissues, suck or consume blood. According to the feeding habit, location and number of worm density the nematode cause various forms of nutritional impact on the infected host.

Arthropods constituting of insects, flies, ticks, mites and fleas are generally ectoparasites. Arthropods inflict animal health through annoyance, blood sucking, skin and tissue damage and most importantly by transmitting pathogens. All these factors associated with arthropod parasitism lead to poor animal health and production despite of balanced nutritional diets.

Nutrition Parasite Interactions

Influence of Nutrition

Protein and energy diet variations have been shown to be influenced by various parameters related to nutrition-parasite interactions. These have variously been dealt in, mostly in sheep followed by some in cattle under experimental controlled conditions. Animals fed on ideal balanced diet are able to mount an immune response that helps to recover from parasitic infections than those deficient in one or more nutrients. A balanced nutritional diet consists of adequate amounts of protein, energy, minerals, vitamins and water. Antibodies that fight invaded parasites are composed of protein. Energy is needed to drive the metabolic functions involved in mounting an immune response. Proper hydration is absolutely necessary for metabolic function. Several minerals and vitamins are directly involved in the immune response. While all are important, a few are more likely to be deficient in the diet than others. The minerals and vitamins most likely to be deficient and/or most likely to produce benefit by supplementation include phosphorus, copper, selenium, zinc, vitamins A and E. Phosphorus is an essential component in energy metabolism and is vital to cell wall integrity. Copper is needed for the formation of antibodies and white blood cells in addition to the production of antioxidant enzymes that protect cell membranes. Selenium is an antioxidant that works in conjunction with vitamin E to protect cell membranes. Zinc is essential for the maintenance of epithelial cells as well as the production of antioxidant enzymes. Vitamin A also has a role in maintenance of epithelial cells that help keep out invaders.

The extent of metabolic impairment in parasitic infection is largely determined by the level of infection and also by host factors such as age, breed, nutritional and immune status. An important factor in pathogenesis of parasitic gastroenteritis is a reduction in feed intake by the host compounded by protein losing gastroenteropathy (van Houtert and Sykes, 1996). Thus, parasitism increases the amino acid demand of gastrointestinal tissue. Peripheral tissues are consequently denied the nutrients required for optimal growth and production. Moreover, there is a direct competition between the immune system and other body tissues for amino acids. Normal animal performance in the face of parasitic infection is possible if the animal is maintained at a high plane of nutrition, especially protein supply (Coop and Kyriazakis, 1999). A simple observation that the animals maintained on a high plane of nutrition withstood ill effects of parasitism to a great extent led to exploration of nutritional management of parasitism in a series of research carried out during last two decades.

There are now convincing evidence that plant based condensed tannin increases the availability of protein in the small intestine of ruminants, and this indirectly improves host resistance and resilience against parasite challenge (Khan *et al.*, 2001) In an experiment, goats given diets containing cassava foliage, containing condensed tannin as well as higher level of protein, had faster growth and better feed conversion in comparison to goats fed grass alone. Interestingly, it was also noticed that the earlier group had lower EPG (egg per gram of faeces), reflecting less worm load than the second group (Sokerya and Preston, 2003). Some of the condensed tannins have antihelmintic properties. Excess protein supplementation has also been shown to reduce worm burden up to 50% in sheep infected with *Trichostrongylus colubriformis* (Bown *et al.*, 1991).

Role of mineral nutrients has also been highlighted in alleviating deleterious effects of gastrointestinal parasitism. The exact mechanism is still unknown. Phosphorus supplementation @ 2.75 rather than 1.88 g/kgDM reduced worm establishment by 90% in sheep (Coop and Field, 1983). Copper therapy using Cu-oxide wire particles (COWP) reduced establishment of *H. contortus* and *Ostertagia circumcincta* by 95% and 65%, respectively but had no effect on the establishment of *T. colubriformis* (Bang et al., 1990). There is also evidence that the outcome of larval challenge may be influenced by dietary molybdenum concentration. In one such study, molybdenum supplementation reduced worm population of *T. vitrinus* and *H. contortus* by 28% and 78%, respectively (Suttle *et al.*, 1992).

Nutritional Status of the Host and Parasitism

During the past several decades considerable research with increased interest has been directed towards investigations on the interactions between the nutritional status of the host and the parasite establishment, rejection, fecundity *vis-à-vis* mechanism of impaired productivity in ruminants. Most studies have been stimulated by the need to develop sustainable approaches to control nematode infections that are less reliant on frequent chemotherapeutic interventions (Barger, 1996, Coop and Holmes, 1996, Knox and Steel, 1996 and Coop and Kyriazakis, 1999).

It has been established that trickle or concurrent infections of gastro-intestinal nematode infections can impair live-weight gain, soft-tissue deposition, skeletal growth, milk and wool production (Sykes, 1984; Parkins and Holmes, 1989; Poppi *et al.*, 1990). It has been established that anorexia is one of the major factors contributing to the reduced performance of parasitized ruminants (Sykes *et al.*, 1988; Mehra *et al.*, 1999). The mechanisms of host dysfunction have shown a key feature to be the increased endogenous loss of protein in the GI-tract due to leakage of plasma protein and from increased exfoliation of gut epithelial cells and mucoprotein secretion. However, in abomasal infections the majority of the endogenous losses are reabsorbed, partly as non-protein nitrogen (Rowe *et al.*, 1988). This recycling of protein has an energy cost and it has been shown using pair-feeding studies that the gross efficiency of use of ME for energy deposition is decreased both by abomasal and intestinal infection (Sykes, 1983). Overall, there is a net movement of protein from productive processes such as meat, bone, milk and wool production into the synthesis of plasma proteins and repair of the gastro-intestinal tract and mucus secretion (Symons, 1985).

Reduction in voluntary feed intake as one of the major factors contributing to the reduced performance of parasitized ruminants is well established, although its mechanism is not fully known (Symons, 1985; Sykes *et al.* 1988). The hypotheses include, alteration in availability of amino acids, changes in flow rates and pH of digesta, alteration in gut peptides or hormones or direct neural effects on the central nervous system.

Studies in cattle experimentally infected with *Ostertagia ostertagi* have shown associations between anorexic condition, elevated blood gastrin concentrations and reduction in the rate of passage of digesta suggesting that the increase in gastrin reduce reticulorumen motility, inducing stasis of ingesta, thus leading to reduction in feed intake. Subsequently, endogenous blood gastrin levels got raised indirectly in worm-free calves by the administration of gastric acid secretion inhibitor, omeprazole, a marked reduction in feed intake was induced (Poppi *et al.*, 1990). The role of two factors was examined by Dynes *et al.* (1998) that may affect depression of feed intake by antagonizing various pathways and monitoring eating patterns. The addition of potent competitive antagonist of peripheral cholecystokinin (CKK) action had no effect on short-term intake suggesting that peripheral CKK is not directly involved in parasite-induced depression of appetite. When the satiety effect of the hypothalamus was blocked through diazepam receptor with benzodiazepine drug short-term feed intake increased significantly in both control and in *T. colubriformis*-infected sheep, suggesting that reduction of feed intake may involve control satiety signals. Although the gastrointestinal tract may be locally damaged there appears to be little effect on protein digestion and absorption *per se* and therefore it may be beneficial to provide additional protein at the duodenum. This could be achieved by increasing overall feed intake or by increasing the proportion of rumen undegradable protein in the diet.

The general consensus from these various studies is that protein intake does not appear to influence initial parasite establishment to naïve sheep, although the pathophysiological consequences are usually more severe in animals on lower planes of protein intake. Animals fed on reduced feed quality during dry season have been reported to support chronic haemonchosis. This observation has been repeated in other tropical areas where a fall in feed quality during the dry season is frequently associated with severe parasitism despite low or negligible larval intake.

Immunity, Parasitism and Nutrition

Host protein and energy nutrition can greatly influence the expression of immunity in cattle, sheep and goats (Bown *et al.*, 1991; Coop *et al.*, 1995), infected with a trickle dose of gastrointestinal nematodes. It was found that supplementation of a hay diet with 'protected' protein (50 or 100 g fish meal per day) affected the rate of worm expulsion after 10 weeks of trickle infection with *T. colubriformis* and that the apparent rate of expulsion was related to the level of supplementation (van Houtert *et al.*, 1995). It was found that no difference existed in the number of worms carried by sheep infected with *H. contortus*, but supplementation of a basal diet with soybean meal had significant effects on worm fecundity (Wallace *et al.*, 1995).

In the above example fishmeal supplementation resulted in an increase in the concentration of mast cell proteinases, and elevation in the levels of circulating eosinophils; however, these were not accompanied by changes in the levels of circulating specific and non-specific antibodies. It is likely that this reflects the minor role of peripheral serum antibodies in the immune response towards these gastrointestinal parasites.

There is evidence that host nutrition can affect the levels of circulating antibodies in bacterial or viral challenges (Sinclair and Reid, 1998). The question to consider is what nutrient(s) are expected to affect the degree of expression of immunity to parasites? Most research has concentrated on the effects of host protein nutrition on their resilience and resistance to gastrointestinal nematode infection. This seems reasonable, since many components of the effector arm of the immune system, such as immunoglobulins, muco-proteins and cellular products such as leukotrienes, are proteinaceous in nature and they would be expected to draw on protein resources especially in quantitative terms i.e., specific amino acids (Lewis and Austen, 1981; Coop and Holmes, 1996). In most instances protein has been dealt within its generic sense, although it is most likely that the requirements of the immune system are higher for some specific amino acids than others (MacRae, 1993). More recent investigations are now considering both protein quantity and quality when addressing its interactions with parasitism.

Significantly less emphasis has been given to the effects of micronutrients such as minerals and vitamins on parasitism, although it is known that the immune system has specific requirements for certain micronutrients such as zinc (Bundy and Golden, 1987; Chandra, 1993). An exception is the investigation, which suggests that an increase in phosphorus supply (from 1.88 to 2.75 g kg-1 DM) decreases mean worm burdens (from 11 000 to 1300) in sheep infected with a trickle dose of *T. vitrinus* over 14 weeks (Coop and Field, 1983). These relationships need further investigation, since the effect of phosphorus supplementation will be influenced by the degree of hypertrophy induced in the small intestine, which results in impaired absorption of P in parasitised animals (Poppi *et al.*, 1990). Trace elements like copper (Bang *et al.*, 1990), molybdenum (Suttle *et al.*, 1992) and selenium (McDonald *et al.*, 1989) can influence host resistance to nematode infection. They may have a direct anthelmintic effect as well as influencing host metabolism and therefore the levels of supplementation and the host's mineral status important. It was demonstrated that administration of copper oxide wire particles to young lambs reduced the establishment of the abomasal nematodes *H. contortus* and *O. circumcincta* (Bang *et al.*, 1990). In contrast, there was no evidence of an increase in worm burdens in lambs, which were hypocupraemic (Hucker and Yong, 1986).

It can be concluded from the above discussion, that there is strong support for the idea that host nutrition can affect the degree of host immunity to parasite infection. Our understanding will improve by investigations that investigate, which effectors of the immune response are affected by host nutrition, and by considering quantitatively the role of specific nutrients in this interaction.

References

Bang, K.S., Familton, A.S. and Sykes, A.R. (1990). *Res. Vet. Sci.*, 49: 132-137.

Barger, I.A. (1996). *Int. J. Parasitol.*, 26: 1001-1007.

Bown, M.D., Poppi, D.P. and Sykes, A.R. (1991). *Amer. J. Agric.*, 42: 253-267.

Bundy, D.A.P. and Golden, M.H.N. (1987). *Parasitology*, 98: 623-635.

Chandra, R.K. (1993). Nutrition and the immune system. *Proc. Nurt. Soc.*, 52: 77-84.

Coop, R.L. and Field, A.C. (1983). *Res. Vet. Sci.*, 35: 175-181.

Coop, R.L. and Holmes, P.H. (1996). *Int. J. Parasitol.*, 26: 951-962.

Coop, R.L. and Kyriazakis, I. (1999). *Vet. Parasitol.*, 84: 187-204.

Coop, R.L., Huntley, J.F. and Smith, W.D. (1995). *Res. Vet. Sci.*, 59: 24-29.

Dynes, R.A., Poppi, D.P., Barrell, G.K. and Sykes, A.R. (1998). *Br. J. Nutr.*, 79: 47-54.

Hucker, D.A. and Yong, W.K. (1986). *Vet. Parasitol.*, 19: 67-76.

Khan, L.P., Knox, M.R., Walkden-Brown, S.W. and Lea, J.M. (2001). *Recent Advances in Asian Nutrion in Australia*, 13: 87-95.

Knox, M. and Steel, J.W. (1996). *Int. J. Parasitol.*, 26: 963-970.

Lewis, R.A. and Austen, K.F. (1981). *Nature*, 293: 103-108.

MacRae, J.C. (1993). *Proc. Nutr. Soc.*, 52: 121-130.

McDonald, J.W., Overend, D.J. and Paynter, D.I. (1989). *Res. Vet. Sci.*, 47: 319-322.

Mehra, U.R., Verma, A.K. Dass, R.S., Sharma, R.L. and Yadav, S.C. (1999). *Vet. Record.*, 145: 699-702.

Parkins, J.J. and Holmes, P.H. (1989). *Nutr. Res. Rev.*, 2: 227-246.

Poppi, D.P., Sykes, A.R. and Dynes, R.A. (1990). *Proc. New Zealand Soc. Anim. Prod.*, 50: 237-243.

Rowe, J.B., Nolan, J.V., de Chaneet, G., Teleni, E. and Holmes, P.H. (1988). *Br. J. Nutr.*, 59: 125-139.

Scrimshaw, N.S., Taylor, E.E. and Gordon, J.E. (1968). *Interactions of Nutrition and Infection.* WHO Monograph 57, pp 329, Geneva : World Health Organization.

Sinclair, M.C. and Reid, H.W. (1998). *Proc. Int. Symp. on* : Metabolic Stress in Dairy Cows. *Br. Soc. Anim. Sci.* Edinburgh, 11 pp.

Smyth, J.D. (1994). Animal Parasitology, Cambrridge University Press, Cambridge, Pp.549

Sokerya, S. and Preston, T.R. (2003). *Livestock Res. Rural Devel.*, 15: 1-14.

Suttle, N.F., Knox, D.P., Jackson, F., Coop, R.L. and Angus, K.W. (1992). *Res. Vet. Sci.*, 52: 230-235.

Sykes, A.R. (1983). Effects of parasitosm on metabolism in the sheep. In: Haresign, W. (Ed.), The Sheep Production. Nottingham Easter School of Agricultural Science, No. 35. Butterworths, London, pp. 317-334.

Sykes, A.R. (1984). *Anim. Prod.*, 59: 155-172.

Sykes, A.R., Poppi, D.P. and Elliot, D.C. (1988). *J. Agric. Sci. Camb.* 110: 531-541.

Symons, L.E.A. (1985). *Adv. Parasitol.*, 24: 103-133.

van Houtert, M.F.J. and Sykes, A.R. (1996). *Int. J. Parasitol.*, 26: 1151-1167.

van Houtert, M.F.J., Barger, I.A., Steel, J.W., Windon, R.G. and Emery, D.L. (1995). *Vet. Parasitol.*, 56: 163-180.

Wallace, D.S., Bairden, K., Duncan, J.L., Fishwick, G., Gill, E.M., Holmes, P.H., McKellar, Q.A., Murray, M., Parkins, J.J. and Stear, M.J. (1995). *Res. Vet. Sci.*, 58: 232-237.

□□□

Animal Nutrition, 2012
eds. Dr. (Mrs.) Usha R. Mehra et al., pp. 651-661
Satish Serial Publishing House e-mail : info@satishserial.com; website : www.satishserial.com

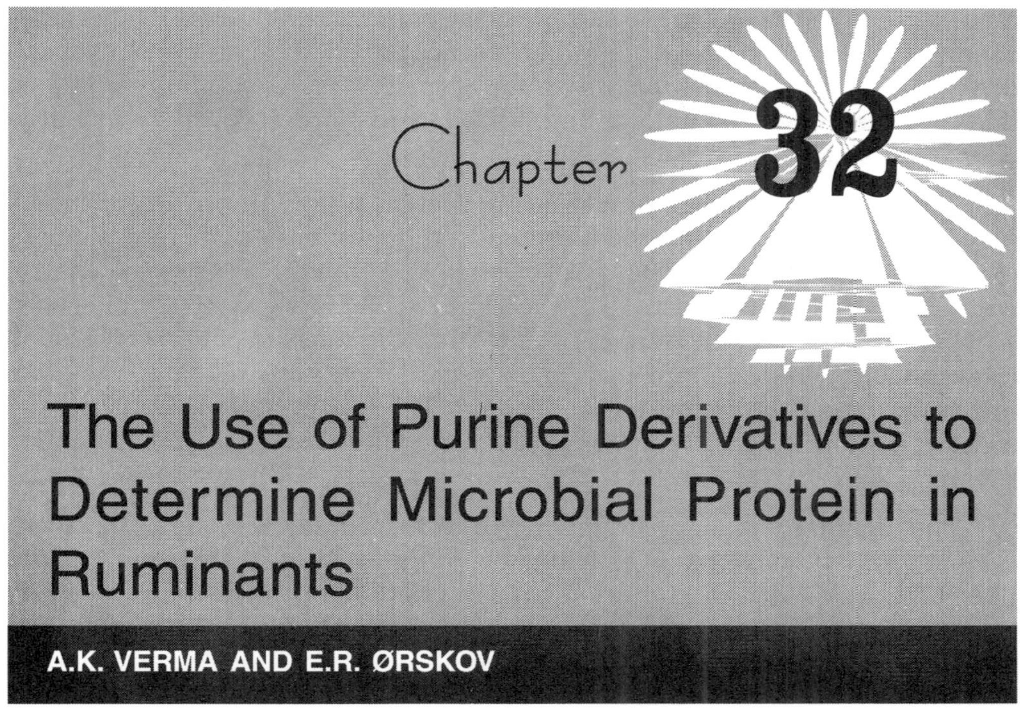

Chapter 32

The Use of Purine Derivatives to Determine Microbial Protein in Ruminants

A.K. VERMA AND E.R. ØRSKOV

Purines are heterocyclic ring structures (nitrogenous bases) with varying functional groups. The purine bases, adenine and guanine, are found in DNA and RNA. Rumen microorganisms have high concentrations of purine containing compounds relative to their concentrations in plants and mammalian cells. Of the total nitrogen present in rumen bacteria, nucleic acids and proteins comprise 13-19% and 75-85%, respectively. The term purine derivatives refer to the sum of allantoin, uric acid, xanthine and hypoxanthine. These are the end products of purine metabolism. All the four compounds are excreted in the urine of sheep, goats, llamas, red deer and camels; but xanthine and hypoxanthine are virtually absent from the urine of cattle, buffaloes and yaks. As the rumen microbes are rich in purines, the amount of purine derivatives in urine can be used as a tool for estimating microbial protein supply to the ruminants.

It is well known fact that microbial protein is by far the largest protein source for ruminant animals. It is also well known that it is not constant but by far the most important parameter is the energy generated from carbohydrate in the anaerobic system in the rumen (see Ørskov 1992). But of course N mainly in the form of ammonia is needed and may in some instances be the limiting factor in which case the animal often responds by less feed intake as feed degradation and digestibility is reduced and rumen retention time increased.

Due to the importance of measuring protein supply in ruminants which may have little relation to protein in the feed due to protein degradability of the feed and more related to energy supply for microbial growth, a lot of work has been carried out as described in detail by Ørskov (1992). The same author also described the dynamic of protein from the feed entering the small intestine which require information on degradation rate and flow rate often measured using the nylon bag technique. The use of abomasal fistulae to measure protein flow is of course not practical for large scale protein evaluation (Ørskov, 2001).

The possibility of using excretion products from nucleic acids, the purine derivatives (PD) was first investigated by Topps & Elliot (1965) using the idea that there was much more nucleic acid in microbial protein than in dietary protein. They also showed that when an intake increased PD excretion increased. The problem was that they could not determine the endogenous excretion as PD is also formed in the turnover of protein from the animal body. As a result there was not much more research done until the development of the intragastric nutrition technique developed by Ørskov *et al.* (1979) when it became possible to feed ruminants on volatile fatty acids by infusion and maintain normal conditions but with no microbial protein produced. It was then possible to get information on aspects of endogenous PD excretion first initiated by Fujihara *et al.* (1987).

Brief Background of Purine Metabolism in Ruminants

Microbial nucleic acids leaving the rumen undergo extensive digestion in the small intestine. No apparent digestion occurs in the abomasum. In the small intestine, purine nucleotides are hydrolyzed into purine nucleoside and free bases. Both forms can be absorbed from the intestine. There have been very few studies on measuring the digestibility of microbial purines. However, it can be regarded as being the same as the digestibility of nucleic acids since purine nucleoside and free bases can be readily absorbed. The digestibility of microbial nucleic acids is about 85%. Purine nucleosides and free bases absorbed from the intestinal lumen are subjected to degradation as well as utilization in the intestinal mucosa. This is where sheep and cattle differ from each other. In cattle, there is a very high activity of xanthine oxidase in the intestinal mucosa, which can convert practically all the absorbed purines into uric acid. The result is that the absorbed purines enter the liver as uric acid and therefore are not available to be incorporated into tissue nucleic acids. In sheep, the activity of xanthine oxidase is negligible and therefore, absorbed purines can enter the liver unchanged and are available for incorporation into the tissue nucleic acids (this process is usually called salvage).

Both the salvage and degradation enzymes are very active and there could be competition for the substrates between salvage and degradation pathways. The result is that, those absorbed purines that have not been incorporated in the tissue nucleic acids are completely converted into their metabolic end products, hypoxanthine, uric acid and allantoin. The PD entering the blood can also be from the degradation of tissue nucleic acids. This fraction is called "endogenous PD". Measurement of the magnitude of endogenous excretion has been made with the aid of the technique of intragastric infusion, or the technique of replacement of digesta entering the small intestine. The endogenous excretion of PD is three times higher in cattle than in sheep per kg of metabolic weight (150 and 530 μmol/kg $W^{0.75}$ per day for sheep and cattle respectively). Cross species comparison is also interesting. Sheep, goats, pigs and humans are very similar in the magnitude of endogenous excretion expressed on basis of metabolic weight. The difference in tissue distribution of xanthine oxidase may be the reason for these species differences. Cattle have high xanthine oxidase activities in most tissues including the blood, whereas sheep have low xanthine oxidase activities in most tissues and none in the blood. The high xanthine oxidase activity will divert more purines released from the tissue nucleic acid degradation away from the salvage pathway into the degradation pathway.

When using the daily excretion of PD to calculate the amount of exogenous purine absorbed by the animal, we need to correct for the contribution from the PD of endogenous origin. In sheep, when we take into account the amount of exogenous purines utilized by the animal, the net endogenous contribution (i.e. the endogenous loss minus exogenous purines utilized) is reduced. Therefore, as the amount of exogenous microbials available to the animal increases, the net endogenous contribution decreases to practically zero. The response curve of PD excretion vs purine absorbed is not linear as shown in the work of Chen *et al.* (1990) and Balcells *et al.* (1992). In cattle, since the exogenous purines are not available for utilization by the animal, the purine loss must be replaced by *de novo* synthesis from amino acids. As a result, there is always a net endogenous contribution to the total excretion in urine. The response curve of PD excretion vs purine absorbed is linear. It is now clear that we need to use different equations for sheep and cattle to calculate the purine absorption from the daily excretion of PD. Two equations were proposed by Chen *et al.* (1990). The studies of Balcells *et al.* (1992) also derived a similar equation for sheep and confirmed the general model for cattle. PD both from endogenous and exogenous sources entering the blood are cleared rapidly. The clearance rate constant is about 30%/hr. Urinary excretion is the primary route for the disposal of these purine end products. In sheep and cattle, uric acid and allantoin, once filtered in the glomerullus, are quantitatively excreted in the urine. There is very little secretion and reabsorption of these compounds in the nephric tubes. Thus the urinary excretion of PD is a function of the plasma concentration and the glomerular filtration rate (GFR). It should be noted that allantoin, uric acid, xanthine and hypoxanthine are all present in sheep urine but only allantoin and uric acid in cattle urine. This may be because in cattle the high activity of xanthine oxidase in the blood and tissues (also kidney) converts xanthine and hypoxanthine into uric acid prior to excretion in the urine.

The ability to determine microbial protein from PD in the urine became great international interest and was taken up by International Atomic Energy Agency Nutrition Group, which has been discussed in detail by Makkar (2004). Trials were conducted with different types of animals in different countries including Spain, Malaysia, Indonesia, Vietnam, Sri Lanka, China Venezuela and Turkey Here it became obvious that buffaloes in particular Pimpa *et al.* (2002) and Yak cattle Long *et al.* (1999) had much lower than predicted PD excretion in comparison to other cattle. Even at fasting the buffaloes showed much lower PD excretion which might indicate lower endogenous excretion but this has now been shown not to be the case. Thanh and Ørskov (2006) fed buffalo calves and cattle calves on milk with no access to solid food i.e. no rumen development and thus no microbial protein produced. When they were compared, there were no differences between cattle calves and buffalo calves in PD excretion but when they were fed on solid food for 2 months which stimulated rumen development the buffalo calves had a PD excretion of about 1/3 of cattle calves. This of course means that the same equation for calculating microbial protein production cannot be used for both species. The more purines are recycled into the rumen in buffaloes than cattle, might be owing to the permeability from blood to rumen or the purines staying in the blood for longer time *i.e.* differences in GFR. Recent work by Thanh and Ørskov (2008) has shown clearly that GFR was considerably lower in buffaloes than cattle showing a higher probability of recycling to the rumen in buffaloes compared to cattle. Whether there are also differences in permeability from blood to rumen is not known. Buffaloes or mature buffaloes also show much lower fasting PD excretion as part of the endogenous PD is recycled to the rumen and destroyed. In other words fasting PD excretion cannot be used to determine endogenous PD production.

Modeling Approach for the Estimation of Rumen Microbial Protein Production

The technique has been developed and used to estimate microbial protein supply in cattle, sheep, buffaloes and goats. Species differences in purine metabolism are attributed to the level of endogenous excretion, the utilization ability of exogenous purines and enzyme profiles which are involved in purine degradation. Chen *et al.* (1990) proposed a general mechanistic model to depict the quantitative relationship between the amount of purine absorbed (X, mmol/d) and the purine derivatives excreted (Y, mmol/d). This model can be applied to sheep, goat, cattle and other species (Fig. 1).

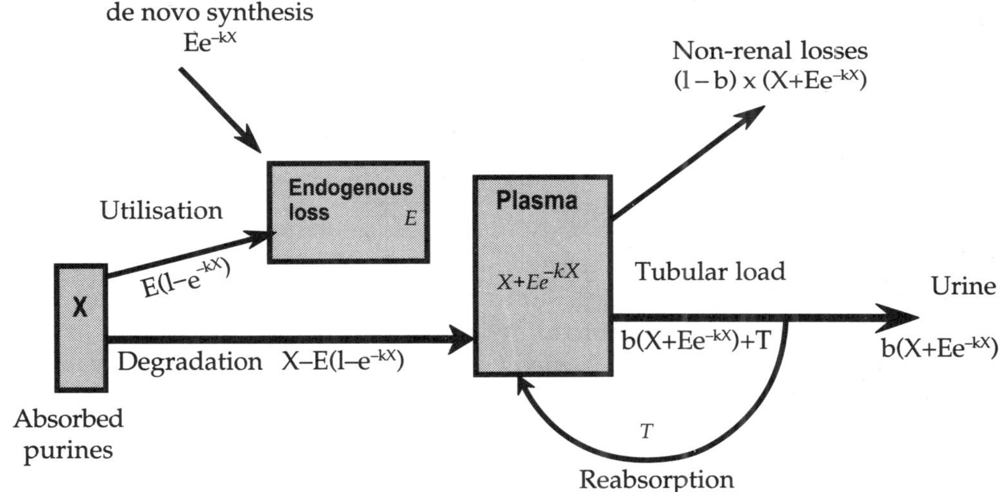

Fig. 1 : A model which describes the quantitative relationship between purine absorption and excretion of purine derivatives in urine (Chen and Ørskov, 2003).

The endogenous production of purine derivatives is denoted as "E" in the diagram. The animal will need to replace the endogenous purine loss by either *de novo* synthesis (creating purines from amino acids) or salvaging preformed purines if available. When no exogenous purines are available, the loss has to be replaced all by *de novo* synthesis. However, when exogenous supply is increased, there is evidence in the literature to show that *de novo* synthesis is reduced and even turned off. For simplicity, the amount of *de novo* synthesis is described in this model as Ee^{-kX}, where X is the exogenous purine supply. Accordingly, the amount of exogenous purines utilized is E $(1-e^{-kX})$, the rest is converted into purine derivatives and enters the plasma. The amount of purine derivatives entering the plasma is $X+ Ee^{-kX}$. This model also assumes a constant partitioning between the renal excretion and non-renal route of disposal. The factor "b" represents the proportion of plasma purine derivatives to be disposed of by renal excretion, thus urinary excretion of purine derivatives: $Y=bX+bEe^{-kX}$, Y is curvilinearly related to X and this model is applicable for small ruminants. When exogenous purine input is zero (X=0), bE becomes the measured endogenous excretion, a constant per $kgW^{0.75}$.

When the model is applied to cattle in which exogenous purine is not available for utilization ($e^{-kX}=1$), the equation becomes Y=bX+bE. Y is linearly related to X. Again, when X=0, bE becomes the measured endogenous excretion. The xanthine oxidase activity in the intestinal mucosa may provide an indication as to whether a linear or curvilinear response would be expected.

PDC Index

Analysis of spot urine samples for purine derivatives and creatinine, and linking the information to feed intake, makes possible to study the nutritional adequacy in ruminant livestock under field conditions. In the absence of total urine collection, Purine dervatives:Creatinine ratio may provide an index to detect differences in excretion of purine derivatives assuming that creatinine excretion depends only on the body mass and is constantly excreted through out the day. The ratio of Purine derivatives:Creatinine (mmol:mmol) concentrations in hourly urine samples (referred to as spot urine) when corrected for metabolic weight to allow comparison between animals is called PDC index (Chen *et al.*, 2003). However, data of the direct (purine derivatives)/(creatinine) ratio can only be compared within the same animal or among animals of the same body weight, since the daily creatinine excretion is a function of body weight.

PDC index = (Purine derivatives)/(Creatinine) x $W^{0.75}$

Where, W is the body weight (kg), (Purine derivatives) and (Creatinine) are their concentrations in urine, in mmol/L. Data of PDC index can be compared among animals of different body weights (but the same breed). By definition, the PDC index and urinary excretion of purine derivatives has a following linear relationship:

Purine derivative excretion = PDC index x C, where, C is the daily creatinine excretion (mmol/kg $W^{0.75}$) for a specific breed of animals, and should have been previously measured using complete urine collection. From this equation, total daily excretion of purine derivatives can be calculated from the PDC index, yet without the need for total urine collection.

Purine Nitrogen Index

During microbial fermentation, part of the dietary nitrogen is converted to ammonia, a proportion of which is captured by rumen microorganisms for the synthesis of microbial protein. The remaining ammonia is absorbed from the rumen and is finally excreted, as a source of nitrogen, in the urine. Purine Nitrogen Index refers to the ratio of purine derivative nitrogen to total nitrogen in urine (Chen *et al.* 1999). This has been proposed as an index of the utilization of nitrogen in the rumen compared to the amount wasted in the urine. If a diet or a dietary regime has poor conversion efficiency, proportionally less dietary nitrogen is converted to microbial protein and more excreted in the urine resulting in a low purine nitrogen index. Endogenous nitrogen output, nitrogen intake, protein degradability, digestibility of protein and inefficiency of absorbed amino acids can all affect the value of purine nitrogen index. Purine nitrogen index could be used as one of the criteria to help and formulate ruminant diets that are biologically more efficient and produce less nitrogen waste. A practical application would be to set an empirical threshold criterion for a specific group of ruminants, and diets with purine nitrogen index values lower than this threshold are graded as unsatisfactory with respect to nitrogen utilization. Even though purine nitrogen index can be used as a tool for rapid feed evaluation in ruminants it has certain limitations. The index does not offer any explanation to the cause of poor efficiency and it is not sensitive for detecting small differences. However the latter limitation could be overcome by using it in a 'grouping' system.

Calculation of microbial protein supply from PD excretion

Method of Calculation

The method to estimate the intestinal flow microbial N from PD excretion was summarized by Chen and Makkar (1993).

Step 1 : the absorption of purines (X mmol/d) is estimated from the PD excretion in the urine (Y, mmol/d) based on a previously established equation, for example, the equations below for sheep and cattle respectively.

For sheep: $Y = 0.84X + (0.150\ W^{0.75}\ e^{-0.25X})$

The calculation of X based on the above non-linear equation can be performed by means of the Newton Raphson iteration process, as shown below:

$$X_{n+1} = X_n - \frac{f(X_n)}{f'(X_n)}$$

Where, $f(X) = 0.84\ X + 0.150\ W^{0.75}\ e^{-0.25X} - Y$ and the derivative of f(X): $f'(X) = 0.84 - 0.038\ W^{0.75}\ e^{-0.25X}$

Given an initial value of $X_1 = Y \div 0.84$ to feed into the above equation to calculate X_2, and so on after 4 iterations, X_5 should have reached a constant value.

For European cattle $Y = 0.85X + (0.385\ W^{0.75})$
Thus, $X = (Y - 0.385 \times W^{0.75}) \div 0.85$

For Zebu cattle $Y = 0.85X + (0.147\ W^{0.75})$
Thus, $X = (Y - 0.147 \times W^{0.75}) \div 0.85$

For other animals, more specific equation for the target animal should be used. In the authors' experience, when the equation developed for European cattle was used for cattle in tropical countries, lower values of microbial N estimate were obtained. This was probably because the endogenous excretion of those animals was lower than the value (0.385 mmol/kg $W^{0.75}$/d) used for European cattle. The equation recently acquired for Zebu cattle may be more suitable.

For lactating cows, the output of PD in the milk can be added to the urinary PD excretion so as to improve the accuracy. Since the PD concentration in milk was rather constant (see discussion later), the milk output of PD can simply be calculated as milk yield times an average concentration previously measured.

Step 2 : Microbial N yield, i.e. the intestinal flow of microbial N, is then calculated using:

$$\text{Microbial N (gN/D)} = \frac{X(\text{mmol/d}) \times 70}{0.116 \times 0.83 \times 1000} = 0.727X$$

The factors used in equation are:

Digestibility of microbial purines is assumed to be 0.83. This is taken as the mean digestibility value for microbial nucleic acids based on observations reported in the literature.

(i) The N content of purines is 70 mg N/mmol.

(ii) The ratio of purine-N: total-N in mixed rumen microbes was measured as 11.6:100 [85].

It should be stated that the ratio of purine-N:total-N may need to be redefined for different feeding regimes or for different animal species, in order to improve accuracy of the calculation. See also http://www-naweb.iaea.org/nafa/aph/purine-cd/html/about/index.html

Calculation of other target parameters

Purine Derivatives in Urine (Cattle & Buffaloes)

PD (mmol/d) = Allantoin (mmol/d) + Uric acid (mmol/d)

Purine Derivatives in Plasma (Cattle & Buffaloes)

PD (mmol/L) = Allantoin (mmol/L) + Uric acid (mmol/L)

Purine Derivatives in Urine (Sheep & Goats)

PD (mmol/d) = Allantoin (mmol/d) + Uric acid (mmol/d) + Xanthine (mmol/d) + Hypo-xanthine (mmol/d)

Purine Derivatives in Plasma (Sheep & Goats)

PD (mmol/L) = Allantoin (mmol/L) + Uric acid (mmol/L) + Xanthine (mmol/L) + Hypo-xanthine (mmol/L)

Purine derivatives:Creatinine (PDC index)

PDC index = [PD] / [Creatinine] x $W^{0.75}$

Where, $W^{0.75}$ represents the metabolic body weight (kg) of the animal. [PD] and [Creatinine] were PD and creatinine concentration in mmol/L in urine.

Purine nitrogen index (PNI)

PNI = Total PD excreted in urine (mmol / d) X 0.056 / Nitrogen excreted in urine (g/d)

Glomerular filtration rate (GFR)

GFR (L/d) = Creatinine excretion in urine (mmol/d) /plasma creatinine concentration (mmol/L)

Renal clearance of purine derivatives

Tubular load of allantoin (mmol/d) = GFR (L/d) x plasma allantoin concentration (mmol/L)

Net re-absorption of allantoin (mmol/d) = Tubular load (mmol/d)-excretion in urine (mmol/d) tubular load of uric acid (mmol/d) = GFR (L/d) x plasma uric acid concentration (mmol/d)

Net re-absorption of uric acid (mmol/d) = Tubular load (mmol/d)-excretion in urine (mmol/d)

Practical Use of PD for Measurement of Microbial Protein

One practical problem with the PD method for determining microbial protein is the necessity for total urine collection and therefore the possibility was assessed with use of creatinine as internal marker. This of course reduces the accuracy as createnine excretion does vary between animals. Spot sampling worked almost as well when the animals were fed in one meal or several meals per day. See also review by Tas and Susenbeth (2007) for details about spot sampling. Another possibility was the use of plasma PD concentration however the rapid renal clearance makes this extremely inaccurate and of little practical value. It has been shown that a higher feeding level will tend to increase net microbial protein production per unit fermented as recorded by

PD excretion, presumably due to lower maintenance for microbes as rumen retention time is increased Chen and Ørskov (2004).

There is still more work needed to determine the practical use of PD. For example since the microbial protein production is influenced by food intake the purine to creatinine ratio in spot urine samples might also be used as a method to predict intake at pasture. More work is required to compare different types of cattle e.g. *Bos indicus* and *Bos taurus* with particular emphasis on determination of GFR.

Acknowledgement

The authors wish to acknowledge the contribution of Dr. X. B. Chen as a large part of the review was based on his earlier work and writing.

References

Balcells, J., Guada, J.A., Castrillo, C. and Gasa, J. (1991). J. Agric. Sci. Camb., 116:309-317.

Chen, X. B., Jayasuriya, M.C.N. and Makkar, H.P.S. (2003). Measurement and application of PD:Creatinine ratio in spot urine samples of ruminants. Development, standardization and validation of nuclear-based technologies for estimating microbial protein supply in ruminant livestock for improving productivity. (H. P. S. Makkar Ed.) IAEA-2003, Vienna.

Chen, X.B. and Orskov, E.R. (2003). Research on urinary excretion of purine derivatives in ruminants : past and future. Development, standardization and validation of nuclear-based technologies for estimating microbial protein supply in ruminant livestock for improving productivity. (H. P. S. Makkar Ed.) IAEA-2003, Vienna.

Chen, X. B., Orskov, E. R. and Hovell F.D. DeB. (1990). *British. J. Nutr.*, 63: 121-129.

Chen, X. B., Hovell, F. D. Deb., Ørskov, E. R. and Brown, D. S. (1990). *Brit J. Nutr.*, 63: 131-142.

Chen, X. B. and Makkar, H.P.S. (1993). Training package. The technique for the estimation of microbial N supply in ruminants from purine derivatives in the urine. Joint FAO/IAEA Division, Rome.

Chen, X. B., Subba, D. B., Orskov, E. R. and Jayasuriya, M. C. N. (1999). IAEA- TECDOC-1093, 97. IAEA Publication, Vienna.

Chen, X.B. and Ørskov, E.R. 2004. Research on urinary excretion of purine derivatives in ruminants past present and future. In: Estimation of microbial protein supply in ruminants using purine derivatives (Eds. H.P.Ș. Makkar and X.B. Chen) FAO/IAEA. Kluwer Academic Publishers, London. pp. 180-210.

Fujihara, T., Ørskov, E. R. and Reeds, P. J. 1987. *J. Agric. Sci. Camb.*, 109:7-12.

Long, R. J. 1999. *J. Agric. Sci. Camb.*, 133: 427-431.

Makkar, H. P. S. 2004. Development, standardisation and validation of nuclear based technologies for estimating microbial protein supply in ruminant livestock for improving productivity. In: Estimation of microbial protein supply in ruminants using purine derivatives (Eds. H.P.S. Makkar and X.B. Chen) FAO/IAEA. Kluwer Academic Publishers, London. pp. 2-13.

Ørskov, E.R. 1992. *Protein Nutrition in Ruminants.* Academic press Ltd ISBN 0-12-528481-2

Ørskov, E.R. 2001. *Trails and Trials in Livestock Research.* Gadjah Mada University Press, Yogyakarta, Indonesia.

Ørskov, E.R., Grubb, D.A., Wenham, G. and Corrigall, W. 1979. *Brit. J. Nutr.,* 41:553-558.

Pimpa, O., Liang, J. B., Balcells, J., Jelan, Z. A. and Abdullah, N. 2002. *Anim. Feed Sci. Technol.,* 104: 191-199.

Thanh, V.T.K. and Ørskov E. R. 2006. *Anim. Sci.,* 82:355-358.

Thanh, V.T.K., Ørskov, E. R. Thanh, N. T. and Susmel, P., 2008. Personnel communication.

Tas, B.M. and Susenbeth, A. 2007. *Livestock Science,* 111: 181-192.

Topps, J.H. and Elliot, R.C. 1965. *Nature,* 2005: 498-499.

□□□

Animal Nutrition, 2012
eds. Dr. (Mrs.) Usha R. Mehra et al., pp. 663-689
Satish Serial Publishing House e-mail : info@satishserial.com; website : www.satishserial.com

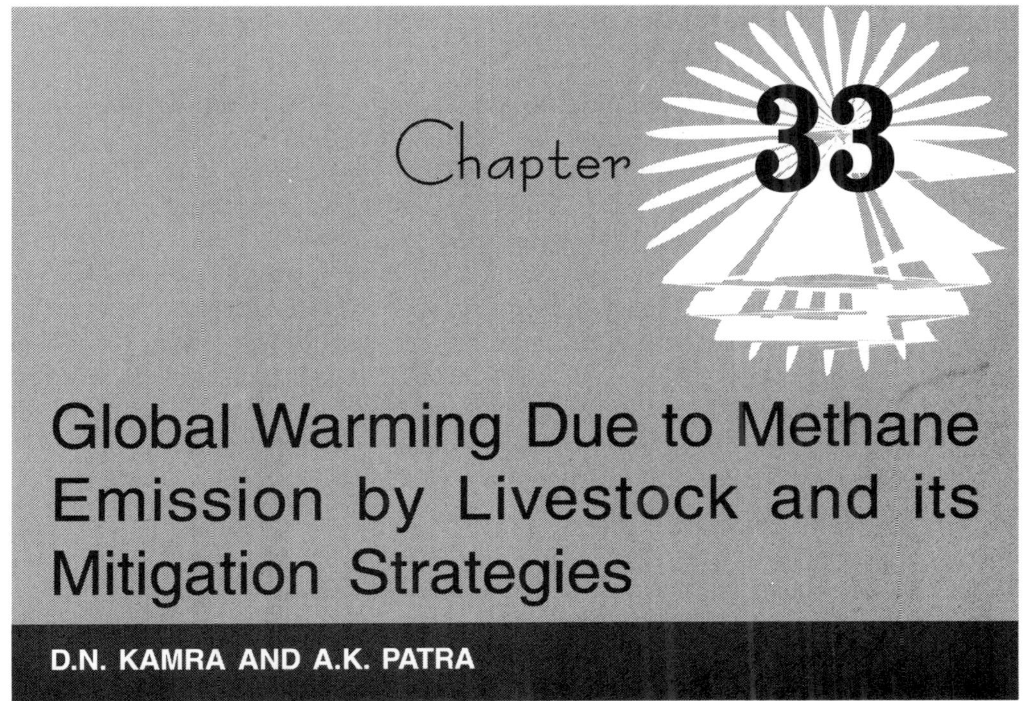

Chapter 33

Global Warming Due to Methane Emission by Livestock and its Mitigation Strategies

D.N. KAMRA AND A.K. PATRA

Global warming is the average increase in temperature of Earth's surface (land and oceans). Global surface temperature increased by 0.74 ± 0.18°C (1.33 ± 0.32°F) from 1906-2005 as per estimates of the Intergovernmental Panel on Climate Change (IPCC), which has been primarily attributed to the anthropogenic greenhouse gas emissions. These facts have also been endorsed by several other scientific/academic bodies through out the globe. A similar increase in the next century (upto 2100) might be as high as 1.1-6.4°C (2-11.5°F). Such a wide variation in the predictions might be due to a large number of uncertainties like different models used for these predictions, volumes of green house gases to be released into the atmosphere, corrective measures to be taken to combat these emissions due to anthropogenic and natural activities *etc.*

As a result of increase in atmospheric temperature and melting of ice on the mountains, the average rise in sea level during the last century has been 1.8 mm per year and during last 10 years, it has been as high as 3.1 mm/year and it is expected to be much higher in the coming years (480 mm in the next century). In addition to that thermal expansion of water also contributes towards this rise in sea level.

Intergovernmental Panel on Climate Change (IPCC) included six gases under the head "greenhouse gases" i.e. carbon dioxide (CO_2), methane (CH_4), nitrous oxide (N_2O), hydrofluorocarbons (HFCs), perfluorocarbons (PFCs) and sulphur hexafluoride (SF_6) (Table 1, IPCC, 1996). The first three are present in the atmosphere and are also produced as a result of agricultural and livestock activities of the human beings. The Global Warming Potential (GWP) of these gases in comparison to carbon dioxide is several times higher like methane and nitrous oxide have 23 and 296 times higher potential for global warming, respectively (IPCC, 2001). Therefore it is essential that their levels in the atmosphere are kept within safe levels. During the last two centuries the levels of two important green house gases like methane and nitrous oxide have risen by 115% and 15%, respectively (IPCC, 1996) which is not a good indication for the environment.

Table 1 : Green house effect gases and their source of production

Gas	GWP*	Source
Agricultural activities		
Carbondioxide	1	Combustion of fossil fuels
Methane	23	Enteric and waste fermentation, emissions from natural gas and oil fields
Nitrous oxide	296	Agricultural and industrial activities
Industrial activities		
Hydrofluorocarbons	12,000	Refrigeration and air conditioning
Perfluorocarbons	2,290	By-product of smelting process
Sulphur hexafluoride	22,200	Insulant in electrical switchgear and transformers

*Global warming potential (IPCC, 2001)

Methanogenesis in the Rumen

In the digestion of feed by the microbes in the rumen, the cofactors like NAD and NADP get reduced to NADH and NADPH and the sugars are partially oxidized to volatile fatty acids. To continue the fermentation, the reduced cofactors get oxidized by transferring hydrogen to carbondioxide (also generated during fermentation of carbohydrates in the rumen) and resulting in the formation of methane. This conversion of carbondioxide and hydrogen to methane is accomplished by methanogenic archaea, a group of microorganisms that is widely distributed in nature and is also responsible for methane synthesis in manure, effluent ponds and soil. Although over 66 species of archaea have been isolated from a range of anaerobic habitats, only a few have been isolated from the rumen (McAllister *et al.*, 1996). *Methanobrevibacter* and *Methanomicrobium* have been found in large numbers in the rumen and small numbers of *Methanosarcina* are also present (Jarvis *et al.*, 2000). However, non-culture methods based on 16S rRNA indicate that there is a far greater diversity of methanogenic archaea in the rumen than has presently been recognized (Whiteford *et al.*, 2001).

If the hydrogen generated during fermentation is not removed from the rumen eco-system, it might inhibit fermentation of feed due to non availability of oxidized cofactors. Thus to continue fermentation in the rumen, hydrogen has to be utilized and methanogenesis is one such process which acts as a hydrogen sink. During this process of methanogenesis, 5-15% of gross energy consumed by the animals is wasted. Therefore inhibition of methane emission by the animals is essential to improve efficiency of feed utilization and protecting the environment from its green house effect.

Methods of Methane Mitigation

Dietary Manipulation

The chemical composition of diet is an important factor which affects rumen fermentation and methane emission by the animals. An experiment in author's laboratory indicated that energy level in diet and the type of roughage used (wheat straw, paddy straw or sugarcane bagasse) affects the extent of methanogenesis significantly while the level of protein was not very important, if it meets the minimum requirement of the animals (Chaterjee *et al.*, 2006). Sugarcane bagasee caused the highest synthesis of methane per unit of digested dry matter and wheat straw the minimum, while methane generation was intermediate with paddy straw as roughage source. Sugarcane bagasse and paddy straw produced 11% and 4% more methane as compared to that on wheat straw.

Methane production was significantly lower in the sheep fed on green sorghum and wheat straw in the ratio of 90:10 as compared to where the ratio was 60:40 (31.5 *vs* 46.9 l/kg DMI). The dry matter intake was similar in both the groups, whereas, dry matter, organic matter, crude protein and nitrogen free extract digestibilities were significantly higher in the former group (Haque *et al.*, 2001). In another experiment three isonitrogenous diets containing mustard cake, sunflower cake and soyabean cake were fed to Murrah buffaloes and it showed that significantly higher methane was emitted (l/d) in soyabean cake group but there was no difference in methane energy loss as percentage of GE and DE. The difference might be due to higher feed intake in the third group where nitrogen source was soyabean cake (Saraswat *et al.*, 2001).

Improvement in the digestibility of lignocellulosic feeds with different treatments also resulted in lower methanogenesis by the animals. Wheat straw treatment with urea (4 kg urea per 100 kg DM) or urea plus calcium hydroxide (3 kg urea + 3 kg calcium hydroxide per 100 kg DM) and stored for 21 days before feeding, reduced methane emission by sheep. Feeding of urea sprinkled wheat straw and without storage time was not able to mitigate methane emission by sheep (Sahoo *et al.*, 2000).

The treatment of straw with urea and urea molasses mineral block lick caused a reduction of 12-15% methane production and the molar proportion of acetate decreased accompanied with an increase in propionate production. On inclusion of green maize and berseem in the ration, methanogenesis decreased significantly (Singh and Mohini, 1999). By increasing the concentrate level in the paddy straw based diet there was a depression in methane production accompanied with an increase in propionate concentration in the rumen liquor.

Beauchemin and McGinn (2006) reported that adding canola oil at the rate of 4.6% of dry matter intake inhibited methane emission by 32% and decreased methane emissions as a per cent of gross energy intake by 21%, but this decrease in methane emission was primarily attributed to reduced feed intake and lower total tract digestibility of feed, especially the fibre component.

Eight oil cakes were tested to study their effect on *in vitro* methanogenesis using a substrate of wheat straw and oil cake in the ratio of 75:25, respectively. Soybean cake containing diet showed the highest and castor bean cake (expeller extracted, EE) the lowest gas production. The methane production was highest with soybean cake followed by cotton seed cake, groundnut cake, mustard seed cake, castor bean cake (solvent extracted, SE), castor bean cake (EE), karanj cake (SE) and karanj cake (EE). *In vitro* true digestibility (IVTD) was highest with soybean meal and ground nut cake. The lowest IVTD was reported with karanj cake (EE) and castor bean cake (EE and SE). The feed with soybean cake showed significantly ($P<0.05$) higher number of holotrichs in comparison to the other groups. Castor bean cake and karanj cake inhibited methanogenesis significantly, but these two oil cakes also affected *in vitro* dry matter degradability of feed adversely, which might be due to the presence of anti-nutritional factors (Kumar *et al.*, 2007).

Fumaric acid is a precursor of propionic acid in the fermentation of feed in the rumen and can act as an alternate sink for consumption of hydrogen generated in the rumen. When used as a feed additive, fumaric acid reduces methane emission, but the reports so far indicate that the results are not consistent and may vary from one laboratory to the other (Wallace, 2004). But fumaric acid does act as an alternate hydrogen sink in the rumen, as its inclusion in the diet increases total VFA concentration, increased propionate proportion and decreased acetate:propionate ratio (Beauchemin and McGinn, 2006), but the levels required to inhibit methanogenesis to a significant extent may cause a drop in pH which might affect feed fermentation adversely. Wallace *et al.* (2006) reported that by encapsulating fumaric acid in a shell of hydrogenated vegetable oil prevented a fall in pH, but retained the ability of inhibiting methanogenesis. Free fumaric acid (10% in the ration) and an equivalent amount of encapsulated fumaric acid decreased methane emission to the extent of 49% and 75% compared to control sheep without supplementation of fumaric acid. The presence of methanogens and other hydrogen utilizing bacteria (propionate producers or fumarate utilizers) stimulate the activity of cellulose degrading bacteria and help in better utilization of feed (Carro and Ranilla, 2003).

The results of the experiments conducted so far indicate that type of diet, feed additives, roughage level and type, oil cakes, residual fatty acids in oil cakes etc. are some of the important properties which affect rumen fermentation and methane emission by the animals. Therefore, it is very important to formulate a diet depending upon the feed resources available with the animal farmer for minimized methane emission.

Microbial Manipulation

Microbial intervention of the rumen eco-system to inhibit methanogenesis must be achieved without adversely affecting the overall microbial process responsible for fibre digestion because this is the key to bioconversion of lignocellulosic feeds to utilizable nutrients for the livestock. The microbial interventions include suppression of methanogenic archaea, protozoa inhibition, reducing hydrogen generation or finding out an alternate hydrogen sink, where hydrogen generated during fermentation can be diverted to some more useful pathway where it can be brought back into the energy cycle through reductive acetogenesis.

Bacteriophages

Rumen fluid contains up to 10^9 bacteriophage/ml (Klieve and Swain 1993) and phages have been identified in many rumen bacterial species (Klieve *et al.*, 1989). Despite viruses having been identified in non-ruminal methanogenic archaea, there have been no studies of natural phage infection in ruminal methanogens. Rumen bacteriophages are in some cases strain specific (Klieve *et al.*, 1991) and if archaeal viruses share this trait, the development of a broadly effective virus-based control for rumen methanogens could be difficult (Klieve and Hegarty 1999). The heterogeneity identified in methanogens by 16S rRNA sequencing has indicated that methanogens colonised the gastrointestinal tract on a number of occasions. Consequently, it is reasonable to expect multiple strains of Archaea will be present in the rumen and this could limit the efficacy of biological control of methanogenesis in the rumen.

Enhanced Acetogenesis

The bacteria which are able to convert two moles of carbon dioxide to one mole of acetate, either autotrophically or heterotrophically, can be classified as reductive acetogens (Prins and Lankhorst, 1977). The heterotrophic acetogens are also known as homo-acetogens as these are able to bioconvert sugar quantitatively into acetate (Ljungdahl, 1986). The autotrophic acetogens convert exogenous carbondioxide and molecular hydrogen (evolved during fermentation) into acetate. Thus autotrophic reductive acetogens can also serve as an alternate hydrogen sink in the rumen microbial eco-system. Reductive acetogens have been observed in lambs about 24 h after birth and accounted for approximately 1% of the acetate produced (Morvan *et al.*, 1994), but activity and number of acetogens decreased rapidly afterwards. In comparison to methanogenesis, reductive acetogenesis has an added advantage that its end product (acetate) is an energy source for the animal, which is synthesized from energy less components (like carbon dioxide and hydrogen). The reductive acetogens are present in the rumen of steers (Leedle and Greening, 1988) along with methanogenic archaea. The presence of only the reductive acetogen is not sufficient for increasing the acetate production in the rumen fermentation, but corresponding inhibition of methanogens is also essentially required (Fievez *et al.*, 1999). A few experiments conducted with methane inhibitors and inoculation with reductive acetogens like *Peptostreptococcus productus* and *Acetitomaculum ruminis* has shown that reductive acetogenesis can be stimulated in *in vitro* rumen fermentation (Greening and Leedle, 1989, Nollet *et al.*, 1997). The same effect could not be reproduced in *in vivo* experiments. The use of 2-bromoethanesulphonic acid along with sodium formate and methanol for the stimulation of reductive acetogenesis has been proposed, but the methanogenic microflora of the rumen adapts itself to the presence of 2-bromoethanesulphonic acid and inhibition of methanogenesis gets reversed (Immig *et al.*, 1996). In another experiment it has been observed that methanogenesis is inhibited when supernatant of *Lacobacillus plantarum* 80 was fed to ruminants along with *Peptostreptococcus productus*. But this effect was reversed within six days, but there was no stimulation of reductive acetogenesis as the composition of volatile fatty acids was not changed in *in vitro* experiments (Nollet *et al.*, 1997). This effect of inhibition of methanogenesis has been attributed to anti-protozoal effect rather than the anti-bacterial effect on fermentation. In addition to the above reductive acetogenic microbes, *Eubacterium limosum* has been isolated which is able to utilize methanol and H_2-CO_2 and generate acetate (Genther *et al.*, 1981).

The results of *in vitro* experiments have shown that reductive acetogenesis can serve as an alternate hydrogen sink in rumen fermentation, but *in vivo* experiments have failed so far. One of the major reasons for its failure might be due to poor affinity of the reaction with molecular hydrogen as it requires higher hydrogen threshold level (1.26 *vs* 0.067 mmole/l) as compared to that required for methanogenesis (Weimer, 1998). Efforts are needed to explore the biochemical pathways which determine the direction of hydrogen transfer either for methane generation or for acetate synthesis. If all the reducing power generated during rumen fermentation is diverted towards reductive acetogenesis, 5-10% of the gross energy intake by the animals can be saved and brought back into the energy cycle of the animals, which otherwise would have been lost in methane generation and released by the animals into the atmosphere. In addition to that it will also help in protecting the environment by reduced release of methane by the animals.

Plant Secondary Metabolites

The term plant secondary metabolite is used to describe a group of chemical compounds found in plants that are not involved in the primary biochemical processes of plant growth and reproduction. These compounds might function as a nutrient store and defense mechanisms which ensures survival of their structure and reproductive elements protecting against insect or pathogen predation or by restricting grazing by herbivores. Several thousand plant secondary metabolites have been reported in various plants and many of them have found their use in traditional Indian and Chinese system of medicine (Kamra *et al.*, 2009). Some of these metabolites, which are able to modify rumen microbial ecosystem for inhibiting methane emission and improving feed utilization, have been reviewed here. As methanogens are attached with ciliate protozoa through an ecto-symbiotic relationship and the extent of methane emission is related to total feed fermentation in the rumen, the effect of plant secondary compounds on ciliate protozoa and other rumen microbes will also be discussed in this chapter.

Saponins

Saponins cover a wide variety of chemical compounds and man has used their properties for centuries. Chemically, saponins are high molecular weight glycosides in which sugars are linked to a triterpene or steroidal aglycone moiety. A large number of saponins could be possible depending upon the modifications of the ring structures of aglycone moieties and the number of sugars added to it. Traditionally saponin-containing plants have been used as soap substitutes.

Effect of Saponins on Ruminal Microbes

Numerous studies have demonstrated that saponins and saponin-containing plants have toxic effects on protozoa. Earliest observation that sarsaponin from *Yucca schidigera* decreased the protozoal population but not bacterial population in *in vitro* continuous culture systems (Valdez *et al.*, 1986). *Yucca schidigera* has been shown to suppress the growth of rumen ciliates *in vitro* (Wallace *et al.*, 1994) and in RUSITEC without affecting dry matter disappearance and other rumen microbial populations (Wang *et al.*, 1998). The butanol extract of *Yucca schidigera* showed anti-protozoal activity and caused defaunation (Makkar *et al.*, 1998; Wang *et al.*, 1998) and the active component has been identified as saponins. Alfalfa saponins isolated by ethanol extraction and partial acid hydrolysis decreased protozoal numbers in the rumen of sheep by 34 and 66% at the inclusion levels of 2 and 4% dietary dry matter, respectively (Lu and Jorgensen, 1987). A methanol extract of *Sapindus rarak* fruit depressed the protozoal population in the rumen of sheep by 57%, a reduction that was attributed to saponins in the extract (Thalib *et al.*, 1996). The berries of *Sapindus mukorossi* (soap nut) extracted in different solvents caused a depression in methane and gas production by 96% and 39%, 20% and 12%, 23% and 0% with ethanol, water and methanol extracts, respectively, as compared to respective controls. The extracts also exhibited antiprotozoal activity resulting in 70-90% lesser protozoa in the treated samples (Agarwal *et al.*, 2006). Saponin like material in the organic phase of a butanol-water mixture of *Sesbania sesban* foliage, a leguminous tree, was found to be inhibitory to protozoal activity (Newbold *et al.*, 1997). However, protozoal activity of *Sesbania sesban* varied with different accessions having different types of saponins but the adaptation of animals to these plants has also been reported (Teferedegne *et al.*, 1999; Wallace *et al.*, 2002). Protozoal activity, as measured by the breakdown of [^{14}C] leucine-labelled *Selenomonas ruminantium* in rumen fluid incubated *in vitro,* was inhibited by the addition of 1% *Yucca schidigera* extract. Similarly, saponins from *Quillaja saponaria* and *Acacia auriculoformis* (Makkar *et al.*, 1998) and soapnut (Kamra *et al.*, 2000) have also shown anti-protozoal activity *in vitro*. Hess *et al.* (2003) studied three saponin rich tropical fruits - *Sapindus saponaria* (12% saponins), *Enterolobium cyclocarpum* (1.9% saponins) and *Pithecellobium saman* (1.7% saponins) supplemented to forage based diets in Rusitec using rumen fluid from faunated and defaunated cow. The *S. saponaria* reduced protozoal count (54%) and daily methane release (20%) without affecting the methanogens in faunated rumen fluid. Further, the effect of *S. saponaria* on methane was more pronounced in defaunated (29%) than faunated (14%) rumen fluid indicating that reduced methane production was not entirely due to associated depression in protozoal count.

In *in vivo* studies, *Y. schidigera* decreased rumen protozoal numbers in heifers (Hristov *et al.*, 1999). A decrease in protozoal numbers was also reported in the rumen of sheep infused with pure alfalfa saponins (Lu and Jorgensen, 1987) or fed saponin-containing plants, including *S. sesban* (Newbold *et al.*, 1997; Odenyo *et al.*, 1997) and *Enterolobium cyclocarpum* (Navas-Camacho *et al.*, 1993). The sensitivity of ciliate protozoa towards saponins might be explained by the presence of sterols in protozoa, which are absent in bacterial membranes. Thus, sterol-binding capability of saponins (Hostettmann and Marston, 1995) most likely caused destruction of protozoal cell membranes.

In addition to protozoa, bacteria and fungi are also influenced by the presence of saponins in the rumen. *Yucca schidigera* extract (1%, v/v) inhibited the growth of *Butyrivibrio fibrisolvens* and *Streptococcus bovis*, while the growth of *Prevotella ruminicola* was stimulated and the growth of *Selenomonas ruminantium* Z108 was unaffected (Wallace *et al.*, 1994). Wang *et al.* (2000) also observed that growth of some bacteria, *Streptococcus bovis, Prevotella bryantii* and *Ruminobacter amylophilus* was reduced as a result of alteration of the cell wall of bacteria, while the growth of *Selenimonas ruminantium* was enhanced in the presence of steroidal saponins. However, some studies with saponin-containing plants showed increased bacterial numbers, presumably as a consequence of inhibition of protozoa (Valdez *et al.*, 1986; Newbold *et al.*, 1997). Steroidal saponins from *Y. schidigera* had no effect on bacterial count in Rusitec; however, inoculating fluid from the fermenter into the medium containing saponins decreased the viable count (Wang *et al.*, 1998). Ruminal fungi, *Neocallimastix frontalis* and *Piromyces rhizinflata*, are also sensitive to *Y. schidigera* saponins (Wang *et al.*, 2000). Wina *et al.* (2005) investigated the effect of saponins containing a methanol extract of *Sapindus rarak* at concentrations of 0, 0.25, 0.5, 1.0, 2.0 and 4.0 mg/ml to an elephant grass and wheat bran (7:3 w/w) diet *in vitro*. Microbial biomass gradually increased with increasing extract from 102.8 (control) to 147.3 at 4 mg/ml and protozoal count was decreased. There was no effect on *Fibrobacter* spp., however, there was a negative effect on *Ruminococcus albus* and *Ruminococcus flavefaciens* at 2 and 4 mg/ml extract. Rumen fungus, *Chytridiomycetes* was reduced at the highest level. The xylanase activity and NDF digestibility decreased at higher levels of extract. In experiment with sheep, Hess *et al.* (2004) reported that supplementation with fruits of *S. saponaria* (250 g/kg concentrate) increased total bacteria count and decreased total ciliate protozoa count in lambs fed basal diets of grass hay or grass and legume mixture (1:2 or 2: 1) along with concentrate (1:3). Daily methane release was reduced by *S. saponaria* supplementation in all basal diets. The digestibilities of organic matter and neutral-detergent fibre were reduced by supplementation with *S. saponaria*. Ruminal fluid ammonia concentration was not significantly affected by the inclusion of *S. saponaria* in the concentrate. *Acacia concinna, Moringa oleifera* and *Sapindus mukorossi/ S. Saponaria* are some of the plants which have high saponin content and are able to inhibit methanogenesis in the rumen and some of them also have anti-protozoal characteristics (Table 2).

One of the problems of using saponins or saponin-containing plants is that anti-protozoal activity was found to be transient (Newbold *et al.*, 1997; Teferedegne *et al.*, 1999). The time dependence of the detoxification process of the saponins was clearly demonstrated in ruminal fluid *in vitro*. However, some of the studies suggested that protozoa *per se* did not develop resistance to these anti-protozoal compounds (Newbold *et al.*, 1997). Therefore, it is possible that bacterial population of the rumen degraded the saponins or saponin-containing plants.

Saponins are degraded in batch cultures of rumen fluid *in vitro* (Makkar and Becker, 1997) although, apparently, the resultant sapogenins, the aglycone remaining after the removal of sugar moiety, are degraded more slowly (Wang *et al.*, 1998). Since the saponins, not the aglycone sapogenins, are toxic to the protozoa, it is likely that cleavage of the sugar moieties of saponins by rumen microbes renders the saponins ineffective to protozoa (Teferedegne *et al.*, 1999). *Fibrobacter succinogenes* apparently deglycosylated the saponins from *Yucca shidigera* (Wang *et al.*, 2000). The observation made by Odenyo *et al.* (1997) that *S. sesban* introduced directly into the rumen remained toxic to protozoa, but not dietary *S. sesban* implying that chewing caused detoxification, perhaps by salivary amylase or that the larger particle size protected saponins from degradation.

Tannins

Tannins are widely distributed in nutritionally important forage trees, shrubs, legumes, cereals and grains that often limit their utilization as feedstuffs. Tannins are polyphenolic compounds of plant origin, which are of two distinct types: hydrolysable tannins : the polymers of gallic acid (gallotannins) or ellagic acid (ellagotannins) with a sugar core which is usually glucose and these tannins are readily hydrolyzed by acids or enzymes into monomeric units. The second type of tannins are the condensed tannins : which are further sub-divided into (a) proanthocyanidins which are di-, tri or polymers of the anthocyanidins and/or catechin flavan-3-ol units and (b) leucoanthocyanidins which are dimers of the flavan-3, 4-diol flavonoids. The flavan-3-ol monomer units are linked by C4-C9 or C4-C6 interflavonoid linkages that give the shape of condensed tannins a polymer chain. The number of monomeric units may vary and this determines the degree of polymerisation from bi-, tri- and tetraflavonoids to higher oligomers. These can then produce an infinite variety of chemical structures, which in turn could produce different biological properties.

Table 2 : Plants containing secondary metabolites and their effect on rumen fermentation characteristics

Botanical Name	Common name	Plant part	Active principles	Effect on rumen fermentation	Reference
Acacia concinna	Shikakai	Seed pulp	Saponins, tannins	Methane inhibition with methanol extract, anti-protozoal activity	Patra *et al.*, 2006b
Allium cepa	Onion	Bulb	Trithiolane, dihydrothiopene, lacrimatory factor (19:1 mixture of Z -and E - propanethial S -oxide), quercicetin and oleanolic acid	No effect on methanogenesis	Patra *et al.*, 2006c
Allium sativum	Garlic	Bulb	Volatile oil - a llicin, diallyl disulfide and diallyl trisulfide	Inhibits methanogenesis, No effect on ciliate protozoa	Patra *et al.*, 2006c; Busquet *et al.*, 2006
Azadirachta indica	Neem	Seed pulp, leaves	Bitter principles - nimbin, nimbidin, azadirachtin	Methane inhibition, protozoa inhibition, Stimulates rumen fibre degrading enzyme activities	Agarwal *et al*, 1991; Patra *et al.*, 2006b
Bergenia crassifolia		Leaves, roots	Tannins	Inhibition of methanogenesis	Jayanegara et al., 2009
Citrus sinensis	Orange	Peels	Terpenoids	No effect on methanogenesis	Kumar , 2007
Coriandrum sativum	Coriander	Leaves and seeds	Essential oils - linalool and geraniol, butylphthalides-pinene neocnidilide, ligustilide and terpinine, flavonoids, coumarins, phthalides and phenolic acids	No effect on methanogenesis and ciliate protozoa	Kamra *et al.*, 2006

Contd...

Emblica officinalis	Amla	Seed pulp	Tannins, chebulinic acid (astringent substance), gallic acid and resin	Inhibits methanogenesis and ciliate protozoa	Patra *et al.*, 2006b
Eucalyptus globulus	Eucalyptus	Oil, leaves	α-pinene, β-pinene, α-phellandrene, 1,8 cineole, limonene, terpinen -4-ol, piperitone and globulol	Inhibition of methanogenesis	Kamra *et al.*, 2006
Foeniculum vulgare	Fennel	Seed	Essential oil - α-pinene, β-pinene, fenchone, trans -anethole, camphene, methy l chavicol, 1,8-cineole and anisic aldehyde	Inhibition of methanogenesis and ciliate protozoa	Patra *et al.*, 2006c
Mentha piperita/ Mentha haplocalyx	Peppermint /Bo he in Chinese and field mint in English	Oil	Menthol, menthone, 1,8 -cineole, methyl acetate, methofuran, isomenthone, α-pinene, trans-sabinene hydrate	Inhibition of methanogenesis and ciliate protozoa	Agarwal *et al.*, 2009
Moringa oleifera	Sahjan	Leaves, seed	Saponins, phenols and tannins	No effect of leaves on methanogenesis	Kamra *et al.*, 2006
Ocimum sanctum	Tulsi	Leaves	Essential oil (euganol, methyleuganol, caryophyllene, terpenes, sequiterpenes), camphor	Enhances rumen methanogenesis	Kamra *et al.*, 2006
Peltiphyllum peltatum		Leaves	Tannins	Inhibition of methanogenesis	Jayanegara et al., 2009
Populus deltoides	Poplar	Leaves	Essential oil, tannins, flavonoids and resin	Inhibition of methanogenesis and ciliate protozoa	Kamra *et al.*, 2006

Contd...

Psidium guajava	Guava	Leaves and fruit	α-selinene, β-caryophyllene, caryophyllene oxide, squalene, selin-11-en-4α-ol, guaijavarin, isoquercetin, hyperin, quercitrin and quercetin-3-O-gentobioside, β-sitosterol, uvaol, oleanolic acid and ursolic acid	Inhibition of methanogenesis and ciliate protozoa	Chaterjee, 2005
Quercus incana	Oak	Leaves	Catechin, hyperin, quajaverin, astragalin, tiliroside, tellimoside, isorhamnetin, kaempferol, triterpenoids, triterpene saponingallic acids	Inhibition of methanogenesis	Kamra *et al.*, 2006
Rheum undulatum		Leaves	Tannins	Inhibition of methanogenesis	Jayanegara et al., 2009
Rhus typhina		Leaves	Tannins	Inhibition of methanogenesis	Jayanegara et al., 2009
Sapindus mukorossi/ S. saponaria	Soapnut, Reetha	Seed pulp	Saponins (mukoroside)	Inhibition of methanogenesis, improve propionate production	Kamra *et al.*, 2000; Hess *et al.*, 2004; Agarwal *et al.*, 2006
Syzygium aromaticum	Clove	Flower buds/oil	Volatile oil- eugenol, pinene acetyleugenol, methyl salicylate, and vanillin, caryophyllene oxide, caryophylla-3(12), 6-dien-4-ol, caryophylla-3(12), gum and oleanolic acid, ellagitannin-eugeniin	Inhibition of methanogenesis, adverse effect on digestibility at high concentration	Patra *et al.*, 2006c

Contd...

Terminalia belerica	Bahera	Seed pulp	Gallic acid, ellagic acid and che bulagic acid, â - sitosterol, ethyl gallate, belleric acid and bellericanin.	Inhibition of methanogenesis and ciliate protozoa	Patra *et al.*, 2006a
Terminalia chebula	Harad	Seed pulp	Tannins, chebulinic acid (astringent substance), gallic acid and resin	Inhibition of methanogenesis and ciliate protozoa	Patra *et al.*, 2006a
Vaccinium vitis - idaea	?	Leaves	Tannins	Inhibition of methanogenesis	Jayanegara et al., 2009
Zingiber officinalis	Ginger		Essential oil - zingerone zingiberene, farnesene, curcumene, linalo ol, gingerol, shogaol, sesquiphellandrene, zingerone sesquiphellandrene	No effect on methane inhibition	Kamra *et al.*, 2006

These polyphenolic polymers are of relatively high molecular weight and have capacity to form complexes with carbohydrates and proteins. Low molecular weight condensed oligomers are more reactive and have higher protein precipitating capacities than high molecular weight polymeric tannins.

Metabolism of Tannins in Rumen

Rumen microbes are able to degrade simple plant phenolic compounds to some extent to counter anti-nutritive effects of tannins of forage origin. Phenolic glycosides such as rutin and naringin and flavonoid ring system of the common plant flavonoids (quercitrin) are readily degraded in rumen by hydrolysis of the glycoside and cleavage of the heterocyclic ring to acetate, butyrate, di- and monohydroxyphenolics and phloroglucinol (Simpson *et al.*, 1969; Lowry and Kennedy, 1996). Some quantitative nutritional trials have shown apparent losses of 29% and 51% of condensed tannins from *Acacia barteri* and *Bauhania varigata*, repectively upto 24 h of fermentation (Makkar *et al.*, 1995; Paul *et al.*, 2006). Similarly, with pure culture studies on tannin degrading bacteria isolated from goats exposed to calliandra tannins were able to reduce tannic acid and condensed tannins from the medium (Wiryawan *et al.*, 1999). This apparent loss could be due to degradation of monomeric, dimeric and oligomeric tannins. However, there is no evidence of cleavage of carbon-carbon bonds of heterocyclic ring system of flavan-3-ols (catechin, epicatechin) that are the monomeric units of condensed tannins and these observations need to be confirmed by definitive experiments on microbial degradation of model condensed tannins. In contrast to condensed tannins, the ester bonds of hydrolysable tannins are cleaved in the rumen by *Selenomonas ruminantium* and *Streptococcus* spp. which produce esterase, tannin acylhydrolase (Nelson *et al.*, 1998) to form metabolites, gallic acid and ellagic acid. Gallic acid is then decarboxylated in the rumen to pyrrogallol and converted to resorcinol and phloroglucinol before cleavage of the phloroglucinol ring to acetate and butyrate by *Eubacterium oxidoreducens, Streptococcus bovis, Syntrophococcus sucromutans* and *Coprococcus* sp. (Krumholz and Bryant, 1986; Murdiati *et al.*, 1992).

Effects of Tannins on Rumen Microbes

Tannins are generally regarded as inhibitory to the growth of microorganism, which might be due to complexing ability of tannins with the cell wall of bacteria causing morphological changes of the cell wall and the extracellular enzymes secreted (Jones *et al.*, 1994). Bae *et al.* (1993) reported that cell associated and extracellular endoglucanase activity of *Fibrobacter succinogenes* were inhibited by condensed tannins (100-400 mg/ml) from *Lotus corniculatus* under *in vitro* conditions. Jones *et al.* (1994) studied the effects of condensed tannins on growth and proteolysis by four strains of ruminal bacteria and observed that growth of proteolytic bacteria (*Butyrivibrio fibrisolvens, Ruminobacter amylophilus* and *Streptococcus bovis*) was reduced by condensed tannins but a strain of *Prevotella ruminicola* was tolerant to condensed tannins from sainfoin (*Onobrychris viciifolia*). Similarly, condensed tannins in *Lotus corniculatus* reduced the populations of *Clostridium proteoclasticum, Butyrivibrio fibrisolvens, Eubacterium* spp. and *Streptococcus bovis* in sheep (Min *et al.,* 2002). Tagari *et al.* (1965) also observed the inhibition of growth of cellulolytic and proteolytic bacteria by carob tannins in artificial rumen.

Effects of tannins on rumen protozoa are variable. Newbold *et al.* (1997) investigated that tannins were not responsible for the anti-protozoal activity of *Sesbania sesban.* McSweeney *et al.* (1998; 2001a,b) showed that Calliandra tannins have inhibitory effects on rumen cellulolytic bacteria including *F. succinogenes* and *Ruminococcus* spp. The Calliandra tannins did not affect the total population of protozoa, fungi and proteolytic bacteria. Although, tannins affected some bacteria, rumen microbial population appeared to adapt and efficiency of microbial protein synthesis (g microbial protein per kg organic matter apparently digested in the rumen) was unaffected. Salem *et al.* (1997) also observed a linear increase in protozoa numbers in rumen fluid of sheep fed on a Lucerne hay based diet by addition of increased proportion of *Acacia cyanophylla* Lindl. foliage, which contained 4.5% condensed tannins. Similarly, condensed tannins in birdsfoot treefoil (*Lotus corniculatus*) and sulla (*Hedysarum coronarium*) increased protozoal numbers in the rumen of sheep (Chiquette *et al.,* 1989; Terrill *et al.,* 1992). However, Makkar *et al.* (1995) reported that quebracho tannin (condensed tannin) significantly reduced the number of total protozoa, entodiniomorphs and holotrichs, the effect being higher on holotrichs, which might increase the efficiency of microbial protein synthesis in the rumen. However, fibre-degrading ability of rumen fungi might be less sensitive to the inhibitory effects of condensed tannins compared to cellulolytic bacteria (McSweeney *et al.,* 1998). Salawu *et al.* (1999) showed that quebracho tannins (condensed tannin) reduced cellulase and xylanase activities of the rumen microbes and total rumen protozoa in sheep fed on grass-barley diet supplemented with 50g quebracho tannin per kg diet. Saravanan (2000) observed 75% reduction in the protozoa number in sheep fed on a diet containing 0.5% condensed tannins obtained from leaf extract of the plant *Uncaria gambier.*

Muhammad *et al.* (1995) tested the effects of tannic acid, ellagic acid, gallic acid and catechin on rumen fungus *Neocallimastix frontalis* strain RE1. All these compounds inhibited cellulolysis and zoospore attachment to cellulose by this fungus. Gallic acid, ellagic acid and catechin were more inhibitory to cellulolysis than tannic acid. However, ellagic acid was most inhibitory to zoospore attachment, perhaps indicating the involvement of different cell-surface receptors in this process.

Inhibition of Methanogenesis

Forages containing condensed tannins have been shown to decrease methane production by the ruminants. Tannins present in *Calliandra calothyrus* reduced nutrient degradation and methane release per gram of organic matter degraded in *in vitro* experiments with rumen simulation technique (RUSITEC) (Hess *et al.*, 2003). Reduced methane production was also observed in RUSITEC as the proportion of sainfoin (*Onobrychis viciifolia*) incubated were increased (McMahon *et al.*, 1999). Woodward *et al.* (2002) investigated the effect of feeding of sulla on methane emission and milk yield in Friesian and Jersey dairy cows. Cows grazing on sulla had higher daily dry matter intake (13.1 vs. 10.7 kg DM) and daily milk solid production (1.07 vs. 0.81 kg) than grazing perennial ryegrass pasture. Total daily methane emission was similar (253.9 vs. 260 g). However, cows fed sulla produced less methane per kg DM intake (19.5 vs. 24.6 g) and per kg milk solid yield (243.3 vs. 327.8 g). Similar trends in methane emission and milk production have been observed in sheep fed lotus silage (Woodward *et al.*, 2001). There was also a 16% reduction in methane production in lambs fed on *Lotus pedunculatus* (lotus), which might be due to the presence of condensed tannins (Waghorn *et al.*, 2002). Another condensed tannins containing forage *Sericea lespedeza* (17.7% CT) decreased methane emission (7.4 vs. 10.6 g/d and 6.9 vs. 16.2 g/kg DMI for *Sericea lespedeza* and crabgrass/tall fescue, respectively) in Angora goats (Puchala *et al.*, 2005). Dry matter intake (1.11 vs. 0.67 kg/d) and digestible DMI (0.71 vs. 0.51 kg/d) were greater for *Sericea lespedeza* than for crabgrass/tall fescue in this study. Tavendale *et al.* (2005) reported that methane production (ml/g DM) at 12 h for *M. sativa* (25 ml) was higher than *L. pedunculatus* (17.6 ml; $P < 0.05$) that contains 10% condensed tannins and after addition of PEG increased methane production for *L. pedunculatus* (17%, $P < 0.001$) but not for *M. sativa*. They also studied the mechanism of inhibitory effects of extractable condensed tannin fractions from *L. pedunculatus* on the common rumen methanogens *Methanobrevibacter ruminantium*, strains YLM-1 and DSM1093. Oligomeric CT fractions were inactive against both the strains, as determined by methane production measurements. The polymeric fraction completely inhibited methane production. Inhibitory effects in broth culture for strain YLM-1 were bacteriostatic, while strain DSM1093 did not recover growth, as indicated by methane production, even upon prolonged incubation. In a plate assay, the zone of inhibition with the polymeric fraction remained after a further week of incubation. Results indicated that CT action on methanogenesis can be attributed to indirect effects via reduced hydrogen production (and presumably reduced forage digestibility) and via direct inhibitory effects on methanogens.

Bergenia crassifolia, Emblica officinalis, Peltiphyllum peltatum, Populus deltoides, Quercus incana, Rheum undulatum, Terminalia belerica, Terminalia chebula and *Vaccinium vitis-idaea* are some other plants containing high tannin contents and have a potential to inhibit *in vitro* as well as *in vivo* methane emission by the rumen microbes (Table 2).

Flavonoids

Flavonoids have been suspected to have anti-nutritional characteristics for ruminants (Van Soest, 1994) and also antibacterial effect, which was found to be more effective against Gram-positive bacterial strains than on Gram-negative (Mirzoeva *et al.*, 1997).

Unlike flavan-3-ols (monomeric units of condensed tannins), the flavonoids of common plants are readily degraded in the rumen by hydrolysis of the glycosides and cleavage of the heterocyclic ring (Lowry and Kennedy, 1996). The products of flavonoid degradation in the rumen include acetate, butyrate, di- and monohydroxyphenolics, and phloroglucinol. The di- and monohydroxyphenolics are probably released from the B ring while phloroglucinol would be derived from the A ring of the flavonoids (Cheng *et al.*, 1969). The degradation products of flavonoids could modify the microbial metabolism in the rumen. The bacterial ring fission of aglycone flavonoids leads to the production of 3,4 dihydroxyphenylacetic acid from isoquercitrin and quercitrin, phenylacetic acid from naringenin (Schneider *et al.*, 1999; Winter *et al.*, 1989). Some of these simple phenolic compounds may interact with the biosynthesis of aromatic amino acids. Analogous molecules, phenylpropanoic acid and phenylacetic acid have been reported to enhance cellulose-degrading bacteria in the rumen (Stack *et al.*, 1983).

Broudiscou *et al.* (2000) studied the effect of thirteen dry plant extracts, selected for their high flavonoid content on rumen fermentation and methanogenesis in continuous cultures of rumen microbes. *Lavandula officinalis* and *Solidago virga-aurea* stimulated fermentation, whereas methanogenesis was decreased with *Equisetum arvense* and *Salvia officinalis*. In another experiment, Broudiscou and Lassalas (2000) studied the effects of *Lavandula officinalis* and *Equisetum arvense* dry extracts, and of isoqercitrin, a flavonoid present in *Equisetum arvense* on fermentation of diets varying in forage contents by rumen microbes in batch culture. The amounts of acetate and propionate produced from 100% hay diet were increased by the plant extracts, strongly by *L. officinalis* (60% and 37%, respectively) and *E. arvense* (59% and 40%, respectively), to a lesser degree by isoquercitrin (29% and 15%, respectively). In dual outflow fermenters receiving a 50:50 hay-barley diet for seven days, the addition of *L. officinalis* appeared to increase the amount of fermented organic matter, while *E. arvense* tended to inhibit methanogenesis (Broudiscou and Lassalas, 2000). *Achillea millefolium* appeared to induce extensive stimulation of microbial metabolism as it increased both degradabilities of crude protein and cell wall constituents and the efficiency and yield of biomass production (Broudiscou *et al.*, 2002).

Essential Oils

Essential oils are steam-volatile or organic-solvent extracts of plants. They are commonly derived from herbs and spices and also present in many plants for their protective role against bacterial, fungal or insect attack. They are mainly cyclic hydrocarbons and their alcohol, aldehyde or ester derivatives.

Essential oils as feed additives in animal nutrition have been reviewed by several researchers (Losa and Brufau, 2001, Wallace *et al.*, 2002). Essential oils were examined many years ago to test their effect on poor palatability in some plant species (Oh *et al.*, 1968). Estell *et al.* (1998) studied the effect of some volatile compounds (camphor, limonene, cis-jasmone, beta-caryophyllene, borneol and alfa-pinene) on the consumption of alfalfa pellets by sheep. Camphor, alfa-pinene and borneol depressed the consumption of alfalfa pellets, whereas, other three compounds had no discernable effect on consumption. Therefore, the essential oils to be used as feed additives should be considered from the point of feed intake and acceptability by the animals.

Wallace *et al.* (2002) investigated the rate of degradation of different protein meals and colonisation of feedstuffs incubated in nylon bags by attached enzyme activity in the presence of essential oils. Of the protein meals tested, essential oil had significant effect only on the breakdown of pea meal, the most rapidly degraded meal. Bacterial proteinase and amylase associated with plant (pea and rapeseed) protein supplement tended to be lower in animals receiving essential oils, while corresponding activities associated with fishmeal were unaffected. Glutamate dehydrogenase activity, a measure of total microbial colonization, associated with grass hay suspended in the bovine rumen was decreased by essential oils, while colonization of the less degradable fibrous substrates, grass silage and barley straw, was unaffected. Carboxymethylcellulase activity, a measure of fibrolytic bacterial population was similar. This indicated that essential oils might suppress the colonization and/or digestion of readily degradable substrates by amylolytic and proteolytic bacteria without affecting fibre digestion (Wallace *et al.*, 2002). Individual essential oils had different effects on mixed ruminal bacteria. Monoterpene hydrocarbons were less toxic and sometimes stimulatory to microbial activity compared to the corresponding oxygenated compounds, the monoterpene alcohols and aldehyde (Oh *et al.*, 1967, 1968). Feeding of 500 mg Ropadiar (containing volatile oil of marjoram) to sheep showed higher concentration of protein in the rumen fluid without affecting the nutrient digestibility

(Kozelov *et al.*, 2001). Total viable count of bacteria was unaffected by essential oil, but hyperammonia producing bacteria (HAP) that include *Clostridium sticklandi* and *Prevotella anaerobius* were decreased by 77% in sheep receiving low protein diet without affecting protozoal numbers or activity (Wallace *et al.*, 2002). HAP bacteria have a high capability to generate NH_3 from amino acids (Wallace *et al.*, 2002). Therefore, the inhibition of HAP bacteria by commercial blend of essential oil mixture decreased rumen ammonia concentration in sheep (Fernandez *et al.*, 1997) and cattle (Newbold *et al.*, 1999). The doses and types of essential oils and type of diet and adaptation to essential oils by rumen microorganism appear to be important to get benefits of their inclusion in the diet. It is known that HAP comprise only around 1% of the rumen bacterial population. Nevertheless, even a small decrease in the rate of NH_3 production might be beneficial nutritionally (Wallace *et al.*, 2002). Whether these effects translate into improved productivity will depend on animal and dietary factors, of which little experimental evidence is available.

Allium sativum, Coriandrum sativum, Eucalyptus globulus, Foeniculum vulgare, Mentha piperita, Ocimum sanctum, Populus deltoides and *Syzygium aromaticum* are some of the plants which contain high concentration of essential oils and are effective against methane emission and protozoa growth in the rumen, but some of them also have adverse effects on degradability of feed and nutrient utilization by the animals (Table 2). The results of *in vivo* experiments with these plants are also variable and need further experimentation before their practical application in the livestock production.

Immunization

Vaccines usually provide a means to control pathogenic infectious microbes and help in improving livestock productivity. Natural development of antibodies by lambs to mixed methanogens has been shown (Baker, 1999) and development of a vaccination strategy to reduce rumen methanogensis is in progress.

Commonwealth Scientific and Industrial Research Organization (CSIRO) Livestock Industries in Australia has a large experience of novel approaches to manipulation of microorganisms in the rumen and holds patents for vaccine technologies targeting the manipulation of rumen protozoa and methanogens. These discoveries made by researchers at the Floreat Laboratory in Perth, Australia in the 1990s are aimed at protozoa to reduce significantly their population in the rumen to free more protein and nutrients for wool production and growth of the livestock. The protozoal vaccine involves administration of the vaccine subcutaneously in the neck region.

Researchers are testing different anti-protozoal vaccine formulations. It is anticipated that a prototype protozoa vaccine formulation will be identified soon, which will then be subjected to a series of field trials before any decision is made about commercial production. Two other vaccine formulations have also been tested in sheep and cattle in CSIRO. Extensive publicity has been given to a vaccine against methanogens being developed in Australia that is claimed to reduce CH_4 production per kilogram of food by 11-23%. This approach shows great promise as it may involve "once-in-a-lifetime" injection and be applicable to all classes of ruminants. It is, however, still at the development and testing stage and is unlikely to be available soon, even for evaluation.

A recent study by Williams *et al.* (2009), it has been a target to identify methanogens present in sheep and develop a vaccine against these prominent methanogens and to study its effect on total methane emission by the animals. They identified five phylotypes of methanogenic archaea which accounted for more than 52% of total methanogens present. A vaccine generated against these five strains was used for vaccination of sheep, which caused an increase in specific immunoglobulin G titers in plasma, saliva and rumen fluid, but methane emission and methanogen numbers were not different in vaccinated and non-vaccinated groups. The methanogenic diversity was greater in vaccinated animals. One interesting finding was that the methogenic microbes usually take more than 4 weeks to get stabilized and care must be taken to carry on experiments for longer duration to get acceptable and repeatable results. The observations of this experiment indicated a necessity of a broad spectrum vaccine representing majority of methanogens present in the rumen to get positive influence on methane emission by the animals.

Potential Research Areas

- *Dietary manipulations* : To screen conventional and non-conventional feed resources for their potential to affect methane emission by the animals.
- *Chemical feed additives* : Methane analogues, unsaturated fatty acids and organic acids, which have minimum side effects on feed utilization and no residues left in the livestock products like meat and milk.
- *Microbial feed additives* : Reductive acetogenic bacteria, yeasts and other microbes which may manipulate rumen fermentation and reduce methane emission.
- *Plant secondary compounds (PSC)* : The results of recent experiments conducted in Rumen-up programme of European Commission and Coordinated Research Project of IAEA indicated that there do exist plants

which have a potential to be used as anti-methaogenic and anti-protozoal agents, but some of them have toxic influence on other microbes of the rumen. Therefore, optimum dose of PSC content in the diet should be standardized in a manner so that inhibition in methane production can be achieved without adversely affecting nutrient utilization.

- *Genomics* : For identifying methanogens and inhibition mechanism of methanogenesis.

References

Agarwal, N., Chandra S., Kumar R., Chaudhary, L.C. and Kamra, D.N. (2009). *Anim. Feed Sci. Technol.,* 148(2-4): 321-327.

Agarwal, N., Kamra, D.N. and Chaudhary, L.C. (2006). *J. Appl. Anim. Res.,* 30: 1-4.

Agarwal, N., Kewalramani, N., Kamra, D.N., Agrawal, D.K. and Nath, K. (1991). *J. Sci. Food Agric.,* 57: 147-150.

Bae, H.D., McAllister, T.A Yanke, L.J., Cheng, K.J. and Muir, A.D. (1993). *Applied Environ. Microbiol.,* 59: 2132-2138.

Baker, S.K. (1999). Biology of rumen methanogens and stimulation of animal immunity. *In.* Meeting the Kyoto Protocol: Implications for the Australian Livestock Industries. (Eds. P.J. Reyenga, S.M. Howden). pp29-37. Bureau of Rural Sciences, Canberra.

Beauchemin, K.A. and McGinn, S.M. (2006). *J. Anim. Sci.,* 84: 1489–1496.

Broudiscou, L.P., Papon, Y. and Broudiscou, A.F. (2002). *Anim. Feed Sci. Technol,* 101: 183-189.

Broudiscou, L.P., Papon, Y. and Broudiscou, A.F. (2000). *Anim. Feed Sci. Technol.,* 87: 263-277.

Broudiscou, L.P. and Lassalas, B. (2000). *Reprod. Nutr. Develop.,* 40: 431-440.

Busquet, M., Calsamiglia, S., Ferret, A. and Kamel, C. (2006). *J. Dairy Sci.,* 89: 761-771.

Carro, M.D. and Ranilla, M.J. (2003). *Brit. J. Nutr.,* 90: 617–623.

Chatterjee, P.N. (2005). Influence of diet and plant secondary compounds on methanogenesis and rumen fermentation pattern. Ph.D. Thesis, IVRI Deemed Univ., Izatnagar, India.

Chatterjee, P.N., Kamra, D.N. and Agarwal, N. (2006). *Indian J. Anim. Nutr.* 23: 72-77.

Cheng, K.J., Jones, G.A., Simpson, F.J. and Bryant, M.P. (1969). *Canadian J. Microbiol.,* 15: 1365-1371.

Chiquette, J., Cheng, K.J., Rode, L.M. and Milligan, L.P. (1989). *Canadian J. Microbiol,* 69: 1031-1039.

Estell, R.E., Fredrikson, E.L., Tellez, M.R., Havstad, K.M., Shupe, W.L., Anderson, D.M. and Remmenga, M.D. (1998). *J. Anim. Sci.,* 76: 228-232.

Fernandez, M., Serrano, E., Frutos, P., Giraldez, F.J., Mantecon, A.R., and Llach, J.R. (1997). Efecto del aditivo CRINA HC sobre la actividad degradativa ruminal en la especie ovina [Effect of CRINA HC supplement upon the rumen degradative activity in sheep]. ITEA, 18 (vol. Extra): 160-162.

Fievez, V., Piattoni, F., Mbanzamihigo, L. and Demeyer, D. (1999). *J. Appl. Anim. Res.*, 16: 1-22.

Genther, S.B.R., Davis, C.L. and Bryant, M.P. (1981). *Appl. Environ. Microbiol.*, 42: 12-19.

Greening, R.C. and Leedle, J.A.Z. (1989). *Arch. Microbiol.*, 151: 399-406.

Haque, N., Saraswat, M.L. and Sahoo. A. (2001). *Indian J. Anim. Sci.*, 71: 797-799.

Haque, N., Saraswat, M.L., Hasah, Q.Z., Bhar, R., Mehra, U.R., Khan, M.Y., Verma, A.K. and Dass, R.S. (2004). *Indian J. Anim. Sci.*, 74: 973-976.

Hess, H.D., M. Kreuzer, T.E. Diaz, C.E. Lascano, J.E. Carulla, C.R. Soliva, and A. Machmuller. (2003). *Anim. Feed Sci. Technol.*, 109(1-4): 79-94.

Hess, H.D., Beuret, R.A., Lotscher, M., Hindrichsen, I.K., Machmüller, A., Carulla, J.E., Lascano, C.E. and Kreuzer, M. (2004). *Anim. Sci.*, 79: 177-189.

Hostettmann, K. and Marston, A. (1995). *Saponins*. Cambridge University Press.

Hristov, A.N., McAllister, T.A., Van Herk, F.H., Cheng, K.J., Newbold, C.J. and Cheeke, P.R. (1999). *J. Anim. Sci.*, 77: 2554-2563.

Immig, I., Demeyer, D., Fiedler, D.M., van Nevel, C. and Mbanzamihigo, L. (1996). *Arch. Anim. Nutr.*, 49: 363-370.

Intergovernmental Panel on Climate Change (IPCC). (1996). Guidelines for national greenhouse gas inventories – Greenhouse gas inventory reference manual. IPCC WGI Technical Support Unit, Bracknell, UK.

Intergovernmental Panel on Climate Change (IPCC). (2001). Climate change 2001: the scientific basis. [Third Assessment Report from Working Group 1. Edited by Houghton, J.T. *et al.*] Cambridge University Press, UK.

Jarvis, G.N., Strompl, C., Burgess, D.M., Skillman, L.C., Moore, E.R.B. and Joblin, K.N. (2000). *Curr. Microbiol.*, 40: 327-332.

Jayanegara, A., Togtokhbayar, N., Makkar, H.P.S. and Becker, K. (2009). *Anim. Feed Sci. Technol.*, 150: 230-237.

Jones, G. A., McAllister, T. A., Muir, A. D. and Cheng, K. J. (1994). *Appl. Environ. Microbiol.*, 60: 1374-1378.

Kamra, D.N., Agarwal, N. and Chaudhary, L.C. (2006). Inhibition of ruminal methanogenesis by tropical plants containing secondary compounds. *International Congress Series* 1293, 156-163.

Kamra, D.N., Perera, A.N.F., Xie, Z.-Q. and Diao, Q.Y. (2009). The use of plant secondary metabolites as medicine and feed additives for eco-friendly livestock production. In : *Harvesting Knowledge – Pharming Opportunities*. Eds. J.R. Scaife and P.E. Vercoe, pp 8-20.

Kamra, D.N., Singh, R., Agarwal, N. and Pathak, N.N. (2000). *Buffalo J.*, 16: 99-104.

Klieve, A. and Hegarty, R.S. (1999). *Aust. J. Agric. Res.*, 50: 1315-1319.

Klieve, A.V., Gregg, K., Bauchop, T. (1991). *Curr. Micro.*, 23: 183-187.

Klieve, A.V., Hudman J.F., Bauchop, T. (1989). *Appl. Env. Micro.*, 55: 1630-1634.

Klieve, A.V., Swain, R.A. (1993). *Appl. Env. Micro.*, 59: 2299-2303.

Kozelov, L., Tliev, F., Profirov, J., Nikolov, IV. S., Ganev, G. Modeva, T. and Krasteva, M. (2001). The effect of supplementing sheep with Ropadiar on digestibility and fermentation in the rumen. *Zhivotnov" dni Nuki*, 38: 152-154.

Krumholz, L.R. and Bryant, M.P. (1986). *Arch. Microbiol.*, 144: 8-14.

Kumar, R. (2007). Effect of plant extracts on *in vitro* methanogenesis and microbial diversity in the rumen of buffalo. Ph.D. Thesis, IVRI Deemed to be University, IVRI, Izatnagar, India.

Kumar, R., Kamra, D.N., Agarwal, N. and Chaudhary, L.C. (2007). *Asian-Aust. J. Anim. Sci.*, 20: 1196-1200.

Leedle, J.A.Z. and Greening, R.C. (1988). *Appl. Env. Micro.* 54: 502-506.

Ljungdahl, L. (1986). *Appl. Environ. Microbiol.*, 40: 415-450.

Losa, R. and Brufau, J. (2001). The use of essential oils in animal nutrition. Feed manufacturing in the Mediterranean region. Improving safety: from feed to ffod. Proceedings of the III Conference of Feed Manufacturers of the Mediterranean organised by ASFAC, 22-24 March, 2000. *Cahiers Options Mediterraneennes*, 54: 39-44.

Lowry, J.B. and Kennedy, P.M. (1996). *Proc. Aust. Soc. Anim. Prod.*, 21:366.

Lu, C.D. and Jorgensen, N.A. (1987). *J. Nutr.*, 117: 919-927.

Makkar, H.P.S. and Becker, K. 1997. Degradation of quillaja saponins by mixed culture of rumen microbes. *Lett. Appl. Microbiol.*, 25: 243-245.

Makkar, H.P.S., Sen, S., Blummel, M. and Becker, K. (1998). *J. Agric. Food Chem.*, 46: 4324-4328.

Makkar, H.P.S.; Blummel, M. and Becker, K. (1995). *J. Sci. Food Agric.* 69: 481-493.

McAllister, T.A., Okine, E.K., Mathison, G.W. and Cheng, K.N. (1996). *Can. J. Anim. Sci.*, 76: 231-243.

McMahon, L.R., Majak, W., McAllister, T.A., Hall, J.W., Jones, G.A., Popp, J.D. and Cheng, K.J. (1999). *Can. J. Anim. Sci.*, 79: 203–212.

McSweeney, C.S., Palmer, B., Bunch, R. and Krause, D.O. (2001b). *J. Appl. Microbiol.*, 90: 78-88.

McSweeney, C.S., Palmer, B., Kennedy, P.M. and Krause, D.O. (1998). *Proc. Aust. Soc. Anim. Prod.*, 22: 289.

McSweeney, C.S., Palmer, B., McNeill, D.M. and Krause, D.O. (2001a). *Anim. Feed Sci. Technol.*, 91: 83-93.

Min, B.R., Attwood, G.T., Reilly, K., Sun, W., Peters, J.S., Barry, T.N. and McNabb, W.C. (2002). *Can. J. Anim. Sci.*, 48:911-921.

Mirzoeva, O.K., Grishanin, R.N. and Calder, P.C. (1997). *Microbial Res.* 152: 239-246.

Morvan, B., Doré, J., Rieu-Lesme, F., Foucat, L., Fonty, G. and Gouet, P. (1994). FEMS *Microbiol. Letters,* 117: 249-256.

Muhammed, S., Stewart, C.S. and Acamovic, T. (1995). *Anim. Sci.*, 60: 550A.

Murdiati, T.B., McSweeny, C.S. and Lowry, J.B. (1992). *Aust. J. Agric. Res.*, 43: 1307-1319.

Navas-Camacho, A., Laredo, M.A., Cuesta, A., Anzola, H. and Leon, J.C. (1993). *Livestock Res. Rural Develop.*, 5: 58-71.

Nelson, K.E., Thonney, M.L., Woolston, T.K., Zinder, S.H. and Pell, A.N. (1998). *Appl. Environ. Microbiol.* 64: 3824-3830.

Newbold, C.J., McIntosh, F.M., Wallace, R.J., Williams, P. and Sutton, J.D. (1999). Effects of essential oils on ammonia production by rumen fluid *in vitro.* Book of Abstracts of VIII Intern. Sump. Protein Metabol. Nutr., P63.

Newbold, C.J., El-Hassan, S.M., Wang, J., Ortega, M.E. and Wallace, R.J. (1997). *Brit. J. Nutr.*, 78: 237-249.

Nollet, L., Mbanzamihigo, L., Demeyer, D. and Verstraete, W. (1997). *Anim. Feed Sci. Technol.*, 71: 47-64.

Odenyo, A., Osuji, P.O. and Karanfil, O. (1997). *Anim. Feed Sci. Technol.*, 67: 169.

Oh, H.K., Jones, M.B. and Longhurst, W.M. (1967). *Appl. Microbiol.*, 15: 777-784.

Oh, H.K., Jones, M.B. and Longhurst, W.M. (1968). *Appl. Microbiol.*, 16: 39-44.

Patra, A.K., Kamra, D.N. and Agarwal, N. (2006a). *Anim. Feed Sci. Technol.*, 128: 276-291.

Patra, A.K., Kamra, D.N. and Agarwal, N. (2006b). *Anim. Nutr. Feed Technol.*, 6: 203-213.

Patra, A.K., Kamra, D.N. and Agarwal, N. (2006c). Effect of spices on rumen fermentattaion, methanogenesis and protozoa counts in *in vitro* gas production test. *International Congress Series,* 1293: 176-179.

Paul, S.S., Kamra, D.N., Sastry, V.R.B. and Sahu, N.P. (2006). *J. Sci. Food Agric.*, 86: 258-270.

Prins, R.A. and Lankhorst, A. (1977). *FEMS Microbiol. Lett.*, 1: 255-258.

Puchala, R., Min B. R., Goetsch A.L. aand Sahlu T. (2005). *J. Anim. Sci.*, 83: 182-186.

Sahoo, B., Sarawat M.L., Haque, N. and Khan, M.Y. (2000). *Small Ruminant Res.*, 35: 13-19.

Salawu, M.B., Acamovic, T., Stewart, C.S. and Hovell, F.D. De, B. (1999). *Anim. Sci.*, 69: 265-274.

Salem, H.B., Nefzaoui, A., Salem, L.B. Tisserand, J.L. Ben-Salem, H. and Ben-Salem, L. (1997). *Anim. Feed Sci. Technol.*, 68: 101-113.

Saraswat, M.L., Haque, N., Sengar, S.S. and Tomar, S.K. (2001). *Indian J. Anim. Sci.*, 71: 363-366.

Saravanan, T.S. (2000). Effect of bromochloromethane on methanogenesis, nutrient utilization and growth rate of lambs. M.V.Sc. thesis, IVRI, Izatnagar, India.

Schneider, H., Schwiertz, A., Collins, M.D. and Blaut, M. (1999). *Arch. Microbiol.*, 171: 81-91.

Simpson, F.J., Jones, G.A. and Wolin, E.A. (1969). *Can. J. Microbiol.*, 15: 972-974.

Singh, G.P. and Mohini, M. (1999). *Indian J. Dairy Biosci.*, 10: 14–19.

Stack, R.J., Hungate and R.E. Opsahl, W.P. (1983). *Appl. Environ. Microbiol.*, 46: 539-544.

Tagari, H., Heins, Y., Tamir, M. and Volcani, R. (1965). *Appl. Microbiol.*, 13: 437-442.

Tavendale, M.H., Meagher, I.P., Pacheco, D., Walker, N., Atwood, G.T. and Subathira, S. (2005). *Anim. Feed Sci.Technol.*, 123/124: 403-419.

Teferedegne, B., McIntosh, F., Osuji, P.O., Odenyo, A., Wallace, R.J. and Newbold, C.J. (1999). *Anim. Feed Sci. Technol.*, 78: 11-20.

Terrill, T.H., Douglas, G.B., Foote, A.G., Purchas, R.W., Wilson, G.F. and Barry, T.N. (1992). *J. Agric. Sci.*, 119: 265-273.

Thalib, A., Widiawati, Y., Hamid, H., Suherman, D. and Sabrani, M. (1996). *Jurnal Ilmu Ternak dan Veteriner*, 2(1): 17-21.

Valdez, F.R., Bush, L.J., Goetsch, A.L. and Owen, F.N. (1986). *J. Dairy Sci.*, 69: 1568-1575.

Van Soest, P.J. (1994). *Nutritional Ecology of the Ruminants*. Second edition, Cornell University Press, Ithaca, USA.

Waghorn, G.C., Tavendale, M.H. and Woodfield, D.R. (2002). *Proc. New Zealand Grassl. Assoc.*, 64: 167-171.

Wallace, R.J. (2004). *Proc. Nutr. Soc.*, 63: 621–629.

Wallace, R.J., McEwan, N. R., McIntosh, F.M., Teferedenge, B. and Newbold, C.J. (2002). *Asian-Aust. J. Anim.*15: 1458-1468.

Wallace, R.J., Arthaud, L. and Newbold, C.J. (1994). *Appl. Environ. Microbiol.*, 60: 1762-1767.

Wallace, R.J., Wood, T.A., Rowe, A., Price, J., Yanez, D.R., Williams, S.P. and Newbold, C.J. (2006). Encapsulated fumaric acid as a means of decreasing ruminal methane emissions. *International Congress Series*, 1293: 148–151.

Wang, Y., McAllister, T.A., Newbold, C.J., Rode, L.M., Cheeke, P.R. and Cheng, K.-J. (1998). *Anim. Feed Sci. Technol.*, 74: 143-153.

Wang, Y., T.A. Mcallister, L.J. Yanke, Z.J. Xu, P.R. Cheeke, and K.J. Cheng. (2000). *J. Sci. Food Agric.*, 80: 2114-2112.

Weimer, P.J. (1998). *J. Anim. Sci.*, 76: 3114-3122.

Whitford, M.F., Teather, R.M. and Forster R.J. (2001). Phylogenetic analysis of methanogens from the bovine rumen. *BMC Microbiology,* www.biomedcentral.com/1471-2180/1/5.

Williams, Y.J., Popovski, S., Rea, S.M., Skillman, L.C., Toovey, A.F., Northwood, K.S. and Wright, A.G. (2009). *Appl. Environ. Microbiol.,* 75 :1860-1866.

Wina, E., Muetzel, S., Hoffmann, E., Makkar, S.P.S. and Becker, K. (2005). *Anim. Feed Sci. Technol.,* 121: 159-174.

Winter, J., Moore, L. H. Dowell, V. R. Jr. and Bokkenheuser, V. D. (1989). *Appl. Environ. Microbiol.,* 55: 1203-1208.

Wiryawan, K.G., Tangendjaja, B., Suryahadi and Brooker, J.D. (1999). Proc. an International Workshop, Adelaide, Australia, 31 May to 2 June, pp.123-126.

Woodward, S.L., Waghorn G.C., Lassey K.R. and Laboyrie, P.G. (2001). *Proc. New Zealand Soc. Anim. Prod.,* 61: 23-26.

Woodward, S.L., Waghorn, G.C., Lassey, K.R. and Laboyric, P.G. (2002). *Proc. New Zealand Soc. Anim. Prod.,* 62: 227-230.

□□□

Animal Nutrition, 2012
eds. Dr. (Mrs.) Usha R. Mehra et al., pp. 691-706
Satish Serial Publishing House e-mail : info@satishserial.com; website : www.satishserial.com

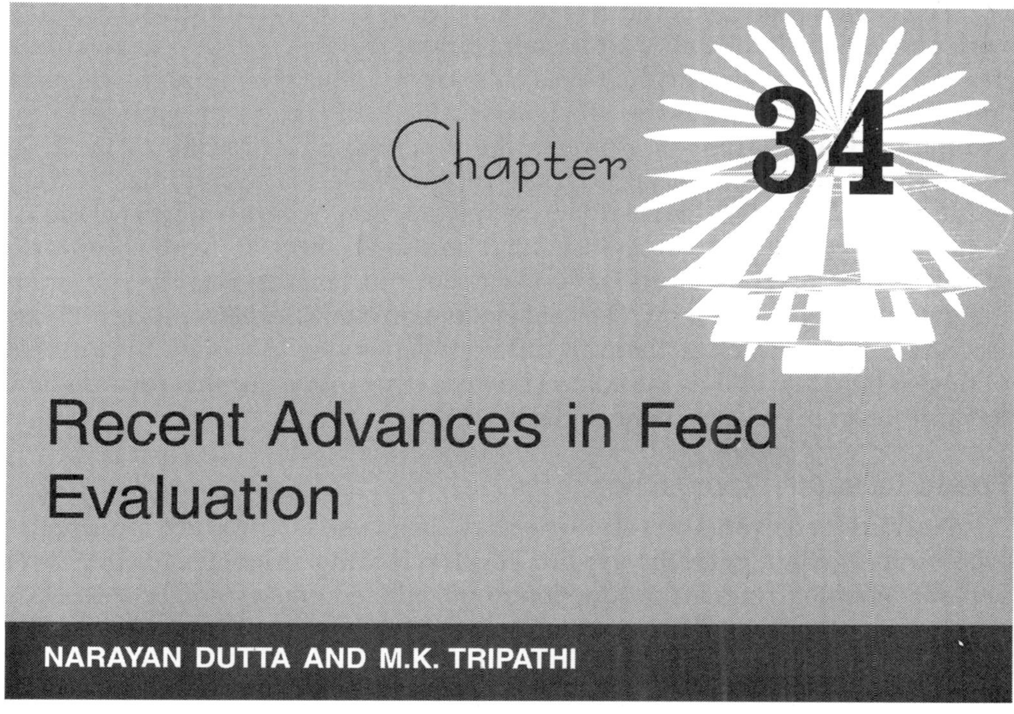

Recent Advances in Feed Evaluation

NARAYAN DUTTA AND M.K. TRIPATHI

Livestock production is a major component of agricultural economy in developing countries like India and goes well beyond direct food production. Though, ruminant production in mixed farming is largely limited by forage quality, which is mainly reflected in low intake and digestibility. Poor nutrition results in low rates of production, reproduction as well as increased susceptibility to different diseases. This is because animals thrive primarily on poor quality roughages (cereal straws and stovers), which are deficient in nutrients (protein and minerals, etc.) essential for microbial fermentation. Consequently, the digestibility and intake of digestible nutrients are very low. These deficiencies can partly be mitigated by supplementing roughage diets with feeds containing the deficient nutrients. Roughage diets and supplements may differ vastly in quality and therefore in the quantity eaten by the animal. A perceptive of the factors which affect rumen degradability of low-quality basal feeds and microbial protein production will assist the nutritionists in formulating diets that will be utilized more efficiently. There are several techniques, which are being used for feed and fodder evaluation.

Feed evaluation concerns the use of methods to describe animal feedstuffs with respect to their ability to sustain different types and levels of animal performance. The feed evaluation goals are to determine specific chemical constituent and optimize the efficiency of feed utilization by animals. Feed evaluation is important to establish the potential of feedstuffs to meet the requirement and need for appropriate supplementation to optimize nutrient requirement for desired level of animal production. Apart from the chemical entities of feed, animal response such as the amount of feed voluntarily consumed, digestion and utilization of major nutrient are also the important indicators of feed evaluation. The feed evaluation characteristics allow different feedstuffs to characterize them in different categories. Accurate information of the feedstuffs provides the correct balance of nutrients for diet formulations to fulfill nutrient requirement of the animal.

Feed-Evaluation Approaches

Various feed evaluation strategies have been used to produce information when put together, could be used to develop feeding strategies for improved and sustainable ruminant production in mixed farming system. It is expected that new methods evolved or modified will give a new dimension to feed evaluation approach.

Indirect Methods for Feed Evaluation

Chemical Composition of Feeds

Henneberg and Stochman, at Weende Experiment Station in Germany, proposed a scheme of chemical analysis of feeds and fodders in 1865. Under this scheme various nutrients that had some common properties were grouped together and analyzed. These nutrients are known as proximate principles of feeds. In this system of analysis, feedstuffs are analyzed into water, crude protein, ether extract, crude fibre, nitrogen free extract and ash. The chemical composition of feeds gives only the potential value of the feed stuffs but it does not give the actual nutritive value of the feed stuffs until the losses of nutrients in faeces, urine, gases etc from animal during digestion, absorption and metabolism are also taken into consideration. Nutrients present in the feed stuffs are not completely available to the body. Large portion of the nutrients are excreted in the faeces because of being not digested in the alimentary tract. This approach proved to be inadequate in feed evaluation.

The chemical analysis of ruminant feeds generally involves estimation of dry matter (DM), organic matter (OM), structural carbohydrates (fibre and non starch polysaccharides; (NSP), soluble carbohydrates, starch and crude protein (CP) content. Evaluation of silage requires further analysis of the pH, organic acid, ammonia nitrogen and true protein content. The DM of feedstuffs is determined by oven drying the samples to a constant weight at 60 or 100°C, while silage DM by distillation after toluene treatment due to high content of volatile organic acids. OM is determined by difference after ashing feed sample at 500°C for 4 hours (AOAC, 2005) that removes carbon (organic matter) and residue can be used for the determination of individual mineral elements of feedstuff.

The widely used method for the analysis of structural constituents of feed is the detergent extraction method of Van Soest *et al.* (1991). This new method proposes to use 0.5 g sample and addition of 50 ml heat stable amylase, the use of sodium sulfite was optional for NDF measurement. Other steps for the estimation of NDF, ADF, lignin and silica were more or less similar to previous procedure. These are gravimetric procedures that involve extraction of feedstuff with neutral detergent solution to leave a fibrous residue known as neutral detergent fibre (NDF) contain predominantly cellulose, hemicellulose and lignin. The residue left after extraction with acid detergent solution contain cellulose and lignin and known as acid detergent fibre (ADF). The exact composition of NDF and ADF residue is not known. The fibre content of feed may be described more accurately by non-starch polysaccharides (NSP) analysis, by quantification of carbohydrates monomers that derived from acid hydrolysis of de-starched samples. The NSP analysis provides detail of the chemical composition of the fibre, the amount present can be quantified more accurately because measured values are independent of feed processing and storage. Recently, Hendrickson *et al.* (2006) suggested enzymatic-chemical procedure of fibre analysis. Hemicellulose, cellulose and lignin contents of feeds, concentrate ingredients, complete concentrates and faeces were analyzed using the Van Soest detergent procedure (analyzing NDF, ADF, and Acid Detergent Lignin (ADL)) and the enzymatic-chemical procedure (analyzing cellulose, soluble and insoluble noncellulosic polysaccharides, and Klason lignin (KL)). Klason lignin is determined as the unhydrolyzed residue remaining after the two-stage sulfuric acid hydrolysis for the determination of total dietary fibre according to the method of (Theander and Westerlund, 1986). The detergent method and the enzymatic-chemical method are equivalent with respect to cellulose. However, soluble hemicellulose in concentrate was partly detected by the detergent procedure, and the procedure is therefore not suitable for all kinds of concentrates. The detergent system detected low hemicellulose contents indicate that a certain percentage of soluble hemicellulose might have been dissolved in neutral detergent solution. However, measuring hemicellulose content in the faeces by the detergent method, in which no significant amounts of residual soluble hemicelluloses are expected, still resulted in lower hemicellulose contents. Cellulose digestibility as determined by the detergent method seems to be quite reliable because the values were close to line of equality when related to the enzymatic-chemically derived data. The detergent system underestimated lignin contents, when determined as ADL and would have even increased the hemicellulose estimate. Weaknesses were found for ADL as a measure for lignin and for both ADL and KL as an indicator of fiber digestibility in comparison where the major variations occur in concentrates and where ingredients with high amounts of soluble hemicellulose or with an uneven lignin distribution and association with fiber are used. The low accuracy of dietary lignin in concentrate-dominated diets to predict fiber digestibility was compared with mainly on forage-dominated diets. Therefore, lignin is only a reliable indicator of fiber digestibility in diets in which the dietary lignin content is mainly supplied by the forage and Klason lignin correlated more closely with the measured fibre digestibility than ADL.

The crude protein content of feedstuffs is usually determined by the Kjeldahl procedure that involves acid digestion and distillation. More recent method of CP estimation is the combustion and determination of released gaseous N. The ammonia N is determined in water extracts by either distillation or use of specific ion-sensitive electrode. These methods measure N and CP content is calculated from the N content multiplied by 6.25 to obtain approximate protein value, assuming that the N is derived from protein containing 16 percent nitrogen.

Near Infrared Reflectance Spectroscopy (NIRS) Techniques

Near infrared reflectance spectroscopy (NIRS) is the recently adopted method for the feed quality evaluation. The NIRS is based on calibrations to define reference methods, and their correlation to absorption of light at different wave lengths in the near infrared region, which is measured by reflectance from sample material. This technique is preferred over traditional laboratory methods because of accuracy, precision, speed and unit cost of analysis. However, technique ultimately relies on a set of standard samples whose composition has been determined by traditional methods. The ability to predict chemical composition using NIRS was very good for residual moisture, starch, ADF, NDF and CP but moderate for CF and ADL and low for ash (De Boever *et al.*, 1997). The NIRS also predicted rumen degradation characteristics and ME value of the feedstuffs. Givens *et al.* (1991) compared the results of three *in-vitro* procedures (rumen-fluid pepsin, pepsin cellulose and neutral detergent - cellulose) with NIRS to predict organic matter digestibility of cereal straw. The NIRS predicted the OMD of cereal straw more accurately than *in-vitro* procedures. However, NIRS predicted OMD and energy values of silages somewhat lower than *in vitro* methods (De Boever *et al.*, 1997). NIRS can predict precise *in-vivo* OMD of silages by developing calibration using second order modified least square regression (Baker *et al.*, 1994). Ngonyamo-Majee *et al.* (2008) used NIRS for breeding trials to develop corn hybrids of desired properties for improved rumen degradability. Kinetic parameters of nutrient degradation were developed as reference method using *in vitro* methods to develop calibration equations of NIRS (Wilman *et al.*, 2000 and Andres *et al.*, 2005). The *in-situ* procedures as reference methods were developed for measurement of indigestible NDF and NIRS predicted precise *in-situ* NDF degradation (Nousiainem *et al.*, 2004). Using NIRS *in-situ* NDF degradation characteristics and developed calibration equations, Nordheim *et al.* (2007) predicted INDF (indigestible NDF estimated using heat stable amylase and inclusive of residual ash) and fractional degradation rate of NDF (kdNDF); but the lag time could not be predicted. To determine the digestibility and ME value of feeds Deaville *et al.* (2008) compared NIRS with laboratory and *in vitro* digestibility measures to predict digestible organic matter in the dry matter (DOMD) and metabolisable energy (ME) contents measured *in vivo* using sheep. Spectral models using the mean spectra of two scans were compared with those using individual spectra (duplicate spectra). Overall NIRS accurately predicted the concentration of chemical components in whole crop cereals apart from crude protein, ammonia-nitrogen, water-soluble carbohydrates, fermentation acids and solubility values. In addition, the spectral models had higher prediction power for *in vivo* DOMD and ME than chemical components or *in vitro* digestion methods. {Overall there was a benefit from the use of duplicate spectra rather than mean spectra and especially for predicting *in vivo* DOMD and ME where the sample population size was smaller}. The spectral models derived, deal equally well with whole crop wheat and whole crop barley and would be of considerable practical value allowing rapid determination of nutritive value of these forages before their use in diets of productive animals.

Indicator Methods for Measuring Digestibility

AIA and Lignin Technique

Apparent digestibility of a feeds and fodders can be estimated using a natural constituent of the feed as an internal indicator or an external indicator. Acid insoluble ash (AIA) or lignin can be used as natural indicator for the estimation of dry-matter intake and digestibility. During the collection period faecal grab samples may be collected at five representative times a day and the feed used in the experiment analysed for AIA/ lignin. The ratio between the concentration of AIA/lignin in the feed and the faeces gives an estimate of digestibility.

Digestibility of DM = 100 - [100 (AIA concentration in diet)/ (AIA concentration in faeces)]

By feeding of external indicator, there is no need of harnessing the animals with faeces bags.

N- Alkanes Technique

Feed evaluation in grazing animals remained an issue for researcher due to difficulties incurred in measurement of intake and digestibility therefore need felt to develop quick and accurate method that should not disturb animal at grazing. The use of N-alkanes have been tried to estimate diet composition of domestic animals (Salt *et al.*, 1992; Duncan *et al.*, 1999 and Hutchings *et al.*, 2000) and of wild herbivores (Bugalho *et al.*, 2001; Hulbert *et al.*, 2001 and Rao *et al.*, 2003). N-alkanes are long-chain saturated hydrocarbons that occur widely in plant cuticles and can be used as internal chemical markers for estimating intake, digestibility and the diet composition in herbivores by recovering them in the faeces as they are chemically inert (Mayes and Dove, 2000; Dove and Mayes, 2005). Since plant species are characterized by different concentrations of N-alkanes, the chemical markers recovered in faeces can be used to identify and quantify the plants ingested by herbivores. The technique is based on long chain n-Alkanes (aliphatic hydrocarbons) estimation that is inherently present in the waxes of plant species. This technique, in contrast to widely used chromic oxide technique, does not require an independent assessment of digestibility, nor does it rely on the quantitative recovery of the dosed n-alkanes as a marker. Alkanes generally show a relatively low reactivity, because their 'C' bonds are relatively stable and cannot be easily broken. The possible role of alkanes as internal markers was also suggested to estimate digestibility. The double alkane method estimates the intake, digestibility and diet composition of grazing and browsing ruminants (Dove and Mayes, 2005) as well as the proportion of organic matter digested and efficiency of microbial protein production in the rumen (Dove *et al.*, 1990). The technique also estimates nutrient composition of diet in animals consuming a feed supplement (Charmley and Dove, 2007). The use of plant wax long chain alcohols in combination with alkanes improve measurement of nutrient composition and intake in grazing sheep (Dove and Charmley, 2008) and the dosing of even chain alkane three times daily minimizes variations in faecal concentration and measured intake, similar to that of directly measurements (Smith *et al.*, 2007). Though the technique is promising but requires complex analysis of plant alkanes and wax long chain alcohols.

Digestibility Estimation for Feed Evaluation

Several methods have been developed to evaluate feedstuffs in terms of digestibility. These are *in vivo, in-sacco* and *in-vitro* methods. The *in-vivo* measurement provides actual measure of digestibility as this represent the response digestive process involved in animal system. However, such trials can not be carried out for all the feedstuffs under different feeding practices because these trails are of more time consuming, labour intensive and thus more expensive. Moreover, facilities for such trials are not available in all laboratories. Therefore number of *in vitro* (batch culture digestibility, enzyme digestibility and gas production) and *in-sacco* (nylon bag digestibility) methods have been developed to estimate digestibility and the extent of ruminal degradation of feed, and variations in response to changes in dietary conditions. These methods are easy, rapid and less expensive hence widely used to generate information about the nature and sensitivity of feed to various changes, and this information is used for the development of mechanistic models of feed quality and diet formulations.

In vitro Technique

In Tilley and Terry (1963) method, substrate is incubated for 48h in rumen inoculum followed by 48h incubation in a pepsin-hydrochloric acid solution. Filtration, drying and ashing procedures are then applied to recover and quantify the unsolubilized dry or organic matter residue. The sequential treatments were designed to mimic ruminal fermentation and abomasal/ intestinal digestion in the animal. *In vitro* digestibilities are calculated as the difference of substrate supplied and recovered in the residue and were correlated well to *in vivo* apparent digestibility in 148 roughages. Further, Goering and Van Soest (1970) replaced the second stage in aforesaid technique by treating the residue obtained after 48h of incubation in rumen inoculum with neutral detergent (ND) solution to get better separation of adherent microbial biomass from the undegraded feed residue than achieved by the pepsin-hydrochloric acid treatment in the original Tilley and Terry (1963) method.

Continuous Culture (in-vitro) Effluent Technique

Simulated rumen fermentation technique was investigated (Barbi *et al.*, 1993) to replace rumen fluid (Rusitec). In this technique continuous flow of culture and effluent is maintained. The sample placed in nylon bags (pore size 25μ) is incubated with rumen fluid in fermenters/reaction vessels for appropriate time depending upon the feed to be tested. The artificial saliva is prepared to simulate the composition of ruminant saliva and flows at a measured flow rate monitored mechanically. The output i.e. effluent and gases are collected in effluent vessel and intact urine bags, respectively (Czerkawski and Breckenridge, 1977). The whole procedure is to simulate continuous culture fermentation of feed that occurs in rumen that accounts for both feed digestibility and gas production. The main drawback of Rusitec was the much lower microbial activity of effluent than that of rumen fluid. Attempts were made to increase microbial activity by decreasing particle size of the feed, increasing feed input and glucose infusion to the Rusitec but these interventions could hardly increase microbial activity and microbial concentration of the effluent flask. By addition of *Selenomonas ruminatium* in continuous cultures; predominant mixed culture of bacteria was maintained up to four months (Van Kessel and Russel, 1996) but methanogens did not persist. Barbi *et al.* (1995) found day to day variations in Rusitec effluent fluid to be similar to that in rumen fluid. The liquid turnover and pH adjustment must be taken into consideration for mixed diets evaluation for ruminants (Fondevela and Perez-Espes, 2008).

Cell Free Enzymes (*in vitro*) Techniques

In this technique, cocktail of cell-free enzymes are used as the source of inocula for *in-vitro* evaluation of feedstuffs. The feed is treated with required concentration of mixed cell-free enzymes for appropriate time and the degradability of feed at different hours of incubation is recorded. This helps in attributing feed value. This technique could overcome the need to maintain experimental animals and provide more consistent inoculum source. To date relatively little has been known to develop means of predicting fermentation dynamics and this approach could be viable for the gas production technique (Rymer *et al.*, 2005) because the enzymes need to be those associated with fermentation.

In vitro Gas-Production Technique

In vitro evaluation of ruminant feeds based on the inoculation of small amounts of substrate with rumen micro-organisms under controlled conditions in the laboratory, is indispensable tools for ruminant nutritionists and rumen microbiologists. These tests are largely free of the disadvantages associated with direct *in vivo* animal experimentation, which is more costly and laborious, more difficult to control and also impractical when only small amounts of feed are available as is often the case in plant breeding programmes. In addition, concerns on animal welfare and ethical issues on use of animals in experiments are increasingly gaining ground. Both factors, practical considerations and ethical reservations, call for further development or improvement of *in vitro* techniques.

Rymer *et al.* (2005) reviewed methodologies used for the measurement of *in vitro* gas production to determine the impact of source of variations on resultant gas production profiles. Under tropical environment where poor quality roughages provide major source of feed energy and animals have a higher rumen pH. The composition of media recommended by Steingass (1983) and Goering and Van Soest (1970) seems to be promising, as these medium maintain a higher final pH. The large source of variation in the gas production is the source of inoculums and activity of the microbial inoculums. To minimize variation in gas production profile the inocula sample should be collected and pooled from more than one animal, the diet and sampling schedule should be designed to minimize variations between runs. Rumen fluid collection from liquid and solid phase before feeding is recommended. The microbial activity of inocula should be determined before inoculation by measuring absorbance at 600 nm after 50 fold dilution of rumen fluid inocula.

Origin of Gas

When a feedstuff is incubated with buffered rumen fluid *in vitro*, the carbohydrates are fermented to short chain fatty acids (SCFA), gases (mainly CO_2 and CH_4) and microbial cells. Gas production is basically the result of fermentation of carbohydrate to acetate, propionate and butyrate. Gas production from protein fermentation is relatively small as compared to carbohydrate fermentation (Wolin, 1960). The contribution of fat to gas production is negligible. The gas produced (CO_2 and CH_4) in this technique is the direct result of fermentation and the indirectly from the buffering of SCFA (CO_2 released from the bicarbonate buffer). For roughages, when bicarbonate buffer is used, about 50% of the total gas is generated from buffering of the SCFAs and the rest is evolved directly from fermentation (Blümmel and Orskov, 1993). At very high molar proportion of propionate (concentrate diets) the amount of CO_2 generated from buffering of SCFA is about 60% of total gas production. Each mmol of SCFA produced from fermentation releases 0.8 - 1.0 mmol of CO_2 from the buffered rumen fluid solution, depending on the amount of phosphate buffer present (Blümmel and Fernandez-Rivera, 2002). Gas is produced mainly when substrate is fermented to acetate and butyrate. Substrate fermentation to propionate yields gas only from buffering of the acid and, therefore relatively lower gas production is associated with the propionate production.

Stoichiometry of Gas Production

An important aspect of gas production in anaerobic system is that stoichiometric laws of fermentation balance can be applied since fermentation products must be derived from substrate incubated. High correlation between stoichiometrically calculated gas and actually recorded values has been reported (Blümmel and Orskov, 1993; Blümmel and Fernandez-Rivera, 2002). The stoichiometric balance allows the theoretical calculation of equilibrated amounts of the products (SCFA and gases) (VanSoest, 1994). If the molar proportion and amount of SCFA are known, the theoretical amounts of CH_4 and CO_2 expected from the rumen fermentation can be calculated.

Implications of the Relationship between Gas and SCFA Production

Short chain fatty acids can provide most or all of the ruminants' energy requirements. *In vitro* gas production can, therefore, be considered as an estimate of the energy potential of a feed. SCFA's are only one of the two major useful products of rumen degradation, the other being microbial biomass (MB). SCFAs and MB are linked in that adenosine triphosphate (ATP) is generated along the SCFA and ATP is a major source of energy for maintenance and growth of rumen microorganism. It is generally assumed that each mmol of acetate, propionate and butyrate results in the production of 2, 3 and 3 mmol of ATP, respectively. Additionally, 1 mmol of ATP is produced with each mmol of CH_4. Thus, 1 mmol of SCFA with 0.65 A, 0.25 P and 0.1 B would yield 2.66 mmol of ATP. It is important to realize that all products, i.e. SCFA, gases and MB must be derived from the degraded feed, which they must balance. A general inverse relationship between SCFA and MBP production per unit substrate degraded has been observed. However, SCFA and gas production is closely related.

OMTDR = SCFA+GAS + MBP

Microbial Protein Supply using Total Urine Excretion of Purine Derivatives

Several methods have been proposed for the estimation of microbial protein synthesized by rumen micro-organisms. Most of them require elaborate cannulation (duodenal canulae to estimate MBP arriving at duodenum) of the animal and expensive instruments for the analysis of the diverse microbial markers (e.g. diaminopimelic acid (DAPA), aminoethylphosphoric acid (AEPA), RNA and amino acid labeled with ^{35}S, ^{32}P, and ^{15}N). Some researchers have recently recognized the need for simpler and non-invasive procedures for the determination of the daily synthesis of microbial protein. Such methods involve the use of either total urinary purine derivatives (PD), i.e. the sum of allantoin, hypoxanthine, xanthine and uric acid or allantoin alone (Dewhurst and Webster, 1988). Purine derivatives are the products of nucleic acid metabolism that are considered to consist chiefly of microbial biomass from rumen and get degraded at duodenal level. The end products of duodenal digestion are converted to urea in liver and directed towards kidney; where it is further converted to allantoin, uric acid, xanthine and hypoxanthine. Depending upon species these PD are reabsorbed and occur in body fluids in different concentrations. The concentration of PD in urine, plasma, milk or saliva thus indicates the nutritional status of ruminant.

These methods are currently being developed such that the ratio of the concentration of either PD or allantoin to creatinine in spot urine or plasma samples or PDC index could be used to diagnose the nutritional status of animals (Chen *et al.*, 1992). Results obtained with these methods are comparable to those obtained with conventional methods. However, because of assumptions about the proportions of purines salvaged and the endogenous contribution, the urinary purine derivatives are good indicators only of relative dietary differences.

In-SACCO (nylon-bag) Feed Evaluation Technique

The nylon-bag technique is a very simple and useful biological tool for *in vivo* animal nutrition studies. This technique provides a means of ranking feeds according to the rate and extent of degradation of various nutrients (Mehrez and Orskov, 1977). It involves incubating samples of feeds in the rumen of fistulated animals for 0 to 72 hours and subsequent determination of the disappearance of the different feed components. The nylon-bag technique is very simple and appropriate method for nutritional evaluation of large number of samples. The nylon-bag technique uses bags (17 x 9 cm) made of nylon mesh (30–50 μm). A sample of known weight is tightly sealed in the nylon bags and placed in the rumen of a fistulated animal. After the required period of time, the sample is removed, washed, dried and weighed. Degradability (or disappearance) of the substrate is determined by the weight loss during the incubation period. The dried residue may also be used for chemical analyses. The pore size of the bags must allow entry of rumen microbes and escape of accumulated gases, and keep solid particle losses to a minimum. The efflux of feed particles from the bags without breakdown by rumen microbes is corrected by using zero-hour bags. These bags are filled with the substrate but are not incubated in the rumen; they are washed and dried in the same way as the incubated bags. Furthermore, the zero-hour bags are used to correct for passage of material from pressure applied to the nylon bags during washing.

The extent of degradation of various feeds using nylon-bag technique depends on various factors viz how the bags are placed in the rumen, particle size of sample vis-à-vis the pore size of the nylon bag, loss of feed particles through the bag cloth (a function of fineness of grinding, cloth pore size and feed material), method of washing, the length of time that the samples are incubated in the rumen and the rumen environment in which degradability is determined. The disappearance (%) may be calculated using the formula:

Disappearance (%) = (A-B) x D – (C-B) x E/ (A-B) x D

Where: A = Weight of the original sample + nylon bag, B = Weight of empty, nylon bag, C = Weight of the sample + nylon bag after incubation, D = Dry matter of feed sample, E = Dry matter of residue sample.

The fermentation kinetics of substrate can be estimated by fitting DM/N disappearance in single exponential equations proposed by Orskov and McDonald (1979) or by McDonald (1981) with and without lag phase.

$Y = a + b\,(1-e^{-ct})$......... Ørskov and McDonald (1979)

$Y = a + b\,(1-e^{-c\,(t-tl)})$..... McDonald (1981) model with lag

Where: Y = degradability at time (t), a = intercept, b = potentially degradable fraction, c = rate of degradation of b, tl = lag time.

In addition, Borderick and Cochran (2000) reviewed available *in-situ* methods used for the estimation of feed and nutrient digestibility in the gastrointestinal tract and recommended standard procedure considering the basal diet fed to animals, bag, sample and animal characteristics, replication, incubation method, rinsing/ bag washing technology and microbial corrections.

Table 1 : Recommended procedure for ruminal *in-situ* trial (Borderick and Cochran, 2000)

Attribute	Recommendation
Basal diet	
Type	60:40 roughage (dry) to concentrate
Level of feeding	Maintenance
Bag	
Material	Polyester
Pore size	40-60 μm
Sample size: surface area	10-15 mg cm^{-2}
Sample grind size	
Concentrates	2 mm
Roughages	2 mm
Animal Species	Adult cattle or sheep (or species of application if used other than cattle or sheep)
Replication	
No of animals	2
No of days	2
No of bags	1
Pre-incubation	None
Incubation conditions	
Position in rumen	Ventral sac (free movement)
Entry/ removal order	If standardized mechanical rinsing is used, sequential removal seems viable. Otherwise, sequential entry followed by removal and rinsing at the same time seems advisable.
Times	Adequate to describe curve
Rinsing	Machine: five 1-min rinses and 2-min spin at the low water setting (~45 l)
Microbial correction	Yes, when residue detected
Standard feed	Yes, if available

Recommendation for *in situ* Procedure for Post Ruminal Digestion

The current application of the mobile bag procedure was recommended by Borderick and Cochran, (2000) for the post ruminal *in-situ* method. A small sample (1.0 -1.5 g for concentrate or ruminally digested material, 0.5 - 1.2 g for forages) into small polyester bag (25 X 40 mm for swine and 35 X 50 mm for cattle) having a pore size of approximately 40-50 µm. For monogastric animals, pre-treatment of samples with acid-pepsin is required before placement in duodenum. Bags are generally collected from the faeces and the rinsing procedure is similar to ruminal *in-situ* procedures.

Direct Method for Feed Evaluation

Determination of Feed Intake and Digestibility Coefficient

Voluntary intake is determined by offering animals a known quantity of feed and determining the amount remaining at the end of the feeding period. Digestion and retention coefficients are determined by collecting all the excreta (mainly urine and faeces) for analyzing feed and excreta samples. The amount of various nutrients absorbed and retained in the body or stored can also be determined by analyzing urine and other products such as milk. It will take about 23-28 days for the evaluation of nutritive value of any feeds. The animals may be offered feed *ad libitum* with minimum of 20–25% uneaten feed. The first 14-21 days of the experiment are preliminary or adaptation period followed by a collection period of 5-7 days during metabolism trial.

Calculations

Voluntary dry-matter intake and apparent dry-matter digestibility of the feed may be calculated as follows:

Average daily dry-matter intake = A – B

Apparent dry-matter digestibility (%) = (A-B-C/A-B) X100

Where:
A = Avg. dry matter offered daily
B = Avg. dry matter refused daily
C = Avg. dry matter voided in faeces daily.

Comparative Feeding Trial

The direct evaluation of unit cost of a feed or its nutritional value as compared to a standard/conventional feed may be made by use of comparative feeding trials and measuring the parameters as said above. By feeding a group of animal (minimum 6 animals in each group) with standard feed and another group of identical animals (in respect of body weight, age, sex, species, breed and production levels etc.) with test feed; information regarding availability of various nutrients, feed cost per unit gain in live weight etc. can be arrived at easily. However, this direct measurement technique rather proves uneconomical and can consider very few feeds at a time.

Nonetheless, a researcher can emanate newer strategies like supplementation of deficient nutrients (e.g. minerals, urea etc.) with a cheaper new feed to reduce cost of production.

Real Time PCR Technique

Most recently, real-time PCR technique has been proposed due to the problem of accuracy in predicting available energy from a total mixed ration which is limited because of variation in digestibility of individual feedstuffs from predicted values in response to associative effects. To overcome this limitation, plant-specific real-time PCR assays can be used to predict the digestion of individual feeds within a total mixed ration (Alexander *et al.*, 2009). In this technique 0.5 g dry matter is incubated in buffered rumen fluid at pH 6.8 or 5.5 for up to 48 h. Regression analysis between DNA disappearance and dry matter disappearance (DMD) of feed under evaluation is used to predict DMD in mixed rations, after plant-specific DNA quantification. The actual DM remaining is compared against the total predicted DM remaining by summing the individual values predicted for individual feedstuff in the mixed rations. The method is accurate and precise in predicting DM remaining (Concordance and Pearson correlations were 0.89 and 0.91, respectively). Difference between coefficients of the actual and total predicted DM ranges from -0.081 to 0.087 or -0.08 to 0.09 when the pH is 6.8 or 5.5, respectively. Furthermore, by analyzing substrate incubated at pH 5.5, the method tested in the presence of an associative effect (reduced pH) known to inhibit fibre digestion but have limited consequence on starch utilization. The method predicted DMD in agreement with the expected results. The DMD is significantly affected by interactions between time and pH or between diet and pH, and DMD was affected by time or diet. This lead to redefined models to more effectively predict the available energy of individual feedstuffs within a total mixed ration.

Low-copy plant genes (less than 10 copies per cell genome) have been detected in the ruminant digestive tract associated only with solid feed residues, and an inverse relationship between plant cell degradation and persistence of plant cell DNA has been observed (Alexander *et al.*, 2004 and Phipps *et al.*, 2003). The unique plant DNA markers may provide the means to estimate the digestibility of specific plant cells within a mixed diet. The real-time PCR assays specific to test feed may be used to estimate dry matter disappearance (DMD) within a diet during fermentation. Microbial DNA, likely to dilute plant DNA to varying extents is determined by the length of fermentation and/or type of fermentation substrate. To account this variation, the amount of feed DNA is quantified in 200 ng of extracted DNA used to calculate the total amount (DM basis) of each feed-specific type of DNA remaining at every point for individual substrates throughout fermentation. These observations are used to determine total DNA disappearance of test substrates.

References

Alexander, T.W., Sharma, R., Deng, M.Y., Whetsell, A.J., Jennings, J.C., Wang, Y., Okine, E., Damgaard, D. and McAllister, T.A. (2004). *J. Biotechnol.*, 112: 255–266.

Alexander, T.W., Wang, Y., Reuter, T., Okine, E.K., Dixon, W.T. and McAllister, T.A. (2009). *Anim. Feed Sci. Technol.*, 149:240-249.

Andres, S., Giraldez, F.J., Gonzaliz, J.S., Pelaez, R., Priets, N. and Calloja, A., (2005). *Austr. J. Agri. Res.*, 56: 187-193.

AOAC (2000). Offical Methods of Analysis of the AOAC International. 17th Edition, Vol. 1-2, AOAC International. Gailtherburg. MD. USA.

Baker, C.W., Givens, D.I. and Deaville, E.R. (1994). *Anim. Feed Sci. Technol.*, 50 :17-26.

Barbi, J.H.T., Owen, E. and Theodorou, M.K. 1993. *Anim. Prod.*, 56: 462A.

Barbi, J.H.T., Owen, E. and Theodorou, M.K. (1995). *Anim. Sci.*, 60: 542A.

Blummel, M. and Fernandez-Rivera, S. (2002). *Anim. Nutr. Feed Technol.*, 2: 93-115.

Blümmel, M. and Ørskov, R.R. 1993. *Anim. Feed Sci. Technol.*, 40: 109-119.

Borderick, G.A. and Cochran, R.C. (2000). In: Feeding System and Feed Evaluation Models. Theodorou, M.K. and France, J. (Eds). CABI publishing, Wallingford, UK. pp.53-85.

Bugalho, M.N., Milne, J.A. and Racey, P.A. (2001). *J. Zool. (London)*, 255: 285-289.

Charley, E and Dove, H. (2007). *Aust. J. Agri. Res.*, 58: 1215-1225.

Chen, X.B., Grubic, G., Orskov, E.R. and Osuji, P.O. (1992). *Anim. Prod.*, 55:185-91.

Czerkawski, J.W. and Grace Breckenridge (1977). *British J. Nutr.*, 38:371.

De Boever, J.L., Cottyn, B.G., De Brabander, D.L., Vanacker, J.M. and Boucque, Ch.V. (1997). *Anim. Feed Sci. Technol.*, 66: 211-222.

Deaville, E.R., Humphries, D.J. and Givens, D.I. (2008). *Anim. Feed Sci. Technol.*, 149: 114-124.

Dove, H and Mayes, R.W. (2005). *Small Rumi. Res.*, 5: 123-139.

Dove, H. and Charmley, E. (2008). *Anim.*, 2: 1474-1485.

Dove, H., Milne, J.A. and Mayes, R.W. (1990). *Proceeding of Newzeland Soc. Anim. Prod.*, 50: 457-459.

Duncan, A.J., Mayes, R.W., Lamb, C.S., Young, S.A. and Castillo, I. (1999). *J. Agri. Sci., Cambridge*, 132: 233-246.

Fondevela, M. and Perez-Espes, B. (2008). *Anim. Feed Sci. Technol.*, 144: 196-211.

Givens, D.I., Baker, C.W., Moss, A.R., and Adamson, A.H. (1991). *Anim. Feed Sci. Technol.,* 35 : 83-94.

Goering, H.K. and VanSoest, P.J. (1970). In: Agricultural Handbook No 379. Agricultural Research Service, US Department of Agriculture, Washington, DC.

Hindrichsen, I. K., Kreuzer, M., Madsen,V. and Bach Knudsen, K.E. (2006). *J. Dairy Sci.,* 89: 2168-2176.

Hulbert, I.A., Iason, G.R., and Mayes, R.W. (2001). *Oecologia.* 129: 197-205.

Hutchings, M.R., Gordon, I.J., Robertson, E., Kyriazakis, I. and Jackson, F. (2000). *J. Agri. Sci.,* 135: 65-75.

Mayes, R.W. and Dove, H. (2000). *Nutr. Res. Reviews,* 13:107-138.

McDonald, I. (1981). *J. Agri. Sci., Cambridge,* 96: 251-252.

Mehrez, A.Z. and Orskov, E.R. (1977). *J. Agri. Sci.,* 88: 645-50.

Menke, K.H. and Steingass, H. (1988.) *Animal Research and Development,* 28: 7-55.

Ngonyamo-Majee, D., Shaver, R.D., Coors, J.G., Sapienzee, D., Correa, C.E.S. and Lauer, J.G. (2008). *Anim. Feed Sci. Technol.,* 142, 247-258.

Nordheim, H., Volden, H., Fystro, G. and Lunnam, T. (2007). *Animal Feed Science and Technology,* 139, 92-108.

Nousiainem, J., Ahvenjarvi, S., Rinni, M., Hellamaki, M. and Huhtanem, P. (2004). *Anim. Feed Sci. Technol.,* 115: 295-311.

Ørskov, E.R. and McDonald, I. (1979). *J. Agri. Sci., Cambridge,* 92: 499-503.

Phipps, R.H., Deaville, E.R. and Maddison, B.C. (2003). *J. Dairy Sci.,* 86: 4070–4078.

Rao, S.J., Iason, G.R., Hulbert, I.A.R., Mayes, R.W. and Racey, P.A. (2003). *Canad. J. Zool.,* 81: 1047-1056.

Rymer, C., Huntington, J.A., Williams, B.A., Givens, D.I. (2005). *Anim. Feed Sci. Technol.,* 123-124: 9-30.

Salt, C.A., Mayes, R.W. and Elston, D.A. (1992). *J. Applied Ecol.,* 29: 378-387.

Smith, D.G., Mayes, R.W., Hallands, T., Cuddeford, D., Yulu, H.H., Maloladrero, C.M. and Gillen, T. (2007). *J. Agri. Sci., Cambridge,* 145: 237-281.

Tilley, J.M.A. and Terry, R.A. (1963). *J. Briti. Grassland Soc.,* 18: 104-111.

Theander, O. and Westerlund, E. A. (1986). *J. Agri. Food Chemi.,* 34:330.

Van Kessel, J.S. and Russel, J.B. (1996). *J. Dairy Sci.,* 79: 1237-1243.

Van Soest, P.J. (1994). In: 2nd ed. Cornell University Press, Ithaca, New York, pp. 272-273.

Van Soest, P.J., Robertson, J. B. and Lewis, B. A. (1991). *J. Dairy Sci.,* 74: 3583-3597.

Wilman, D., Field, M., Lister, S.J. and Givens, D.I. (2000). *Anim. Feed Sci. Technol.,* 88: 135-151.

Wolin, M.J. (1960). *J. Dairy Sci.,* 43: 1452-1459.

□□□

Animal Nutrition, 2012
eds. Dr. (Mrs.) Usha R. Mehra et al., pp. 707-733
Satish Serial Publishing House e-mail : info@satishserial.com; website : www.satishserial.com

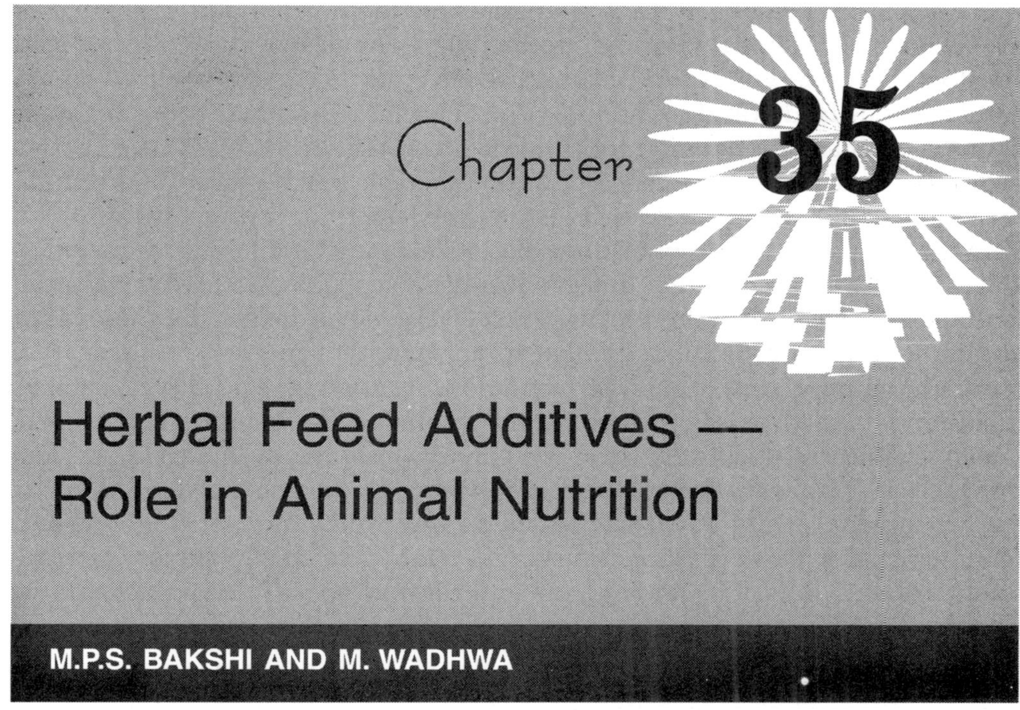

Herbal Feed Additives — Role in Animal Nutrition

M.P.S. BAKSHI AND M. WADHWA

The ruminants can convert low quality feeds and non-protein nitrogen into high quality protein. The plant carbohydrates (NPN) and nitrogenous compounds are fermented in the rumen to volatile fatty acids and microbial biomass, which provides energy and protein to the animal. However, rumen fermentation also produces methane (a loss of 2-12% of the GE consumed), a potent greenhouse gas and ammonia. The efficiency of rumen metabolism can have a profound effect on the production efficiency of the animal and the output of waste products polluting the environment. Efforts are afoot to develop technologies, which help in improving productivity of ruminants, without having much impact on the environment. There are many feed additives/supplements, which have specific and desirable rumen-modulating properties like better gas profile (less methane), preventing growth of the bacteria responsible for ruminant lactic acidosis, potent inhibitors of gut pathogenic bacteria, more favourable end-products (propionate), and less dietary protein breakdown in the rumen. Therefore, strong need based research should be conducted to find safer rumen-modulating feed additives to achieve full potential of production, health and environmental benefits.

Antibiotics have been used in animals for therapeutic and prophylactic use as well as for improving the productivity. The use of antibiotics as feed additives began in 1940's and became universal practice in animal production. Antibiotics as feed additives help to control bacterial and parasitic infections, enhance animal productivity and improve feed efficiency, but cause serious negative impacts i.e. emergence of antibiotic-resistant bacteria. The routine feeding of four antibiotics to livestock, i.e. bacitracin zinc, spiramycin, virginiamycin and tylosin phosphate, has been banned in the European Union since July 1999, because this practice has been suspected to favour bacterial pathogens resistance to these drugs (EC, 2003). Nevertheless the removal of antibiotic growth-promoters has led to an increased interest in alternative means of manipulating rumen fermentation. A number of additives, such as ionophores and probiotics, have been introduced into ruminant nutrition, mostly to improve feed utilization with an ultimate aim of increasing animal production (Nagaraja, 1995). Currently, there is a strong debate about the safety aspects of chemical additives as they may be carcinogenic and teratogenic. For these reasons, consumers tend to be suspicious of chemical additives and thus the demand for natural and socially more acceptable additives has been intensified.

The use of herbs (flowering plant whose stem does not become woody) in livestock production and reproduction is as old as the ancient history and the earliest mention of the medicinal use of soma plant was found in the Rigveda, which is believed to have been written between 2000 and 1400 B.C. Ayurved, in fact, is the foundation of the ancient medical science of India, in which a section has been devoted to the veterinary therapeutics (Pashu chikitsa). The drugs of plant origin have formed a predominant part of the Hindu and Unani medicine and the curative powers of certain herbs were well known. Greeks were the first to be perfect in the field of medicine. A Greek herbal specialist: Hippocrates was known to have an extensive record of about 400 herbal plants. The secrets of herbal medicines were soon passed over to the adventurous Romans, who used the herbal remedies better than any other people. Romans have contributed widely to the field of herbs by developing several unique drugs and medicines. There is undying belief that herbs are free of undesirable side effects on the animal system.

For years, humans suffering from malaria were cured by the extract from the bark of cincona tree (quinine). It has been replaced by the extract of wormwood shrub. One of active ingredient of wormwood is thujone having properties similar to tetra-hydro-cannabinol, it is also active agent in marijuana. Black walnut extract has been effective for parasitic and fungal infections. Neem (*Azadirachta indica*) has been used since ages in India to provide health care to livestock. It cures gastric disorders viz. diarrhoea, dysentery, hyperacidity, antidiabetic, strong wormicide and cure GIT ulcers. Neem leaves (contain nimbin, nimbinae, nimbandiol, nimbolide) are carminative and aids digestion. The supplementation of neem leaf powder resulted in significant improvement in daily DM intake and daily live weight gain in calves (Kukde *et al.*, 1999). Cranberry juice containing benzoic acid has been used for a number of years as an aid in combating urinary infection and kills pathogens.

Spices (aromatic substance of vegetative origin) such as fennel, anise have been successfully used to stimulate feed intake, improve digestion, milk production and decrease flatulence in pigs and cattle. Spice rosemary has been reported to possess antioxidant property and have better stability than BHA and BHT. Mixture of various herbs marketed commercially as galactogogues and stomachics were found to depress rumen as well as circulatory biogenic amines. The cellulolytic bacterial population, total VFA production, propionate concentration and milk yield were increased considerably in cows (Singh *et al.*, 1991). Onion and garlic supplementation resulted in significant increase in daily feed intake, decrease in rumen NH_3-N, while TVFA were significantly increased in Zaraibi goats. Wawrzynczak *et al.* (2000) observed higher feed intake, significant higher daily weight gain and improved feed conversion efficiency in the calves fed 1.0 per cent herbs (*Mentha piperita, Thymus vulgaris, Salvia officinalis, Viola tricolor, Chamomilla* recutita and *Urtica dioica*) supplemented in concentrate. Culinary additives like turmeric, coriander seeds, ginger and bitter gourd (bitter in nature due to the presence of caffeine, alkaloids and berberine) are bactericidal, germicidal, anti viral, anti inflammatory, detoxifying and rejuvenating in nature.

The evaluation of various herbal feed additives [Shatavar (*Asparagus racemosus),* Jiwanti (*Leptidenia reticulata*), Bhringraj (*Eclipta alba*), Mustak (*Cyperus scariosus*), Jeera (*Cumin seed*), Saunf (*Fochieulim vulgare*), Kutki (*Picrorrhiza kurro*), Chitrak (*Plumbago zeylanica*) and Soe (*Ancthum sowa)*] by *in vitro* gas production technique revealed that bhringraj *(Eclipta alba),* kutki *(Kutaki picorrhiza)* and jeera *(Cuminum cyminum)* supplemented individually at 0.4% of the substrate, improved the digestibility of nutrients significantly (Bakshi *et al.*, 2005). Further, combination of *Asparagus racemosus, Leptidenia reticulata, Eclipta alba* in 3:1:2 ratio, supplemented @ 0.4% of the DM intake also improved the nutrient utilization significantly in buffalo calves (Bakshi and Wadhwa, 2004), and suggested further exploitation, for improving the production status of dairy cows. Results also revealed that supplementation of herbs beyond 0.4 % showed no additional benefits as far as utilization of nutrients was concerned. Wadhwa and Bakshi (2006) reported that improvement in digestibility could be due to significant improvement in the activities of carboxymethyl cellulase, filter paper degrading activity and that of xylanase, when the diet was supplemented with *Kutaki picorrhiza* as compared to un-supplemented diet or diet supplemented with other herbal feed additives (*Eclipta alba* or mixture of *Eclipta alba* and *Kutaki picorrhiza* in 1:1 ratio). The higher activity of most of the microbial enzymes in the rumen of the animals fed diet supplemented with *Kutaki picorrhiza* resulted in higher availability of the end products of digestion leading to significantly higher microbial protein synthesis in the rumen. However, no alteration in the rumen volume and outflow rate was observed, though dilution rate was improved in groups where *Kutaki picorrhiza* or combination of *Kutaki picorrhiza* and *Eclipta alba* were supplemented. However, *in vivo* studies revealed that *Kutaki picorrhiza, Eclipta alba* or combination of *Kutaki picorrhiza* and *Eclipta alba* in 1:1 ratio supplemented @ 0.4% of diet for 30 days only (thereafter withdrawn) in a 77 day growth trial did not have,any beneficial effect on the DM intake, digestibility of nutrients, N-retention, biochemical changes in the rumen, nutritive value and performance of buffalo calves (Neelam Rani *et al.,* 2006).

Herbal feed additives could either influence feeding pattern, or influence the growth of favourable microorganisms in the rumen, or stimulate the secretion of various digestive enzymes, which in turn may improve the efficiency of utilization of nutrients or stimulate the milk secretory tissue, resulting in improved productive and reproductive performance of dairy animals. The success of herbs in animal system can be attributed to the presence of variety of plant secondary metabolites (PSM)/compounds (Fig 1.), which provide protection against predators, pathogens and environmental stress (Iason, 2005). Some are toxic to animals, but others may not be, and indeed many have been used to manipulate gut function in both ruminants and non ruminants (Greathead, 2003). The dietary manipulation and other strategies like impact of plant secondary metabolites to mitigate the enteric methane production and in turn on nutrient utilization have been reviewed extensively (Bakshi and Wadhwa 2009; Wadhwa and Bakshi 2009 and Bakshi and Wadhwa 2011[a,b]). Broadly, these compounds fall into six categories; essential oils, organosulphurs, saponins, polyphenols, organic acids and oligosaccharides.

Essential oils

The term essential is derived from 'essence' means liquid perfume providing specific flavours and odours to many plants. These are found throughout the plant, including roots, bark, flowers, petals, leaves, fruit bodies and stems (Hirasa and Takemasa, 1998). Their concentration within plants vary due to stage of growth, plant health (Dudareva *et al.,* 2004) and environmental factors such as light, temperature and moisture stress (Gershenzon *et al.,* 2000).

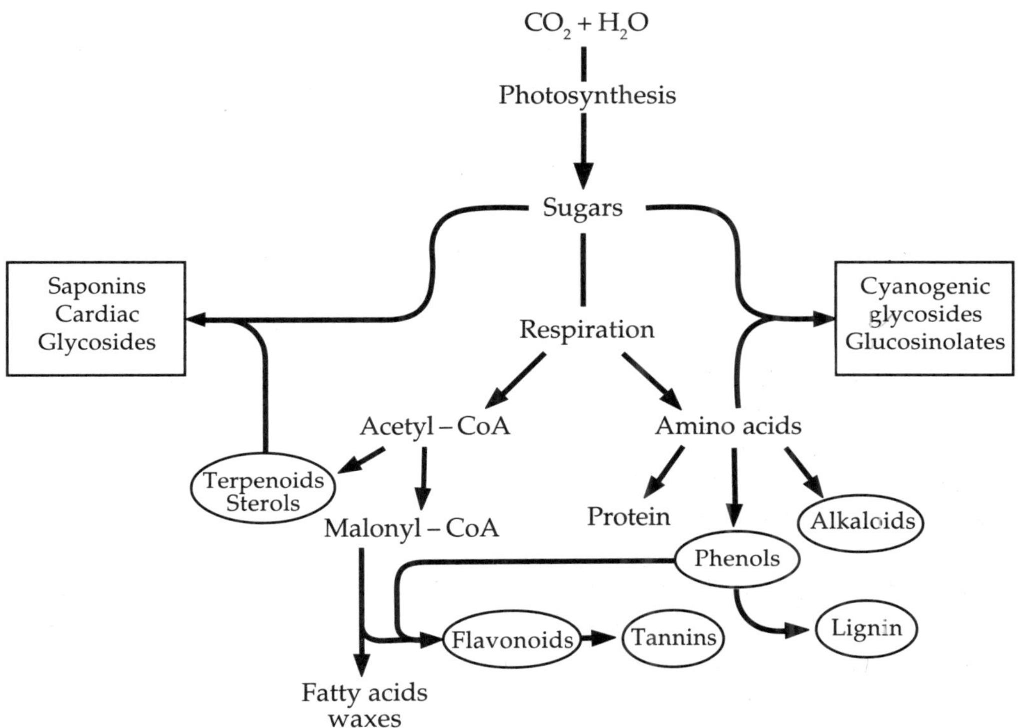

Fig. 1 : Secondary metabolites are derived from primary metabolites

The essential oils (EO) are aromatic steam volatile or organic solvent extracted compounds from plants, made up of alcohol, ester or aldehyde derivatives of terpenoids (monoterpenoids and sesquiterpenoids) and phenylpropanoids (Calsamiglia *et al.*, 2007). These 2 groups originate from different precursors of primary metabolism and are synthesized through different pathways (Fig 2). Terpenoids are highly diversified group of plant metabolites and about 15000 different compounds have been reported (Gershenzon and Croteau, 1991). These are characterized by isoperene unit (C_5H_8) present in a compound. Some plants have phenylpropnoids in significant numbers and refer to 3 carbon chain attached to an benzene ring (Fig. 3).

Possible modes of action

The EO has antimicrobial activities against both gram-negative and gram-positive bacteria (Table 1) and fungicidal properties (Calsamiglia *et al.*, 2007). It has been suggested that gram-negative bacteria tended to have a higher resistance to essential oils than gram-positive bacteria (Chao *et al.*, 2000). The EO, due to the hydrophobic nature and affinity for lipids, accumulate in the

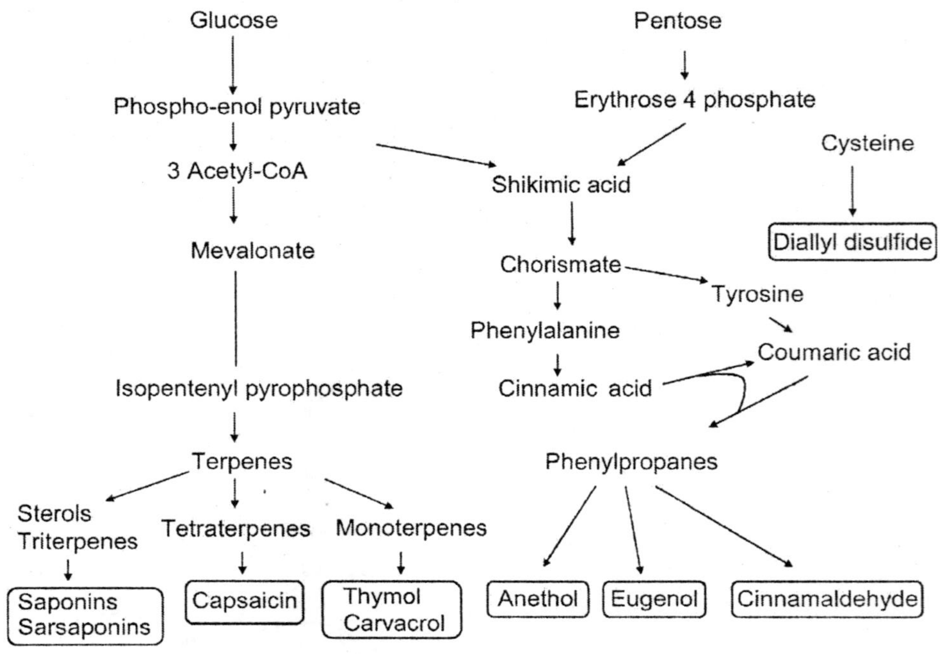

Fig. 2 : Metabolic pathways of the biosynthesis of the main plant extract active components.

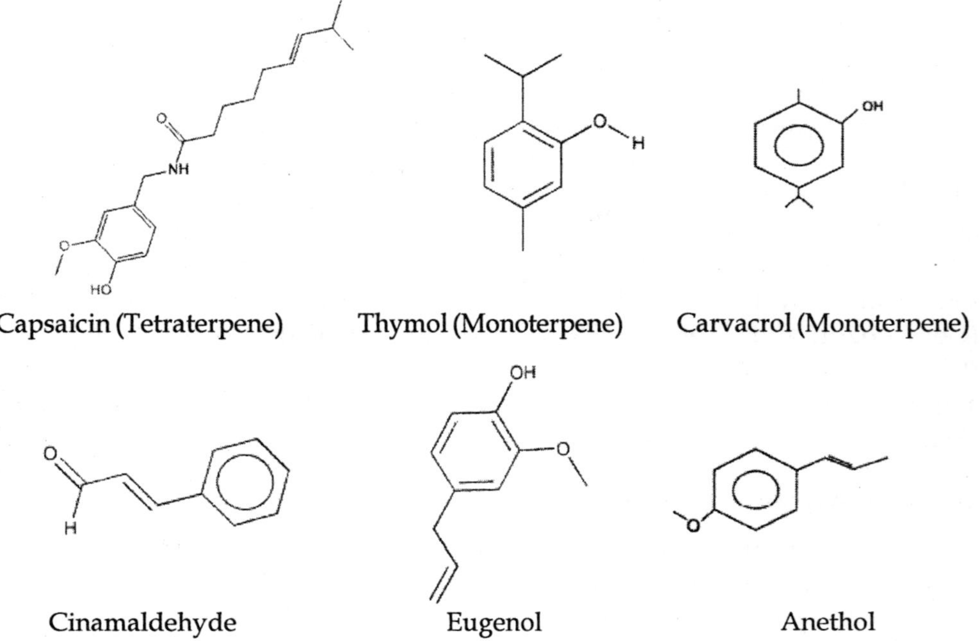

Fig. 3 : Phenylpropnoids

lipid bilayer of bacterial cell membranes and disrupt their integrity either directly or by denaturating the membrane proteins, causing increased membrane permeability leading to leakage of cytoplasmic enzymes and metabolites, which effects tran's membrane ionic gradient. Bacteria can counter balance these effects by using ionic pumps, but large amount of energy are diverted, resulting in the depletion of the proton-motive force across cell membrane, decreased ATP synthesis slowing microbial growth and may cause cell death (Burt, 2004). Structure-function relationships associated with polar groups, number of double bonds, molecular size and molecular solubility have marked effects on their activities (Kamel, 2001). Juven *et al.* (1994) reported that antimicrobial action of essential oils (thymol, CIN, GAR) increased as pH decreased from 7.0 to 5.5 indicating that effect of essential oils on microbial fermentation is pH dependent.

Effects of essential oils

A commercial blend of EO (BEO) depressed the activity of "hyper-ammonia-producing" bacteria like *Peptostreptococcus anaerobius, Clostridium sticklandii* and *Prevotella ruminicola,* species (McIntosh *et al.,* 2003) without affecting the activity of proteinase and peptidase. The BEO did not effect specific bacterial colonization of starch-rich substrates (Duval *et al.,* 2007) and protozoal population or their activity (Benchaar *et al.,* 2006, 2007). However, Patra et al. (2006[a,b]) reported that the ethanol and methanol extracts of clove decreased while that of onion, ginger and garlic increased the protozoa numbers. The EO inhibit deamination and methanogenesis resulting in lower NH_3-N, methane and flatulence, reduces acetate and increases propionate and butyrate concentrations. Different levels of essential oils like carvacrol (Oregano sps), cinnamin oil (Cinnamin) and garlic oil (Alliums) were selected to assess their effect on methane production (Lamba *et al.,* 2009). The net gas production, irrespective of the level used, varied significantly between 127.6 (cinnamin oil) to 184.7 ml/gDM/24h (carvacrol). The methane production was lowest in garlic oil. However,a contribution of methane to net gas production was lowest in carvacrol supplemented diet followed by garlic oil. Partitioning factor was observed to be highest for cinnamin oil, supplemented diet. The NGP, CH_4 production and TOMD decreased linearly, while the partitioning factor increased with increase in the level of essential oil, irrespective of nature of oil. However, the increase in level of oil beyond 2% was unable to improve these parameters. These observations clearly indicated that supplementation of essential oil beyond 2% would not provide any additional benefits. Patra *et al.* (2006[a,b]) reported the effect of spices on *in vitro* gas production and found that ethanol and methanol extracts of clove and garlic and methanol extract of fennel inhibited methane production. However, water extracts of these products and all extracts of onion and ginger had no effect on methane production. Total VFA's were higher on inclusion of extracts of garlic and onion. All extracts of garlic and methanol extract of fennel decreased molar proportion of acetate and A:P ratio. Methanol and ethanol extracts of clove decreased DM degradability.

Increase DM intake, ruminal true OM and N digestibility's (Yang *et al.*, 2007), total tract ADF and starch digestibility (Benchaar *et al.*, 2006), improved feed conversion efficiency, milk yield and fat yield (Kung *et al.*, 2008) in dairy cows. EO decrease stress to the animals (Hosoda *et al.*, 2006), act as antioxidant (Cheel *et al.*, 2005) and antinociceptive (Viana *et al.*, 2000). Stimulate the immune system, thereby enhancing the resistance of animals to inflammatory and infectious diseases. Concha *et al.* (1996) showed that the extract of ginseng root stimulated *in vitro* activities of neutrophills and lymphocytes from bovine peripheral blood and milk. Body weight and body condition score were unaffected by treatment. There was no beneficial effect of supplementing EO in prepartum dairy cows. The response to EO is dependent on the roughage to concentrate ratio, type of feedstuff and type and level of EO used.

Organosulphur compounds

Garlic (*Allium sativum*) is the most extensively investigated from human health point of view. It has been used medicinally since ages, contains sulphur-containing compounds like glutamyl-S-allyl-l-cysteins and S-allyll- cysteine sulphoxides (alliin) in intact garlic, which are converted into thiosulphinates (such as allicin) through enzymic reactions when raw garlic is cut or crushed (Stoll and Seebeck, 1948). Thus, a wide range of different organosulphur compounds are produced during the processing of garlic (Kodera *et al.*, 2002). The garlic oil (GAR) has a wide spectrum antibacterial activity against gram positive and negative bacteria, fungi, parasites and viruses (Reuter *et al.*, 1996). GAR have four active components i.e. allicin (ALL), diallyl sulphide (DAS), diallyl disulphide (DADS) and allyl mercaptan (ALM). DADS and ALM resulted in similar but mild effects than GAR suggesting synergistic effects between different compounds present in GAR. It has been suggested that the antimicrobial potency of allyl sulphides of garlic oil increases with each addition of S atom (Reuter *et al.*, 1996; O'Gara *et al.*, 2000), reason for DADS to show stronger effects compared to DAS. The main antimicrobial mechanism appears to be related to its capacity to interact with the sulfhydryl group (–SH) of the active compounds. The active compounds help in liver detoxification by increasing the production of glutathione transferase and provide immunity by increasing the activity of macrophage and lymphocytes. The strong antibacterial properties of these compounds may serve to inhibit the bacterial conversion of nitrate to nitrite in the rumen and may reduce the formation of nitrosamines, which are carcinogenic (Naganawa *et al.*, 1996). GAR, DAD

Table 1 : Essential oils with microbial activity, their main active components, and susceptible microorganisms.

Essential oil of	Name	Active components	Susceptible microorganisms	References
Allium sativum	Garlic	Allicin, diallyl sulfite	*Enterpathogenic bacteria*	Ross *et al.*, 2001
Anethum graveolens	Dill	Limonene, carvone	Gram- positive and gram-negative bacteria	Deans and Ritchie, 1987
Capsicum annum	Paprika	Capsaicin	Gram-positive and gram-negative bacteria	Deans and Ritchie, 1987
Cinnamomum cassia	Cassia	Cinnamaldehyde	*Escherichia coli, Staphylococcus aureus, Listeria monocytogenes, Salmonella enteritidis*	Ouattara *et al.*, 1997; Mahmoud, 1994; Smith-Palmer *et al.*, 1998
Juniperus oxycedrus	Juniper	Cadinene, pinene	*Aeromonas sobria, Enterococcus fecalis, Staph. aureus*	Hammer *et al.*, 1999
Melaleuca alternifolia	Tea tree	Terpinen-4-ol	*Staph. aureus, E. coli*, Gram-positive and gram-negative bacteria	Chao and Young, 2000; Cox *et al.*, 2001
Origanum vulgare	Oregano	Carvacrol, thymol	Gram-positive and gram negative bacteria	Sivropoulou *et al.*, 1996; Dorman and Deans, 2000
Pimpinella anisum	Anise	Anethol	*Aeromonas hydrophila, Brevibacterium linens, Brochothrics theromosphacta*	Deans and Ritchie, 1987
Rosmarinus officinalis	Rosemary	1.8- Cineole	*Staph. aureus, L. monocytogenes Campylobacter jejuni*	Ouattara *et al.*,1997; Smith-Palmer *et al.*, 1998
Syzygium aromaticum	Clove	Eugenol	*E. coli, Staph. aureus, L. Monocytogenes, S. enteritidis, C. jejuni*	Quattara *et al.*, 1997; Smith-Palmer *et al.*,1998
Thymus vulgaris	Thyme	Thymol, carvacrol	*Salmonella typhimurium, Staph. aureus, Aspergillus flavus*	Juven *et al.*, 1944; Quattara *et al.*, 1997; Mahmoud, 1994
Zingiber officinale	Ginger	Zingiberene, zingerone	Gram-positive and gram negative bacteria	Chao and Young, 2000

and ALM have the ability to decrease methane production by direct inhibition of rumen methanogenesis archaea (through inhibition of hydroxy methyl glutaryl (HMG) CoA reductase, which is responsible for catalyzing the synthesis of sphenoid alcohol, a constituent of the lipids in the cell membrane of methanogens), which may help to improve the efficiency of energy use in the rumen. The excess hydrogen produced by a direct inhibition of methane production results in increased concentrations of other hydrogen sinks such as propionate and butyrate without affecting nutrient digestibility.

Saponins

Saponins are found in many plants, lower marine animals and some bacteria (Riguera, 1997; Yoshiki *et al.*, 1998). The name is derived from Latin word 'sapo' which means the plant containing frothing agent which form stable foam in aqueous solutions similar to soaps. Since ages the roots of soapwort plant (Genus *Saponaria*, Family *Caryophyllaceae*) were used as soap. Saponins are also found in the family *Sapindaceae*, genus *Sapindus* (soapberry or soapnut), and in the families *Aceraceae* (maples) and *Hippocastanaceae* (horse chestnuts). These are found in leaves, stems, roots, bulbs, blossom, and fruit. Commercial formulations of plant-derived saponins occur in different parts of the plants such as the bark of *Quillaja saponaria*; trunk and root of *Yucca schidigera*; fruit of *Sapindus saponaria* and *Sapindus rarak*; seed and leaf of *Camellia cinensis*. These are often bitter to taste and some are toxic to cold-blooded organisms and insects at particular concentrations.

Structure

Saponins are high molecular weight glycosides made up of glycon (sugars) and a hydrophobic aglycone (sapogenin) moiety. The sugar may be glucose, galactose, arabinose, xylose or glucuronic acid, while sapogenin may be neutral (containing steroids) or acidic (containing triterpenoids). The saponins that have one sugar molecule attached at the C3 position are monodesmoside saponins, and those that have an additional sugar moiety at the C26 or C28 position are bidesmoside saponins. The diversity and complexity of saponin structures arises from the variability of the aglycon structure, the nature of the side chains and the position of attachment of these moieties on the aglycone. The type of linkage and the sugar composition of the saponin are directly related to their biological activity (Chwalek *et al.*, 2004; Jung *et al.*, 2004).

Mode of action

The saponins are poorly absorbed from the digestive tract (Cheeke, 1996), thereby effect the activity and population of enteric microorganisms. Protozoa counts in rumen fluid decreased with higher doses of sarsaponins from

Y. Schidigera (Pen *et al.*, 2006) and with saponin rich plants or fruits (Kamra *et al.*, 2000; Agarwal *et al.*, 2006). The detergent action of saponins kills rumen protozoa and identified as possible defaunating agents in the rumen (Newbold *et al.*, 1997). The susceptibility of ruminal ciliate protozoa to saponins is probably expected due to the presence of cholesterol in eukaryotic (including protozoa) cells membranes, but absent in prokaryotic bacterial cells, as saponins exhibit an affinity towards cholesterol (Klita *et al.*, 1996). Permeability is altered by the formation of a micelle-like aggregation of saponins and cholesterol (Seeman, 1974). Suppression or elimination of protozoa may enhance the flow of microbial protein from the rumen, increase the efficiency of feed utilization, and improve the nutrition of the animal, provided that the loss of protozoa does not impair the fiber breakdown (Newbold *et al.*, 1997). On the other hand, high doses of saponin are known to cause damage to the villi tips of the intestinal epithelium (Gee *et al.*, 1996); this would impair the digestive capability of the animal as the absorptive area is decreased and mucosal enzyme production is suppressed. This could lead to lower feed efficiency and weight gain (Ilsley *et al.*, 2005).

Growth of cellulolytic bacteria has been decreased (Ningrat *et al.*, 2002), increased (Thalib *et al.*, 1996) or unaffected (Wina *et al.*, 2006) by the presence of *S. rarak* saponins. Some *Butyrivibrio* and *Bacteroides* strains are capable of degrading alfalfa saponins (Gutierrez and Davis, 1962). Makkar and Becker (1997) observed 100% disappearance of *Quillaja* saponin after 24 h of incubation and concluded that it was due to degradation by rumen microbes, thus the microbes get immuned to the effect of saponins. Odenyo *et al.* (1997) observed that 300 g/day of *S. sesban* introduced directly into the rumen remained toxic to protozoa, but when the same amount incorporated into the diet, *S. sesban* was ineffective. This suggests that chewing causes detoxification by salivary amylase and it may be responsible for the differences in the *in-vitro* and *in-vivo* studies.

Effects of saponins on the rumen fermentation

The effects of saponins on total ruminal VFA production and molar proportions are variable. Some studies have observed increased propionate production at the expense of acetate and butyrate production, whilst others have seen no effect. It may be either due to saponin type and concentration; composition of the diet e.g. diet rich in grain or starch improved the proportion of propionate (Liu *et al.*, 2003) in contrast to fibrous diets or mixed forages (Hess *et al.*, 2003[a,b]).

The glycol component binds ammonia, and the sapogenin fraction may affect ammonia concentration indirectly via their toxicity to gram positive bacteria and rumen ciliate protozoa (Wallace *et al.*, 1994; Ryan *et al.*, 1997) or by suppressing peptidase-producing bacteria (Wallace *et al.*, 1994; Wang *et al.*, 2000). One of the reasons for the lower ammonia levels could be the higher incorporation of ammonia, peptide or amino acids into microbial protein (Makkar *et al.*, 1998). The other reason, inhibition of bacterial lysis, is probably partially responsible for decreased ruminal ammonia concentrations observed in defaunated animals (Hristov *et al.*, 1999).

The effects of saponins or saponins extracts on the microbial protein synthesis (MPS) are not consistent. It may be due to differences in the chemical composition and inclusion rate of the saponins or type of diet (Goetsch and Owens, 1985). Sarsaponin increased the digestion of sorghum silage and other fibrous feeds but apparently decreased the digestion of cereal and protein meals. Similarly Santoso *et al.* (2004[a]) found no significant effect of *Y. schidigera* on the efficiency of MPS in sheep fed timothy silage diets whereas yucca significantly stimulated EMPS, when the diet was timothy hay.

Effect on methanogens

Given the detrimental effect of saponins on protozoa and that around 25% of ruminal methanogens live in association with protozoa (Newbold *et al.*, 1997), the potential effect of saponins on methanogenic archea and methane production in the rumen is of great interest. The elimination of ciliate protozoa, from the rumen, reduced methane emission by 30 to 45% (Ushida *et al.*, 1986; Lila *et al.*, 2005). The reduction of methane emission in response to *Y. schidigera* extract (Santoso *et al.*, 2004[b]), *S. saponaria* (Hess *et al.*, 2003a, 2004) and *S. rarak* (Ningrat *et al.*, 2002) is due to utilization of hydrogen produced by protozoa by methanogenic bacteria (Stumm and Zwart, 1986; Ushida *et al.*, 1997). Inclusion of tea saponins (TS) significantly reduced methane production in faunated rumen fluid, but not in the defaunated rumen fluid, suggesting that inhibition of methanogenesis by TS was primarily due to their anti-protozoal activity. However, results are not consistent, which may be due to different basal diets, saponin concentration and adaptation period used (Wang *et al.*, 1998; Hess *et al.*, 2003[b]). *In vitro* fermentation experiments using the ruminal fluid of Holstein cows (Pen *et al.*, 2006) demonstrated that *Yucca schidigera* extract (YSE) decreased methane production whereas *Quillaja saponaria* extract (QSE) did not. Protozoal numbers decreased in both cases (56% with YSE, 41% with QSE). The chemical nature of the saponins may be responsible for the differing activities.

Tannins

Tannins originated from the French word *tan* means the bark of the holm oak and other trees used in tanning. The tannins are widely distributed among trees, shrubs and herbaceous leguminous plants especially in new leaves and flowers (McLeod, 1974; Perevolotsky, 1994). High temperatures, water stress, extreme light intensity and poor soil quality increase the tannin content of plants (Van Soest, 1994).

These are high molecular weight phenolic compounds, divided into two groups: the hydrolysable (HT) and the condensed tannins (CT). The HTs are made up of a carbohydrate core whose hydroxyl groups are esterified with phenolic acids, mainly Gallic and hexahydroxydiphenic acid (Fig. 4&5). The CTs or proanthocyanidins, are non-branched polymers of flavonoids units (flavan-3-ol, flavan-3, 4-diol), and usually have a higher molecular weight (1000-20000 Da) than the HT (500-3000 Da). Rana *et al.* (2006) evaluated 12 leaves of forest trees of semi hilly arid zone and observed that HT content varied between 1.4 to 15.1% while the CT content varied between 0.4 to 4.6%. Majority of the tree leaves selected had moderate levels (2-5%) of net tannins. Leaves of *Carrisa* had the highest, whereas the leaves of *Anogeissus* had the lowest concentration of CT.

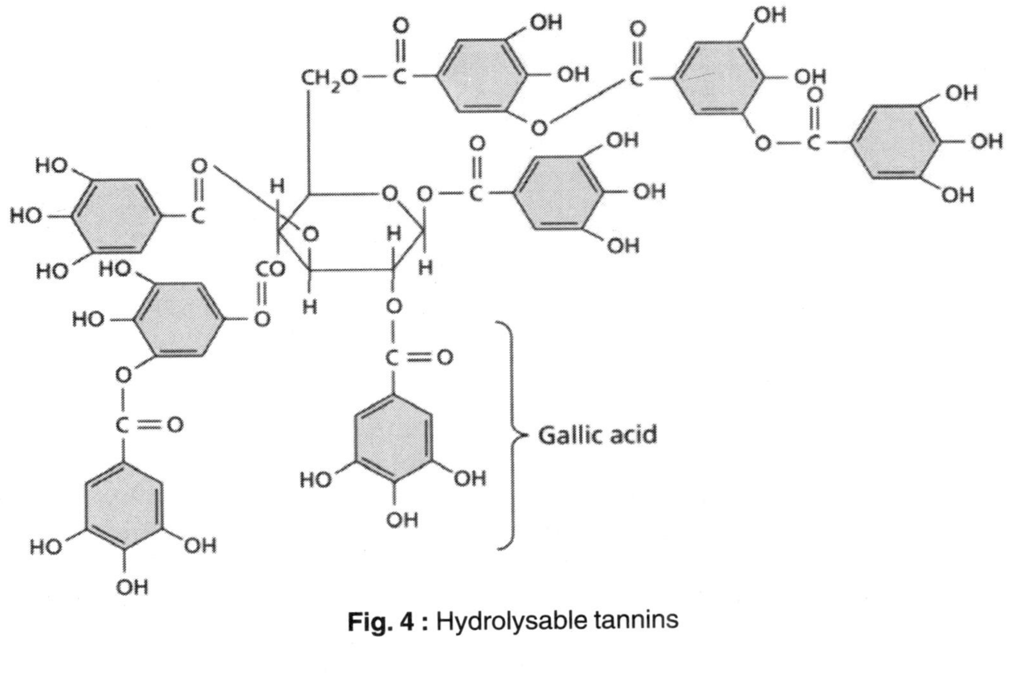

Fig. 4 : Hydrolysable tannins

Mode of action

Tannins reduce ruminal degradation of different dietary components by substrate privation (McMahon *et al.*, 2000), enzyme inhibition (Jones *et al.*, 1994) and direct action on rumen microorganisms by altering the permeability of their membranes (Scalbert, 1991). Tannins prevent or at least interfere with the attachment of rumen microorganisms to plant cell walls, which is essential for degradation to occur (McAllister *et al.*, 1994[a]). Further, the formation of complexes with proteins (rich in proline), and carbohydrates renders these nutrients inaccessible to microorganisms (Mueller-Harvey and McAllan, 1992). Tannins also act as chelating agents, and this can reduce the availability of certain metallic ions necessary for the metabolism of rumen microorganisms (Scalbert, 1991).

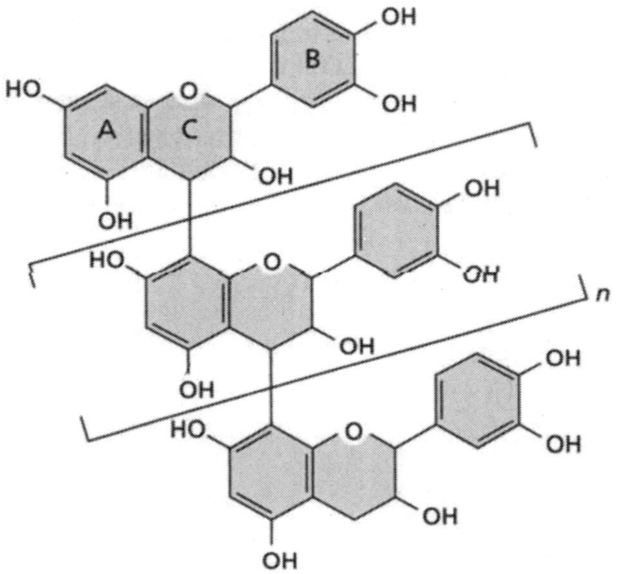

Fig. 5 : Condense tannins

Some rumen microbes can tolerate tannins (O'Donovan and Brooker, 2001). Several species of the ruminal microbiota respond to the presence of tannins by changing their morphology. Chiquette *et al.* (1988) observed a thick glycocalyx on ruminal bacterial walls in response to high levels of CT. Among the bacteria able to use HT are *Streptococcus caprinus* (*S. gallolyticus*), which produces pyrogallol (a product of tannic acid degradation) when gallate decarboxylase activity increases (O'Donovan and Brooker, 2001). The degradation of CT has not been demonstrated even *in vitro* (McSweeney *et al.*, 2001).

Effect of tannins

Tannins can be beneficial or detrimental to ruminants, depending on type and quantity consumed, the compound's structure, molecular weight, and physiology of the consuming species (Hagerman and Butler, 1991).

Voluntary feed intake

The consumption of plant species with high CT or HT contents (>5% of DM) significantly depresses feed intake, while medium or low consumption (<5% of DM) did not affect voluntary feed intake (Barry and Manley, 1984; Waghorn *et al.*, 1994). Three main mechanisms have been suggested to explain the negative effects of high tannin concentrations on voluntary feed intake: reduction in feed palatability, slowing of digestion, and development of conditioned aversions.

Digestibility of the diet

Tannins mainly reduce the digestibility of proteins, but they also affect other feed components to different degrees (Kumar and Singh, 1984). Their main effect on proteins is based on their ability to form hydrogen bonds that are stable between pH 3.5 and 8. These complexes-stable at rumen pH-dissociate when the pH falls below 3.5 (as in abomasum, pH 2.5-3) or is greater than 8 as in the duodenum (McLeod, 1974; Mueller-Harvey and McAllan, 1992). The evidence that tannins reduce the digestibility of feed is the increase in faecal-N excretion with the increase in dietary tannin content. Silanikove *et al.* (1994) reported that CT inhibits the activity of trypsin and amylase. The consequences of tannin ingestion include increased secretion of endogenous proteins such as salivary glycoproteins, mucus and digestive enzymes, and increased desquamation of intestinal cells (Waghorn, 1996), resulting in increased metabolic faecal-N.

After their dissociation from proteins in the abomasum at pH <3.5, the tannins might once again bind to dietary proteins in the intestine as the pH at the beginning of the intestine is (˜5.5) and therefore impede digestion (Blytt *et al.*, 1988). Changes in the permeability of the intestinal wall caused by the reaction between tannins and the membrane proteins of the intestinal mucosal cells, and the resulting reduction in intestinal absorption, may also be responsible for reduced intestinal digestibility (McLeod, 1974; Silanikove *et al.*, 2001). These tests do not take into account factors such as the presence of bile salts (Blytt *et al.*, 1988), which could act as detergents and prevent the binding of tannins to digestive enzymes. The CTs inhibit the activity of hemicellulases than cellulases (Waghorn, 1996). This is possibly due to the fact that the latter are associated with bacterial cell walls while the hemicellulases are extracellular and therefore more sensitive (Van Soest, 1994). This explains the greater reduction in the degradability of hemicellulose in the presence of tannins (Barry and Manley, 1984; Waghorn *et al.*, 1994; Hervás *et al.*, 2003). Bakshi and Wadhwa (2004) reported the adverse effects of condensed tannins on the digestibility of nutrients (correlation coefficient for DM, NDF and CP was -0.71, -0.79 and -0.64, respectively), whereas hydrolysable tannins showed no such adverse affect (correlation coefficient for DM, NDF and CP were, 0.56, 0.46 and 0.4, respectively).

Methane inhibition

Condensed tannins can reduce enteric methane emissions from ruminants (Puchala *et al.*, 2005). The reduction in methane was confounded with changes in forage quality. Carulla *et al.* (2005) reported that feeding *Acacia mearnsii* (black wattle tree) extract (2.5% of DMI) to sheep decreased methane/kg of DM intake by approximately 12%. The affinity of condensed tannins for protozoa and methanogens may be particularly important due to the symbiotic role these populations have on methane production (McAllister *et al.*, 1996).

Animal production

Tannins in several types of forage can have beneficial effects in moderate amounts (Waghorn and McNabb, 2003). The high dietary concentrations of condensed tannins could negatively affect animal performance and may even possibly be toxic (Hervas *et al.*, 2003). The intake of CT @ 1.0- 4.0% of DM improves the digestive utilization of feed by ruminants, mainly because of a reduction in ruminal protein degradation and, as a consequence, a greater availability of essential amino acids for absorption in the small intestine (Barry and McNabb, 1999; Min *et al.*, 2003). Driedger and Hartfield (1972) report increases in nitrogen retention in lambs fed soya bean meal treated with HT.

Wang *et al.* (1996[a]) observed that the grazing of *L. corniculatus* (CT 3.4% of DM) reduced feed intake but increased the gain in liveweight, carcass weight, and dressing percentage. Montossi *et al.* (1996) observed a 23% improvement in liveweight gain and wool production by 10%, when lambs grazed *Holcus lanatus* (CT 4.2% of DM). Wang *et al.* (1996[b]) reported an increase of 21% milk production during mid and late lactation, increase in the efficiency of milk production, increased protein and lactose production, and a decrease in the fat content of the milk in sheep fed *L. corniculatus* (CT 4.4% of DM). With respect to the effect of CT on reproductive efficiency, Min *et al.* (1999) observed that sheep grazing *L. corniculatus* (CT 1.7% of DM) increased their production of lambs by 25% due to increased rates of ovulation and a subsequently increased lambing percentage, possibly related to protein utilization.

Bloat prevention

It is well documented that bloat occurs when grazing ruminants consume large quantities of leguminous plants. However, when these animals graze on leguminous plants containing CT (for example *Onobrychis viciifolia*) this does not occur (Barry and McNabb, 1999; McMahon *et al.*, 2000). The substitution of a small amount (approximately 10%) of ingested alfalfa DM by *Onobrychis viciifolia* provides unquestionable benefits in the prevention of bloat (McMahon *et al.*, 1999 and 2000).

Internal parasites

The tannins of numerous plant species help to control certain internal parasites of animals, for example the nematode *Trichostrongylus colubriformis* (Butter *et al.*, 2000). It is speculated that the positive effect on the host animal might be associated with a direct negative effect on the parasites plus an indirect effect in the form of increased availability and digestive utilization of protein (Min and Hart, 2003).

Toxicity

It has long been known that the toxicity of tannins is related to their molecular size (McLeod, 1974) as tannins with high molecular weight cannot be absorbed. This might explain the high toxicity of low molecular weight HT from *Quercus* species in rats, while the larger, high molecular weight CT of *Lespedeza cuneata* seem not to be toxic.

Blend of plant secondary metabolites

Extracts of garlic, cassium, anise, oregano, capsicum, yucca, and a combination of these extracts were evaluated in continuous culture fermenters inoculated with ruminal fluid from cows fed diets containing 60:40 forage to concentrate ratio. Extracts were dosed at a level approximating 150mg/ animal/day. Total VFA concentration was unaffected by treatment, but molar proportions of acetate increased when anise, oregano and capsicum were dosed; whereas, propionate decreased for yucca, anise, oregano and capsicum compared with control (no extracts) and the blend. Because the energy available for microbial growth was similar across treatments, the authors assumed that utilisation of peptides, amino acids and ammonia-N by rumen micro-organisms was similar across treatments. Therefore, changes in the concentration of nitrogen fractions were attributed to changes in the proteolytic, peptidolytic and deaminase activity of the mixed population of ruminal microbes. Anise increased protein degradation; whereas, garlic and yucca appeared to inhibit degradation. Lower concentrations of peptide N observed for oregano and extracts may indicate that these extracts accelerated the degradation of peptides to amino acids or that they reduced the rate of proteolysis or both. It was concluded that the use of some extracts individually performed better than a mixture, suggesting that antagonistic effects (clearly seen in peptide degradation) or interactions among individual additives occur. This may, in fact, negate an overall benefit for using a blend without a clear understanding of mode of action on rumen protein and energy metabolism.

Cinnamaldehyde (1g/cow per day; 43 mg/kg of DMI), quebracho condensed tannin extract (150 g/cow per day; 0.64% of DMI, providing 0.45% of condensed tannins), and *Yucca schidigera* saponin extract (60 g/ cow per day; 2,750 mg/ kg of DMI, providing 275 mg/ kg of saponins) exerted negligible effects on digestion, rumen microbial fermentation, protozoal numbers, milk production, and milk composition. Even though CIN has been reported to modulate rumen microbial fermentation *in vitro* at high dosage rates, results from this study suggest that it may be a challenge to achieve such effects *in vivo*. The lack of effects of these plant extracts may be due to the adaptation of ruminal microbes, to bacterial degradation of these compounds, or both (Benchaar *et al.,* 2008).

Organic acids

Some organic acids used as feed additives were found to be potent agent for rumen manipulation. Intermediates of the citric acid cycle accumulate in plant tissue and may represent as much as 10% of the DM of grasses (Stout *et al.,* 1967). Some of the forages like alfalfa, bermuda grass and tall fescue are rich in malate. It can contribute up to 1.5% of the DM of mature grasses (Bohman *et al.,* 1983) and between 2.9 and 4.5% of DM in different alfalfa varieties at 42 d of maturity (Callaway *et al.,* 1997). The intra-ruminal malate concentrations between 0.03 and 10 mM increased lactate uptake by *S. ruminantium* in a dose-response fashion, and the 10 mM level was the most stimulatory. However, release of this organic acid in the rumen may be dependent on at least some plant cell wall digestion. *In vitro* studies have shown that 7.5 mM malate is completely fermented within 10 to 24 h by mixed ruminal microorganisms (Callaway and Martin, 1997; Martin, 1998). Martin *et al* (1999) reported that there was linear increase in pH and acetate at increased level of malate (80 g/d) in cattle consuming high grain diet. Malate was more effective in lactate utilization than fumarate or aspartate. Collectively, these results suggest that selecting for and incorporating forage varieties that are high in malate may improve rumen fermentation. Malate can be a good alternative to antimicrobial compounds for curing acidosis because there is no risk of developing antibiotic resistance or having unwanted residues appearing in either meat or milk products.

Supplementation of medium chain fatty acids (carprylic and capric acid @ 5% of diet) selectively decreased the fibre digesting bacteria and so fibre digestibility. Amongst the medium chain fatty acids, carpic acid decreased the xylan digestion but not the caprylic acid. But long chain fatty acids had no apparent effect on fibre digestion (Ushida *et al.,* 1992) in sheep. Starch and pectin digestion was not affected by medium chain fatty acids (Ushida *et al.,* 1991). Fatty acids, especially from grass lipid had no inhibitory effect on activity of the fibrolytic bacteria (Hino and Nagatake, 1993). The grass lipids also contain β-carotene, which stimulate fibre digestion. So these two contrasting characters of grass lipids need careful consideration for manipulation.

Oligosaccharides

Oligosaccharides are constituted by two to ten units of sugar monomers (glucose, fructose, galactose, mannose, etc.). The best known are mannan oligosaccharides (MOS), galacto-oligosaccharides (GOS), fructo-oligosaccharides (FOS), xylo-oligosaccharides (XOS) and raffinose oligosaccharides (ROS).

Carbohydrates are important surface entities of many animal cells; they project from the cell surface and form the antigenic determinants of certain cell types. Bacteria (including pathogens) recognize these sugars and have receptors which allow them to attach, colonize and, in the case of pathogens cause disease in the animal. Mannose specific lectins (glycoprotein, protein fimbriae on the bacterial surface), are utilized by many gastrointestinal pathogens as a means of attachment to the gut epithelium. One way to prevent pathogens from causing disease is to prevent them from attaching to the epithelial cells in the gut. MOS has been successfully used to prevent this attachment by providing the bacteria a mannose-rich receptor that serves to occupy the binding sites on the bacteria and prevent colonization. Several studies have been conducted examining the role of mannans and their derivatives on binding of pathogens to epithelial cells in the GI tract. MOS causes agglutination of bacteria. Trials in species ranging from dogs, poultry, to pigs, calves and heifers have demonstrated reductions in pathogens such as *E. coli, Salmonella, Clostridia* and *Vibrio* sp. Unlike many feed additives, MOS is not affected by heat. Heating MOS to 121°C for 20 minutes had no adverse effects on any of the parameters examined. MOS are obtained from cell walls of yeasts, copra or palm kernel meal.

In addition to positive responses in terms of pathogen control, MOS supplementation modulates the immune function in a number of species ranging from turkeys to dogs, pigs and calves. Savage *et al.* (1996) found bile IgA and plasma IgG levels to be greater in birds supplemented with MOS compared to unsupplemented birds. In sows receiving MOS, higher concentrations of colostrum IgG and IgM were noted compared to unsupplemented sows. In addition, the piglets from supplemented sows were significantly heavier at weaning. MOS had a lower incidence of respiratory disease than unsupplemented calves (Newman *et al.*, 1993). Nonspecific cellular immunity has also been positively influenced enhanced macrophage activity. An overall improvement in performance of over 17% has been observed in summarizing over 12 trials conducted with MOS from Alltech, Inc.

The GOS are known to suppress ammonia producing bacteria, and stimulate the production of *Bifidobactrium* which has the ability to assimilate ammonia as an N source. GOS supplemented diets as compared to controls resulted in 10% reduction in CH_4 production. GOS may have enhanced propionate producers such as *Selenomonas*, *Succinomonas* and *Megasphaera*, while the growth of acetate producers (*Rumininococcus*, *Butyrivibrio*) may have been inhibited. Since propionate production competes with methanogenesis for available hydrogen, the increased molar production of propionate resulted in lower methane emission. These are readily fermented in the rumen and may have negative influence on fiber digestibility, especially that of hemicellulose. However, GOS are not digestible in non ruminants. When ruminants consume excess dietary nitrate, an acute and subclinical toxicity of nitrate occurs due to ruminal nitrite accumulation causing methemoglobin formation in blood. GOS were reported to decrease rumen methanogenesis and blood methemoglobinemia in nitrate-treated sheep. When GOS was administered with nitrate, blood methemoglobin levels tended to decrease compared to that in the administration of nitrate alone, possibly due to the abatement of ruminal and plasma nitrite accumulation by GOS.

Infusion with 0.6% SBOS in the ileum increased the amount of CD4 cells T-lymphocytes and the concentration of serum IgG and IgA. SBOS could improve cell-mediated and humoral immunity in sheep when infused in different parts of the gastrointestinal tract. The immune-stimulatory activities of SBOS in sheep observed in this study could be explained by the following facts. Firstly, SBOS can selectively stimulate the proliferation of beneficial bacteria that synthesize abundant nutrients such as vitamins and amino acids which are essential for the growth and development of immune organs. Secondly, SBOS can stimulate the proliferation of intestinal bifidobacteria which can stimulate the secretion of secretory IgA by immune cells in the intestinal mucosa. Thirdly, SBOS have toxin-, virus- and fungi-binding properties and can act as immune-adjuvant of these exogenous antigens to enhance B T-lymphocytes-mediated immunity.

Caution

Many herbs are extremely dangerous and should not be used without critical identification. The similarities between comfrey a well known herb for arthritis treatment and foxglove have proved fatal. Another herb ephedra can also be very dangerous.

Critical issues

- As herbs (PSM) possess different chemical and physical properties, they have different fermentation characteristics and hence, effects on animal health.

- Optimal levels of inclusion in diets yet to be established for most animal species.
- The optimum level may vary depending on the physiological status of the animal.
- Interactions between the active components need to be elucidated.
- Pre-biotic oligosaccharides may antagonize the effects of antibiotics.
- Type of feedstuffs offered, roughage to concentrate ratio in the diet and production potential (milk, meat and wool) of the animal may affect the response to PSM.
- Most of the studies are based on *in vitro* fermentation; similar results may not be obtained in *in-vivo* studies, under field conditions.
- The possible adaptation of rumen microbes to the herbal feed additive may limit the utility of an herb (PSM) on the performance of animals.
- The duration of supplementation of herbs and specific withdrawal periods needs to be investigated.
- Due to the growing focus on food safety, it is imperative to explore alternatives to antimicrobial compounds to address the acidosis problem.
- Practical formulations and economics are yet to be worked out.
- Mode of supplementation (powdered herb or crude extract or active component extract or pure active component) needs to be worked out.

References

Agarwal, N., Kamra, D. N., Chaudhary, L. C. and Patra, A. K. (2006). *J. Appl. Anim. Res.,* 30:1-4.

Bakshi, M. P. S. and Wadhwa, M. (2004). *Bubalus bubalis., J. Buffalo Sci. Tech.,* 10: 65-70.

Bakshi, M. P. S., Neelam Rani, Wadhwa, M. and Kaushal, S. (2005). *Indian J. Anim.Nutr.,* 21: 249-53.

Bakshi, M.P.S. and Wadhwa, M. (2009). Pakistan J. Zool. 9 (Supple 2).

Bakshi, M.P.S. and Wadhwa, M. (2011[a]). Significance of Plant Secondary Metabolites in Relation to Methane Production by Ruminants. *Proc. Anim. Nutr. Assoc. Conf.* held at Bhubaneshwar, pp. 25-28.

Bakshi, M.P.S. and Wadhwa, M. (2011[b]). Role of phytogenics in mitigation of enteric methane production and performance of animals. In Nutritional Interventions for clean and green livestock production, (Chaturvedi, V.B., Dutta, N., Verma, A.K., Singh, P. and Kamra, D.N. (Eds.) held at IVRI Feb. 3-23. pp. 180-184.

Barry, T.N. and Manley, T.R. (1984). *Br. J. Nutr.,* 51: 493-504.

Barry, T.N. and Mcnab, W.C. (1999). *Br. J. Nutr.*, 81: 263-72.

Benchaar, C., Calsamiglia, S., Chaves, A.V., Fraser, G.R., Colombatto, D., McAllister, T.A. and Beauchemin, K.A. (2008). Anim. Feed Sci. Technol. 145 : 209-228.

Benchaar, C., Petit, H.V., Berthiaume, R., Ouellet, D.R., Chiquette, J. and Chouinard, P.Y. (2007). *J. Dairy. Sci.*, 90: 886-897.

Benchaar, C., Petit, H.V., Berthiaume, R., Whyte, T.D. and Chouinard, P.Y. (2006). *J. Dairy. Sci.*, 89: 4652-64.

Blytt, H.J., Guscar, T.K. and Butler, L.G. (1988). *J. Chem. Ecol.*, 14: 1455-65.

Bohman, V. R., Horn, F. P., Stewart, B. A., Mathers, A.C. and Grunes, D.L. (1983). *J. Anim. Sci.* 57:1352-1363.

Burt, S. (2004). *Int. J. Food Microbiol.*, 94: 223-53.

Butter, N.L., Dawson, J.M., Wakelin, D., Buttery, P.J. (2000). *J. Agric. Sci.*, 134: 89-99.

Callaway, T. R., and Martin, S.A. (1997). *J. Dairy Sci.* 80: 1126-1135.

Callaway, T. R., Martin, S. A., Wampler, J.L., Hill, N.S., Gill G.M. (1997). *J. Dairy Sci.* 80: 1651-1655.

Calsamiglia, S., Busquet, M., Cardozo, P.W., Castillejos, L. and Ferret, A. (2007). *J. Dairy Sci.* 90: 2580-2595.

Carulla, J. E., Kreuzer, M., Machmuller, A. and Hess, H. D. (2005). *Aust. J. Agric. Res.* 56: 961-970.

Chao, S. C. and Young, D. G. (2000). *J. Essential Oil Res.* 12: 639-49.

Chao, S.C., Young, D.G. and Oberg, C.J. (2000). *J. Essential Oil Res.*, 12: 639-49.

Cheeke, P.R. (1996). *Adv. Exp. Med. Biol.*, 405: 377-85.

Cheel, J., Theoduloz, C., Rodriiguez, J. and Schmeda-Hirschmann, G. (2005). *J. Agric. Food Chem.* 53: 2511-17.

Chwalek, M., Ple, K. and Voutquenne-Nazabadioko, L. (2004). *Chem. Pharm. Bull.*, 52: 965-71.

Concha, C., Hu, S.and Holmberg, O. (1996). *Vet. Res.* 27:107-15.

Cox, S.D., Mann, C.M. and Markam, J.L. (2001). *J. Appl. Microbiol.*, 91: 492-97.

Deans, S. G. and Ritchie, G. (1987). *Int. J. Food Microbiol.* 5: 165-80.

Dorman, H. J. D. and Deans, S.G. (2000). *J. Appl. Microbiol.*, 88: 308-16.

Driedger, A. and Hatfield, E. (1972). *J. Anim. Sci.*, 34: 465-68.

Dudareva, N., Pichersky, E. and Gershenzon, J. (2004). *Plant Physiol.*, 135: 1893-1902.

Duval. S.M., McEwan N.R., Graham R.C., Wallace R.J. and Newbold C.J. 2007. *J. Appl. Microb.* ISSN 1364-72.

EC. 2003. European Commission, *Official J. Eur. Commun.*, L268: 29-43.

Gee, J.M., Wal, J.M., Miller, K., Atkinson, H., Grigoriadou, F., Wijnands, M.V.W., Penniks, A.H., Wortley, G. and Johnson, I.T. 1996. *Toxicology* 117: 219-28.

Gershenzon, J., and Croteau, R.B. 1991. *Terpenoids.*, pp165-219.

Gershenzon, J., Mc Conkey, M.E. and Croteau, R.B. 2000. *Plant Physiol.*, 22: 205-13.

Goetsch, A.L. and Owens, F.N. 1985. *J. Dairy Sci.*, 68: 2377-84.

Greathead, H. (2003). *Proc. Nutr. Soc.*, 62: 279-90.

Gutierrez, J.D. and Davis, R.E. (1962). *J. Anim. Sci.*, 21: 819-23.

Hagerman, A.E. and Butler, L.G. (1991). In: *Herbivores: their interactions with secondary plant metabolites*, Vol I: The chemical participants, (Rosenthal G.A. and Berenbaum M.R., eds.), Academic Press, NY (USA), pp. 355-388.

Hammer, K.A., Carson, C.F. and Riley, T.V. (1999). *J. Appl. Microbiol.*86: 985-90.

Hervás, G., Frutos, P., Giráldez, F.J., Mantecón, A.R., Álvarez Del Pino, M.C. (2003). *Anim. Feed Sci. Technol.*, 109: 65-78.

Hess, H.D., Beuret, R.A., Lotscher, M., Hindrichsen, I.K., Machmuller, A., Carulla, J.E., Lascano, C.E., Kreuzer, M. (2004). *J. Anim. Sci.*, 79: 177-89.

Hess, H.D., Kreuzer, M., Diaz, T.E., Lascano, C.E., Carulla, J.E., Soliva, C.R., Machmuller, A. (2003[a]). *Anim. Feed Sci. Technol.*, 109: 79-94.

Hess, H.D., Monsalve, L.M., Lascano, C.E., Carulla, J.E., Diaz, T.E., Kreuzer, M. (2003[b]). *Aust. J. Agric. Res.*, 54: 703-13.

Hino, T. and Nagatake, Y. (1993). *Anim. Feed Sci. Technol.*, 64: 121-28.

Hirasa, K., and Takemasa, M. (1998). *Spice Science Technology*, Marcel Dekker, Inc., New York.

Hosoda, K., Kuramoto, K., Eruden, B., Nishida, T. and Shioya. S. (2006). *Asian-Austr. J. Anim. Sci.* 19: 35-41.

Iason, G. (2005) *Proc. Nutr. Soc.*, 64: 123-31.

Ilsley, S.E., Miller, H.M. and Kamel, C. (2005). *J. Anim. Sci.* 83: 82-88.

Jones, G.A., McAllister, T.A., Muir, A.D. and Cheng, K.J. (1994). *Appl. Environ. Microb.*, 60: 1374-78.

Jung, H.J., Lee, C.O., Lee, K.T., Choi, J. and Park, H.J. (2004). *Biol. Pharm. Bull.*, 27: 744-47.

Juven, B. J., Kanner, J., Schved, F., and Weisslowicz, H. (1994). *J. App. Bact.*, 76: 626-31.

Kamel, C. (2001). *Recent Adv. Anim. Nutr.*, 135-50.

Kamra, D. N., Singh, R., Chaudhary, L. C., Aggarwal, N. and Pathak, N. N. (2000). *Buffalo J.*, 16: 99-104.

Klita, P.T., Mathison, G.W., Fenton, T.W. and Hardin, R.T. (1996). *J. Anim. Sci.* 74: 1144-56.

Kodera, Y., Suzuki, A., Imada, I., Kasuga, S., Sumioka, I., Kanezawa, A., Fujikawa, M., Nagae, S., Masamoto, M. (2002). *J. Agric. Food Chem.*, 50: 622-32.

Kukde, R.J., Kalaskur, S.R. and Nimbalkar, R.V. (1999). *Pashudhan,* 14: 5.

Kumar, R. and Singh, M. (1984). *J. Agr. Food Chem.*, 32: 447-53.

Kung, L. Jr., Williams, P., Schmidt, R. J. and Hu, W. (2008). *J. Dairy Sci.* 91: 4793-4800.

Lamba, J.S., Wadhwa, M. and Bakshi, M.P.S. (2009). *Asian-Aust. J.Anim.Sci.* (In Press).

Lila, Z.A., Mohammed, N., Kandam S., Mitsunori, K., and Itabashi, H. (2005). *Asian-Aust. J. Anim. Sci.*, 18: 1746-51.

Liu, J.Y., Yuan, W.Z., Ye, J. and Wu, Y. (2003). *Proc. Sixth Internl. Symp. Nutr. Herbi. Merida,* Mexico.

Mahmoud, A. L. E. (1994). *Lett. Appl. Microbiol.*, 19: 110-13.

Makkar, H.P.S. and Becker, K. (1997). *Lett. Appl. Microbiol.*, 25: 243-45.

Makkar, H.P.S., Sen, S., Blummel, M. and Becker, K. (1998). *J. Agric. Food Chem.*, 46: 4324-28.

Martin, S.A. (1998). *J. Anim. Sci.*, 65: 9-15.

Martin, S.A., Streeter, M.N., Nisbet, D.S., Hill, G. and Williams, S.E. (1999). *J. Anim. Sci.*, 77: 1008-15.

McAllister, T.A., Bae, H.D., Jones, G.A. and Cheng, K.J. (1994[a]). *J. Anim. Sci.*, 72: 3004-18.

McAllister, T.A., Okine, E.K., Mathison, G.W. and Cheng, K.J. (1996). *Can. J. Anim. Sci.*, 76: 231-243.

McLeod, M.N. (1974). *Nutr. Abstr. Rev.*, 44: 803-12.

McMahon, L.R., Majak, W., Mcallister, T.A., Hall, J.W., Jones, G.A., Popp, J.D. and Cheng, K.J. (1999). *Can. J. Anim. Sci.*, 79: 203-12.

McMahon, L.R., McAllister, T.A., Berg, B.P., Majak, W., Acharya, S.N., Popp, J.D., Coulman, B.E., Wang, Y. and Cheng, K.J. (2000). *Can. J. Plant Sci.*, 80: 469-85.

McSweeney, C.S., Palmer, B., Mcneill, D.M. and Krause, D.O. (2001). *Anim. Feed Sci. Technol.*, 91: 83-93.

Min, B.R. and Hart, S.P. (2003). *J. Anim. Sci.*, 81: E102-E109.

Min, B.R., Mcnabb, W.C., Barry, T.N., Kemp, P.D., Waghorn, G.C. and Mcdonald, M.F. (1999) *J. Agric. Sci.*, 132: 323-34.

Montossi, F.M., Hodgson, J., Morris, S.T. and Risso, D.F. (1996). *Proc. NZ. Soc. Anim. Prod.*, 56: 118-21.

Mueller-Harvey, I. and McAllan, A.B. (1992). In: *Advances in plant cell biochemistry and biotechnology,* Vol. 1 (Morrison I.M., ed.). JAI Press Ltd., London (UK), pp. 151-17.

Naganawa, R., Iwata, N., Ishikawa, K., Fukudua, H., Fujino, T. and Suzuki, A. (1996). *Appl. Environ. Microbiol.*, 62: 4238-42.

Nagaraja, T.G., (1995). In: *Biotechnology in Animal Feeds and Animals Feeding.* Wallace, R.J., Chesson, A. (Eds.), VCH Verlagsgesellschaft, Weinheim, pp. 173-204.

Neelam Rani, Wadhwa, M., Kaushal, S. and Bakshi, M.P.S. (2006). *Anim. Nutr. Feed Technol.*, 6: 147-51.

Newbold, C.J., ElHassan, S.M., Wang, J., Ortega, M.E. and Wallace, R.J. (1997). *Br. J. Nutr.*, 78: 237-49.

Newman, K.E., Jacques, K.A. and Buede, R. (1993). *J. Anim. Sci.* 71: 271.

Ningrat, R.W.S., Garnsworthy, P.C. and Newbold, C.J. (2002). *Reprod. Nutr. Dev.*, 42: (Suppl. 1): S82.

O'Donovan, L. and Brooker, J.D. (2001). *Microbiol.*, 147: 1025-33.

O'Gara, E. A., Hill, D. J., and Maslin, D.J. (2000). *Appl. Enviorn. Microbiol.*, 66: 2269-73.

Odenyo, A.A., Osuji, P.O. and Karanfil, O. components, and susceptible microorganisms.

(1997). *Anim. Feed Sci. Technol.*, 67: 169-80.

Ouattara, B., Simard, R. E., Holley, R. A., Piette, G.J.P. and Be´gin, A. (1997). *Int. J. Food Microbiol.* 37: 155-62.

Patra, A. K., Kamra, D. N. and Aggarwal, N. (2006[a]). *Anim. Feed sci. Technol.*, 128: 276-91.

Patra, A. K., Kamra, D. N. and Aggarwal, N. (2006[b]). *Internl. Cong. Ser.*, 1293: 176-79.

Pen, B., Sar, C., Mwenya, B., Kuwaki, K., Morikawa, R. and Takahashi, J. (2006). *Anim Feed Sci. Technol.*, 129:175-86.

Perevolotsky, A. (1994). *Oikos.*, 71: 333-40.

Pinares-Patin˜ O.C.S., Ulyatt, M. J., Waghorn, G. C., Lassey, K. R., Barry, T. N., Holmes, C. W. and Johnson, D. E. (2003). *J. Agric. Sci.* 140: 215-26.

Puchala, R., Min, B.R., Goetsch, A.L. and Sahlu, T. (2005). *J. Anim. Sci.*, 83: 182-86.

Rana, K.K., Wadhwa, M. and Bakshi, M.P.S. (2006). *Asian-Aust. J. Anim. Sci.*, 19: 1134-38.

Reuter, H.D., Koch, J.P. and Lawson, L. (1996). In *Garlic, the science and therapeutic application of Allium sativa L. and related species.*, H.P. Koch and L.D. Lawson ed. PP 135-12, Williams and Wilkins, Baltimore, MD.

Riguera, R. 1997. *J. Mar. Biotechnol.*, 5: 187-93.

Ross, Z. M., O'Gara, E. A., Hill, D. J., Sleightholme, H. V. and Maslin, D. J. (2001). *Appl. Environ. Microbiol.*, 67: 475-80.

Ryan, J. P., Quinn, T., and Leek, B. L. (1997). *J. Dairy Sci.*, 81: 3222-30.

Santoso, B., Mwenya, B., Sar, C., Gamo, Y., Kobayashi, T., Morikawa, R. and Takahash, J. (2004[a]). *J. Anim. Sci.*, 75: 525-31.

Santoso, B., Mwenya, B., Sar, C., Gamo,Y., Kobayashi, T., Morikawa, R., Kimura, K., Mizukoshi, H. and Takahashi, J. (2004[b]). *Livest. Prod. Sci.*, 91: 209-17.

Savage, T. F., Cotter, P. F. and Zakrzewska, E. I. (1996). *Poult. Sci.* 75: 143 (abstr.).

Seeman, P. (1974). *Fed. Proc.*, 33: 2116-24.

Silanikove, N., Nitsan, Z. and Perevolotsky, A. (1994). *J. Agric. Food Chem.*, 42: 2844-47.

Silanikove, N., Perevolotsky, A. and Provenza, F.D. (2001). *Anim. Feed Sci. Technol.*, 91: 69-81.

Singh, N., Kumari, R., Yadav, R.S., Akbar, M.A. and Sengupta, B.P. (1991). *Indian Vet Med J.*, 15: 20-24.

Sivropoulou, A., Papanikolaou, E., Nikolaou, C., Kokkini, S., Lanaras, T. and Arsenakis, M. (1996). *J. Agric. Food Chem.*, 44: 1202-1205.

Smith-Palmer, A., Stewart, J. and Fyfe, L. (1998). *Lett. Appl. Microbiol.*, 26:118-22.

Stoll, A. and Seebeck, E. (1948). *Helv. Chim. Acta.*, 31: 189-210.

Stout, P.R., Brownell, J. and Burau, R.G. (1967). *Agron. J.* 59: 21-24.

Stumm, C.K. and Zwart, K.B. (1986). *Microbiol. Sci.*, 3: 100-105.

Thalib, A., Widiawatii, Y., Hamid, H., Suherman, D. and Sabrani, M. (1996). *J. Ilmu Ternak dan Vertiner.*, 2: 17-20.

Ushida, K., Kojima, Y. and Kawashima, R. (1991). *Anim. Sci. Tech.*, 62: 870-74.

Ushida, K., Miyazaki, A. and Kawashima, R. (1986). *Jpn. J. Zootech. Sci.*, 57: 71-77.

Ushida, K., Tokura, M., Takenaka, A., and Itabashi, H. (1997). In *Rumen Microbes and Digestive Physiology in Ruminants.* R. Onodera, H. Itabashi, K. Ushida, H. Yano, and Y. Sasaki, eds. PP 209-20. Japan Scientific Societies Press, Tokyo and S. Karger AG Basel, Switzerland.

Ushida, K., Umeda, M., Kishigami, R. and Kojima, Y. (1992). *Anim. Sci. Tech.*, 63: 591-97.

Van Soest, P.J. (ed.), (1994). *Nutritional ecology of the ruminant,* 2nd ed. Cornell Univ Press. Ithaca, NY, USA. 476 p.

Viana, G.S.B., Vale, T.G., Pinho, R.S.N. and Matos. F.J.A. (2000). *J. Ethnopharmacol.* 70: 323-27.

Wadhwa, M. and Bakshi, M.P.S. (2006). *Indian J. Anim. Nutr.*, 23: 102-109.

Wadhwa, M. and Bakshi, M.P.S. (2009). Animal agriculture and green house gas emission: Mitigation strategres. Proc. World Comf. Anim. Nutr. Assoc. (Eds. Pattanaik, A.K., Verma, A.K., Kamra, D.N. and Sharma, K.). pp. 119-122.

Wadhwa, M. Hundal, J.S., Kaur, K. and Bakshi, M.P.S. (2010). Effect of essential oils dissolved on different solvents on in vitro methane production. Proc. 4th Intl. Comf. Greenhouse gases and Animal Agriculture, pp. 157. held at Banff. Canada.

Waghorn, G. (1996). *Proc. Canadian Soc. Anim. Sci. Annual Meeting*, Lethbridge, Canada (Rode L.M., ed.). pp. 175-94.

Waghorn, G.C. and McNabb, W.C. (2003). *Proc. Nutr. Soc.*, 62: 383-92.

Waghorn, G.C., Shelton, I.D. and McNabb, W.C. (1994[a]). *J. Agric. Sci.*, 123: 99-107.

Wallace, R.J., Arthaud, L. and Newbold, C.J. (1994). *Appl. Environ. Microbiol.*, 60: 1762-67.

Wang, Y., Douglas, G.B., Waghorn, G.C., Barry, T.N. and Foote, A.G. (1996[a]). *J. Agric. Sci.*, 126: 353-62.

Wang, Y., McAllister, T.A., Yanke, L.J., Xu, Z.J., Cheeke, P.R. and Cheng, K.J. (2000). *J. Sci. Food Agric.*, 80: 2114-22.

Wang, Y., Waghorn, G.C., McNabb, W.C., Barry, T.N., Hedley, M.J. and Shelton, I.D. (1996[b]). *J. Agric. Sci.*, 127: 413-21.

Wang,Y., McAllister, T.A., Newbold, C.J., Rode, L.M., Cheeke, P.R. and Cheng, K.J. (1998). *Anim. Feed Sci. Technol.*, 74: 143-53.

Wawrzynczak, S., Kraszewski, J., Wawryznski, M. and Kozlowski, J. (2000). *Ann. Anim. Sci. Roczniki-Naukowe-Zootechniki* 27: 133-42.

Wina, E., Muetzel, S. and Becker, K. (2006). *J. Appl. Microbiol.*, 100: 114-22.

Yang, W.Z., Benchaar, C., Ametaj, B.N., Chaves, A.V., He, M.L. and McAllister, T.A. (2007). *J. Dairy Sci.* 90: 5671-81.

Yoshiki, Y., Kudou, S. and Okubo, K. (1998). *Biosci. Biotech. Biochem,.* 62: 2291-99.

□□□

Animal Nutrition, 2012
eds. Dr. (Mrs.) Usha R. Mehra et al., pp. 735-752
Satish Serial Publishing House e-mail : info@satishserial.com; website : www.satishserial.com

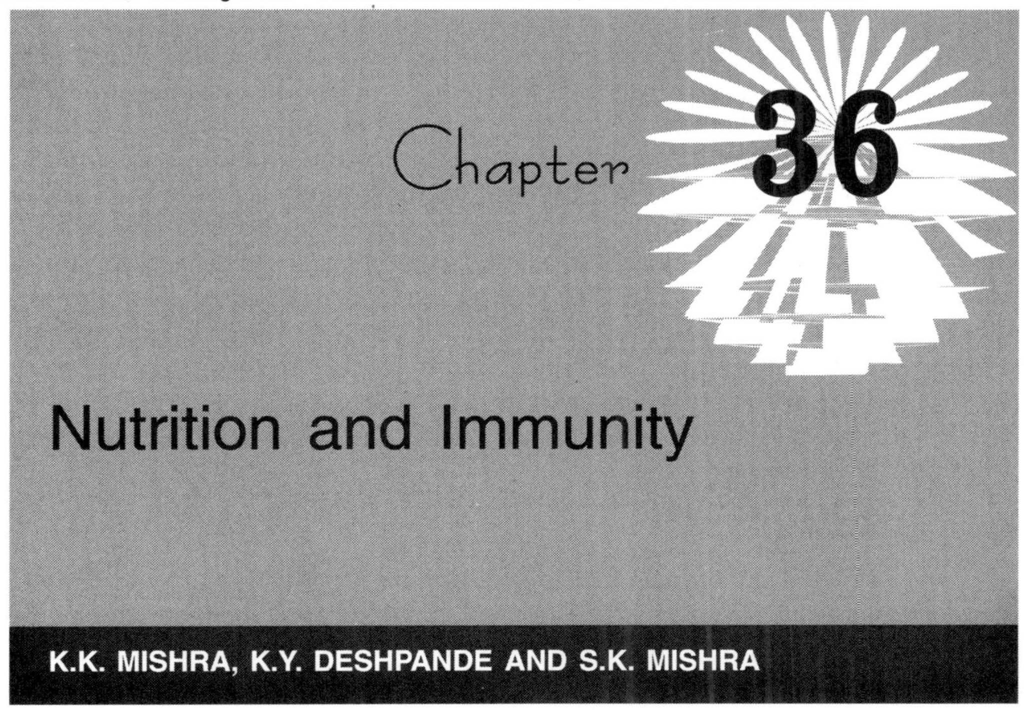

Chapter 36

Nutrition and Immunity

K.K. MISHRA, K.Y. DESHPANDE AND S.K. MISHRA

Nutrition has inclusive role in several physiological processes in the body. Hence, it is obvious that nutrition has important implications to immunity and incidence of diseases in animals. Though assumed since ages, it is only in recent years that specific mechanisms by which nutrients affect immunity have become known. The foundations for Nutritional Immunology emerged in the early 1800s with the finding that severe malnutrition would lead to thymic atrophy and for most of that century; all evidence for a relationship between malnutrition and the immune system was based on anatomical findings. After the discovery of vitamins, it became evident that essential nutrients have an important role in host resistance. Vitamin A is commonly known as the "anti-infective" vitamin. Many attempts have been made to use vitamin A therapeutically during infectious diseases. With the development of knowledge about the functions of immune system, it was proposed that malnutrition depresses humoral immunity by reducing the production of antibodies to vaccines and cell mediated immunity by inducing allergy to intra-dermal tests. Abraham E. Axelrod and his students initiated the systematic studies of immuno-nutritional inter-relationships in laboratory animals in 1947 followed by numerous studies and the field of nutritional immunology was well established by the late 1970s. Since the immune response requires rapid synthesis of proteins for immune cells and immune products, the immune system is particularly sensitive to a nutrient deficiency. Synthesis of these proteins is directly or indirectly affected by most nutrient deficiencies including vitamins and trace minerals. Other nutrients like vitamin A and D regulate the immune response or act as antioxidants to protect immune cells and other cells from the toxic effects of a wide variety of enzymes and chemicals used by the immune cells to destroy bacteria and infected cells. The immune system has especially high requirements for antioxidant nutrients as compared to other systems in the body. These nutrients are quickly depleted when animals are stressed e.g. when suffering from infectious diseases. To comprehend the inter-relationship between nutrition and immunity, a brief account on types of immunity is discussed ahead.

Types of Immunity

Innate immunity: It consists of several anatomic, physiologic, and cellular components. Innate immunity is a non-selective immune system. It does not modify itself depending upon the type of pathogen challenge. Instead, it prevents infection by targeting general properties of pathogens. It includes epithelial tissue which covers body surfaces (example skin or hide, hoof, cornea) and lines body cavities (respiratory, urogenital, gastrointestinal), secretions that block (mucus) or washout (saliva, tears) infectious agents, cells in blood and tissue that engulf, kill and digest infectious microorganisms (phagocytes) and include macrophages, monocytes, and neutrophils. Epithelial tissues act as a physical barrier to keep infectious agents from entering the body. Breaks in this covering layer caused by physical damage or by nutrient deficiencies such as vitamin A and zinc can result in infectious agents gaining access to the body. Phagocytes continually circulate through blood and migrate into tissues in search of invading pathogens. The cellular component of innate immunity identifies pathogens by their presentation of distinct pathogen-associated molecular patterns (PAMPs). Specifically, pathogens contain molecules not typically found in mammalian cells and via such strategies; the cells of the innate system are able to recognize foreign cells (Forsberg and Wang, 2006). Many antimicrobial compounds in body fluids and secretions are frequently affected by stress. Apart from these, normal microbial flora can compete with disease causing organisms, thereby holding them in check but are less effective in stressed animals. The term innate immunity implies that it is stable or unwavering. However, this is not the case. Although always present to some degree, innate immunity is regulated and may be strengthened or weakened by plane of nutrition.

Specific or acquired immunity: Exposure to a foreign substance (antigen) results in the development of immune cells and antibodies specific against that particular antigen only. It takes time for the specific immunity to develop and therefore is effective in preventing infection only if the animal was previously exposed to that antigen. It is also important for recovery from many infections. The foreign substance (antigen) may be a live virus or bacteria but need not be infective or alive to induce immunity. Weakened or dead viruses or bacteria, and even specific fragments of pathogens or pieces of their DNA can be used in vaccines to induce immunity with reduced risk of disease. This exposure to the antigen triggers growth and development of two types of blood cells specific for eliminating the antigen which are the T-cells (cell-mediated immunity) and the B-cells responsible for antibody production (humoral immunity).

T-cells secrete numerous chemicals such as interleukins and interferon, which help to regulate the entire immune system as needed and increase effectiveness of other immune cells including phagocytes and B-cells. Some T-cells directly destroy target cells. Antibodies are secreted by B-cells and found in blood plasma, nasal secretions and other fluids. Because of their fairly large size, they cannot enter into cells. Hence, are not effective against intracellular pathogens. All antibodies act by binding to the foreign substance which in many cases prevents the virus or bacteria from replicating or being infective. Apart from this, it makes much easier for other immune products or cells to destroy the pathogen. Vaccines may be designed to stimulate primarily an antibody response or an increase in cell-mediated immunity, depending on which type of immune response is most effective against a specific pathogen. All immune mechanisms are neither affected equally by a nutrient deficiency nor does it always affect the same mechanism equally for different antigens. Deficient animals may have adequate antibody responses to some antigens or vaccines, while depressed antibody responses to other antigens. Under practical conditions, deficient animals may be more susceptible to some but not all disease causing organisms. After challenge by a pathogen, a systemic acute phase or inflammatory response results which is considered to be the foundation of non-specific immunity. Antibody titers developing as a result of the humoral response are not a direct burden on the animal's pool of nutrients. Hence, they are nutritionally inconsequential. It is only the systemic acute phase response that has nutritional consequences for the animal and is associated with a shift in nutrients use away from skeletal muscle accretion and towards hepatic secretion of acute phase proteins as well as cellular and macromolecule turnover.

Effect of Nutritional Status on Resistance to Infection

Disease-resistance of stressed animals can be improved by good nutrition by helping to counteract the suppression of the immune system caused by stress hormones and by providing nutrients essential for maintaining and activating the immune system. In general, diets containing relatively low or high levels of dietary proteins adversely affect immunity to infection compared to diets with moderate protein levels. Vitamins A and D within the ranges that are normally fed are important in immunity regulation. Vitamin A deficiency reduces resistance to all types of disease, including parasites. Vitamin A supplementation is essential for cattle fed grain based diets. Under practical conditions, vitamin D deficiency is unlikely to be a concern even when cattle are not supplemented, unless they also do not have access to sunlight.

Antioxidant nutrients are crucial to the immune response, becoming rapidly depleted during infection. The amount of antioxidant nutrients in the diet determines the antioxidant status of the animal. These key nutrients include dietary antioxidants such as carotenes, vitamin E and vitamin A, and trace minerals such as selenium, zinc, copper and manganese used to synthesize antioxidant enzymes. Antioxidants protect immune cells and surrounding tissues from damage caused by the immune response, which otherwise would damage the animal as much or more than the disease organisms. Antioxidants help to maintain the effectiveness of phagocytes, which are the first- line of defense against invading pathogens. If phagocytes are deficient in antioxidants, microbial killing is ineffective. Vitamin E is currently the most important antioxidant in feedlot diets. Supplementation with vitamin E has been reported to improve growth, feed efficiency, morbidity and antibody titers of feedlot cattle, but not consistently (Secrist *et al.*, 1997). Magnesium and phosphorus are the most important macro minerals associated with the immune response and their supplementation levels influence the immune status of the animal and mortality.

Trace minerals have important functions as components of vital proteins. Young growing animals are depositing protein at high rates and are therefore more vulnerable to trace element deficiencies than older animals. Copper, zinc, manganese and selenium are also required for the production of antioxidant enzymes. Deficiencies of copper and selenium impair the ability of bovine phagocytes to kill invading microorganisms. A zinc deficiency increases nonspecific infections, and inhibits normal healing of wounds. It is well known that B-vitamins and vitamin C affect immunity and resistance to stress. Cattle are unusual in that most B-vitamins are supplied by microbial synthesis in the rumen, rather than the diet. In fact, dietary B-vitamins are usually degraded in the rumen. The combination of stress and low intake can result in low availability of B-vitamins, which may affect rumen microbes and/or the animal itself. In spite of the fact that B-vitamin requirements of cattle are not known, and that dietary B-vitamins are partially or extensively degraded in the rumen, B-vitamin supplementation of diets has been reported to improve performance.

It is extremely important to distinguish between the effects of nutrition on immunological function in adults from those upon neonatal or developing organisms. Insufficient availability of essential nutrients is a more critical factor in young animals than in adults since young animals undergo rapid growth and development and are subjected to a higher degree of physiological stress. Therefore, nutritional deficiencies which might not result in an impaired immune response in adult animals might cause notable dysfunction in the developing fetus or neonate, rendering it more susceptible to a variety of infectious agents. If the essential nutrient deficiency occurs during a critical period of development or embryogenesis, the capacity for normal immune ontogenesis may be permanently compromised. Consequently, even prolonged periods of subsequent nutritional rehabilitation in such animals may not result in an acceptable level of immunological function (Gershwin *et al.*, 1987).

Malnutrition and Immunity Development

A number of attempts have been made to reproduce dietary conditions in experimental animals similar to those of malnourished animal populations. While it is difficult to duplicate such dietary deficiencies, empirical studies in animals allow one to observe precisely and serially the effects of early nutritional deficiencies and also allow for specific antigenic challenge. The results in turn, have helped to elucidate the role of specific nutrients in the immunodeficiency observed in animals. Several mechanisms for the immunodeficiency observed in animals fed restricted levels of protein and calories during development have been suggested (Srivastava *et al.*, 1981). Abnormal metabolism of nucleotides and nucleosides occurs in both thymus and spleen of neonatal offspring of rats experiencing dietary deprivation e.g. thymocytes and splenocytes from the malnourished rats have altered intracellular levels of ATP, ADP, cAMP, 5′AMP and adenosine, suggesting that such metabolic alterations may be fundamental to the immunodeficiency observed in animals deprived of essential nutrients during critical periods of development. This further proves that protein energy under nutrition early in life can modulate the metabolism of mRNA and hence protein synthesis in lymphoidal tissues. How far these changes influence the immune responsiveness of the animal is not known yet.

Impaired histidine metabolism (amination) may in part be responsible for the immunodeficiency of protein-calorie under nutrition (Enwonwu, 1986).

It has been established in several experimental animals that protein calorie under nutrition can result in a marked increase in the free histidine pool in several tissues due to increased synthesis of the amine. Some functional subsets of T-lymphocytes have a greater density of histamine receptors than other lymphocytes (Plaut *et al.* 1980) and the cytolytic activity of the former is inhibited by histamine through a histamine induced increase in cAMP. Histamine can also have a suppressive effect on lymphocyte proliferation, which is due to a histamine induced increase in prostaglandins or a histamine induced reduction in interleukin-2 production and activity (Gershwin *et al.* 1987).

Protein Deficiency during Peri-natal Immunogenesis

The protein malnutrition poses significant hindrance to immunogenesis. The studies have shown that immune responsiveness of rodents deprived of protein during gestation is markedly altered. Feeding rats protein deficient diet for 4 days prior to mating and then throughout gestation results in a delay in the appearance of IgG_{2B} in malnourished offspring (Olusi *et al.*, 1980). Even after nutritional rehabilitation for 4 months with a high protein diet, IgG levels in serum are significantly lower in formerly malnourished offspring. Offspring born to dams that are fed a diet deficient in protein for 3 months prior to gestation have a prolonged period of reduced immune function (Gebhardt and Newberne, 1974). Thus, protein deficiency alone can impair immune responsiveness for prolonged periods, perhaps permanently, if imposed during critical periods of development of immune system.

Vitamin Deficiencies during Peri-natal Immunogenesis

Vitamin deficiency during development and its influence upon the ontogenesis of intact immune function has been investigated rather sporadically. Nonetheless, the potential importance of such deficiencies is becoming apparent as methodology to detect marginal degrees of deficiency is being developed. Laboratory animals fed vitamin A deficient diets are more vulnerable to natural or experimentally induced infections (Nauss and Newberne, 1985) and are characterized by low macrophage activity, impaired antigen-stimulated lymphocyte trapping in lymph nodes and a reduced response to polyclonal mitogens. Vitamin A deficiency imposed in mice during the last third of pregnancy and continued until weeks postnatal has been reported to result in marked immunological dysfunction like impaired delayed hypersensitivity response to skin antigens such as dinitrofluorobenzene and reduced serum IgM responses to a protein antigen (Smith *et al.*, 1987). Detailed studies on effect of vitamins deficiency on immunity development in neonates are warranted to improve our understanding of these subtle mechanisms.

Mineral Deficiencies during peri-natal Immunogenesis

Insufficient trace metals during critical periods of immune development can have profound and deleterious impact on ability of the host to respond to pathogenic challenge.

Zinc: It is the most comprehensively studied of all minerals with regard to its effect upon the development of the immune response. Effects of Zinc deficiency on immune functions include increased susceptibility to infection (hypogammaglobulinemia), abnormal cell mediated immunity, depressed cytotoxicity, depressed levels of natural killer cell activity, circulating thymic hormones and depressed/retarded growth of lymphoid organs during fetal or early post-natal deprivation (especially T- dependant tissues) and mobility of B-cell surface markers (Gershwin *et al.,* 1987). Deficiency of zinc imposed in mice beginning at parturition and continuing throughout the postnatal period results in profound abrogation of a number of immune functions. Such post-natal zinc deprived mice experienced a selective retardation of lymphoid organ growth, most notably the thymus (Beach *et al.,* 1979). A number of immune parameters are also reported to be altered by postnatal zinc deprivation like depressed *in vitro* blast transformation response to mitogens (Con A and PHA), decreased direct plaque-forming cell response to SRBC immunization and a highly aberrant serum immunoglobulin profile like elevated levels of IgG and no detectable IgM, IgG_{2A} or IgA (Beach *et al.,* 1980). Even marginal dietary deprivation of zinc during postnatal development has been associated with a significant degree of impairment of immunological function and has been reported to be passed on to F_2 and F_3 generations, although of a lesser magnitude than that seen in first generation offspring (Beach *et al.,* 1983). Gestational zinc deficiency results in a retardation of B-cell development *in utero,* which persists into the neonatal and young adult period in spite of nutritional repletion.

Copper: Dietary copper deficiency in experimental animals can result in decreased resistance to tumor challenge and an increased susceptibility to bacterial infections (Jones and Suttle, 1981). Dietary copper deficiency can result in an impaired neutrophilic function, decreased bactericidal activity and increased infection rates in sheep and cattle. In mice, a copper deficient diet imposed from the time of parturition throughout the early postnatal period results in a reduced mixed lymphocyte reaction response, decreased antibody response to SRBC, a reduction in lymphocyte stimulation by Concanavalin A low cytochrome oxidase and Cu, Zn-superoxide dismutase activities along with small thymus glands, enlarged spleen and liver when compared to copper-adequate mice (Prohaska *et al.,* 1983). Spleens of the copper deficient mice are characterized by a high number of B cells and a low number of T cells along with the reduction in T cell number mainly occurring due to a reduction in the number of T helper cells (Lukasewycz *et al.*, 1985). Alterations in splenocyte membranes due in part to lipid peroxidative damage secondary to low Cu, Zn superoxide dismutase activity has been implicated as one of the primary lesions. *In vitro,* copper deficiency resu1ts in reduction in splenocyte production of Interleukin 1 and T- cell replacing factor. It is possible that some of the immune defects observed in copper deficient animals may be the result of reductions in hormonal signals.

Iron: Piglets are naturally deficient in iron at birth as compared to neonates of other species. Thumps are the classical example wherein, iron deficient newborn piglets become susceptible to various infections due to general weakness and microcytic hypochromic anemia (reduced RBCs and haemoglobin). The low iron in sow's milk (0.5-1 ppm), high litter size, rearing on cement floors, weaning at an early age, inherent low stores of iron, a comparatively higher growth rate (5 times birth weight at 3 weeks age; thus higher iron requirement than neonates of other species) and iron deficiency in dam etc. predispose the piglet to thumps or piglet anemia. The reduced oxygen carrying capacity of blood (10g Hb/100 ml blood at birth to 3-4g at 3 weeks age), and general anemia, weakness depresses the immune system of piglets. However, pasting of dams teats with ferrous sulphate or parenteral administration of iron dextran (150-200mg I/M at 2-3 days age) revives the piglets and reduces the percentage of runts in a litter. Prenatal and early postnatal iron deficiency may cause long-term impairment of humoral immunity in rats. Natural killer cell activity is also significantly impaired in rat pups subjected to iron deficiency during gestation and lactation (Sherman and Lockwood, 1987). It is still not clear whether this effect of perinatal iron deficiency on natural killer cell activity is reversible with postnatal iron supplementation.

Selenium: Mice exposed to selenium deficiency during gestation, lactation and post weaning development have low IgM and IgG antibody responses to SRBC, while mice exposed to the deficient diet only during post-weaning development have a normal IgM response but a reduced IgG response (Mulhern *et al.*, 1985). Deficient mice have normal cell-mediated lympholysis apart from mixed lymphocyte and mitogenic responses. Bursa development in birds has been reported to be retarded by selenium deficiency, with bursa weights being 50% lower in the selenium deficient chicks compared to controls (Marsh *et al.*, 1986). Impaired humoral immune response to SRBC in 2 week old selenium-deficient chicks also has been reported. There is no report on the reversibility of the above immune defects associated with developmental selenium deficiency.

Effect of Specific Nutrients on Immunity in Animals

A lot of researches within the past decade have been done, describing how individual nutrients affect immunity. A general mechanism by which nutrients support the immune system is, probably, via provision of antioxidants. Immune cells are characterized by high levels of reactive oxygen species (ROS) which are used, in part, to kill ingested pathogens. As a result, immune cells are susceptible to ROS-mediated cellular damage (Chew and Park, 2004). Nutrients with anti-oxidant properties (carotenes, vitamin E, vitamin C, zinc, and selenium), therefore, support immunity. Complex inter-relationships exist between certain micronutrients, immune function and disease resistance in cattle. Several micronutrients have been shown to influence immune responses. The relationship between deficiencies of some micronutrients and disease resistance is less clear. A number of studies have indicated that Cr supplementation may improve cell-mediated and humoral immune response as well as resistance to respiratory infections. Deficiencies of Cu, Se, vitamin E and Co in cattle reduce the ability of isolated neutrophils to kill yeast and/or bacteria. Cu deficiency reduces antibody production, but cell-mediated immunity is generally not altered. However, Cu deficiency reduces production of interferon and tumour necrosis factor by mononuclear cells. Low vitamin E and/or Se status leads to increased susceptibility of dairy cows to intramammary infections. Marginal Zn deficiency does not impair antibody production in laboratory animals or lymphocyte responsiveness to mitogen stimulation in ruminants. Co deficiency has been associated with reduced resistance to parasitic infections. It is well documented that vitamin A-deficient animals are more susceptible to various types of infections. â-carotene, possibly via its antioxidant properties, may affect immune function and disease resistance independent of its role as a precursor of vitamin A. Given below is a brief summary of how individual nutrients affect immune function in ruminants.

Carotenoids: Disease resistance is also a function of cell differentiation. One of the primary functions of vitamin A is to maintain proper epithelial tissue differentiation and prevent epithelial keratinization apart from maintaining cellularity of lymphoid organs, enhance phagocyte activity and for enhancing both cellular and humoral immunity. Carotenoids are plant pigments and anti-oxidants, which include â-carotene, lutein, canthaxanthin, lycopene, and astaxanthin (Chew and Park, 2004). While, carotenoids (*i.e.* â-carotene) have traditionally been viewed as a source of vitamin A, studies have shown that carotenoids have immunostimulatory properties independent of their roles as precursors of vitamin A. Immunostimulatory properties of carotenoids have been recorded like canthaxanthin increased mitogen-stimulated lymphocyte proliferation in rats (Bendich and Shapiro, 1986). There are also many others documented mechanisms by which carotenoids, independent of vitamin A, benefit immunity. In ruminants, for example, supplementation with β-carotene at dry-off has been shown to reduce mammary gland infections (Chew, 1987). It also increases lymphocyte blastogenesis and increases neutrophil killing activity.

Vitamin A: It has been implicated as an essential dietary component in host resistance to infectious disease. Vitamin A has numerous roles in the immune system. Animals deficient in vitamin A have impaired innate immunity, including loss of mucosal barrier integrity and decreased numbers and/or function of innate immune phagocytic and natural killer cells. Lymphocyte homing, immunoglobulin A (IgA) responses in the mucosa and T-dependent antibody responses are decreased in vitamin A-deficient animals. Vitamin A is also required for the balance of T regulatory (Treg) and T helper (Th) 17 cells in mucosal tissues (Duriancik and Hoag, 2010), regulation of antigen presenting cells, maintaining dendritic cells and as a key modulator of TGF beta which can suppress several cytokines. Vitamin A deficiency affects both humoral and cellular immunity in the mucosa and modulation of dendritic cells is likely an important mechanism through which vitamin A deficiency affects mucosal immune responses against infection.

Vitamin D: Low levels of Vitamin D have been associated with development of autoimmune disorders like systemic lupus erythematosus (Bartley, 2010), the reason being that a low vitamin D level hinders the ability of the macrophages to produce activated 1-25 dihydroxyvitamin at sites of inflammation which has important immuno-regulatory functions including down-regulation of antigen-presenting cells such as dendritic cells. Under the influence of 1-25Dihydroxyvitamin D, these dendritic cells become tolerogenic as opposed to immunogenic and abrogate an immune response at early stages.

Vitamin E and Selenium: Vitamin E and Se serve essential and complimentary functions in support of the immune system in ruminant animals which is mainly related to anti-oxidation. They act synergistically wherein, vitamin E is considered as first line of defense and selenium containing enzyme, glutathione peroxidase is second line of defense to curb the free radicals that damage the epithelium or body lipids and fat soluble vitamins. Most consistent effects on the ruminant immune system have been shown with these two nutrients. Feeding elevated levels of Se to ruminant animals reduces incidence of diseases including intra-mammary infections (Smith *et al.*, 1984); since Se enhances neutrophil killing activity while Se deficiency increases neutrophil adherence affects ability of neutrophils to attack and sequester pathogen (Spears, 2000). Peripartum reduction in neutrophil superoxide anion production and impaired IL-1 production by monocytes is reported to be prevented by Vitamin E while its supplementation increases lymphocyte proliferation. Se and vitamin E increase antibody responses of dairy cattle. Injection of Se either alone or in combination with vitamin E significantly improves the production of specific antibodies against *E. coli* (Parnousis *et al.*, 2001) and the production of specific antibodies is reported to be greater after the administration of Se alone. Feeding vitamins E and C can protect the phagocytic function and surrounding tissues because Vitamin C helps to regenerate vitamin E by reducing vitamin E radicals formed when vitamin E scavenges oxygen radicals. Protection of cells from free radical oxidation, reduction the detrimental effects of certain eicosanoids and enhancement of humoral and cellular immune responses in disease and stress are the important roles of Vitamins A, E, C and carotenoids.

Omega-3 and omega-6 fatty acids: Dietary fatty acids can affect immunity through the production of the cytokines (Lessard *et al.*, 2004). A mechanism by which fatty acids affect immunity is through production of eicosenoids (*e.g.*prostaglandins) and leukotrienes. Diets rich in the omega-6 fatty acids such as linoleic acid lead to the formation of arachidonic acid, whereas, diets rich in the omega-3 fatty acids such as linolenic acid (flaxseed, and fish oils) lead to the formation of eicosapentaenoic acid (EPA). Eicosenoids synthesized from arachidonic acid tend to have strong inflammatory potential, whereas, those synthesized from EPA have lesser potential. Hence, inflammatory reactions and production of pro-inflammatory cytokines including IL-1, IL-6, and TNF-alpha can be reduced by feeding fatty acid mixtures which are enriched in the omega-3 fatty acids (Forsberg and Wang, 2006). EPA has modulating action on production of eicosinoids from arachidonic acid and thus plays major role in prevention of heart diseases. Diets enriched in the omega-3s have been introduced into the pet food as a strategy to reduce inflammation and a product with by-pass of high omega-3/ omega-6 ratios is available for improving reproduction in dairy cattle. However, there is not enough proof on the value of modifying fatty acids in ruminants as a strategy to benefit immunity.

Chromium (Cr): Its supplementation may improve cell-mediated and humoral immune response as well as resistance to respiratory infections in stressed cattle. The supplementation of Cr to dairy cattle in a biologically-available form like Cr-amino acid complex or Cr-yeast results in increased Con-A induced blastogenesis in peri-parturient cattle and increased development of titer to ovalbumin immunization and IBRV antigen (Burton *et al.*, 1994). Supplementation of stressed calves with high-Cr yeast increased antibody production in response to human red blood cells. Cr, fed as a chelate increases IgG_2 antibody response to tetanus toxoid (Fladyna *et al.*, 2003). A common finding among studies which have detected a benefit to Cr supplementation is the presence of a stress factor like shipping, parturition, weaning etc and hence, alleviating stress-associated immunosuppression may be one of the mechanisms by which Cr acts. The requirement of Cr increases in stress conditions or during infections. Cr^{3+} has been found to increase glucose tolerance in rats and organic Cr in brewer's yeast (chelate) has been termed as glucose tolerance factor (GTF). However, Cr supplementation has not been proved to be beneficial during immune stress in pigs.

Copper (Cu): Experimental models of Cu deficiency often fail to increase incidence of disease although it is well known that natural Cu deficiency increases susceptibility of ruminant animals to disease (Spears, 2000). Several studies have investigated effects of Cu on immunity in ruminant animals. Some studies have shown that supplementation of Cu-deficient diets augments markers of immune function, whereas others do not. It should not be surprising that Cu supports immunity as it is associated with many proteins. Copper-containing ceruloplasmin serves as a protective antioxidant and is a necessary component of the acute phase response. A copper deficiency reduces the amount of ceruloplasmin, which is released during an inflammatory stress. Cu has been shown to increase neutrophil killing activity of a common mold *Candida albicans*. Low Cu status has been reported to reduce mitogens stimulated blastogenesis following weaning and IBRV challenge and enhance cell mediated immunity (DTH-response) (Ward *et al.*, 1997). There is a lack of studies which directly implicate Cu in immune function. Apart from this, copper is instrumental to maintain normal osteoblastic activity, collagen and elastin formation, normal maturation of RBCs, normal hair and wool pigmentation (integral part of polyphenyl oxidase that is required for conversion of tyrosine to melanin and incorporation of 2-S group in keratin).

Zinc (Zn): It plays an essential role as an immunonutrient as it is associated with over 300 proteins (Rink and Gabriel, 2000). Clearly, a Zn deficiency has opportunity to impact a large number of cellular events which might compromise immunity e.g., Zn plays an important role in transcriptional control. Cells deficient in Zn have reduced ability to proliferate. The immune response requires rapid proliferation of cells (e.g.T and B-lymphocytes) in response to specific antigens. Zn deficiency prevents this aspect of immunity from developing. Zn deficiencies thwarts wound healing, impose bone deformities and causes severe skin lesions at extremities in chicks. The acid-base balance in body fluids is maintained by Zn containing enzyme carbonic anhydrase. Zn is also known to maintain reproductive function in animals. Marginal Zn deficiency has little effect on immune function in ruminants, but Zn supplementation may be beneficial.

Iron (Fe): It is an essential micro-nutrient and required for adequate erythropoietic function, oxidative metabolism and cellular immune responses. During infection, iron is removed from the circulation by macrophages and sequestered into compartments which are nutritionally unavailable to bacteria and parasites. Macrophages involved in recycling iron from erythrocytes limit the release of the recycled iron, thus lowering the extra cellular iron concentration and under the influence of cytokines; macrophages infected by intracellular microbes inhibit their multiplication by moving iron from the phagosomes to cytoplasmic ferritin (Ganj, 2009). As part of their host defense repertoire, neutrophils accumulating in infected tissues secrete proteins that chelate various forms of iron. Increased mortality and morbidity occurs in a variety of diseases when the iron lost from circulation is replenished by injections or very high dietary supplementation. On the other end, the iron deficiency also affects the tissue respiration process as iron is integral part of many important enzymes e.g. cytochrome, cytochrome oxidase, peroxidase and catalase. This may leave the tissue susceptible to free radical attack during stress and infections.

Mangnese (Mn): Its requirement by the gastrointestinal tract, lungs and several other tissues in the birds are increased during an immune response since manganese serves as a cofactor of superoxide dismutase and ameliorates damage induced by the immune response itself.

Nucleotides: They are the monomeric precursors units of RNA and DNA. Animals have a continuous requirement for nucleotides, especially for systems that present a high risk of cell turnover, like the immune system (Schaller, 2004). Nucleotides may become semi-essential nutrients under certain circumstances (e.g. weaning period) because endogenous synthesis may be insufficient to sustain normal function. In this case the immune function depends upon dietary nucleotide sources. Dietary supplementation with nucleotides has already been used in animals and humans with proved health benefits. Nucleotides have been shown to improve biological markers of the immune response in puppies and helped to attain an improved overall health status (Romano *et al.*, 2006) and promote intestinal growth and maturation in young rats (Dauy *et al.*, 1994). There are proven benefits of dietary supplementation with nucleotides especially in highly replicating tissues like those of gastrointestinal tract, immune system, etc. In the case of the immune system, dietary supplementation have shown an increase both in humoral immunity (increase in Ig concentration for several vaccines increase of unspecific IgM and IgA values) (Schaller, 2004) and in cellular immunity (increase in lymphocyte proliferation, increase in NK cells and IL-2) (Carver *et al.*,1991).

Nutrition vis-α-vis Immunity Development in Poultry

Response of poultry to a disease challenge is highly influenced by nutrients. The development and maturation of the immune system of young poultry fed nutritionally deficient diets is also compromised. It is essential to ensure that poultry diets contain enough of a specific nutrient to ensure the desired growth, feed conversion and immune response, but not too much so as to impair the immune function either directly or indirectly. Several nutrients (sodium, chloride, zinc, methionine, valine, threonine, vitamin A, riboflavin, pantothenic acid, pyridoxine and selenium) are considered essential to proper immune function and when deficient in the diet, have been shown to have a negative effect on the immunological response in the bird (Butcher and Miles, 2002).

A well-nourished bird is immunologically more competent and better able to cope with disease challenges than a poorly nourished bird. Normally, during such a challenge nutrients are shunted away from growth. Defense mechanisms take priority in a disease challenge and these nutrients help the bird's system overcome the challenge. For example, body proteins are broken down and amino acids are shunted away from growth and are used by specific cells to synthesize critical proteins allowing the bird to mount a successful immune response to a particular disease challenge. There is increase in numbers of Lymphoid cells, acute phase proteins and antibodies through the use of amino acids. The immune system of the bird can be influenced by nutrition in several ways like anatomical development of lymphoid tissues, mucus production, synthesis of immunologically active substances, cellular proliferation, cellular activation and movement, intracellular killing of pathogens and modulation and regulation of the immune process (Butcher and Miles, 2002). A change in feed intake leads to a change in nutrient and energy intake. However, young poultry in today's commercial poultry industry are usually not subjected to diets which are severely limited in nutrients and energy. Most of the literature data suggests that dietary concentrations of most nutrients necessary for optimal growth, are also necessary for optimal immuno-competence. However, when a diet is deficient in protein or amino acids, the concentration of circulating antibodies to a specific challenge organism is low.

Dietary arginine concentration of 1.25% of the diet supports the proper immune system functions in healthy chicks (Kidd et al., 2001) and plays a very important role as a potent immunological modulator through production of nitric oxide via cellular metabolic pathway (Collier and Vallance, 1989). Additional improvements in immunity include improved thymic weight and function, enhanced lymphocyte mitogenesis, improved immunity against tumors and enhanced wound healing (Efron and Barbul, 1998; Evoy *et al.*, 1998).

Low mineral level in the feed has been associated with a reduced humoral immune response in poultry. For example broilers fed diets deficient in sodium or chloride, have lower antibody concentrations. The balance between sodium and chloride in the diet is important because a high chloride concentration in relation to that of sodium may result in a reduced immune response (Butcher and Miles, 2002). Increased dietary supplementation of certain nutrients, above that needed for maximum growth and feed efficiency is beneficial for the immune response, even though most nutrients required by the immune system are present in the diet in sufficient concentrations. Vitamins A, E and C as well as the amino acids methionine and valine have been shown to benefit immune function when added to the diet of poultry at higher concentrations than are required to maximize growth and feed efficiency. Vitamin A has been reported to reduce mortality in chicks infected with coccidial oocysts. The omega 3 and 6 fatty acids are also beneficial for the immune system at higher than normal concentrations in the diet. But too much of some nutrients may also be harmful to the immune system e.g. too much dietary methionine suppresses the immune system which is evident before changes in growth and feed consumption are detected.

It is well known that deficiencies of vitamin E and selenium will inhibit the immune response in poultry. Vitamin E has been referred to be an immune system booster and exerts a complementary effect on the immune system of poultry by inhibiting the synthesis of prostaglandins produced in the cells following the oxidation of cellular membranes and is responsible for inhibiting the inflammation and immune response. Vitamin E affects the development and maintenance of immuno-competence through multiple factors like by acting directly on the immune cell or by indirectly altering metabolic and endocrine parameters, which in turn influence immune function (Gershwin *et al.*, 1985). Selenium along with vitamin E helps tissues in protecting biological membranes from oxidative damage. Vitamin E is very important in preventing peroxidation of fatty acid which acts as immunoregulatory molecules by mediating cellular communication, membrane fluidity and second messenger elaboration (Klasing, 1997). Another potential immunoregulatory mechanism that is associated with vitamin E is the modulation of arachidonic metabolism via cyclooxygenase and lipoxygenase pathways (Blumberg, 1994) which lead to the synthesis of prostaglandins and leukotrienes respectively. Among the trace minerals commonly used in poultry, Zn and Mn are of particular interest in broiler chickens because of their metabolic involvement in growth, skeletal integrity, enzyme activities, and immune competence. Zinc is also important in wound healing, thymic function and proliferation of lymphocytes and thus, assisting the bird's immune system to overcome a challenge. Often, higher levels of Zn and Mn are supplemented in diets for enhancing immune response in chicken because both minerals are responsible for sustained activity of superoxide dismutase that is vital for macrophage and heterophil integrity (Cook-Mills and Fraker, 1993). The immune response measured as antibody titers to sheep RBC increases significantly with higher Zn (80 ppm) supplementation and cell-mediated immune response to phytohemagglutinin with Mn level at 120 ppm. However, fortification of diets with excess minerals may cause antagonism, affecting mineral bioavailability and masking the advantages of supplementation.

Researchers have traditionally focused on the effects of known nutrients and studied their effects on various aspects of immunity. Use of feed additives or nutraceuticles to enhance immune function presents itself as a new strategy in maintaining health and nutrition of livestock as well as poultry. Nowadays, the trend and focus is entirely on revealing novel ways for manipulating immune functions and to possibly enhance it *in vivo* which appears as an interface between nutrition and immunity with added knowledge of immuno-regulation. There are multiple on-going researches in nutritional immunological aspects and are likely to yield exciting new findings in the coming time.

References

Bartley J. (2010). *Expert Rev. Anti Infect. Ther.*, 8(12):1359-69.

Beach, R.S., Gershwin, M.E. and Hurley, L. S. (1979). *Develop. Comp. Immunol.*, 3: 725-735.

Beach, R.S., Gershwin, M.E., Makashoima, R.K. and Hurley, L.S. (1980). *J. Nutr.*, 110: 805-815.

Beach, R.S., Gershwin, M.E. and Hurley, L .S. (1983). *Am. J. Clin. Nutr.*, 38: 579-590.

Bendich, A. and Shapiro, S.S. (1986). *J. Nutr.*, 116:2254-2262.

Blumberg, J. (1994). Vitamins. *In: Diet, Nutrition, and Immunity. R. A. Forse, ed. CRC Press, Baca Raton, FL.* Pp. 234-247.

Burton, J.L., Mallard, D.A. and Mowat, D.N. (1994). *Can. J. Anim. Sci.*, 58:148-151.

Butchers, G D and Miles, R D. (2002). Interrelationship of Nutrition and Immunity. In: VM139 series of the Veterinary Medicine-Large Animal Clinical Sciences Department, Florida Cooperative Extension Service, Institute of Food and Agricultural Sciences, University of Florida.

Carver, J.D., Pimentel, B., Cox, W., Barness, L.A. (1991) *Pediatrics.* 88: 359-363.

Chew, B.P. (1987). *J. Anim. Sci.* 70:2732-2743.

Chew, B.P. and J.S. Park. (2004). *J. Nutr.*, 134:257S-261S.

Collier, J. and Vallance, P. (1989). *Trends Pharmacol. Sci.*, 10:427-431.

Cook-Mills, J.M. and Fraker, P.J. (1993). The role of metals in the production of toxic oxygen metabolites by mononuclear phagocytes. In: Cunningham R (ed) Nutrient modulation of the immune response. Marcel Dekker, New York, pp 127–140.

Dauy, R., Quan, R.and Gil, A. (1994). *J. Nutr.*, 124 (8 Suppl): 1436S-1441S.

Duriancik, D. M. and. Hoag, K. A. (2010). *Cell. Immunol.*, 265(2): 156–163.

Efron, D. T. and Barbul, A. (1998). *Curr. Opin. Clin. Nutr. Metab. Care*, 1:531-538.

Enwonwu, C. (1986). *Nutr. Res.*, 6: 337-348.

Evoy, D., Lieberman, M. D., Fahey, T. J. and Daly, J. M. (1998). *Nutr.*,14:611-617.

Faldyna, M., Pechova, A. and Krejci, J. (2003). J. Vet. Med. B. *Infect. Dis. Vet. Pub. Health*, 7:326-331.

Forsberg, N. E. and Wang, Y. (2006). Nutrition and Immunity in Dairy Cattle: Implications to Hemorrhagic Bowel Syndrome. Paper presented at Mid-South Ruminant Nutrition Conference. pp 11-20.

Ganz, T. (2009). *Curr Opin Immunol.*, 21(1): 63–67.

Gerbhardt, B.M. and Newberne, P. M.(1974). *J. Immunol.*, 26: 489-495.

Gershwin, M., Beach, R.and Hurley, L.(1985).The potent impact of nutritional factors on immune response. In: *Nutrition and Immunity. Academic Press, New York, NY.* Pp. 1-7.

Gershwin, M.E., Keen, C. L., Fletcher, M. P. and Hurley, L.S. (1987). *Proc. Nutr. Soc. Aust., 12: 1-10.*

Jones, D. G. and Suttle N. F. (1981). *Res. Vet. Sci.*, 31: 145-151.

Kidd, M. T., Peebles, E. D., Whitmarsh, S. K., Yeatman, J. B. and Wideman, R. F. Jr. (2001). *Poultry Sci.*, 80:1535-1542.

Klasing, K.C.(1997). Interaction between nutrition and infectious disease. In: *Diseases of Poultry, B. W. Calnek, ed. Iowa State University Press, Ames, IA.* Pp., 73-80.

Lessard, M., Gagnon, N., Godson, D.L. and Petit, H.V. (2004). *J. Dairy Sci.*, 87:2197-2210.

Lukasewcyz, O.A. Prohaska, J. R., Meyer, S.G., Schmidtke, J.R. Hatfield, S.M and marder, P. (1985). *Infect. Immun.*, 48: 644-647.

Marsh, J.A., Combs, G.F., Whitacre, M.E. and Dietert, R.R. (1986). *Proc. Soc. Exp. Bio. Med.*, 182:425-436.

Mulhern, S.A., Taylor, G.L., Magruder, L.E. and Vessey, A.R. (1985). *Nutr. Res.*, 5: 201-210.

Nauss, K. M. and Newberne, P.M. (1985). *J. Nutr.*, 115: 1316-1324.

Olusi, S. O., Thurman, G.B. and Goldstein, A.L. (1980). *Clin. Immunol. Immunopath.*, 15 : 687-691.

Parnousis, N., Roubies, N. Karatzias, H., Frydas, S. and Papasteriadis, A. (2001). *Vet. Rec.*, 149:643-646.

Plaut, M., Marone, G., Thomas, L.L. and Lichtenstein, L.M. (1980). *Adv. Cyclic Nucleotide Res.*, 12: 107-116.

Rink, L., and Gabriel, P. (2000). *Proc. Nutr. Soc.*, 59:541-552.

Prohaska, J.R., Downing, S. W. and Lukasewycz, O. A. (1983). *J. Nutr.*, 113: 1583-1590.

Romano, V., Martinez-Puig, D., Torre, C., Iraculis, N. Vilaseca, L. and Chetrit. I.C. (2006). Dietary Nucleotides Improve The Immune System Of Puppies at Weaning. In: *American Academy of Veterinary Nutrition (2006).*

Schaller J., Kuchan J., Thomas D.L., Cordle C.T., Winship T.R., Buck R.H., Baggs G.E. and Wheeler, J.G. (2004). *Pediatric Res.*, 56:W6,883-890

Secrist, D.S., Owens, F.N. and Gill, D.R. (1997). *Proc. Anim. Sci.*, 13:47-54.

Sherman, A. R. and Lockwood, J.F. (1987). *J. Nutr.*, 117: 567.

Smith, L.K., Harrison, J.H., Hancock, D.D., Todhunter, D.A. and Conrad, H.R. (1984). *J. Dairy Sci.*, 67:1293-1300.

Smith, S. M., Levy, N. S. and Hayes, C. E. (1987). *J. Nutr.*, 117: 857-865.

Spears, J.W. (2000). *Proc. Nutr. Soc.*, 59:587-594.

Srivastava, U S, Rakshit A K, Seebag , M, Omoloko, C and Thakur, M L. (1981). *Nutr. Reports Intntl.*, 23:1035.

Ward, J.D., Gengelbach, G.P. and Spears, J.W. (1997). *J. Anim. Sci.*, 75:1400-1408.

□□□

Animal Nutrition, 2012
eds. Dr. (Mrs.) Usha R. Mehra et al., pp. 753-770
Satish Serial Publishing House e-mail : info@satishserial.com; website : www.satishserial.com

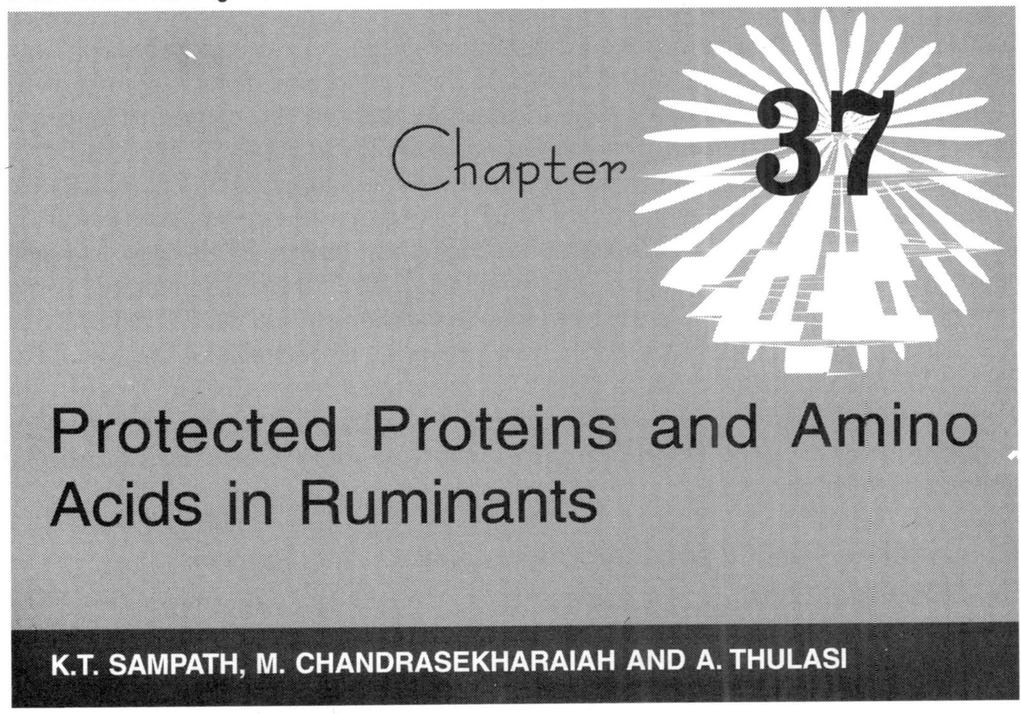

Chapter 37

Protected Proteins and Amino Acids in Ruminants

K.T. SAMPATH, M. CHANDRASEKHARAIAH AND A. THULASI

Ruminants derive their requirements of amino acids from two radically different sources. One is from the microbial protein synthesized in the rumen and the other is from the feed offered to the animal. The microbial protein is synthesized from nitrogenous feed material, which is fermented in the rumen i.e. the rumen degradable protein (RDP). The microbes use end products of fermentation such as ammonia, peptides and amino acids as building blocks for their own body proteins. These microorganisms are digested in the lower tract and provide amino acids. Some of the protein in the feed escape fermentation in the rumen i.e. undegradable protein (UDP) and reaches the hind gut, digested and provide amino acids, which are also absorbed through the gut wall in to the blood stream. The combination of amino acids derived from the two sources constitutes total supply to the animal.

Microbial protein synthesized in the rumen provides 60-70 percent of protein requirement of the ruminants under normal physiological condition. However, since the microbial protein synthesis is energy dependent process, deficiency of dietary energy especially during early part of the lactation, which is not uncommon, result in correspondingly lower synthesis of bacterial protein in the rumen leading to reduced availability of protein for milk production. Therefore, for sustaining higher level of milk yield and faster growth rate, ruminants need more dietary protein than the flora in the rumen can utilize. However, higher dietary protein intake especially RDP often results in increasing loss of ammonia from the rumen. Excess ammonia is converted in to urea in the liver, the major part of which is excreted through urine resulting in the loss of dietary protein part. Increased ammonia levels also leads to reduced fertility besides causing stress on the liver. Adequate protein supply to high yielding cows without stress from excess ammonia can be ensured by decreasing the degradability of dietary proteins. Experimental studies have shown that if the protein degradation in the rumen is controlled, it results in better utilization of proteins by ruminants. This has lead to the development of techniques to protect greater proportion of dietary proteins from the degradation in the rumen.

Ruminant Feedstuffs and their Degradability in the Rumen

Ruminants consume a wide variety of proteins and non protein nitrogen sources. From the work carried out in different laboratories during last few years, the protein degradability values of a large number of feeds are available now. Various methods (*in vivo, in vitro, in situ*) have been employed for the estimation of degradability of proteins in the rumen with their own limitations. Of the different methods, *in situ* nylon bag technique, which involves the suspension of feed materials in the rumen of fistulated animals is generally accepted method (Mehrez and Orskov, 1977; Orskov and McDonald, 1979). Mean protein degradability values of feed stuffs obtained by different techniques and their RDP and UDP content derived from these values for out flow rate in the range of 4 to 6% per hour is given in Table 1.

Table 1 : Crude protein (CP), Rumen degradable protein (RDP) and undegradable protein (UDP) / bypass protein content of feeds and fodders

Feedstuffs	Degradability (%)	CP	RDP	UDP (bypass protein)
Concentrates		**gram per kg dry matter**		
Bajra	32	120	38	82
Barley	79	100	79	21
Brewers grains	47	260	122	138
Coconut cake (solvent extracted)	23	270	62	208
Coconut cake (expeller)	72	240	173	67
Corn gluten meal (60% CP)	21	600	126	474

contd....

Corn gluten meal (40% CP)	37	400	148	252
Cotton seed	46	170	78	92
Cotton seed cake	51	350	179	171
Cotton seed cake (solvent extracted)	38	360	137	223
Distillers dried grain	46	290	133	157
Gingelly / sesame / til cake	76	350	266	84
Groundnut cake (expellar)	70	450	315	135
Groundnut cake (Deoiled / solvent extracted)	85	480	408	72
Horse gram	57	240	137	103
Jowar	20	100	20	80
Karanja cake	54	320	173	147
Kokam cake	12	140	17	123
Linseed cake	58	280	162	118
Mahua seed cake	57	185	105	80
Maize bran	37	160	59	101
Maize grain	30	90	27	67
Mustard cake	75	350	263	87
Neem seed kernel cake	56	386	217	169
Niger cake	74	330	244	86
Oats	84	100	84	16
Rice bran	65	140	91	49
Rice bran extraction	40	160	64	96
Rice broken	32	110	35	75
Rice polish	51	120	61	59
Rubber seed cake	72	280	202	78
Safflower cake	64	220	141	79
Salseed meal	30	90	27	63
Silk cotton seed cake	78	370	289	81
Soyabean meal extractions	60	460	276	184
Sunflower meal	55	300	165	135
Roughages				
Alfalfa, dehydrated	40	200	80	120
Alfalfa fresh (*Medicago sativa*)	76	200	152	48
Berseem (*Trifolium alexndrium*)	49	259	127	132
Grass hay	45	29	13	16
Guninea grass	40	82	33	49
Maize early cut	58	165	96	69
Oats (*Avena Sativa*)	52	126	65	61
Para grass	48	71	34	37
Rice straw	38	40	15	25
Subabul (*Leucaena leucocephola*)	32	250	80	170
Sugar cane tops, chaffed, ensiled	15	68	10	58
Wheat straw	55	33	18	15

It can be seen from Table 1 that some of the feed stuffs have ruminal degradability value of more than 60% and are poor sources of UDP/bypass protein. It is difficult to obtain absolute protein degradability values for a wide variety of feedstuffs. Several factors introduce considerable variations into what is supposed to be standard for comparison. It is more realistic therefore to determine the relative RDP and UDP values. These values rank the protein sources and diets relative to one another. The commonly used feedstuffs can be divided into three categories depending up on their degradability in the rumen.

1. Feedstuffs of high ruminal degradability (degradability values ranging from 61 to 100 percent).
2. Feedstuffs of medium ruminal degradability (degradability values ranging from 31 to 60 percent).
3. Feedstuffs of low ruminal degradability (degradability values ranging from 0 to 30 percent).

From the available data, the feedstuffs falling under these categories are given in Table 2.

Table 2 : Feedstuffs of low, medium and high degradability.

Feedstuffs of low degradability (< 30 %)	Feedstuffs of medium degradability (30-60%)	Feedstuffs of high degradability (> 60 %)
Concentrates		
Kokam cake	Bajra	Safflower cake
Jowar	Rice broken	Rice bran
Corn gluten meal (60% CP)	Corn gluten meal (40% CP)	Groundnut cake (expellar)
Coconut cake (solvent extracted)	Maize bran	Coconut cake (expeller)
Maize grain	Cotton seed cake (solvent extracted)	Rubber seed cake
Salseed meal	Rice bran extraction	Niger cake
	Cotton seed	Mustard cake
	Distillers dried grain	Gingelly / sesame / til cake
	Brewers grains	Silk cotton seed cake
	Cotton seed cake	Barley
	Rice polish	Oats
	Karanja cake	Groundnut cake (Deoiled / solvent extracted)
	Sunflower meal	
	Neem seed kernel cake	
	Horse gram	
	Mahua seed cake	
	Linseed cake	
	Soyabean meal extractions	

contd....

Roughages		
Sugar cane tops, chaffed, ensiled	Subabul (*Leucaena leucocephola*) Rice straw Alfalfa, dehydrated Guninea grass Grass hay Para grass Berseem (*Trifolium alexndrium*) Oats (*Avena Sativa*) Wheat straw Maize early cut	Alfalfa fresh (*Medicago sativa*)

Protection of Proteins from Degradation in the Rumen

Results of the studies conducted by McDonald (1948) which revealed that soluble dietary proteins are extensively degraded to ammonia in the rumen and the subsequent observations that protein or amino acids administrated postruminally resulted in greater nitrogen retention as compared to those administrated directly in the rumen, led to attempts to find ways protecting soluble, high quality dietary proteins from microbial degradation with in the rumen. Several approaches have been tried to protect the dietary protein from ruminal degradation. They include closure of esophageal groove, post ruminal infusion, physical processing, heat treatment, chemical treatments viz., formaldehyde treatment and tannic acid treatment, non enzymatic browning technique and using of acids, alkalies, alcohol and metal ions. There are also reports indicating the effectiveness of calcium soaps of long chain fatty acids in protecting the proteins from ruminal degradation.

Closure of Oesophageal Groove

The oesophageal groove is a muscular fold extending downwards from the cardia to the abomasum on the wall of the reticulum. It comprises the end of the thoracic esophagus, the muscular fold itself and also the reticulo omasal orifice. When closed, the groove forms a tube carrying swallowed fluid directly through the omasal orifice into the abomasum. The oesophageal groove cease to function in matured animals. Although rumen bypass of nutrients by closure of oesophageal groove has resulted in significant improvement in growth rate and feed efficiency, practical methods for stimulating the reflex have not been evolved.

Physical Processing

Alterations in the physical form influence the behaviour of the feed particles in the rumen environment. The most often applied way of changing the physical form of the diet is grinding. Increasing the surface area will usually increase the rate of degradability, but the reduced particle size may reduce the retention time in the rumen resulting in increased bypass.

Heat Treatment

Subjecting certain feeds to controlled higher heat decreases the solubility of proteins by creating cross linkages within and among peptide chains to carbohydrates, thus lowering their susceptibility to rumen degradation. However, high temperature and extended heating times render protein less digestible through Maillard reaction between sugar aldehyde groups and free amino groups thus lowering the digestibility of constituent amino acids. In general, the beneficial effects of reduced rate of degradation in rumen appear to be greater than the reduced whole tract protein digestibility caused by limited heat damage. Walli (1996) and Walli *et al.* (2000) observed 150°C for 2 hrs as the optimum temperature- time combination. Sampath *et al.* (1997) reported that the ruminal protein degradability of groundnut cake was reduced by 35% and 45% due to heat treatment for 2 hrs and 3 hours at 130°C, respectively. Further, they observed that heat treatment at that temperature and time duration did not have any negative effect on *in vivo* apparent CP digestibility. Walli and Sirohi (2004) reported that the roasting of soybean at 130°C for 30minutes protects its protein substantially.

Chemical Treatment

Certain chemical agents form reversible cross linkages with amino and amide groups which decreases solubility of proteins at the pH of the rumen. Chemically treated proteins are subsequently made available to the host animal by destruction of these linkages in acidic abomasum. Agents investigated include aldehydes and tanning materials.

Formaldehyde Treatment

Formaldehyde (1 to 1.5 g per 100g CP) treatment has been used to reduce the protein degradability of highly degradable cakes and also to study the impact of its feed on the productive response of dairy animals (Gupta and Walli, 1987; Bhagwat and Srivastava, 1993; Kumar and Walli, 1994; Tiwari and Yadav, 1994; Pratihar and Walli, 1995; Ramachandra and Sampath, 1995; Chatterjee and Walli, 2003a). Chatterjee and Walli (2003b) also optimized the formaldehyde as 1.0 to 1.2g/100g CP for the treatment of mustard and groundnut cakes at which level protein degradability is substantially reduced without having adverse effect on post ruminal degradability.

Tannic Acid Treatment

The presence of tannins in food sources for monogastric animals, is generally viewed adversely. However, in ruminants, tannins can induce beneficial effects. For example, in sheep and cattle higher retention of nitrogen has been observed with low to moderate levels of tannins in forages. In these cases, the lower apparent and true digestibility of nitrogen was compensated for by reduced urinary loss of nitrogen. Moderate levels of tannins (less than 4%) in forage legumes can have beneficial responses in ruminants, resulting in higher growth rates and milk yield. However, even in ruminants, levels of tannins exceeding 6% of the diet affect growth rates and milk yield. Several mechanisms have been suggested to explain how tannins influence protein utilization by ruminants:

One mechanism postulated is that tannins complex proteins at the pH of the rumen (5 to 7) and protect them from microbial enzymes. Subsequently, these complexes dissociate in contact with gastric (pH 2.5-3.5) and pancreatic (pH 8) secretions. High quality dietary proteins would be protected, at least in part, from degradation in the rumen and would then be digested more effectively in the intestine. However, even when released, tannins are still biologically active and can react with digestive enzymes or other proteins. In non-ruminants, tannins decrease intestinal absorption of amino acids (especially methionine) and reduce growth. Tannin-protein complexes that are strong enough to survive in the environment of the rumen may not be broken down and digested in the lower tract.

Another hypothesis is that tannins may increase efficiency in nitrogen recycling to the rumen. Tannins lower the rate of protein degradation and deamination in the rumen resulting in lower rumen ammonia concentration. This results in lower plasma urea nitrogen (PUN). Lower PUN means lower urinary nitrogen excretion with less wastage of nitrogen. Larger amounts of nitrogen are recycled because tannins stimulate increased saliva production. In diets based on tanniniferous forages, nitrogen rumen outflow is often larger than nitrogen intake. Several studies have reported an increase in protein flow when moderate doses of tannins were used. This has been attributed to increased rumen escape of dietary proteins, increase in microbial protein flow (up to 28% in sheep). The larger microbial flow could be the result of increased saliva production, increased rumen turnover rate, and hence, increased microbial outflow, increased nitrogen recycling to the rumen.

Other Methods

Non enzymatic browning technique involves the mixing of a protein source with xylose sugar or sucrose and heating it. (Chalupa, 1975; Stern, 1984 ; Cleale *et al.*, 1986; Winowiski and Stern, 1987).

Using metal ions involves using of Zinc salts (Gaynor *et al.*, 1988).

Using corn protein zein involves the protein supplement or the amino acid coated with zein by mixing it with zein along with binding agent and extrusion (Vandehar *et al.*, 1987).

Using acids and alkalis such as acetic acid, propionic acid and hydrochloric acid (Waltz and Loerch, 1986; Khorasani *et al.*, 1989) and sodium hydroxide (Bowman *et al.*, 1988; Mir *et al.*,1984; Gould *et al.*, 1976).

Using alcohols (ethanol, propanol, isopropanol) with or without addition of heat (Lynch *et al.*, 1987; Lynch *et al.*, 1988).

Genetic Engineering Approach

Alfalfa and other forage legumes are high in protein but deficient in S-amino acids cysteine and methionine. The protein content of forage legumes can be improved for feeding of ruminants by introducing into them the functional genes encoding the proteins rich in sulfur amino acids that are ruminally stable. The delta - and beta-zein proteins contain proportionately high levels of S-amino acids. Bagga *et al.* (2004) in their preliminary studies, transformed alfalfa with CaMV 35S-beta-zein and CaMV 35S-delta-zein gene constructs individually and in combination. The results indicate that as in tobacco both the beta - and the delta -zeins accumulate in the leaves of alfalfa and that the co-expression of the two zein genes has a stabilizing effect on the delta -zein. However, the level of accumulation of the zeins in alfalfa leaves is not high enough to make a significant change in the methionine levels. The data on rumen incubation experiments have demonstrated that the zeins are completely stable in the rumen of cows and thus qualify as the suitable rumen bypass protein that is rich in methionine.

Effect of Protected Protein Supplements on Growth, Milk Production and Reproduction

Milk Production

Sampath *et al.* (1997) studied the effect of formaldehyde treated groundnut (GN) cake in the concentrate mixture of lactating animals on milk production. Fourteen cows whose previous lactation yield was 8 to 10 kg/d were divided into two groups of seven cows each and fed Ragi straw and iso-caloric concentrate mixtures with RDP:UDP in the ratio of 65:35 (Group I) and 50:50 (group II) from 15th day after calving upto 36 weeks. The average yield of fat corrected milk per day per cow was significantly higher in group fed formaldehyde treated groundnut cake (9.40 kg) than in group which received untreated groundnut cake (7.80 kg) and also the decline in milk yield with progress of lactation was much slower in group II. A similar experiment of short duration (four months), on paddy straw based diet also yielded, similar results (Ramachandra and Sampath, 1995).

A study conducted on crossbred kids and lactating goats fed formaldehyde treated mustard cake (Sahoo, 2002) revealed that the growth rate increased significantly (47.5 vs 62.9 g/d) showing a 32.3% increase over control, and the milk yield also increased significantly from 1306 g/d in control group to 1439 g/d in formaldehyde treated group. Garg *et al.* (2002) studied the effect of feeding rumen protected nutrients on milk production in crossbred cows and observed an increase in milk yield, fat and protein and the net average daily income was increased by Rs. 9.61 on feeding 1.0 kg protected (Formaldehyde) sunflower meal in lactating cows. The effect of feeding rumen bypass protein in the form of formaldehyde treated mustard cake protein on milk yield and milk composition in Murrah buffaloes was determined by Chatterjee and Walli (2003b). The average daily yield of protein, fat, SNF and total solids were significantly higher, the feed cost was lower, indicating that the diet containing formaldehyde treated mustard cake was more economical than the control diet containing untreated mustard cake. Increased milk yield, fat and FCM percentages were observed by Garg *et al* (2003) with formaldehyde treated protein supplement in crossbred cows, with no significant effect on the level of protein percentage in milk. Average net daily income increased by Rs. 9.44 upon feeding 1.0 kg protected rapeseed meal in lactating cows. Supplementation of 1.0 kg protected protein in the ration of dairy cows is found to be economical compared to feeding similar quantities of untreated meal. Sahoo and Walli (2005) studied, the effect of feeding formaldehyde-treated mustard cake together with molasses as energy source on milk yield of lactating goats. The average milk yield and 4% FCM yield were higher ($P<0.05$) in the protected protein-fed groups. The overall increase in milk and FCM yields, as a result of feeding protected protein, was 10.18 and 8.67% over the control group. Feeding of formaldehyde-treated mustard proved beneficial for lactating goats, however, additional energy supplement such as molasses, irrespective of feeding bypass protein, had no added advantage in terms of milk production and profit generation. Supplementation of 1.0 kg protected protein in the form of formaldehyde treated rapeseed meal in the ration of low yielding cows was found to be economical, compared to feeding a similar quantity of untreated protein meal on paddy straw based rations (Garg *et al.*, 2005).

Walli and Sirohi (2004), while supplementing the diet with roasted soyabean and untreated soyabean seed in crushed form found that the increase in milk and FCM yield was around 8% in lactating crossbred cows. The lower response was perhaps due to the fact that the time-temperature combination of roasting was not optimum for soyabean, which requires to be worked out.

Walli and Sirohi (2004) also reported 15% increase in milk yield on feeding of formaldehyde-protected mustard-cake to crossbred cows. The increase in feed intake was non significant in the animals fed treated cake.

Growth

Sampath *et al.* (1996) did not observe any effect on growth rate in crossbred calves fed formaldehyde treated groundnut cake. Pachauri *et al.* (1999) also reported that inclusion of formaldehyde treated groundnut cake replacing untreated groundnut cake did not have any additional positive effect on body weight gain and UDP was not important for calves growing at a rate of 450-485g per day. A significant increase in growth rate was observed in goat kids, on feeding formaldehyde treated groundnut cake (Mudgal and Sengar, 1980) and on feeding of formaldehyde treated mustard cake (Sahoo and Walli, 2001). Feeding of formaldehyde treated GN cake resulted in increase in the growth rate of crossbred claves (Kumar and Walli, 1994). Similarly, the feeding of formaldehyde treated mustard cake gave significant increase in growth performance of buffalo calves. The feeding of bypass protein in the form of formaldehyde treated mustard cake can be proven economically beneficial for raising of buffalo calves (Chatterjee and Walli, 2003b) on wheat straw based rations.

Reproduction

Protein nutrition can affect reproduction through toxic effects of ammonia and it's metabolites on gametes and early embryos, through deficiencies of amino acids and by exacerbations of negative balances of energy. Excess degradable protein acts through some unidentified mechanism to decrease uterine pH during luteal phase which may play a role to reduce fertility. Energy cost of detoxifying large amounts of ammonia to urea may aggravate an existing post partum energy shortage. Higher UDP in late dry period improves post partum performance and also reduces metabolic disorders.

Limited studies were carried out in India on the effect of bypass protein supplement on male and female reproduction performance. Supplementation of formaldehyde treated GNC in place of untreated GNC in the concentrate mixture of crossbred cows on paddy straw based ration improved the production and reproductive performance economically (Mishra *et al.*, 2006).

Beneficial Aspects of Feeding Protein of Low Degradability to Ruminants

In ruminants, the microbial protein synthesized in the rumen is the major protein source utilized for body functions. However, higher growth rates and milk production levels require higher protein than usually provided from microbial protein alone. Supplementation with undegradable dietary protein may enhance growth rate and milk production, especially under such conditions. Egan (1988) explained that the enhanced growth or milk production is mediated by

- Dietary protein intact or as peptide delivered to the lower tract can improve the amino acid availability for lean tissue,
- Slow degradation of proteins can result in more constant N supply to the rumen which may improve the supply of NH_3 and possibly peptides for the growth and fermentative activity of rumen micro-organisms, thus improving the supply of microbial protein to the lower tract,
- The extra amino acids absorbed as a result of feeding more ruminal escape protein may be used with high efficiency as an amino acid source for the body protein synthesis, but they may also alter the hormonal balance e.g. between growth hormone and insulin and improve growth through lean tissue growth. Similarly, beneficial effects of UDP supplementation to cows in early lactation could also be due to alteration in the hormonal concentration of insulin and the growth hormone apart from providing more amino acids to the mammary gland. Lower insulin and higher growth hormone levels are likely to favour tissue mobilization of fat and increase milk production.

Limiting Amino Acids

Methionine and Lysine are often reported to be first limiting or co-limiting amino acids for milk production. Feeding of bypass protein sources that supply these limiting amino acids post ruminally may result in increased milk production. Limited numbers of studies have been carried out in India on the amino acid content of feedstuffs as well as its post ruminal availability in ruminants. The essential amino acid content in different ruminant feedstuffs has been determined by Chandrasekharaiah *et al.* (2003). The limiting amino acid content in bypass protein fractions of different feedstuffs have also been determined (Sampath *et al.*, 2002; Sampath *et al.*, 2003). It was observed from the results of these studies that bypass protein content of copra cake (coconut cake), silk worm pupae meal, safflower cake, maize gluten meal, sunflower cake and cotton seed cake are rich in one or both of these limiting amino acids. One full lactation trial was conducted in buffaloes fed with rations such as control (T_0) and two experimental groups (T_1-High Undegradable protein (UDP) low in limiting amino acids and T_2 – High UDP high in limiting amino acids) and the results indicated that experimental ration having high UDP rich in limiting amino acids could improve the quality and quantity of milk production in buffaloes (Dahiya *et al.*, 2007a,b). The better production response observed in some of the studies with sunflower cake and cottonseed cake reported above may also be attributed to these limiting amino acids. On the basis of large number of trials conducted elsewhere, it has been observed that the milk production could increase by adding 12 g of rumen protected methonine and lysine. Research is needed to improve diet formulation models to balance for amino acid requirements and to quantify the potential to reduce protein feeding when using protected amino acid.

Rumen Protected Amino Acids

Amino acids can be added directly to the diets of monogastric animals to overcome nutritional deficiencies. However, free-form amino acids are rapidly degraded by rumen bacteria and are of little or no practical benefit in alleviating amino acid deficiencies for ruminants. Amino acid must be either modified or protected in some way so that they are not susceptible to rumen degradation. Several methods have been used to develop commercial rumen protected amino acid (RPAA) products. However, it must be ensured that amino acid protected from ruminal degradation is still available for intestinal absorption.

The beneficial responses obtained when free amino acids or high quality protein were infused post ruminally have stimulated interest in developing methods of protecting amino acids from ruminal degradation so that increased quantities would pass to the small intestine and be available for absorption. Protection of protein and amino acids has been attempted by heat, chemical treatment, by formation of amino acid analogs or derivatives and by encapsulation. Supplemental dietary amino acids for ruminants need to be provided in a form that will prevent their microbial or chemical degradation in the rumen and facilitate their absorption in a biologically available form. A variety of approaches has been used to achieve delivery of amino acids or their bio-equivalent chemical analogs at the absorption sites. These efforts have focused primarily on methionine and lysine, because these amino acids have been identified as ones that may limit growth and milk or milk protein production in ruminants under several dietary conditions.

The rumen-protected forms of amino acids can be grouped into two general categories. The first includes analogs, derivatives, or polymeric compounds of the amino acids. The main amino acid analogs or derivatives that have been evaluated for their ability to resist microbial degradation are methionine hydroxy analog (MHA), N-(hydroxyl methyl)-DL-methionine calcium, and mono plus di-N-(hydroxyl methyl)-L-lysine calcium. Many other analogs, derivatives, and polymeric forms of methionine and lysine have been evaluated for stability in the rumen by *in vitro* and *in vivo* techniques. The second category is the encapsulated amino acids, which have been developed in several forms. In the early preparations amino acids were embedded in matrixes of protein or fat treated with formaldehyde. These preparations were partly stable in the rumen, and the post ruminal release of amino acids was poor. In addition, they carried only small amounts of amino acids. These problems have been resolved by using polymeric compounds to overcoat cores composed primarily of amino acid(s) and small amounts of other ingredients. Polymeric coatings are usually pH-sensitive and are designed to maintain their structural integrity at the pH normally encountered in the rumen. The lower pH of the abomasum triggers breakdown of the coating allowing release of amino acids for absorption.

A potential problem is that amino acid can be over-protected. Complexes that are extremely inert in the rumen can be indigestible in the small intestine as well. Therefore, a tradeoff exists between good ruminal protection and bioavailability. Effectiveness of an encapsulated rumen-protected methionine compound (RPMet) in delivering methionine postruminally is determined by an increase in plasma methionine concentration. RPMet consisted of DL-methionine cores coated with a pH-sensitive polymer to protect them from ruminal breakdown. The RPMet contained 79% DL-methionine. The methionine was released when the low pH of the abomasum caused the coating to rupture.

Commercial RPMet Products

Met-Plus™ (Nisso America, Inc.), this is an example of a lipid-protected product. It is a matrix compound that contains 65% DL-Met embedded in a mixture of calcium salts of long-chain fatty acids, lauric acid, and butylated hydroxyl toluene (BHT); BHT is a preservative for the fatty acids. However, like other lipid-coated products, the technology relies on achieving a balance between ruminal protection vs. intestinal release so as to maximize the amount of methionine available for intestinal absorption while minimizing losses in the rumen and in faeces.

Mepron® M85 (Degussa Corporation, Germany), this is an example of a surface-coated, carbohydrate-protected product. The small pellets have a diameter of 1.8 mm, a length of 3-4 mm and an approximate density of 1.2 g/cm^3. The pellets consist of a core of Met and starch coated with several thin layers of ethyl cellulose and stearic acid. The final product contains a minimum of 85% DL-Met, and approximately 8.5% non-structural carbohydrates, 3.5% NDF, 1.5 % ash, 1.0% moisture, and 0.5% crude fat. The technology is a combination of coating materials and application that allows for a large payload of Met. Because enzymatic digestion of the ethyl cellulose is minimal, degradation of the product occurs primarily through physical action and abrasion. The result is a product that results in a slow degradation in the rumen and a slow release of Met in the intestine.

Smartamine™ M (Adisseo, Inc., Antony France), this is an example of a lipid/pH-sensitive polymer-protected product. It is a surface-coated product that contains a minimum of 75% DL-Met. The small 2-mm pellets consist of a core of DL-Met plus ethyl cellulose which is covered with a coat of stearic acid containing small droplets of poly 2-vinylpyridine-co-styrene. The copolymer contributes 3% by weight of the final product. The presence of the copolymer appears to alter the stereochemistry of the stearic acid such that the surface-coating becomes enhanced in its resistance to ruminal degradation. The presence of the copolymer, as a result of its solubilization at low pH, also allows for rapid release of the Met in the abomasum.

Effect on Milk Production

Responses to methionine/lysine supplementation in milk yield have been more variable. Some researchers have observed increased milk production with methionine/lysine supplementation whereas others have not. Milk fat content is generally not affected by amino acid supplementation. However, methionine and its hydroxy-analog (MHA) have been used to increase ruminal fibre digestion and alleviate milk fat depression. Therefore, methionine that is not fully protected from ruminal degradation may contribute to increased milk fat synthesis. Methionine is also used by the body in fat metabolism and synthesis. Therefore, the response to amino acid supplementation, in particular, methionine, can be affected by stage of lactation, animal body condition, and diet.

The favorable *in vivo* protection and release characteristics combined with increased plasma amino acid concentration, milk protein content and milk production obtained in studies conducted by Rogers *et al.* (1987) indicated that rumen protected methionine (Rpmet) and rumen protected lysine (Rplys) were effective in delivering methionine and lysine post ruminally in lactating dairy cows. Lysine appeared to improve the utilization of methionine. This fact implied that lysine was used more extensively and could be more limiting for milk production than methionine. In addition to this lysine must be present at greater than 6.5% of the digestible protein for supplemental methionine to elicit a positive response. However, the proportion of amino acids in digesta vary when different diets are fed, which makes it difficult to determine which amino acid is limiting.

Robert *et al.* (1996a) found that protected methionine significantly increased milk protein content and milk protein yield. Robert *et al.* (1996b) also observed that when graded levels of protected lysine was supplemented, there was a significant increase in milk protein content and milk protein yield. Han *et al.* (1996) also found that there was an increase in the total milk yield, total milk protein and fat in Holstein cows fed with rumen protected lysine.

Rumen protected amino acids should generally be safe for administration to the animal. A balance should also be achieved so that amino acids protected from ruminal degradation are available for intestinal absorption. In addition these compounds should be stable when pelleted and when incorporated into silage based total mixed ration (TMR), where PH could be in the acidic range. There have been difficulties in the production technology and where, when and how much of the protected nutrients can be incorporated in the diet (Robinson, 1996).

The influence of rumen-protected protein supplemented with the amino acids lysine (Lys), methionine (Met) and histidine (His) added either as a powder or in the form of rumen-protected tablets to the rumen of dairy cows on the yield, composition and technological suitability of milk was determined by Trinacty *et al.* (2006). Average milk yield in the control cows was significantly lower than in treated cows. Protein, fat and lactose contents were unaffected by the treatment. Protein yield was lower in the control cows. The increase in milk protein yield in treated cows was followed closely by progressive increases in casein content. The content of short and medium chain fatty acids were higher and the proportion of C 18: 1, C18:2, C18:30 and C20:1 was lower in the control animals. The proportion of UFA (both MUFA and PUFA) was increased and that of SFA in milk ($P < 0.05$) was decreased in the treated animals.

The concept of RPAA supplementation has been with us for a long time. In the near future, several commercial sources of rumen protected lysine and methionine will be available to dairy producers. In numerous studies, amino acid supplementation has been shown to be effective in improving milk yield and/or milk protein synthesis. Additionally, RPAA provides dairy producers with the opportunity for more flexibility in their feeding systems. The improvement in nitrogen utilization place RPAA as products that fit well in modern environmentally sensitive production systems. Effective use of RPAA technology as well as "bypass" proteins requires knowledge of amount and amino acid composition of rumen microbial protein, precise amino acid requirements of the cow and an effective delivery system for supplemental amino acid.

At present, the rumen degradability of protein in many feeds and the amino acid composition in the RUP fraction in the some feeds has been elucidated (Erasmus *et al*, 1994; Sampath, 1990). More research is needed to bridge the knowledge on ruminal degradability, intestinal digestibility, composition of nitrogenous feeds, requirements of amino acids, efficiency of absorption and utilization of amino acid. The feeding of rumen protected amino acids holds an elusive promise of enabling the strategic improvement of supply and balance of absorbed amino acid to support metabolic requirements. An added feature of rumen protected amino acids is that they permit the amino acid requirement to be met with less total N in the diet, resulting in higher efficiency of N utilization consequently, they may improve the sustainability of dairying. The practice of feeding protected proteins will only be successful in affecting the animal performance if the proteins / amino acids are not over protected and the animal has the metabolic capacity to respond to increased amino acid supply.

References

Bagga, S., Armendaris, A., Klypina, N; Ray, I., Ghoshroy, S; Endress, M., Sutton, D., Kemp, J.D., Sengupta Gopalan, C. (2004). *Plant Sci.*, 166(2): 273-283.

Bhagwat S.R. and Srivastava A. (1993,). *Indian J. Anim. Sci.*, 46(6):237-240.

Bowman, J.M. Grieve, P.G., Buchnan, Smith, J.G. and Macleod, G.K. (1988). *J. Dairy Sci.*, 71: 982-989.

Chalupa, W. (1975). *J. Dairy Sci.*, 58: 1198-1218.

Chalupa, W. and Sniffen, C. (2006). 21st Annual Southwest Nutrition & Management Conference February 23-24, Tempe, AZ – 96 -109.

Chandrasekharaiah, M., Sampath, K.T., and Thulasi, A. (2003). *Indian J. Anim. Sci.*, 73:305-307.

Chatterjee, A. and Walli, T.K. (2003 a). *Indian J. Anim. Nutr.*, 20(2): 143-148.

Chatterjee and Walli (2003b). *Indian J. Dairy Sci.*, 56: 4-24.

Cleale, R. M., Klopfenstein, T.J., Britton. R.A. and Satterlee, L.D (1986). *J. Anim. Sci.*, 63 (Supplement): 139.

Dahiya, S.S., Chandrasekharaiah, M, Sharma, M.L, Thulasi, A, Punia, B.S and Sampath, K.T. (2007a). In Proceedings of International Tropical Animal Nutrition Conference (Tropnutricon-2007) held at National Dairy Research Institute, Karnal, 4 -7, October 2007. p 10. Abstract No. FR 18.

Dahiya, S.S, Chandrasekharaiah, M, Sharma, M.L, Thulasi, A, Punia, B.S and Sampath, K.T. (2007b). In Proceedings of International Tropical Animal Nutrition Conference (Tropnutricon-2007) held at National Dairy Research Institute, Karnal, 4 -7, October 2007. p 11. Abstract No. FR 19.

Egan, A.R. (1988). In: Fibrous crop residues in animal feed. Kiran Singh and J.B. Schiere (eds.) ICAR. New Delhi, India.

Eramus, L.J., Botha, P.M. and Meissner, H.H. (1994). *J. Dairy Sci.*, 77: 3655-3665.

Garg M.R. Sherasia P.L., Bhanderi, B.M., Gulati, S.K. and Scott, T.W. (2002). *Indian J. Anim. Nutr.* 19: 3, 191-198.

Garg, M. R., Sherasia, P.L., Bhanderi, B. M., Gulati, S.K. and Scott, T.W. (2005). *Anim. Nutr. Feed Technol.*, 5(1): 1-8.

Garg, M. R., Sherasia, P.L., Bhanderi, B. M., Gulati, S.K. and Scott, T.W. (2003). *Indian J. Dairy Sci.*, 56(4): 218-22.

Gaynor, P.J., Montgomery, M.J. and Holmes, C.R. (1988). *J. Dairy Sci.*, 71: 2175-2180.

Gould, D.H. and Macgregor, J.J. (1976). Symposium on Cross linking: 31, Eds. M. Friedman, Plenum Publications, New York.

Gupta, H.K. and Walli, T.K. (1987). *Indian J. Anim. Nutr.*, 4: 94-99.

Han,I.K., Choi, Y.J., Ha., J.K., Ku, Y.G., Lee, H.S. and Lee, S.S. (1996). *Asian Austr. J. Anim. Sci.*, 9 (3)287-294.

Khorasani, G.R., Robinson, P.H. and Kennel. (1989). *J. Dairy Sci.*, 72:2074-2080.

Kumar, V. and Walli, T.K. (1994). Indian J. Anim. Nutr., 4: 29-33.

Lynch, G.L., Berger, L.L. Merchens, N.R. Fahey, G,C., and Baker, E.C., (1987). *J. Anim. Sci.*, 65: 1617-1625.

Lynch , G.L., Vander Aar , P.J. Berger, L.L., Fahey, G,C., and Merchens, N.R. (1988). *J. Dairy Sci.*, 71: 2416-2427.

Mc Donald, I.W. (1948). *Biochem. J.*, 52: 584-587.

Mehrez, A. Z. and Orskov , E.R. (1977). *J. Agric. Sci., Cambridge*, 88:645-650.

Mir, A., Macleod, G.K., Buchnan Smith, J.G. and Grovum, W.L. (1984). *Canadian J. Anim. Sci.*, 64: 853-865.

Mishra, B.B., Swain, R. K., Sahu, B.K. and Samantaray, D.P. (2006). *Anim. Nutr. Feed Technol.*, 6(1): 123-133.

Mudgal, V.D. and Sengar, S.S. (1980). *J. Nucl. Agric. Bio.*, 9:19.

Orskov, E.R. and McDonald, (1979). *J. Agric. Sci. Cambridge.*, 92: 499-503.

Pachauri, V.C., Majumdar, A.B and Mahanta, S.K. (1999). *Indian J. Anim. Sci.*, 69(3): 197-198.

Pratihar, S.K. and Walli, T.K. (1995). Proceedings of VIII ANRW Conference, Mumbai. pp. 95.

Ramachandra, K. S. and Sampath, K.T. (1995). *Indian J. Anim. Nutr.*, 12:1-6.

Robert, J.C., Sloan, B.K. and Denis, C. (1996a). *J. Dairy Sci.*, 79 (suppl), 1:194.

Robert, J.C., Sloan, B.K. and Noziere, C. (1996b). *J. Dairy Sci.*, 79 (suppl), 1:194.

Robinson, P.H. (1996). *Anim. Feed Sci. Technol.*, 59:81-86.

Rogers, J.A., Pierce Sandnec, S.D., Papas, A.M., Polon, C.E., Snifefen, C.J., Muscat, T.V., Staples, C.R. and Clark, J.H. (1989). *J. Dairy Sci.*, 42 :1800-1817.

Sahoo, B. and Walli, T.K. (2005). *Indian J. Dairy Sci.*, 58(3): 184-190.

Sahoo, B. and Walli, T.K. (2001). Proc. of X Anim. Nutr. Conf., Karnal, India.

Sampath, K.T., Prasad, C.S., Ramachandra, K.S., Sundareshan, K.. and Subba Rao, *A.* (1996). *Indian J. Anim. Sci.*, 13(1):1-6.

Sampath, K.T., Prasad, C.S., Ramachandra, K.S., Sunderashan, K. and Subbarao, A. (1997). *Indian J. Anim. Sci.*, 67: 706-708.

Sampath, K.T., Chandrasekharaiah, M. and Thulasi, A. (2002). *Indian J. Anim. Sci.*, 55 (2) 93-96.

Sampath, K.T., Chandrasekharaiah, M. and Thulasi, A (2003). *Indian J. Anim. Sci.*, 73 (10): 76-80.

Sampath, K.T. (1990). *Dairy Guide.* 43-44.

Stern, M.D. (1984). *Canadian J. Anim. Sci.*, 64: (Supplement 1): 468.

Tiwari, D.P. and Yadav, L.S. (1994). *Indian J. Anim. Sci.*, 64: 6:625-679.

Trinacty, J., Krizova, L., Hadrova, S., Hanus, O., Janstova, B., Vorlova, L., Drakova, M. (2006). *J. Anim. Feed Sci.*, 15 (1): 3-15.

Vandehar, M.J., Flakoll, P.J., Bertz, D.C. and Njssen, S. (1987). *J. Anim. Sci.* 65 (Suppl. 1): 501.

Walli, T.K. and Sirohi, S.K. (2004). Proceedings of IV Biennial conference of ANA at Kolkata, Nov 20- 22, 2002 pp. 151-59.

Walli, T.K. (1996). Final report NDRI NDDB Technology Mission Collaborative Project, NDRI, Karnal.

Walli, T.K., Dass, M.M., Rai, S.N. and Garg, M.R. (2000). *Indian J. Dairy Sci.*, 57 (5): 361-368.

Waltz, D. M. and Loerch, S.C. (1986). *J. Anim. Sci.*, 63: 879-887.

Winowiski, T.S. and Stern, M.D. (1987). *J. Anim. Sci.*, 65(Suppl. 1): 468.

□□□

Animal Nutrition, 2012
eds. Dr. (Mrs.) Usha R. Mehra et al., pp. 771-793
Satish Serial Publishing House e-mail : info@satishserial.com; website : www.satishserial.com

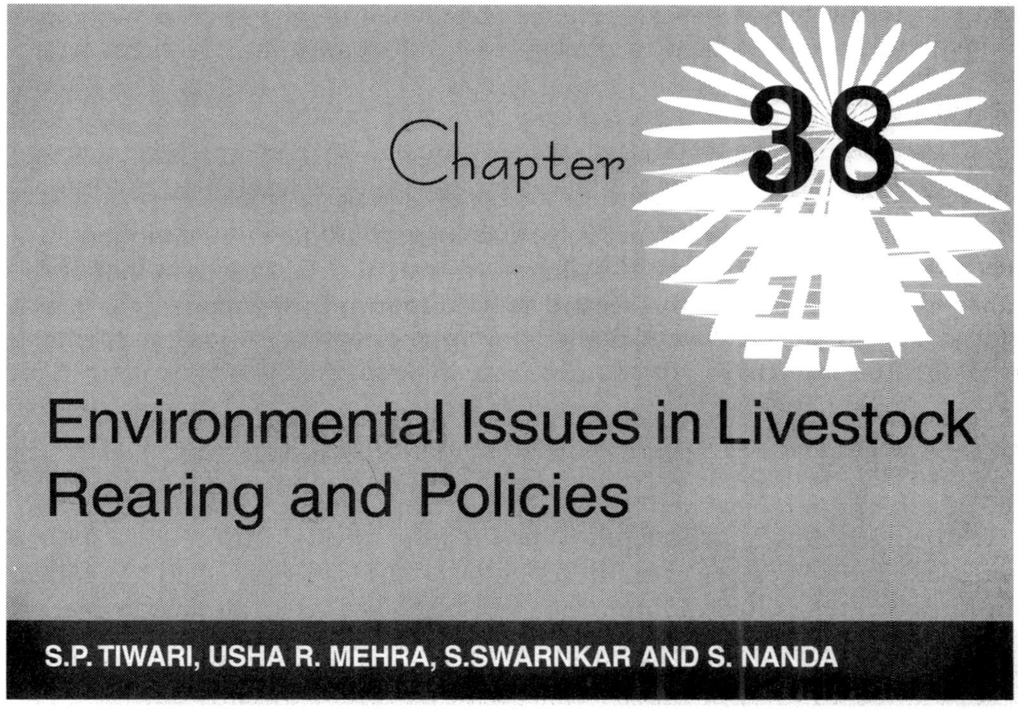

Chapter 38

Environmental Issues in Livestock Rearing and Policies

S.P. TIWARI, USHA R. MEHRA, S.SWARNKAR AND S. NANDA

The atmosphere is fundamental to life on earth. Besides providing the air we breathe, it regulates temperature and distributes water. It is not only a part of key processes such as carbon, nitrogen and oxygen cycles, but also protects life from harmful radiation. These functions are orchestrated, in a fragile dynamic equilibrium, by a complex physics and chemistry. There is increasing evidence that human activity is altering the mechanisms of the atmosphere.

In the following sections, the anthropogenic processes of climate change and air pollution along with role of livestock in these processes (excluding the ozone hole) have been focused. The contribution of the livestock sector to these processes is not well known. At each step of the livestock production process, substances contributing to climate change or air pollution, are emitted into the atmosphere or their sequestration in other reservoirs is hampered. Such changes are either the direct effect of livestock rearing or indirect contributions from steps involved with the marketed animal product. This chapter describes the contribution of livestock production to these emissions and provides a critical assessment of mitigation strategies such as emissions reduction measures related to changes in livestock farming practices.

Air Pollution

"The addition of substances to the atmosphere that result in direct damage to the environment, human health and quality of life is termed air pollution".

The direct warming impact is highest for carbon dioxide simply because its concentration and the emitted quantities are much higher than that of the other gases. Methane is the second most important greenhouse gas. Once emitted, it remains in the atmosphere for approximately 9-15 years. Methane is about 21 times more effective in trapping heat in the atmosphere than carbon dioxide over a 100 year period. Nitrous oxide, a third greenhouse gas with important direct warming potential, is present in the atmosphere in extremely small amounts. However, it is 296 times more effective than carbon dioxide in trapping heat and has a very long atmospheric lifetime (114 years). Livestock activities emit considerable amounts of these three gases. Direct emissions from livestock come from the respiratory process of all animals in the form of carbon dioxide. Ruminants and to a minor extent also monogastrics, emit methane as part of their digestive process, which involves microbial fermentation of fibrous feeds. Animal manure also emits gases such as methane, nitrous oxides, ammonia and carbon dioxide, depending on the way they are produced (solid, liquid) and managed (collection, storage, spreading). Livestock also affect the carbon balance of land used for pasture or feed crops, and thus indirectly contribute to releasing large amounts of carbon into the atmosphere.

In addition, greenhouse gases are also emitted from fossil fuel used in the production process, from marketing of livestock products. Some of the indirect effects are difficult to estimate, as land use related emissions vary widely, depending on biophysical factors as soil, vegetation and climate as well as on human practices.

Relative Greenhouse Gas Contributions Along the Food

Carbon Dioxide

Livestock account for 9 percent of global anthropogenic emissions .When deforestation for pasture and feedcrop land and pasture degradation are taken into account, livestock-related emissions of carbon dioxide are an important component of the global total (some 9 percent). Although small by comparison to Land use, land use change and forestry (LULUCF), the livestock food chain is becoming more fossil fuel intensive, which will increase carbon dioxide emissions from livestock production. As ruminant production (based on traditional local feed resources) shifts to intensive monogastrics (based on food transported over long distances), there is a corresponding shift away from solar energy harnessed by photosynthesis, to fossil fuels.

Methane

Livestock account for 35-40 percent of global anthropogenic emissions. The leading role of livestock, in methane emissions, has long been a well-established fact. Together, enteric fermentation and manure represent some 80 percent of agricultural methane emissions and about 35-40 percent of the total anthropogenic methane emissions. With the decline of ruminant livestock in relative terms, and the overall trend towards higher productivity in ruminant production, it is unlikely that the importance of enteric fermentation will increase further. However, methane emissions from animal manure, although much lower in absolute terms, are considerable and growing rapidly.

Nitrous Oxide

Livestock account for 65 percent of global anthropogenic emissions .Livestock activities contribute substantially to the emission of nitrous oxide, the most potent of the three major greenhouse gases. They contribute almost two-thirds of all anthropogenic N_2O emissions, and 75-80 percent of agricultural emissions. Current trends suggest that this level will substantially increase over the coming decades.

Ammonia

Livestock account for 64 percent of global anthropogenic emissions. Global anthropogenic atmospheric emission of ammonia has recently been estimated to be 47 milliontonnesN (Galloway *et al.*, 2004). Some 94 percent of this is produced by the agricultural sector. The livestock sector contributes about 68 percent of the agriculture share, mainly from deposited and applied manure. The resulting air and environmental pollution (mainly eutrophication, also odour) is more a local or regional environmental problem than a global one. Indeed, similar levels of N depositions can have substantially different environ mental effects depending on the type of eco-system they affect.

The stinging smell over entire landscapes around livestock facilities is partly due to ammonia emission. Ammonia volatilization (nitrified in the soil after deposition) is among the most important causes of acidifying wet and dry atmospheric deposition, and a large part of it originates from livestock excreta.

Livestock's Contribution to the Net Release of Carbon

The net additions of carbon to the atmosphere are estimated to be 4.5 and 6.5 billion tonnes per year. Mostly, the burning of fossil fuel and land-use changes, which destroy organic carbon in the soil, are responsible. The respiration of livestock makes up only a very small part of the net release of carbon. It can be attributed to the livestock sector. Much more is released indirectly by other channels including:

- burning fossil fuel to produce mineral fertilizers used in feed production;
- methane release from the breakdown of fertilizers and from animal manure;
- land-use changes for feed production and for grazing;
- land degradation;
- fossil fuel use during feed and animal production; and
- fossil fuel use in production and transport of processed and refrigerated animal products.

Carbon Emissions from Feed Production

Fossil fuel use in manufacturing fertilizer may emit 41 million tonnes of CO_2 per year. A large share of the world's crop production is fed to animals, either directly or as agro-industrial by-products. Mineral N fertilizer is applied to much of the corresponding cropland, especially in the case of high-energy crops such as maize, used in the production of concentrate feed. The gaseous emissions caused by fertilizer manufacturing should, therefore, be considered among the emissions for which the animal food chain is responsible. This high proportion of N fertilizer going to animal feed is largely owing to maize, which covers large areas in temperate and tropical climates and demands high doses of nitrogen fertilizer. More than half of total maize production is used as feed. In fact maize is the crop, highest in nitrogen fertilizer consumption. Other feed crops are also important consumers of chemical N fertilizer. Grains like barley and sorghum receive large amounts of nitrogen fertilizer. Despite the fact that some oil crops are associated with N fixing organisms themselves ,their intensive production often makes use of nitrogen fertilizer. Such crops predominantly used as animal feed, including rapeseed, soybean and sunflower, garner considerable amounts of N-fertilizer . This results in an estimated annual emission of CO_2 of more than 40 million tonnes at this initial stage of the animal food chain.

On-farm Fossil Fuel use may emit 90 million tonnes CO_2 per year

The share of energy consumption accounted for, by the different stages of livestock production varies widely, depending on the intensity of livestock production (Sainz, 2003). In modern production systems the bulk of the energy is spent on production of feed, forage for ruminants or concentrate feed for poultry or pigs. The significant of energy are also spent on seed, herbicides/

pesticides, diesel for machinery (for land preparation, harvesting, transport) and electricity (irrigation pumps, drying, heating, etc.). On-farm use of fossil fuel by intensive systems produces CO_2 emissions probably even larger than those from chemical N fertilizer for feed.

The share of electricity is larger for intensive monogastrics production (mainly for heating, cooling and ventilation), which uses larger amounts of fossil fuel in feed transportation. However, more than half the energy expenditure during livestock production is for feed production (nearly all in the case of intensive beef operations). We have already considered the contribution of fertilizer production to the energy input for feed: in intensive systems, the combined energy-use for seed and herbicide/pesticide production and fossil fuel for machinery generally exceeds that for fertilizer production.

Related Land use changes may emit 2.4 billion tonnes of CO_2 per year

Land use in the various parts of the world is continually changing. Changes in land use have an impact in carbon fluxes, and many of the land-use changes involve livestock, either occupying land (as pasture or arable land for feed crops) or releasing land for other purposes.

A forest contains more carbon than does a field of annual crops or pasture, and so when forests are harvested, or worse, burned, large amounts of carbon are released from the vegetation and soil to the atmosphere. The net reduction in carbon stocks is not simply equal to the net CO_2 flux from the cleared area. Reality is more complex: forest clearing can produce a complex pattern of net fluxes that change direction over time. The calculation of carbon fluxes owing to forest conversion is, in many ways, the most complex of the emissions inventory components. Estimates of emissions from forest clearing vary because of multiple uncertainties: annual forest clearing rates, the fate of the cleared land, the amounts of carbon contained in different ecosystems, the modes by which CO_2 is released (e.g., burning or decay).

In view of this, and of worldwide trends in extensive livestock production and in cropland for feed production we can realistically estimate that "livestock induced" emissions from deforestation amount to roughly 2.4 billion tonnes of CO_2 per year.

Livestock-releases from cultivated soils may total 28 million tonnes CO_2 per year

Soils are the largest carbon reservoir of the terrestrial carbon cycle. The estimated total amount of carbon stored in soils is about 1100 to 1600 billion tones (Sundquist, 1993). Hence even relatively small changes in carbon stored in the soil could make a significant impact on the global carbon balance.

Further soil carbon losses can be induced by management practices. Under appropriate management practices (such as zero tillage) agricultural soils can serve as a carbon sink and may increasingly do so in future Currently, however, their role as carbon sinks is globally insignificant.

Order-of-magnitude indications can be made by using an average loss rate from soil in a rather temperate climate with moderate to low organic matter content that is somewhere between the loss rate reported for zero and conventional tillage: Assuming an annual loss rate of 100 kg CO_2 per hectare per year (covering temperate brown soil CO_2 loss, and excluding emissions originating from crop residues), the approximately 1.8 million km^2 of arable land cultivated with maize, wheat and soybean for feed would add an annual CO_2 flux of some 18 million tonnes to the livestock balance.

Tropical soils have lower average carbon content (IPCC 2001b), and therefore lower emissions. On the other hand, the considerable expansion of large-scale feed cropping, not only into uncultivated areas, but also into previous pastureland or subsistence cropping, may increase CO_2 emission. In addition, practices such as soil liming contribute to emissions. Soil liming is a common practice in more intensively cultivated tropical areas because of soil acidity. To the extent that these emissions concern cropland for feed production they should be attributed to the livestock sector. Often only crop residues and by-products are used for feeding, in which case a share of emissions corresponding to the value fraction of the commodity should be attributed to livestock.

Another way livestock contributes to gas emissions from cropland is through methane emissions from rice cultivation, globally recognized as an important source of methane.

Releases from livestock-induced desertification of pastures may total 100 million tonnes CO_2 per year

Livestock also play a role in desertification .Where desertification is occurring, degradation often results in reduced productivity or reduced vegetation cover, which produce a change in the carbon and nutrient stocks and cycling of the system. This seems to result in a small reduction in above ground carbon stocks and a slight decline in carbon fixation.

Lal (2001) estimated the carbon loss as a result of desertification. Assuming a loss of 8-12 tonnes of soil carbon per hectare on a desertified land area of 1 billion hectares (UNEP, 1991), the total historic loss would amount to 8-12 billion tonnes of soil carbon. Similarly, degradation of above ground vegetation has led to an estimated carbon loss of 10-16 tonnes per hectare a historic total of 10-16 billion tonnes. Thus, the total C loss as a consequence of desertification may be 18-28 billion tonnes of carbon (FAO, 2004b). Livestock's contribution to this total is difficult to estimate, but it is undoubtedly high: livestock occupies about two-thirds of the global dry land area, and the rate of desertification has been estimated to be higher under pasture than under other land uses (3.2 million hectares per year against 2.5 million hectares per year for cropland, UNEP, 1991). Considering only soil carbon loss (i.e. about 10 tonnes of carbon per hectare), pasture desertification-induced oxidation of carbon would result in CO_2 emissions in the order of 100 million tonnes of CO_2 per year.

Carbon Emissions from Livestock Rearing

Respiration by livestock is not a net source of CO_2

Humans and livestock now account for about a quarter of the total terrestrial animal biomass. Based on animal numbers and live weights, the total livestock biomass amounts to some 0.7 billion tonnes (FAO, 2005b).

According to the function established by Muller and Schneider (1985, cited by Ni *et al.*, 1999), the carbon dioxide from the respiratory process of livestock amount to some 3 billion tonnes of CO_2 or 0.8 billion tonnes of carbon. Cattle alone account for more than half of the total carbon dioxide emissions from respiration.

However, emissions from livestock respiration are part of a rapidly cycling biological system, livestock respiration is not considered to be a net source under the Kyoto Protocol. Applying these emission factors to the livestock numbers in each production system gives an estimate for total global emissions of methane from enteric fermentation 86 million tonnes CH_4 annually.

Methane released from Animal Manure may total 18 million tonnes per year

The anaerobic decomposition of organic material in livestock manure also releases methane. This occurs mostly when manure is managed in liquid form, such as in lagoons or holding tanks. Lagoon systems are typical for most large scale pig operations and also for large dairy operations. Globally, methane emissions from anaerobic decomposition of manure have been estimated to total just over 10 million tonnes, or some 4 percent of global anthropogenic methane emissions (US-EPA, 2005). Although of much lesser magnitude than emissions from enteric fermentation, emissions from manure are much higher than those originating from burning residues and similar to the lower estimate of the badly known emissions originating from rice cultivation.

As a species, pig production contributes the largest share, followed by dairy. Developing countries such as China and India would not be very far behind. China has the largest country-level methane emission from manure in the world, mainly from pigs. At a global level, emissions from pig manure represent almost half of total livestock manure emissions.

Carbon Emissions from Livestock Processing and Refrigerated Transport

CO_2 emissions from livestock processing may total several million tonnes per year

Since mostly products from intensive systems are being processed, Diesel is used mainly for transport of products to the processing facilities. Transport-related emissions for milk are high, owing to large volumes and low utilization of transport capacity. In addition, large amounts of energy are used to pasteurize milk and transform it into cheese and dried milk, making the dairy sector responsible for the second highest CO_2 emissions from food processing in Minnesota. The largest emissions result from soybean processing and are a result of physical and chemical methods to separate the crude soy oil and soybean meal from the raw beans. Considering the value fractions of these two commodities (Chapagain and Hoekstra, 2004) some two-thirds of these soy-processing emissions can be attributed to the livestock sector. Thus, the majority of CO_2 emissions related to energy consumption from processing Minnesota's agricultural production can be ascribed to the livestock sector.

Minnesota can be considered a "hotspot" because of its CO_2 emissions from livestock processing and cannot, in light of the above remarks on the variability of energy efficiency and sources, be used as a basis for deriving a global estimate.

Overall, livestock activities contribute an estimated 18 percent to total anthropogenic green-house gas emissions from the five major sectors for greenhouse gas reporting: energy, industry, waste, land use, land use change and forestry (LULUCF) and agriculture. Considering the last two sectors only, livestock's share is over 50 percent. For the agriculture sector alone, livestock constitute nearly 80 percent of all emissions.

Water Pollution

A major driver of use and pollution

The livestock sector is a key player in increasing water use and water depletion. The water used by the livestock sector is over 8 percent of global human water use. The major part of this water is in fact used for irrigation of feed crops, representing 7 percent of the global water use. The water used for product processing and drinking and servicing is insignificant at global level (less than 1 percent of the global water), but it may be of local importance in dry areas (livestock drinking requirements represent 23 percent of total water use in Botswana).

Apart from livestock's use of water for drinking, water is used for irrigating pastures and cropland for feed production. Considerable amounts of water are used in processing of meat and milk in particular. Through the compacting effect of grazing and hoof action on the soil, livestock also have a determining, and often negative, impact on water infiltration and the speed of water movement across the landscape. Livestock play an important role in water quality through the release of nutrients, pathogens and other substances into waterways, mainly from intensive livestock operations.

The contribution of the livestock sector to water depletion is not easily quantified with our current knowledge but there is strong evidence that the sector is a major driver. The volume of water evapotranspired by feed crops represents a significant share (at 15 percent) of the water depleted every year.

Water pollution figures from the United States, the world's largest economy and fourth largest land area, may give some indication of the livestock sector's importance. In the United States, livestock are responsible for an estimated 55 percent of erosion, 37 percent of the pesticides applied, 50 percent of the volume of antibiotics consumed and for 32 percent of the nitrogen load and 33 percent of the phosphorus load into fresh-water resources. Although the effective load into freshwater resources is not assessed for sediments, pesticides, antibiotics, heavy metals or biological contaminants, livestock are likely to have a major role in these pollution processes. Livestock land use and management (especially of animal wastes) appear to be the main mechanism through which livestock contribute to the water depletion process.

Biodiversity

Livestock are a key factor in loss of species

Livestock affect biodiversity in many direct and indirect ways, most of which are difficult to quantify. Livestock and wildlife interact in grazing areas, often negatively, sometimes positively. Livestock help to maintain some of the open grassland ecosystems in their traditional state, but health concerns pose new threats to wild-life. Pasture expansion, often at the expense of forest, has vast negative consequences on some of the most valuable ecosystems in Latin America, while rangeland degradation affects biodiversity on all continents. Crop area expansion and intensification for livestock feed undoubtedly affect biodiversity negatively, sometimes with dramatic consequences (soybean expansion into tropical forests). Water pollution and ammonia emissions, mainly from industrial livestock production, compromise biodiversity, often drastically in the case of aquatic life. Livestock's important contribution to climate change will clearly have repercussions on biodiversity, while the historic role of livestock as a driver and facilitator of invasions by alien species continues.

Livestock now account for about 20 percent of the total terrestrial animal biomass, and occupies a vast area that was once habitat for wildlife. Further, livestock determine, to a significant extent, the nitrogen and phosphorus flows. The fact that the livestock sector is industrializing, in a number of concentrated locations, separates the sector from its land base and interrupts the nutrient flows between land and livestock, creating problems of depletion at the sources (land vegetation and soil) and problems of pollution at the sinks (animal wastes, increasingly disposed of into waterways instead of back on the land). Pollution, as well as overfishing for feed, leads to an increasingly strong impact of livestock on the biodiversity of marine ecosystems.

Species, Products and Production Systems

There are huge differences in environmental impact between the different forms of livestock production, and even the species.

Cattle provide a multitude of products and services, including beef, milk, and traction. In mixed farming systems, cattle are usually well integrated in nutrient flows and can have a positive environmental impact. In developing countries, cattle and buffaloes still provide animal draught for field operations, and in some areas, animal traction is on the increase (parts of sub-Saharan Africa) so that animals substitute for potential fossil fuel use. Livestock also use crop-residues some of which would otherwise be burned, thus making net contributions to environmental objectives. However, cattle in extensive livestock production in developing countries are often only of marginal productivity.

As a result, the vast majority of feed is spent on the animal's maintenance, leading to resource inefficiencies and high levels of environmental damage per unit of output.

The dairy sector is much better connected to land than is the case for other forms of market- oriented production. Most milk operations tend to be close to areas of feed supply because of their daily demand for fibrous feed, and so they are predominantly well integrated with nutrient flows, although excessive use of nitrogen fertilizer on dairy farms is one of the main causes of high nitrate levels in surface water in Organization for Economic Cooperation and Development (OECD) countries. There is a risk of soil and water contamination by large-scale dairy operations, as witnessed by "dairy colonies" in South Asia, and by industrial-type operations in North America and increasingly also in China. Dairy production is also labour intensive and less subjected to economies of scale. Therefore, dairy is the livestock commodity where small-scale or family-based operations can resist market pressures for longer than is the case for poultry or pork. Beef is produced in a wide range of intensities and scales. At both ends of the intensity spectrum there is considerable environmental damage. On the extensive side, cattle are instrumental in degradation of vast grassland areas and are a contributing factor to deforestation (pasture conversion), and the resulting carbon emissions, biodiversity losses and negative impacts on water flows and quality. On the intensive side, feedlots are often vastly beyond the capacity of surrounding land to absorb nutrients. While in the feedlot stage the conversion of concentrate feed into beef is far less efficient than into poultry or pork, and therefore beef has significantly higher resource requirements per unit than pork or poultry. However, taking the total life cycle into account, including the grazing phase, concentrate feed per kilogram of growth is lower for beef than for non-ruminant systems (CAST, 1999).

The production of sheep and goats is usually extensive. Except for small pockets with feed lots in Near East and North America, intensive production based on feed concentrate barely exists. The capacity of small ruminants, in particular goats to grow and reproduce under conditions otherwise unsuitable for any form of agricultural production-makes them useful and very often essential to poor farmers pushed into these environments for lack of alternative livelihoods. Because of their adaptive grazing, sheep and goats have extended their reach further into arid, steep and otherwise marginal territory than cattle. The browsing of goats affects land cover and the potential for forest re-growth. Under overstocked conditions, they are particularly damaging to the environment, through degradation of vegetative cover and soil. However, the low economic value of sheep and goat production means that it does not usually lead directly to mechanized large scale deforestation, as is the case for cattle ranching in Brazil.

Extensive pig production, based on use of household waste and agro industrial byproducts, performs a number of useful environmental functions by turning biomass of no commercial value and that otherwise would be waste - into -value animal protein. However, extensive systems are incapable of meeting the surging urban demand in many developing countries, not only in terms of volume but also in sanitary and other quality standards. The ensuing shift towards larger-scale grain-based industrial systems has been associated with geographic concentration, to such extents that land/livestock balances have become very unfavourable, leading to nutrient overload of soils and water pollution. China is a prime example of these trends. Furthermore, most industrial pig production in the tropics and sub-tropics uses waste-flushing systems involving large amounts of water. This becomes the main polluting agent, exacerbating negative environmental impact.

Poultry production has been the species most subject to structural change. In (OECD) countries, production is almost entirely industrial, while in developing countries it is already predominantly industrial. Although industrial poultry production is entirely based on feed grains and other high value feed material, it is the most efficient form of production of food of animal origin (with the exception of some forms of aquaculture), and has the lowest land requirements per unit of output. Poultry manure is of high nutrient content, relatively easy to manage and widely used as fertilizer and sometimes as feed. Other than for feed crop production, the environmental damage, though perhaps locally important, is of a much lower scale than for the other species.

In conclusion, livestock-environment interactions are often diffuse and indirect; and damage occurs at both the high and low end of the intensity spectrum, but is probably highest for beef and lowest for poultry.

What Needs to be done (Policies)

The future of the livestock environment interface will depend on the balance of two competing demands that are for animal food products on one hand and for environmental services on the other. Both demands are driven by the same factors: increasing populations and increasing incomes and urbanization. The natural resource base within which they must be accommodated is finite. Therefore, the considerable expansion of the livestock sector, required by expanding demand must be accomplished while substantially reducing livestock's environmental impact. In this section we put forward perspectives as to how this can be achieved, compared to a backdrop of "business as usual."

The growth in demand for animal products over the coming decades will be significant. Although the annual growth rate will be somewhat slower than in recent decades, the growth in absolute volume will be vast. Global production of meat is projected to more than double from 229 million tons in 1999/2001 to 465 million tonnes in 2050, and that of milk to increase from 580 to 1043 million tonnes (FAO, 2006a). The bulk of the growth in meat and in milk production will occur in developing countries (FAO, 2006a). Among the meat products, poultry will be the commodity of choice for reasons of acceptance across cultures and technical efficiency in relation to feed concentrates.

(I) Business as usual leads to mounting problems

In the absence of major corrective measures, the environmental impact of livestock production will worsen dramatically. If production doubles, without any reduction in environmental measures per unit of production, environmental damage will double.

Taking into account likely changes in the structure of the industry, while there has been no attempt to quantify the environmental impacts of livestock, it is probably safe to state that under a "business as usual"scenario:

- The livestock production will continue to grow, leading to large areas with high nitrogen and phosphorus surpluses, concentrated discharge of toxic materials, polluting and contaminating land, ground and surface water; and destroying terrestrial and aquatic biodiversity. Continued geographic concentration, with large scale commercial production is growing but with less intensive, widely scattered small holder production, will exacerbate the risk of emerging and traditional zoonotic diseases.
- Demand for feed crops will grow, causing a further conversion of natural habitats into cropland in some places, notably Latin America. The factors that slowed use of feed grain in the period 1985 to 2005, including European Union (EU) agricultural policy reform, drastic structural changes in the previous socialist countries of Eastern Europe and CIS, and the global shift to poultry as efficient converters of feed crops, are likely to wane (FAO, 2006a); therefore feed grain use is projected to expand more with output growth in livestock products. The pressure on crop agriculture to expand and intensify will remain high; and so the associated environmental impacts, in terms of water depletion, climate change and biodiversity loss, will grow.
- Livestock's contribution to anthropogenic greenhouse gas specially nitrous oxide emissions will increase, raising the already significant contribution to global climate change; and
- Livestock induced degradation of the world's arid and semi-arid lands will continue, again contributing significantly to climate change, water depletion and biodiversity losses, and sometimes leading to irreversible loss of productivity. The person deriving a living from livestock will continue to extract the little they can from dwindling common property resources while facing growing marginalization.

(II) Consumers may drive change towards a sustainable livestock sector

These "business as usual" trends lead to disaster and should be diverted into more beneficial paths. Growing economies and populations with increasing scarcity of environmental resources and rising environmental problems are translating into demand for environmental services. This demand will broaden from factors, such as reducing the nuisance factors of flies and odours, to the intermediate demands of clean air and water, to the broader, longer term environmental concerns, including climate change, biodiversity, etc. Locally markets will develop for such services but globally, this is more uncertain although promising models (example carbon trading or debt-for-nature swaps) already exist.

The conflicting demands for animal products and environmental services has been established in some developing countries, and is poised to grow in most developing countries over the coming decades. Consumers are probably ready to use growing voice to exert pressure for change and may be willing to absorb the inevitable price increases. The development of markets for organic products and other forms of ecolabelling are precursors of this trend, as are the tendency towards vegetarianism within developed countries and the trend towards healthier diets.

(III) Encouraging efficiency through adequate market prices

Resource use efficiency is the key to shrink livestock's long shadow. Number of tested and successful technical options are available to mitigate environmental impacts, which can be used in resource management, in crop and livestock production, and in post harvest reduction of losses. However, they will require adequate price signals, reflecting the scarcities of production factors, and correcting the distortions that provide insufficient incentives for efficient resource use.

Prices of land, water and feed resources used for livestock production do not reflect true scarcities. This leads to an overuse of these resources by the livestock sector and to major inefficiencies in the production process. Any future policy to protect the environment will have to introduce adequate market pricing for the main inputs.

In particular, water is grossly under priced in most countries. The development of water markets and different types of cost recovery may be suitable mechanisms to correct the situation. In case of land, introduction and adjustment of grazing fees and lease rates, and improved institutional arrangements for controlled and equitable access may be suggested. Further, removal of price support at product level (i.e. the production subsidies for livestock products in the majority of industrialized countries) is likely to improve technical efficiency.

(IV)Correcting for environmental externalities

Although removal of price distortions at input and product level is useful to enhance technical efficiency of natural resource use in the livestock production process, this may often not be sufficient.

i. Environmental externalities, both negative and positive, need to be explicitly factored into the policy framework, through application of the "provider gets polluter pays" principle. Correcting for the same will lead livestock producers into management choices that are less costly to the environment.

ii. Livestock holders who provide environmental services need to be compensated, either by the immediate beneficiary (such as with improved water quantity and quality for down- stream users) or by the general public. Examples of actions include land management, use of vegetative covers that maintain or restore biodiversity; or the sequestration of carbon in stable organic matter in the soil through pasture management. Managing grasslands to reduce runoff and increase infiltration can greatly reduce sedimentation of water reservoirs. Compensation schemes need to be developed between water and electricity providers and grazers.

iii. Livestock holders who emit waste into waterways or release ammonia into the environment must be held accountable and pay for the damage, to move them to less polluting practices. Applying the polluter pays principle should not present in surmountable problems in situations like these, given that increasing demand for livestock products provides the potential for adequate profits, and that there is an increasing demand for milk and meat produced in a sustainable way. It will be difficult to apply this principle to methane emissions from single cows owned on an Indian mixed farm of half a hectare. However, for most waste emissions in intensive production units, a combination of disincentives and regulation is most appropriate approach.

iv. Taxation of environmental damage and incentives for environmental should be applied in future, which will tackle local externalities and transboundary impacts, through application of international treaties, underlying regulatory frameworks and market mechanisms. Government policies may be required to provide incentives for institutional innovation in this regard.

(V) Technological change

In industrial and mixed production systems, the gap between levels of productivity and levels that are technically attainable indicates that by adopting intensifying technologies important efficiency gains can be realized. With extensive grazing, this is more difficult and sometimes impossible under marginal conditions with severe resource constraints, where current low productivity may be the maximum that can be achieved. Intensification would be possible only on a limited area, estimated at about 10 percent of the total pasture area (Pretty *et al.*, 2000).

i. Correcting for distortions and externalities will bring closer to prices for both inputs and outputs that reflect the true scarcities of production factors and natural resources used. These changed prices will induce technological change that will make better use of resources, and limit pollution and waste.

ii. For now, lack of improved production technologies is not a problem. Given the large market and policy failures, under which the livestock sector operates, there is still a huge progress that can be achieved from wide adoption of existing tried and tested technologies. However, research and development of new technologies suited to more conducive policy frameworks is needed.

iii. Technological change needs to make optimal use of land and water as the most important production factors for livestock, including feed production. Research and development for feed crop production need to further increase yields and factor efficiency.

iv. In the livestock sector, the quest for increasing efficiencies mainly falls on feeding, breeding and animal health. The modern feeding techniques, in production systems that are already industrial but technologically not very advanced, can help to reduce feed grain consumption significantly perhaps by as much as 20 percent of total feed grain use (assuming that half of the yield gap between top feed performers and world averages can be closed). Such improvements would include the use of optimized rations, enzymes and artificial amino acids. Further savings could come with advanced animal genotypes. While research into technological advances for commercial and industrial livestock production have been left to private sector, the public sector needs to assume a proactive role with regard to natural resource management, and in reducing market barriers for small producers.

(VI) Reducing the environmental and social impacts of intensive production

An estimated 80 percent of total livestock sector growth comes from industrial production systems. The environmental problems created by industrial systems do not derive from their large scale or their production intensity, but from their geographical location and concentration. In extreme cases, size may be a problem: sometimes units are so large (a few hundred thousand pigs, for example) that waste disposal will always be a problem, no matter where these units are put.

i. Industrial systems are often located in a way that prevents sustainable waste management. Crop production and livestock activities are being increasingly separated, so that sufficient land to safely dispose of waste is not available nearby. So far, environmental concerns have not often been a factor shaping the regional distribution of livestock production. Easy access to input and product markets, and relative costs of land and labour have so far been the major deter factors. For developing countries, the concentration of industrial units in per urban environments is typical because of infrastructure constraints. In developed countries, there is certainly a move towards rural environments but this often seems to be motivated by an attempt to hide these places away, rather than addressing the fundamental environmental concerns. However, **limitations on livestock densities** (as introduced by the EU) have been a strong factor in arriving at a better balance between livestock and the surrounding ecosystem.

ii. To bring the waste generated into line with capacity of accessible land to absorb, industrial livestock must be located as near as cropland without creating problems of nutrient loading. Location should not be decided by geographically concentrating production units in areas favoured by market access, or feed availability. Suitable policy options include **zoning and licensing, mandatory nutrient management plans, and facilitation of contractual agreements between livestock producers and crop farmers.**

iii. (a) Spatially decentralized livestock sector will create sufficient opportunities and incentives for recycling livestock waste on land. For the medium term future, the preferred option is **the reintegration of crop and livestock activities**. Policies need to drive the decentralization of industrial and intensive livestock away from consumption centers and ports, towards rural areas with nutrient demand. Such policies must comprise regulatory and incentive frameworks. Regulations are needed to deal with heavy metal and drug residue issues at the feed and waste levels, and with other public health aspects such as food-borne pathogens. (b) Spatially decentralized livestock activities can also offer substantial social benefits for rural area with limited alternative employment and growth opportunities.

Incentives need to accompany these regulations, such as **lower taxes** for establishment of commercial production units in nutrient deficit areas, eventually **subsidies** for relocation of large scale enterprises.

iv. Where decentralization cannot be achieved, industrial systems need to have **systems of zero emission** in place, with full waste treatment, including **biogas digestion** and **processing of manure** for use as fertilizer. With current technology these systems will be costly and energy intensive, but biogas, where technology is improving fast, might be an attractive option.

v. To address the environmental impacts associated with production of grain, oil and protein feed; the principles and instruments that have been developed to control environmental issues should be widely applied. They include **integrated pest management** and **soil management** and **fertilization plans**.

vi. To reduce pressure on marine capture fisheries, development of alternatives to the use of fishmeal as feed, for example by using synthetic amino acids is also needed.

vii. The shift to intensive production systems is accompanied by increasing size of operation, driven by economies of scale. Despite an overall growth of the sector, this is only achieved at the cost of pushing numerous small and middle scale producers and other agents out of business. The trend is observed in all countries following the path of intensification: in the EU and North America from as early as the 1960s, and in emerging economies since the 1980s and 1990s. This trend raises social issues of rural emigration and wealth concentration. **Diversification within and outside the agricultural sector** and **social safety nets** are some of the policies developed to address these issues.

(VII) Reorienting extensive grazing towards provision of environmental services

i. Grazing systems need to intensify, in areas where the agro-ecological potential so permits, particularly for dairy production, and nutrient balances are still negative. Excess nutrient loading is a major issue in grass based dairy farming. Reductions in the number of livestock sometimes show quite positive results.

   However, the vast majority of extensive grazing lands are of low productivity. Grazing occupies 26 percent of the terrestrial surface but the contribution of extensive grazing systems to total meat production is very small with less than 9 percent. In areas with little potential for intensification, extensive grazing systems currently provide little in terms of productive output and have high costs in terms of environmental damage (water flows, soil losses, carbon, biodiversity). With increasing demand for environmental services, survival of little productive extensive systems is doubtful, unless they include the provision of environmental services as an important and predominant purpose rather than mere production or subsistence. This can be facilitated **by payments for environmental services or other incentives** to enable livestock producers to make the transition. The value of marginal land is changing and that this change will accelerate. In the past, livestock occupied vast territories because there was no possible alternative use, i.e. the land had no opportunity costs; this made marginally productive activities, such as extensive grazing, profitable.

ii. Water-related services should be grown significantly in future, with local service provision schemes to be widely applied. With suitable incentives, grazers will agree to reduce and more carefully manage grazing pressure, and in certain sensitive areas to abandon grazing activities altogether.

iii. Biodiversity related services (e.g. species and landscape conservation) are complex to manage, because of major methodological issues in the valuation of biodiversity. **Tourism revenues** can be used to help grazers to cohabit with wildlife. Care needs to be taken that such payments for biodiversity extend beyond the attractive" species -mammals and other species interesting to tourists and include biodiversity at large.

iv. Carbon sequestration services, through adjustments in grazing management or abandonment of pastures is difficult, but given the potential of the world's vast grazing lands to sequester large amounts of carbon and to reduce emissions, mechanisms must be developed and deployed to use this potentially cost-effective avenue to address climate change. International agreements will require adaptation so they include **carbon sequestration through Land Use, Land Use Change and Forestry (LULUCF)** and the **expansion of market mechanisms**.

v. As the scarcity of environmental resources increases, so does their value. When functioning market mechanisms can be devised, the demand for environmental services could compete livestock production in more marginal areas where the stocking rate (and hence the gross revenues) would be only one third of the global average.

   This is easier for land under private property and more difficult under common property, particularly where large numbers of impoverished herders or smallholders depend on such land.

vi. Grazing access should be restricted and managed to make livestock production a secondary output, and environmental services primary one. This is already happening in the Alps and other areas in Europe or North America, which are both environmentally vulnerable and precious in environmental terms.

vii. Payment for environmental services should occur at local, national and international level, depending on the nature of the service like water and soil conservation are local goods whereas biodiversity and carbon are global goods.

viii. The large areas degraded as a result of poor management and grazing pressure can be restored if countries realize the immense damage resulting from "laisser faire" and the equally important potential gains from a process guided more consciously by environmental considerations. This transition depends on the relative value of productive potential of a given area, compared with its potential for environmental service provision (Lipper *et al.*, 2006). The lower the agricultural productivity (e.g. poor soil, steep slope) and higher the potential for environmental service provision (e.g. watershed protection), change will be easier.

Degraded grazing areas fit the bill, particularly in humid, hilly or mountainous areas of developing countries, but this change will still require appropriate institutional arrangement for sellers and buyers of environmental services, at the local, national and global scale. Hence, developing such schemes needs to be given priority.

A shift from current "extractive" grazing practices to environmental service oriented grazing ,alternative employment generation and outmigration and **social safety nets** are some of the more obvious policy needs. Establishment of social safety nets for these populations, can be as an international obligation, especially where economic potential for other sectors is limited, and global assets such as biodiversity or climate are concerned. Such measures, **combined with payments for environmental services,** could facilitate the transition from mining of marginal grazing lands to a more sustainable use of these vast areas.

According to a new report published by the United Nations Food and Agriculture Organization, the livestock sector generates more greenhouse gas emissions as measured in CO_2 equivalent-18 percent than transport. It is also a major source of land and water degradation. Says Henning Steinfeld, Chief of FAO's Livestock Information and Policy Branch and senior author of the report: "Livestock are one of the most significant contributors to today's most serious environmental problems. Urgent action is required to remedy the situation." With increased prosperity, people are consuming more meat and dairy products every year. Global meat production is projected to more than double from 229 million tonnes in 1999/2001 to 465 million tonnes in 2050, while milk output is set to climb from 580 to 1043 million tonnes.

Long Shadow

The global livestock sector is growing faster than any other agricultural sub-sector. It provides livelihoods to about 1.3 billion people and contributes about 40 percent to global agricultural output. For many poor farmers in developing countries livestock are also a source of renewable energy for draft and an essential source of organic fertilizer for their crops.

But such rapid growth exacts a steep environmental price, according to the FAO report, *Livestock's Long Shadow-Environmental Issues and Options.* "The environmental costs per unit of livestock production must be cut by one half, just to avoid the level of damage worsening beyond its present level," it warns. When emissions from land use and land use change are included, the livestock sector accounts for 9 percent of CO_2 deriving from human-related activities, but produces a much larger share of even more harmful greenhouse gases. It generates 65 percent of human-related nitrous oxide, which has 296 times the Global Warming Potential (GWP) of CO_2. Most of this comes from manure. And it accounts for respectively 37 percent of all human-induced methane (23 times as warming as CO_2), which is largely produced by the digestive system of ruminants, and 64 percent of ammonia, which contributes significantly to acid rain. Livestock now use 30 percent of the earth's entire land surface, mostly permanent pasture but also including 33 percent of the global arable land used to produce feed for livestock, the report notes. As forests are cleared to create new pastures, it is a major driver of deforestation, especially in Latin America where, for example, some 70 percent of former forests in the Amazon have been turned over to grazing.

Land and Water

At the same time herds cause wide-scale land degradation, with about 20 percent of pastures considered as degraded through overgrazing, compaction and erosion. This figure is even higher in the dry lands where inappropriate policies and inadequate livestock management contribute to advancing desertification. The livestock business is among the most damaging sectors to the earth's increasingly scarce water resources, contributing among other things to water pollution, euthropication and the degeneration of coral reefs. The major polluting agents are animal wastes, antibiotics and hormones, chemicals from tanneries, fertilizers and the pesticides used to spray feed crops. Widespread overgrazing disturbs water cycles, reducing replenishment of above and below ground water resources. Significant amounts of water are withdrawn for the production of feed. Livestock are estimated to be the main inland source of phosphorous and nitrogen contamination of the South China Sea, contributing to biodiversity loss in marine ecosystems. Meat and dairy animals now account for about 20 percent of all terrestrial animal biomass. Livestock's presence in vast tracts of land and its demand for feed crops also contribute to biodiversity loss; 15 out of 24 important ecosystem services are assessed as in decline, with livestock identified as a culprit.

Remedies

The report, which was produced with the support of the multi-institutional Livestock, Environment and Development (LEAD) Initiative, proposes explicitly to consider these environmental costs and suggests a number of ways of remedying the situation, including:

Land degradation-controlling access and removing obstacles to mobility on common pastures. Use of soil conservation methods and silvopastoralism, together with controlled livestock exclusion from sensitive areas; payment schemes for environmental services in livestock-based land use to help, reduce and reverse land degradation.

Atmosphere and climate-increasing the efficiency of livestock production and feed crop agriculture. Improving animal's diets to reduce enteric fermentation and consequent methane emissions, and setting up biogas plant initiatives to recycle manure.

Water-improving the efficiency of irrigation systems. Introducing full-cost pricing for water together with taxes to discourage large-scale livestock concentration close to cities.

Reference

CAST (1999). Animal Agriculture and Global Food Supply Council for Agricultural Science and Technology *(CAST) ISBN* 1-887383-17-4, July 1999, 92 pp.

FAO (2004b). Biodiversity for Food Security. *World Food World Soils Resources Reports* 102, (Available at *www.fao.org/docrep/007/y5738e/y5738e00.htm).*

FAO, (2005b). *State of the world's forests*. FAO, Rome. 153 pp.

FAO, (2006a). *World agriculture: towards 2030/2050, Interim Report.* Rome.

Galloway, J.N., Aber, J.D., Erisman, J.W., Seitzinger, S.P., Howarth, R.W., Cowling, E.B. and Cosby, B.J. (2003). *Bioscience*, 53(4): 341–356.

IPCC (2001b). Climate change 2001: The scientific basis.Contribution of Working Group I to the Third Assessment Report of the Intergovernmental Panel on Climate Change [J.T. Houghton, Y. Ding, D.J. Griggs, M. Noguer, P.J. van der Linden, X. Dai, K. Maskell & C.A. Johnson, eds.]. *Cambridge, UK and New York, Cambridge University Press. 881 pp.*

Lal, R., (2001). *Adv. Agron.*, 76: 1–30.

Lipper, L., Pingali, P.L. and Zurek, M. (2006). *Less-favoured areas: Looking beyond agriculture towards ecosystem services. Agricultural and Development Economics Division (ESA) Working Paper, forthcoming. Rome, FAO.*

Muller, W. & Schneider, B. (1985). *Tieraztliche Umschau 40, 274–280.*

Ni, J-Q., Hendriks, J., Coenegrachts, J. & Vinckier, C. (1999). *Atmospheric Environ.*, 33: 3691–3696.

Pretty, J.N., Brett, C., Gee, D., Hine, R.E., Mason, C.F., Morison, J.I.L., Raven, H., Rayment, M.D. and van der Bijl, G. (2000). *Agricul. Systems*, 65(2): 113–136.

Sainz, R. (2003). Framework for calculating fossil fuel use in livestock systems. Livestock, Environment and Development initiative report. (Available at *ftp://ftp.fao.org/docrep/nonfao/LEAD/X6100E/X6100E00.*

Sundquist, E.T. (1993). Science, 259: 934–941.

UNEP (1991). *Status of desertification and implementation of the United Nations Plan of Action to combat desertification. United Nations Environment Programme, Nairobi. 79 pp.*

US-EPA. (2005a). Mid-Atlantic Integrated Assessment (MAIA), (Available at http://www.epa.gov/maia/html/ about.html).

□□□

Animal Nutrition, 2012
eds. Dr. (Mrs.) Usha R. Mehra et al., pp. 795-810
Satish Serial Publishing House e-mail : info@satishserial.com; website : www.satishserial.com

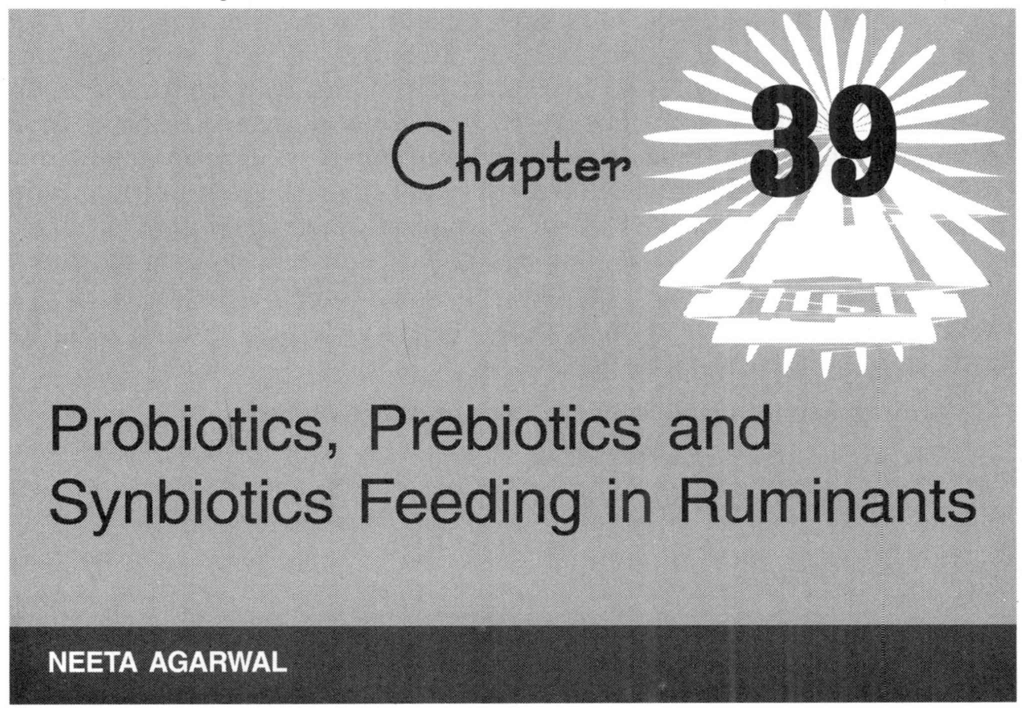

Probiotics, Prebiotics and Synbiotics Feeding in Ruminants

NEETA AGARWAL

The gastrointestinal tract (GIT) of a newly born is completely sterile (Cusnie *et a1.*, 1981) but when it comes in the contact of outer environment, its mother, other animals or feed, the GIT of young one get infested with the microbes which colonize rapidly in the gastrointestinal tract within 24 h. The microbial eco-system of GI tract consists of both harmful and beneficial microbes. This microbial environment inside the gastrointestinal tract dictates the overall performance of the animals by contributing to the nutrient utilization, protecting them from various diseases. Since long back workers are making efforts to optimize the animal production by providing an efficient microbial eco-system in the GIT. Use of antibiotics as feed additive to suppress the harmful microbes was challenged due to their harmful effects. Later the antibiotics were replaced by probiotics which is a highly acceptable strategy and later on use of prebiotics and synbiotics as feed additives to modify microbial eco-system in GI has come up.

Probiotics

The history of probiotics is a century old strategy when Metchnikoff in 1907 realized that the longevity of Bulgarian peasants were related with large consumption of milk fermented with *Lactobacillus acidophilus*.

Since then the microorganism supplemented in the diet (probiotics) has been explained in many ways. The term "Probiotic" (a Greek word meaning "For life") was first of all used by Parker (1974) and he described it as the organisms/substances that contribute to intestinal microbial balance. Later on Fuller (1989) redefined it as "a live microbial feed supplement that beneficially affects the host animal by improving its intestinal microbial balance". Later on US Food and Drug Administration (FDA) in 1989 used the term direct-fed microbes (DFM) instead of probiotic and the manufacturers were directed to write (DFM) on their products (Miles and Bootwalla, 1991). Probiotic feeding has no clinical side effects and therefore is widely accepted Furrie *et al.* (2006). Probiotics acts through;

i) Suppression of viable count of undesirable microbes,

ii) Iimproved immune system and

iii) Alteration of microbial metabolism (Fuller, 1989)

Types of Probiotics

The commonly used probiotic cultures for the feeding of animals belong to *Lactobacillus* sps., *Bacteroides* sps., *Bifidobacterium* sps., *Bacillus* sps., *Pediococcus* sps., *Propionibacterium* sps., *Streptococcus* sps., *Clostridium* sps., *Enterococcus* sps which are mainly effective in pre-ruminant calves, pig and chicken, whereas, in adult ruminants yeast (*Saccharomyces cerevisiae*) and Amaferm (*A.orygae*) are more effective (Fullar *et al.*, 1999). However, the probiotics are highly sps. Specific and host specific therefore it is preferred to use in combination. A large number of microbial cultures have been tested in different species of farm animals, among which lactic acid producing bacteria and yeast are the most commonly used probiotics. (Timmerman *et al.*, 2005).

Probiotics of Rumen Origin

The source of probiotics plays significant role in getting a good response. The cultures isolated from the host itself seem to be very effective as the probiotics fed to the animal is from the same environment and therefore have good chance of survival. But for such approach, first one has to select the microbe as per the requirement. For example in rumen the activity of microcrystalline cellulase (a key enzyme for the degradation of crystalline cellulose) is very low as compared to endoglucanase activity (acts on amorphous cellulose) and it has been reported that by increasing the fibre in the diet, the activity of microcrystalline cellulase decreased (Kamra *et al.*, 2003, Agarwal *et al.*, 2004). To increase the activity of this particular enzyme in the rumen a cellulolytic bacteria rich in microcrystalline cellulase activity was selected from the isolates from the buffalo rumen and grown in the laboratory.

To improve the fibre degradation, the use of isolates from the rumen with high cellulose activity can be used as feed additive (Agarwal *et al.,* 2000).

Rumen fungi are more efficient in fibre degradation because rumen cellulolytic bacteria are protease negative (Agarwal *et al.,* 2000), whereas, rumen fungi have both cellulolytic and proteolytic avtivity (Mountfort and Orpin 1994). Administration of the rumen fungal isolates can be used as probiotics (Paul *et al.,* 2004a,b).

Selection of Probiotic

A microbial culture, to become an efficient feed additive has to operate under heavy environmental stress therefore selection of the cultures should be made on the basis of following characteristics.

- It should fall in the category of generally being recognized as safe (GARS) according to FDA.
- A viable product can be formed at industrial scale.
- It should be stable and viable during long storage and field conditions.
- It should have capability to survive (if not grow) in the GI tract.
- It must produce beneficial effect to host animal.

Selection of a microbe to be used as probiotic is a vital step towards this approach. It is well accepted that live lactic acid bacteria do exert beneficial effects on the health when taken orally but it is also true that not all probiotic bacteria are equal (Dekker *et al.,* 2007). Even different strains of same species might not show similar response. For the screening of microbial cultures for their efficiency to be a potential probiotic, *in vitro* systems are useful and rapid. But for using in vitro system, mode of action of the cultures should be known, like the efficiency of lactic acid bacteria to compete with the coliform bacteria is tested in *in vitro* culture system by using nonpathogenic *E. coli.* The potential of *S. cervisiae* cultures to improve feed degradability can be screened by using in vitro system (Agarwal *et al.,* 2000). Screening of various microbial cultures for their resistance to the GIT environment like, high concentration of volatile fatty acids, bile salts, low pH, various enzymes etc is a prerequisite to select a potent probiotic culture (Agarwal *et al.,* 2000). Mode of feeding is also one of the important aspects to be considered to get good response of probiotic. Feeding of live culture is better than the feeding of lyophilized culture (Scholten *et al.,* 1999), because the dried culture has to rejuvenate in the GIT for biological expression, whereas, live cultures start working as soon as they enter the GIT. A simple method for the production of probiotic has been developed in the author's laboratory (Kamra et al 2002). For the feeding of *L. acidophilus* and *S. cerevisiae,* maize grain or wheat bran (common ingredients of the concentrate mixture) was mixed with equal amount of water and inoculated with 24h old live culture of the probiotic (*S. cerevisiae* or *L. acidophilus*) and incubated at room temperature for overnight. The 24h old fermented feed was ready to feed the animal and a small portion of the fermented feed can be used as inoculum for the fresh feed. The technique was quite simple and can be used in the field conditions.

Probiotic and Production

Chesson and Wallace (1996) reported increases growth rate and milk production (production response) by fungal feed additives in older animals. The effect of feeding yeast culture has been consistently positive on the total bacterial count and cellulolytic bacterial count. *S. cerevisiae* also supports growth of anaerobic fungus. Feeding of *S. cerevisiae* resulted in improvement of digestibility and hence production of the animals (Kamra *et al.*, 2002). Singh *et al.* (1998) grew *S. cerevisae* on agar and the cells were collected by washing with sterilized normal saline and fed to the calves. Significant improvement in feed intake, feed conversion efficiency and growth performance by oral administration of probiotics was reported in chicken, sheep, goat cattle (Casey *et al.*, 2007). Improvement in milk yield, milk fat and protein contents by probiotic feeding has been reported in sheep (Kritas *et al.*, 2006), sow (Alexopoules *et al.*, 2004) and dairy cows (Yu *et al.*, 2007). The effect of fungal cultures on milk yield has been worked out by many workers and it has been found that it is very much affected by the diet and stage of lactation. Williams and Newbold *et al.* (1990) after doing a series of experiments, summarized that the average improvement in milk yield was 4.3% with AO and 5.1 % with yeast. Wallace and Newbold (1993) on the basis of data of other workers gave an average improvement of 7.5% in milk yield. Pasupathy *et al.* (2001) demonstrated higher DM intake with no change in nutrient digestibility and immune status of dogs fed on diet supplemented with *L. acidophilus* strain 15 @ 2x106-107 cfu/animal. The source of probiotic plays significant role in getting good response. The cultures isolated from the host itself seem to be very effective as the probiotic fed to the animal is from the same environment and therefore have good chance of survival. Chevaux and Mazzia-Fabre (2007) conducted trials on 1000 goats and sheep using ruminant specific *S. cerevisiae* I-1077 as a supplement and demonstrated about 9% increase in milk yield (ranging from 4 to 15%) in goat and 7 to 11% in sheep without any change in the milk composition. The increase in milk yield was attributed to the increased feed conversion efficiency of the animals since fibre digestion and nitrogen metabolism were improved significantly.

Probiotic and Health

Chesson and Wallace (1996) explained, lactic acid bacteria in young calves can prevent colonization of pathogens by reducing pH, secreting metabolites and competing for nutrients (health response). Gonzalez *et al.* (1993) considered *L. acidophilus* as a potential biotherapeutic treatment for selected infections. There was no improvement in body weight gain, feed conversion efficiency and occurrence of diarrhoea in preweaning calves (Cruywagen *et al.*, 1995), however the calves fed on *L. acidiphilus* maintained body weight until 2 weeks of age whereas control calves lost body weight during that period. But some overlapping may be there. Bae *et al.* (2003) reported antagonistic effect of *L. helveticus* against Salmonella infection. Increased *Lactobacillus* and reduced Enterococci and Clostridium perfinges count was observed in dogs fed on diet with 0.5g freeze dried *L. animalis* strain 4. In an experiment conducted at Indian Veterinary Research Institute the supplementation of lactic acid bacteria (a mixture of *Lactobacillus acidophilus, L. jugarti* and *L. casei*) significantly reduced incidence of diarrhoea in comparison to control animals. In the first 4 weeks of age the incidence of diarrhea was reduced to 50% and between 5-8 weeks of age it was reduced to less than 15% of the control animals (Ramaswami *et al.*, 2005). Chevaux and Mazzia-Fabre (2007) reported increased faecal Lactobacilli and decreased *E. coli* count by feeding ruminant specific *S. cerevisiae* I-1077 in goat and sheep. In majority of studies the probiotics used are either single strain or combination of two strains but Rolfe (2000) suggested that multiple probiotic strains may be more useful than a single strain because they can proliferate more lactic acid bacteria than single strain. Use of lactate utilizers like *Megasphaera elsdenii* and Propioni-bacterium as probiotic can prevent lactate accumulation in the rumen during transition of low to high concentration diets (Kung and Hession, 1995) thus can be beneficial for the animals suffering from acidosis. Propionibacterium is also helpful in supplying glucose through propionate production. According to Huntington (2000) about 67% glucose comes from propionate in growing ruminants and lactating cows.

Increased in the number of lymphocytes and lymphoid cells was reported in the piglets fed *L. acidophilus* as feed additive (Babinska *et al.*, 2005). The precise mechanisms of immune modulation by probiotics are not very clear but they are known to influence both non-specific and specific immune responses in animal models and in humans (Guarner and Malagelada, 2003).

Anticholesterol activity of probiotics has also been observed in many studies. Lowered cholesterol levels by feeding of various strains of lactobacilli were demonstrated by Umeki *et al.* (2004). The different proposed mechanisms for lowering of cholesterol are, binding of bacteria with cholesterol with increased faecal excretion, assimilation of cholesterol molecule, and deconjugation of bile acids with increased rate of bile acid excretion (Taylor and Williams, 1998).

Probiotic and Methane

Enteric methane produced by the ruminants as a result of fermentation of feed in the rumen is of great concern due to its high global warming potential contributing significantly to the environmental pollution. Production of methane in ruminants is also responsible for 2-12% loss of dietary energy. It is a big challenge for the nutritionist and rumen microbiologist to combat this problem. Few *in vivo* trials have been conducted by using yeast as feed supplement to reduce methane production but the results are inconsistent. Mwenya *et al.* (2004) demonstrated 10% decrease in methane production per day by including 0.4% yeast extract based on *Trichosporon sericeum* in a basal hay and 30% concentrate diet in sheep but this inhibition was attributed to the decrease in feed intake. There was non significant 3% reduction in methane production in sheep when expressed in terms of proportion of dry matter intake. Inconsistency in the response of yeast culture was also demonstrated by Newbold and Rade (2006) using Rumen Simulating fermentors to screen the strains of *S. cerevisiae* as probiotic to inhibit methane production. The reduction in methane production ranged from 0 to 58% and therefore they attributed this variation to the strain of *S. cerevisiae*. The probable ways of yeast to inhibit methane production are by (1) increasing butyrate or propionate production (Lila *et al.*, 2004); (2) by reducing protozoa numbers thus affecting adversely the methanogens associated with the protozoa (Newbold *et al.*, 1998); (3) by stimulating growth of acetogens which utilize hydrogen thus diverting hydrogen towards acetate production (Chaucheyras *et al.*, 1995); and (4) by improving animal productivity (Bruno *et al.*, 2005), but these channels have to be confirmed. A lactate utilizer Propioni bacterium produces propionate, therefore, its feeding as probiotic will reduce acetate to propionate ratio which will lead to decreased methane production. Propioni bacterium has multi-facet activities, helping in preventing acidosis by utilizing lactate, supplying glucose through propionate and reducing methanogenesis by reducing acetate to propionate ratio thus reducing dietary energy loss in the form of methane. But the results are not fully supporting this hypothesis as Ghorbani *et al.* (2002) reported no effect on ruminal concentrations of L-lactate, total VFA, propionate, isobutyrate, and isovalerate, or the ratio of acetate to propionate by feeding of Propionibacterium or Propionibacterium and *E. faecium* in cattle but Kim *et al.* (2000) observed increased propionate production in the rumen of steer by feeding of *P. acidipropionici*. The data indicate that use of propionibacterium can be explored as a probiotic for the ruminants.

Prebiotics

The history of prebiotics is not as old as probiotics, as it is about five decades back when lactulose was used as food supplement for infants (MacGillivray *et al.*, 1959), but in livestock it is at its infantry stage. Roberfroid (2000) defined prebiotics as "nondigestible food ingredients that beneficially affect the host by selectively stimulating the growth and/or activity of one or a limited number of bacteria (probiotics) in the gastrointestinal tract and thereby exert a health-promoting effect". Gibson *et al.* (2004) updated the definition of prebiotic as "a selectively fermented ingredient that allows specific changes both in the composition and/or activity in the gastrointestinal microflora that confers benefits upon host wellbeing and health". One should not confuse with the fibre because though both are typically non-digestible carbohydrates, and both are typically fermented by gut bacteria. However, a prebiotic differs from fibre in that the former is selectively associated with only beneficial members of the gut microbial community. Based on functional characteristics, prebiotics are closely linked with the probiotic concept than the fibre one. Some manufacturers refer prebiotics as fibre, because the latter is more familiar to consumers. A prebiotic is a non digestible food ingredient and also heat resistant so that is not degraded during cooking process. It reaches the intestine without being affected by digestion process and stimulate the growth of bio-cultures beneficial to the animal. The increase in the activity of healthy bacteria like *bifidobacteria, lactobacilli* etc. in the gut and increase resistance to invading pathogensis are called prebiotic effect. An ideal prebiotic is that which should; 1. Neither hydrolyzed nor absorbed in the upper part of gastrointestinal tract, 2. Function as a substrate for one or limited number of potentially beneficial bacteria and 3. Have capability to make the microbial eco-system healthier, 4. Beneficially modulate host defense system 5. Result in a beneficial effect on health of the host (Guarner, 2006). The prebiotics which have scientifically proven evidences are inulin, oligofructose, lactulose, galactooligosaccharides and synthetic fructooligosaccharides (FOS). The chemical structure of these oligosaccharides prevents them from digestion. Inulin type fructans are also called as colonic bifid because they are neither digested nor absorbed in the upper part of gastrointestinal tract due to the ß-configuration of the anomeric C-2 in their fructose and thus reach as such in the lower part of the gut and act as substrate for the endogenous bacteria thus providing the host nutrients directly in the form of energy and metabolic products. The resistant starches, sugar alcohols and difructose anhydride are also some known prebiotics. Some prebiotics which are still under investigations are xylooligosaccharides, sugar alcohols (lactitol, sorbitol and maltito), palatinose, soyoligosaccharides, pecticoligosaccharides, glucooligosaccharides, isomaltooliosaccharides and gentiooligosaccharides. The good sources of prebiotics are leeks, artichokes, garlic, onions, wheat, wheat products, oat, soybean, chicory, asparagus, bananas and among these sources chicory roots are the richest source of inulin. The inulin present in garlic is also highly active. The inulinase activity of *Streptococcus spp*. was tested using different sources of inulin including a pure product but highest activity was found with garlic powder as a source of inulin (Sharma *et al*., 2006). Prebiotics being low in calories is well suited for diabetic also Isomalt, which work as a prebiotic is a commonly used sugar replacer. In the four-week study on Isomalt, the ingredient was found to stimulate bifidobacteria in a group of 20 people. The finished products like bread, chocolate, yogurt also contain prebiotics as one of the ingredient. In addition, the prebiotics like oligofructose, rich in reducing sugars are involved in Maillard reaction resulting in pleasant aroma which can increase the palatability of the product. The prebiotics (inulin and oligofructose) used for animal nutrition is mainly derived from the chicory (*Cichorium intybus*) roots. Chicory inulin-type fructans contain >70% inulin (comprised of chains of both low and high degree of polymerization), sugars, organic acids, proteins, and minerals.

Competitive expulsion of harmful bacteria from the GI tract by using the sugars specifically utilized by only useful bacteria is an another approach of prebiotic. Vaux *et al.* (2002) evaluated few sugars as prebiotics. E. coli are present in good number in rumen as well as in intestine and are responsible for food borne diseases and E. coli 0157:H7 is the predominant strain. It was found that E. coli ferment sorbitol very slowly whereas; good number of sorbitol fermenting bacteria are there in the rumen. It was demonstrated that the inclusion of sorbitol in the medium containing rumen liquour inoculated with E. coli 0157:H7, the E. coli washed out within 72 hr, but with the sterile rumen liquour broth some growth of sorbitol fermenting mutants appeared. The authors obtained similar results with L-arabinose, trehalose and rhamnose also. It was suggested that the use of combination of such competitive sugars can be a better approach for competitive expulsion of pathogens from the rumen.

Effect of Prebiotic on Animal Health

As discussed above the prebiotics stimulates the growth of the useful bacteria of gut, therefore the effects showed by probiotic feeding are also presented by prebiotics feeding. Some of the commonly reported effects of prebiotics are like improvement in digestion, immune status, mineral absorption and overall health of the animal. The stimulatory effect of prebiotic on the microbes having health promoting effects like biofidobacteria and lactobacilli has been documented in several studies (Gibson and Roberfroid, 1995). Male Wistar rats (253±11 g BW) were fed on diet supplemented with galactooligosaccharides (GOS), long-chain fructooligosaccharides (lcFOS), and acidified oligosaccharides (AOS) for three weeks resulted in increased in lactobacilli and bifidobacteria in colon content and faeces as compared to control (Meer *et al.*, 2008). The Holstein heifer calves were fed on diet supplemented with either antibiotic (0.220g oxytetracycline/kg and 0.441g neomycin base/kg) or prebiotic supplement (PB; 20 g/day Prebio Support™, Meiji Feed Co., Ltd. Tokyo, Japan) which contain fermentation products of *Lactobacillus gasseri* and *Propionibacterium freudenreichi* ET-3 from day 2 to 8 week of age. The animal health was judged by assigning scour (diarrhea), respiratory and general appearance score, lymphocyte count IgA and microbial population analysis. There was no difference in the health status of the animals of all the three groups, except that the faecal lactobacilli count was higher in prebiotic fed group (Heinrichs *et al.*, 2009). The authors were of the opinion that since the animals were in very good health status therefore there was no scope of further improvement. The impact of prebiotic feeding can be better observed in the stressed animals. Improvement in growth rate and feed conversion efficiency, with better consistency of faeces in inulin and oligofructose fed preruminant calves as compared to control was demonstrated by Van Leeuwen and Verdonk (2004). The authors were of the opinion that the dietary inulin is effective only in preruminant calves because it is completely fermented by the rumen microbial eco-system.

Improvement in body weight gain by feeding of prebiotics in calves was reported by Heinnichs *et al.* (2003) and Denovan *et al.* (2002). Lower faecal egg count and improved liveweight gain in chicory grazed ewes and their lambs as compared to grass grazed ewes and was reported by Athanasiadou *et al.* (2007). Improvement in immune status of pigs by feeding Brewers yeast containing mannan oligosaccharides (White *et al.*, 2002) and in mice by feeding fructo-oligosaccharides (Hosono *et al.*, 2003) was observed. Comparison among the chicory (CH), mannan-oligosaccharides (MO) and chicory + mannan-oligosaccharides (CM) fed groups of seniour dogs (pointers 8-11 years old and beagles 9-11 years old) revealed increased in the population size of faecal bifidobacteria in all the three groups but lowering of faecal *E. coli* was reported only in MO fed group as compared to control (Grieshop *et al.*, 2004). Nielsen et al (2009) demonstrated that the organic lambs allowed to graze chicory plot (3% or 6% of total grazing area) disliked chicory and because of less chicory intake there was no beneficial effect.

The indirect role of Inulin-type fructans in improving immune system, especially the intestinal immune functions by targeting gut associated lymphoid tissue has been demonstrated by Guarner (2005). The four groups of dogs fed on diet supplemented with 1% chicory (CH), 1% mannon-oligosaccharides (MO), 1% CH + 1% MO (CM) and no supplementation, respectively, resulted in increased neutrophil concentration in CH and CM fed groups and decreased peripheral lymphocytes concentration in CH and MOS fed groups (Grieshop *et al.*, 2004).

Prebiotic: Bile Salts Metabolism

Bile salts play a critical role in the absorption of dietary lipids and maintaining the cholesterol homeostasis in the body. The effect of prebiotic feeding has also been investigated by many workers but the response was variable. Like supplementation of diet with oligofructose resulted in decrease in plasma cholesterol in rats (Fiordaliso *et al.*, 1995), whereas, in lean rats there was no difference (kok *et al.*, 1996). Meer *et al.*, (2003) reported increased serum lathosterol concentration in rats fed on prebiotic supplemented diet. Lathosterol is an intermediate of cholesterol synthesis, therefore increase in cholesterol level can be postulated. The authors have not estimated cholesterol.

Prebiotic and Mineral Absorption

The role of prebiotics in improvement of mineral absorption consequently improvement in bone mineral contents resulting in better bone structure has been demonstrated in many studies. The probable mode of actions are, availability of more substrate for the bacteria resulting in higher production of short chain fatty acids which leads to increased solubility of minerals; due to more of fermentative products the proliferation of enterocytes is stimulated thus providing more surface area for the absorption of minerals, increased expression of calcium binding proteins; gut health is improved due to stabilization of gut microflora; due to the proliferation of bacteria there is more release of growth factors as few bacterial species secrete plyamines (Scholz-Ahrens *et al.*, 2007). The work conducted on calcium supplementation revealed that calcium supplementation alone is not much beneficial because increased dietary calcium slower down the absorption of magnesium and other minerals which are important components of bone structure but when calcium is supplemented with prebiotic, the absorption of calcium and other minerals is also stimulated (Scholz-Ahrens *et al.*, 2002; Scholz-Ahrens and Schrezenmeir, 2002). Effect of prebiotic on mineral absorption also depends on the type of prebiotic, as observed by Afsana *et al.* (2003) who reported better response with difructose as compared to fructooligosaccharides in iron deficiency. Again it has been demonstrated that use of combination of prebiotics is more effective as compared to single. Younes *et al.* (2001) demonstrated increased calcium and magnesium absorption with inulin + resistant starch or inulin + fructooligosaccharides of high degree of polymerization as compared to either of the prebiotics alone.

Synbiotics

A synbiotic is the product where probiotics is combined with prebiotics and prebiotic selectively favours the probiotic. Synbiotic is the most effective intestinal-health products where probiotic and prebiotic have synergistic effect. Technically the product containing prebiotic which supports the growth of probiotic should fall in this categaory e.g. a combination of *Bifidobacterium spp.* (probiotic) and frucooligosccharides (prebiotic) where prebiotic favours the growth of probiotic. But the product containing prebiotic and *Lactobacillus* spp. is also being justified to be termed as synbiotic since the former stimulate the growth of *Bifidobacterium* in the GI tract on one hand and *Lactobacillus* affects microbial community favourably on the other hand. Since both probiotics and prebiotics induced beneficiary effects in human and animals by modulating gastrointestinal microbial eco-system, there combination add to this beneficiary effects of both probiotics and prebiotics.

Synbiotics combine probiotics and prebiotics to improve the survival rate, proliferation of beneficial bacteria in the gastrointestinal tract and ensure that they reach the colon in adequate numbers. Probiotics alone are vulnerable to the gastrointestinal tract environment like pH, bile salts, enzymes etc. and they also have to compete with resident bacteria in the gastrointestinal tract. However, with a prebiotic as a food substrate, the probiotic cells have better chance of surviving and proliferating as the competition for food with the native microbes is less. The selection of probiotic and prebiotic is an important step to get positive expression of the additive. Bielecka *et al.* (2002), screened 30 strains of *Bifidobacterium spp.* (probiotic) *in vitro* for their efficiency to utilize FOS and low polymerized inulin (prebiotic). Out of 30 only 18 were effective and they selected best 3 strains along with FOS for *in vivo* study in rats. Though bifidogenic effect was there in probiotic, prebiotic and synbiotic, but coliform bacteria was significantly low only in FOS fed group, however there was no change in the gut microbial community. Shim *et al.* (2005) reported decreased population of E. coli and increased population of *Lactobacilli* in piglets fed synbiotic.

Importance of nutritional management has also been emphasized in the medical science. Synbiotic therapy has shown promising results in preventing infectious complications. Combinations of *Lactobacillus sps., Biofidobacterium spp.* as probiotics and galactooligosccharides and oat as prebiotics have been successfully used as synbiotic therapy in the postoperative patients to prevent infection (Nomoto *et al.*, 2008). Administration of inulin with the probiotic *Bifidobacterium longum* to the rats suffering from colon carcinogenesis had additional inhibitory effect as compared to administration of inulin or *B. longum* separately (Rowland *et al.*, 1998). Administration of synbiotic is also helpful in preventing number of serious diseases like: food allergies, ulcerous colitis, constipation, diarrhoea, cancers, gastrointestinal infections due to its suppressive effect on putrefactive process in the stomach and intestines. Since both probiotics and prebiotics are effective in improving immune status of the animals, therefore, the combination of the two in symbiotic has additional benefit in improving immune status but the response of synbiotic depend on the specific combination of prebiotic and strain of probiotic. Roller *et al.* (2004) used probiotic (*L. rhamnosus* GG and *B. lactis* Bb 12), prebiotic (inulin enriched with oligofructose), and symbiotic (combination of probiotic and prebiotic) in rats to compare the immune status of the three groups and found best response of rats to symbiotic. *In vitro* study indicated anti-cholesterol activity of synbiotic comprising of *Lactobacillus casei* strain and the prebiotics FOS and maltodextrin (Liong and Shah, 2005).

Feeding of synbiotic containing inulin from chicory root, *L. acodophilus, L. bulgaricus, B. bifidum, B. longum* and *S. thermophilus* enhanced nutrient utilization by improving the activities of digestive enzymes in rats (Yang *et al.,* 2005). Favourable changes in rumen fermentation were observed in Holstein cows fed on a symbiotic (probioic yeast with prebiotic galacto-oligosaccharides) (Mwenya *et al.,* 2005). Shim *et al.* (2005) reported improved digestibility of DM, CP, crude ash and absorption of Ca and P and also significantly increased pre-weaning body weight gain of the piglets fed on diet supplemented with synbiotic as compared to control.

In general probiotics, prebiotics and synbiotics are effective in the stressed animals only. The stress might be nutritional, like deficiency or excess of nutrients; environmental, like thermal, moisture, sanitary conditions etc; emotional; like weaning, transport, change in pen mates etc; diseases both infectious and metabolic; reproductive and productive like parturition, milk production etc. When an animal is in stress, its microbial eco-system of gastrointestinal tract get disturbed and at this stage to re-establish the normal microflora, these feed additives are very effective. From the above discussion it is evident that the all the three groups of feed additives (probiotics, prebiotics and synbiotics) are beneficial for human and animals. But for the expression of these feed additives in the biological system, one should be conscious about the selection of additive for a specific breed. Due to the structural and functional complexity of the microbial eco-system of GI tract, use of combination of strains and other substances (prebiotics) has always being preferred.

Future Research Needs

Though lot of work has been done to extract the maximum benefit from these feed additives but still there is scope of research in this field. Further research must in the following directions.

1. Isolation and characterization of more species specific bacterial strains which can be used as feed additive to have beneficial effect.
2. Identification of more substances from the cheap sources as cost effective prebiotic.
3. Development of disease specific products.
4. There is a big gap in the knowledge of GIT microbial eco-system and to formulate an effective feed additive this gap has to be filled. Therefore there is a strong need to work on structural and functional analysis of the GIT microbial communities of different breeds by using advanced molecular techniques like metagenomics, DNA microarray, DGGE etc.

References

Afsana, K., Shiga, K., Ishizuka S. and Hara H. (2003). Nutr., 133: 355360.

Agarwal, N., Saxena, J., Saha, S., Chaudhary, L.C. and Kamra, D.N. (2004). *Bubalus bubalis*, III, 81-90.

Agarwal, N., Kamra, D.N., Chaudhary, L.C., Agarwal, I., Sahoo, A. and Pathak, N.N. (2002). *Letters in Applied Microbiology*, 34 : 329-336.

Agarwal, N., Agarwal, I., Kamra, D.N. and Chaudhary, L.C. (2000). *J. Appl. Anim. Res.*, 18: 73-80.

Agarwal, N., Kamra, D. N., Chaudhary, L.C., Sahoo, A. and Pathak, N.N. (2000). *Letter Appl. Microbiol.*, 31: 270-273.

Alexopoulos, C., Georgoulakis, I.E., Tzivara, A., Kritas, S.K., Siochu, A. and S.C. Kyriakis, (2004). *J. Anim. Physiol. Anim. Nutr.* 88, 381-392.

Athanasiadou, S., Gray, D., Younie, D., Tzamaloukas, O., Jackson, F. and Kyriazakis, I. (2007). *Parasitology*, 134: 299-307.

Babinska, I., Rotkiewicz, T. and Otrocka-Domagala, I.P. (2005). *Journal of Veterinary Science*, 8: 29-35.

Bae, J. S., Jung-Ryul Byun, and Yung-Ho, Yoon. (2003). *Asian-Aust. J. Anim. Sci.*, 16: 430-434.

Biagi, G., Cipollini, I., Pompei, A., Zaghini, G. and Matteuzzi, D. (2007). *Veterinary Microbiology*, 124:160-165.

Bielecka, Maria, Biedrzycka, Elzbieta, and Majkowska, Anna. (2002). *Food Research International*, 35: 125131

Cabrera, E.J.I., mendoza, M.G.D., Aranda, I.E., Gareia-Bojalil, C., Bareena, G.R. and Ramos, J.J.A. (2000). *Anim. Feed Sci. Technol.*, 83 : 49-55.

Casey, P.G., Gardiner, G.E., Casey, G., Bradshaw, B., Lawlor, P.G., Lynch, P.B., Leonard, F.C., Stanton, C., Ross, R.P., Fitzgerald, G.F. and Hill, C. (2007). *Applied Environ. Microb.*, 73: 1858-1863.

Chaucheyras, F., Fonty, G., Bertin, G. and Gouet, G. (1995). *Curro. Microbiol.*, 31: 201-205.

Chesson, A. and Wallace, J. (1996). Part 3: microbial feed additives for ruminants. *Feed Compounder*, 16: 14-17.

Chevaux, Eric and Mazzia-Fabre, Marina. (2007). *Feed Mix*, 17.

Chou, Lan-Szu, and Weimer, Bart. (1998). *J. Dairy Sci.*, 82: 23-31.

Cruywagen, C.W., Jordaan, Ina, and Venter, L. (1996). *J. Dairy Sci.*, 79: 483-486.

Dekker, J., Collett, M., Prasad, J. and Gopal, P. (2007). *Forum of Nutrition*, 60: 196-208.

Donovan, D.C., Franklin, S.T., Chase, C.C.L.,Hippen,A.R., (2002). *J. Dairy Sci.*, 85:947-950.

Fiordaliso, M., Kok, N., Desager, J.P., Goethals, F., Deboyser, D., Roberfroid, M., Delzenne, N. (1995). *Lipids*, 30: 163-167.

Fuller, R. (1989). *J. App. Bacteriol.*, 66: 365-378.

Furrie, E., Senok, A.C., Frank, D.N. and Sullivan, K.E. (2006). *Clinical Immunology*, 121: 19-22.

Ghorbani, G.R., Morgavi, D.P., Beauchemin, K.A. and Leedle, J.A.Z. (2002). *J. Anim. Sci.*, 80:1977-1986.

Gibson, G.R., Prober, H.M., Rastall, R., Van loo, J.A.E. and Roberfroid, M.B. (2004). *Nutrition Research Reviews*, 17: 259-275.

Gonzalez, S.N., Apella, M.C., Romero, C., Nader de Macias, M.E. and Oliver, G. (1993). *J. Food Protection*, 56: 773-776.

Grieshop, C.M., Flickinger, E.A., Bruce, K.J., Patil, A.R., Czarnecki-Maulden, G.L., and Fahey G.C. Jr. (2004). *Arch. Anim. Nutr.*, 58:483-493.

Guarner, F. (2005). *Br. J. Nutr.*, 93(suppl. 1): S61-S65.

Guarner, F. (2006). *Digestion*, 73 (Suppl. 1): 5-12.

Guarner, F. and Malagelada, J.R. 2003. *Digestion*, 73: (suppl. 1): 5-12.

Heinrichs, A.J., Jones, C.M., Elizondo-Salazar, J.A. and Terrill, S.J. (2009). *Livestock Science*, 125: 149-151.

Heinrichs, A.J., Jones, C.M., Heinrichs, B.S. (2003). *J. Dairy Sci.* 86: 4064-4069.

Hosono, A., Ozawa, A., Kato, R., Ohnishi, Y.,Nakanishi, Y., Kimura, T., Nakamura, R., (2003). *Biosci. Biotechnol. Biochem.* 64: 758-764.

Huntington, G. B. (2000). *Feedstuffs*, 1213:23.

Kamra, D.N., Chaudhary, L.C., Agarwal, N., Singh, R. and Pathak, N.N. (2002). *Indian J. Anim. Sci.*, 72: 472-475.

Kamra, D.N., Saha, S., Bhatt, N., Chaudhary, L.C., and Agarwal, N. (2003). *Asian Aust. J. Anim. Sci.*, 16 : 374-379.

Kim, S.W., Standorf, D.G., Roman-Rosario, H., Yokoyama, M.T. and Rust, S.R. (2000). *J. Anim. Sci.*, 78 (Suppl. 1): 292.

Kok, N., Roberfroid, M. and Delzenne, N. (1996). *Metabolism*, 45: 1547-1550.

Kritas, S.K., Govaris, A., Christodoulopouls G. and Burriel, A.R. (2006) *J. Vet. Med. Ser.*, 53: 170-173.

Kung, Jr., L., and Hession, A.O. (1995). *J. Anim. Sci.*, 73:250-256.

Liong, M.T. and Shah, N.P. (2005). *Applied and Environmental Microbiology*, 71: 1745-1753.

MacGillivray, P.C., Finlay, H.V.L. and Binns, T.B. (1959). *Scott. Med. J.*, 4:18-29.

McGinn, S.M., Beauchemin, K.A., Coates, T. and , Colombatto, D. (2004). *J. Anim. Sci.*, 82: 3346-3356.

Meer, H. van, Boehm, G., Stellaard, F., Vriesema, A., Knol, J., Havinga, R. Pieter, J.S. and Henkjan, J.V. (2008). *J. Physiol. Gastrointest. Liver Physiol.*, 294: G540-G547.

Metchnikoff E. (1907). The prolongation of life. Optimistic studie. Butterworth-Heinemann. London.

Miles, R.D., and Bootwalla, S.M. (1991). Direct-fed microbials in avian. Page 117 in Direct-Fed Microbials in Animal Production: A Review of Literature. Nat. Feed Ingred. Assoc., West Des Moines, IA.

Mounfort, D.O. and Orpin, C.G. (1994). Anaerobic Fungi. Marcel Dekker, Inc., New York, USA.

Mwenya, B., Santosa, S.C., Gamo, Y., Kobayashi, T., Takahashi, J. (2004). *Anim Feed Sci. Technol.*, 115: 313-326.

Nielsen, B.K., Thamsborg, S.M., Hansen, H., Ranvig, H. and Høgh-Jensen, H. (2009). *Livestock Science*, 125: 66-73.

Nomoto, Koji. (2008). *Indian J. Exp. Biol.*, 46: 567-561.

Parker, R.B. (1974). Animal Nutrition and Health (Dec.): 4-8.

Pasupathy, K., Sahoo A. and Pathak N.N. (2001). *Archives of Animal Nutrition*, 3: 243-253.

Paul, S.S., Kamra, D.N., Sastry, V.R.B., Sahu, N.P. and Agarwal, N. (2004a). *Anim. Feed Sci. Technol.*, 115 (1-2) : 143-157.

Paul, S.S., Kamra, D.N., Sastry, V.R.B., Sahu, N.P. and Agarwal, N. (2004b). *Nutr. Repro. Develop.*, 44: 313-319

Ramaswami, N., Chaudhary, L.C., Agarwal, N. and Kamra, D.N. (2005). *Asian Aust. J. Anim. Sci.* 18: 1110-1115.

Rawland, I.R., Rumney C.J., Coutts J.T. and Lievense L.C. (1998). *Carcinogenesis*, 19: 281-285.

Roberfroid, M.B. (2000). Prebiotics and probiotics: are they functional foods? *Am. J. Clin. Nutr.*, 71: 6 Suppl:1682S7S.

Rolfe, R.D., (2000). *J. Nutr.*, 130: 396S-402S.

Roller, M., Rechkemmer, G. and Watzl, B. (2004). *J. Nutr.*, 134: 153-156.

Sahu, N.P., Kamra, D.N. and Paul, S.S. (2004). *Asian Aust. J. Anim. Sci.*, 17(2): 199-202.

Scholten, R.H.J., van der Peet-Schwering, C.M.C., Verstegen, M.W.A., den-Hartog, L.A., Schrama, J.W. and Vesseur, P.C. (1999). *Anim. Feed Sci. Technol.* 82, 1-19.

Scholz-Ahrens, K.E., Ade, P., Marten, B., Weber, P., Timm, W., Ail, Y., Glüer, Claus-C. and Schrezenmeir, J. (2007). *J. Nutr.,* 137: 838S-846S.

Scholz-Ahrens, K.E, Açil, Y, and Schrezenmeir, J. (2002). *Br. J. Nutr.,* 88: 365-378.

Scholz-Ahrens, K.E. and Schrezenmeir, J. (2002). *Br. J. Nutr.,* 87: Suppl 2:S17986.

Shim, S.B. (2005). Effects of prebiotics, probiotics and synbiotics in the diet of young pigs. PhD. Thesis, Animal Nutrition Group, Wageningen institute of Animal Sciences, Wageningen University and Research Centre, Wageningen, The Netherlands.

Singh, R., Chaudhary L.C., Kamra D.N. and Pathak N.N. (1998). *Asian-Aus. J. Anim. Sci.* 11: 268-271.

Taylor, G.R.J. and Williams, C.M. (1998). *Br. J. Nutr.,* 80: S225-S230.

Timmerman, H.M., Mulder, L:, Everts, H., van Espen, D.C. van der Wal, E., Klaassen, G. Rouwers, S.M.G., Hartemink, R., Rombouts, F.M. and Beynen, A.C. (2005). *J. Dairy Sci.,* 88: 2154-2165.

Van Leeuwen, P. and, Verdonk, J.M.A.J. (2004). The gastro-intestinal degradation of inulin preparations and their effects on production performance and gut microflora in calves. Animal Sciences Group Wagingen UR, Lelystad, Netherlands, Project nr 825.20552.02, Report No: 04/100287:1-31.

Vaux, Albane de, Morrison, Mark, and Hutkins Robert, W. (2002). *Appl. and Environ. Microbiol.,* p. 519-524.

Wallace, R.J. and Newbold, C.J. (1993). Rumen fermentation and its manipulation: The development of yeast cultures as feed additives. In Biotechnology in the feed Industry (T.P. Lyons, ed.), Alltech Technical Publications, Nicholasville, Kentucky, pp. 173-192.

White, L.A., Newman, M.C., Cromwell, G.L. and Lindemann, M.D. (2002). *J. Anim. Sci.,* 80: 2619-2628.

Williams, P.E.V., and C.J. Newbold, (1990). Rumen probiosis: The effect of novel microorganisms on rumen fermentation and ruminant productivity. P. 211 In: In Recent Advances in Animal Nutrition. W. Haresign and D.J.A. Pole (eds.). Butterworths, London, England.

Yang, S.C., Chen, J.Y., Shang, H.F., Cheng, T.Y., Tsou, S.C. and Chen, J.R. (2005). *World J. Gastroenterology,* 11: 7413-7417.

Younes, H., Coudray, C., Bellanger, J., Demigne, C., Rayssiguier, Y., and Remesy, C. (2001). *Br. J. Nutr.,* 86: 479-485.

Yu, P., Huber, J.T., Theurer, C.B., Chen, K.H., Nussio, L.G. and Wu, Z. (1997). *J. Dairy Sci.,* 80: 3293-3297.

□□□

About the Editor

Dr. (Mrs.) Usha R. Mehra (Chief Editor), Born on June 18, 1944, at Lucknow U.P. Dr. (Mrs.) Usha R. Mehra did her post-graduation from Bareilly college, Bareilly in 1964 and Doctorate in Animal Nutrition from Indian Veterinary Research Institute, Izatnagar in 1968. She started her research career in 1968 from Indian Veterinary Research Institute, Izatnagar and served the institute for four decades in various capacities till her superannuation as Head and Professor Cum Director, Centre of Advanced Studies in Animal Nutrition. Dr. U.K. Mehra is a distinguished Animal Nutritionist and contributed more specifically in the area of urea molasses mineral block, liquid diet, bypass protein sources, microbial growth and VFA production. She has developed several technologies and patent on Cold process technology for the preparation of Urea Molasses Mineral Block (UMMB) has already been granted and applied for registration of Threshing cum Treatment Machine. She supervised several externally funded research schemes, name few SIDA/IAEA - UNDP scheme, NDDB-IVRI project, CGP NATP project, and Cass fund schemes etc. She was bestowed with several prestigious awards like Hari Om Ashram Trust Award (Twice), Punjab Rao Deshmukh Best Woman Agricultural Scientist Award, Rafi Ahmed Kidwai Award, and Woman Empowerment and Livelihood Award. She has published 180 research papers to her credit in National and International Journals of high repute. She has also contributed many book chapters on various aspects of animal nutrition. She was deputed abroad by Govt. of India to serve as an expert in Nigeria. She was also awarded SIDA/IAEA fellowship for advanced studies in biochemical techniques at Hannah Research Institute Scotland U.K. She visited several countries like Scotland, Switzerland, United Kingdom, United States of America, Germany, Norway, Denmark, Singapore, Malaysia, Mauritius and Mexico *etc*. In recognition of her scientific work she was elected fellow of National Academy of Agricultural Sciences and Animal Nutrition Association. She is a life member of several important Academic bodies, Research Panels, Research Advisory committees and Board of Management. She provided dynamic leadership to ANA as its President from 2003 to 2006.

Dr. Putan Singh (Editor), Born on October 31. 1960 at Village-Bhuria, Post-Kachura, District-Sitapur, U.P. Dr. Putan Singh did his B.Sc. (Ag & AH) in 1984 from Chandra Shekhar Azad University of Agriculture and Technology, Kanpur and M. Sc. and Doctorate in Animal Nutrition from Indian Veterinary Research Institute (IVRI), Izatnagar, Bareilly in 1987 and 1991, respectively. He got IVRI Junior and Senior Research Fellowships for his Master and Doctorate Research Work. He started his research career in ARS in June 11, 1991 as Scientist from NAARM, Hyderabad & subsequently after foundation course and subject matter training he joined IVRI, Izatnagar & Mukteshwar, Kumaon and he became Scientist (Sr. Scale) in 1995. Thereafter, he moved to IVRI, Izatnagar in 1995 and became

Senior Scientist and Principal Scientist in 2000 and 2008, respectively. Dr. Singh has been given an additional responsibility of Co-ordinator, Farm & Estate Section, IVRI, Izatnagar in October, 2009. Dr. Singh also received FAO/IAEA Joint sponsorship with UPM/MARDI for Training Workshop at Malaysia in 2002. He has the honour of receiving appreciation award from ISEE, New Delhi in 2009 and honour of award from Director *cum* Vice-Chancellor, IVRI, Izatnagar in 2010. He became the member of Extension Council of the Institute in 2010. Since 1992, he worked as Co-PI and PI in several institutes and externally funded research projects viz. AICRP, ICAR *Ad hoc* Schemes. NATP, NATP (CGP) and NATCOM besides contractual research project. He has contributed more than 100 publications in reputed research journals, technical bulletins, compendia and books. He has developed several processing methods and technologies and submitted patents and registration of two Threshing cum Feed Treatment Machine and Pashu Choeolater. He has also supervised several MVSc and PhD students and successfully organized few short courses for personnel of National Agricultural Research System. He is a life member of ANA and several other professional societies and associations. Dr. Singh is widely acclaimed for his significant contributions as the treasurer and secretary of the ANA. He has honour to become member of organizing committee of the ANA World conference, which was held successfully at NASC complex, New Delhi in February 2009.

Dr. A.K. Verma (Editor), Born on August 31, 1962 at Village Pasana, District Sultanpur of U.P. Dr. Ashok Kumar Verma did his BSc Ag (Honours) from Kanpur University, Kanpur in 1982, MSc (Ag) in Animal Nutrition from Govind Ballabh Pant University of Agriculture and Technology, Pantnagar in 1985 and PhD in Animal Nutrition from Indian Veterinary Research Institute, Izatnagar in 1991. He started his research career in 1991 as a Scientist in Animal Nutrition Division of IVRI and presently working as Principal Scientist. Dr. A.K. Verma is a distinguished Animal Nutritionist and contributed in the area of urea molasses liquid diet, bypass protein sources and estimation of microbial protein production in ruminant livestock. He acquired training on Near Infrared Reflectance Spectroscopy at Scottish Agriculture College, U.K. under FAO/AHRD programme in 1998. He was awarded coveted Wellcome Travelling Post Doctoral Research Fellowship in 2001 for two years by The Wellcome Trust; U.K. He is recipient of prestigious Hari Om Ashram Trust Award of ICAR, Fellowship of Animal Nutrition Association (FANA) and National Academy of Agricultural Sciences (FNAAS), New Delhi. He is one of the Editors of Animal Nutrition and Feed Technology, the official journal of Animal Nutrition Association. He is General Secretary and a life member of ANA and various other professional societies. He is an experienced academician and researcher having published more than 85 research papers in various National and International Journals of high impact factor and presented papers in conferences and symposia. He has taught and guided many MVSc and Ph.D. students in the discipline of Animal Nutrition.